A NEW SHORT TEXTBOOK OF

MEDICINE

NEW SHORT TEXTBOOK SERIES

A NEW SHORT TEXTBOOK OF

MEDICINE

Edited by

P. JOHN REES
MD FRCP

Consultant Physician, Guy's Hospital, London
Senior Lecturer in Medicine, United Medical and Dental
Schools of Guy's and St Thomas's Hospitals, London

JOHN R. TROUNCE
MD FRCP

Professor Emeritus of Clinical Pharmacology
United Medical and Dental Schools of Guy's and St Thomas's Hospitals, London
Consultant Physician Emeritus, Guy's Hospital, London

Edward Arnold
A division of Hodder & Stoughton
LONDON   BALTIMORE   MELBOURNE   AUCKLAND

© 1988 P. John Rees and John R. Trounce

First published as *A Short Textbook of Medicine* by
Hodder and Stoughton 1962
First published as *A New Short Textbook of Medicine* 1988

British Library in Cataloguing in Publication Data

Rees, P. John
    A new short textbook of medicine
    1. Medicine
    I. Title   II. Trounce, John R.
    610.

    ISBN 0-340-41774-9

Typeset in 10/12pt Palatino by The Alden Press London Northampton
and Oxford.
Printed and bound in Great·Britain for Edward Arnold, the educational,
academic and medical publishing division of Hodder and Stoughton
Limited, 41 Bedford Square, London WC1B 3DQ by Butler & Tanner
Ltd, Frome and London.

Contents

Contributors

S. Cohen CBE, PhD, FRCPath, MD, FRS
Professor Emeritus of Clinical Pathology
United Medical and Dental Schools
Guy's Hospital
London

R. Grahame MD, FRCP
Consultant Physician
Department of Rheumatology
Guy's Hospital
London

T.J. Hamblin FRCP, FRCPath
Consultant Haematologist
Royal Victoria Hospital
Bournemouth

B.H. Hicks MD, FRCP
Senior Lecturer, Consultant Physician
Department of Endocrinology
Guy's Hospital
London

M.D. O'Brien MD, FRCP
Consultant Physician
Department of Neurology
Guy's Hospital
London

M.E. Pembrey MD, FRCP
Professor of Paediatric Genetics
Institute of Child Health
Guilford Street
London

P.J. Rees MD, FRCP
Senior Lecturer, Consultant Physician
United Medical and Dental Schools
Guy's Hospital
London

G.W. Scott MD, FRCP
Consultant Physician
Department of Chest Medicine
Guy's Hospital
London

G.E. Sladen DM, FRCP
Consultant Physician
Department of Gastroenterology
Guy's Hospital
London

D. Taube MD, MRCP
Consultant Physician
Department of Renal Medicine
King's College Hospital
Denmark Hill
London

A.D. Timmis MD, MRCP
Consultant Cardiologist
London Chest Hospital
Bonner Road
London

J.R. Trounce MD, FRCP
Professor Emeritus of Clinical Pharmacology
United Medical and Dental Schools
Guy's Hospital
London

J.P. Watson MD, FRCP, FRCPsych, DPH, DCH
Professor of Psychiatry
United Medical and Dental Schools
Guy's Hospital
London

R.S. Wells MD, FRCP
Consultant Physician
Department of Dermatology
Guy's Hospital
London

G.B. Wyatt FRCP, FFCM, DCH, DTM&H
Senior Lecturer, Honorary Consultant Physician
Liverpool School of Tropical Medicine
Pembroke Place
Liverpool

Preface

The Short Textbook of Medicine was first published in 1962 and it has been regularly updated since then. However, this new edition contains much more extensive changes than before, and represents a virtually complete re-write of the whole book. This takes into account the major advances that have occurred in medicine and is designed to take undergraduate and postgraduate students through the whole range of medical conditions and prepare them for all those changes which are likely in the future.

The new edition has a change in editors and a new format, and in addition, there are six completely new authors for the sections on Cardiology, Gastroenterology, Haematology, Nephrology, Tropical Diseases and Infectious Diseases. This brings a fresh outlook into the new edition, since these chapters have been totally rewritten. All the other chapters have had extensive revision, and two new chapters have been added, on Medicine in Old Age and on Nutrition. There is also an introductory chapter on Medicine in Today's World, putting into perspective medicine as practised in western countries with that seen in less well developed countries. On this same aspect, the chapter on Tropical Medicine deals with the common tropical diseases, with a particular concentration on those conditions which may be imported into western countries.

The number of illustrations, diagrams and tables has been increased in the new edition, and is particularly prominent and useful in the chapter on disorders of the cardiovascular system. There is now a more attractive layout to the new Short Textbook of Medicine. The double column format with slightly larger pages allows easier reading, with generous use of sub-headings to guide the reader through the text. For the most part, the sub-headings have been standardized to keep the format uniform through different chapters.

These radical changes have produced something approaching a new textbook, rather than a revised edition of the old Short Textbook, and in recognition of this, the title has been changed to "A New Short Textbook of Medicine". We believe this provides a clear and stimulating account of general medicine, with an emphasis on practical management. It has been rewritten primarily to serve medical students through their clinical years to qualifying examinations and well beyond. It will also prove useful for postgraduate students, and for all those in related disciplines, such as dentists, nurses and physiotherapists who require a concise and up-to-date textbook of medicine.

1988

PJR
JRT

1
Medicine in Today's World

This textbook has contributions dealing with infectious and tropical diseases but it reflects largely the state of medical knowledge and management in developed countries. Medicine has changed greatly since the first edition of the *Short Textbook of Medicine* in 1962. It will continue to change at an even faster pace over the working life of students who use this edition. New concepts and new diseases will emerge and there will be new developments in investigative tools and in treatment. The ability to deal with these changes will need continuing education after qualification. Evidence of such further education is already required in some countries, and many assess the competence of their doctors at regular intervals. Doctors owe it to their patients to maintain and advance their knowledge in this way and increased public awareness and litigation is likely to demand it more widely.

The current distribution of health care throughout the world is very uneven. One quarter of the world's population lives in developed countries, where four fifths of the total income is consumed. The expenditure on health care is similarly uneven or even more exaggerated. The plight of millions in North Africa who are suffering as a result of droughts has shown the world the extent of the defects in basic care for millions of people in these areas. The doctor-to-population ratio varies a hundred-fold between different countries, and within most countries, developed and developing, there is an urban bias in resources. The priorities for health vary greatly according to local conditions. The distribution of resources on health is traditionally in the hands of politicians who must decide the relative benefit of twenty million pounds spent on a country-wide immunization campaign or on a single military aircraft. The medical profession cannot afford to ignore the responsibility of trying to influence decisions on health care spending, nationally and internationally.

The World Health Organization has set as its target the development of a universal reasonable standard of health care by the end of the century. This declaration of 'Health for all by the year 2000' was made at the Alma Ata conference in Asia in 1978. The achievement of such an aim will depend upon the development of primary health care concentrating on nutrition, sanitation, immunization, child care and the provision of basic treatment.

In parallel with these needs, technology dominates most medical advances in the developed world. Advances in molecular biology improve our ability to diagnose and to treat, new imaging techniques extend our vision. The rate of increase in spending on health, which spiralled through the 1960s, 70s and early 80s, has now slowed. Continued escalation would have committed the total gross national products of countries such as the United Kingdom or the USA to health care. Arguments will continue about the level of health spending and its distribution, but the necessity for limitation has become widely accepted. In the presence of this limitation it will be the duty of medical staff to use the available resources economically and efficiently. There is no ethical reason why doctors should fail to take account of economic factors in their decisions on management of their patients.

The technical developments in medicine must not be allowed to obscure its basic skills. These skills include clinical abilities of history taking, examination, communication and caring. Medicine involves the treatment of patients not diseases, and the place to learn medicine is at the bedside or at the clinic. Medical textbooks such as this fill in the background knowledge, which must then be used to manage patients as individuals, not rigidly to a formula.

The speed of change in diseases themselves is demonstrated by the eradication of smallpox and the emergence of new diseases such as the acquired immune deficiency syndrome (AIDS). Previous editions of this textbook did not deal with AIDS. These new challenges will change our social as well as our medical lives: the most important part of the management of AIDS as this new edition is published relates to health education of the community, while intensive research continues to find preventive and curative treatment.

In the past century, the major advances in reduction of disease have come from public health measures involving nutrition, sanitation and immunization. The major causes of death in the UK have strong associations with smoking, yet we have achieved little in our efforts to persuade our population to give up the habit. The efforts of doctors in the future must include all aspects of medicine. Doctors are in the best position to help in decisions on resource distribution, on health education, and on areas for technological development as well as more traditional fields. The challenges of medicine, new and old, offer an exciting future for the doctor of today.

2
Disorders of the Cardiovascular System

During this century the pattern of cardiovascular disease in the industrialized world has changed considerably. Syphilitic and tuberculous involvement of the cardiovascular system is now rare, and the incidence of rheumatic disease is declining. Myocardial and conducting tissue disease, on the other hand, are being diagnosed more frequently and the importance of arterial hypertension is well recognized. Nevertheless, it is coronary artery disease that has emerged as the major cardiovascular disorder of the present era. Indeed, this 'modern epidemic' has long been the single most common cause of premature death in Europe and North America.

Symptoms of heart disease

Chest pain

Common cardiovascular causes of chest pain are myocardial ischaemia, pericarditis and aortic dissection.
1 Myocardial ischaemia
This results from an imbalance between myocardial oxygen supply and demand and produces pain called *angina* (Table 2.1). Angina is usually a symptom of coronary artery disease which impedes myocardial oxygen supply. The history is diagnostic if the location of the pain, its character, its relation to exertion and its duration are typical. The patient describes retrosternal pain which may radiate into the arms, the throat or the jaw. It has a constricting character, is provoked by exertion and relieved rapidly by rest. When coronary occlusion produces myocardial infarction the pain is similar in location and character but is usually more severe and more prolonged.
2 Pericarditis
This condition also causes central chest pain which is

sharp in character and aggravated by deep inspiration, cough or postural changes. It may last several days.
3 Aortic dissection
This produces tearing pain in either the front or the back of the chest. The onset is abrupt, unlike the crescendo quality of ischaemic cardiac pain.

Dyspnoea

Dyspnoea is an abnormal awareness of breathing occurring either at rest or at an expectedly low level of exertion. Left heart failure is the major cardiac cause. The elevated left atrial pressure that characterizes left heart failure (see page 18) produces a corresponding elevation of the pulmonary capillary pressure. This increases transudation into the lungs, which become oedematous and stiff. The extra effort required to ventilate the stiff lungs causes dyspnoea. Cardiac dyspnoea is usually provoked

Table 2.1 Causes of angina

Impaired myocardial oxygen supply
Coronary artery disease:
    atherosclerosis
    arteritis in connective tissue disorders
    syphilis
Coronary artery spasm
Congenital coronary artery disease:
    arteriovenous fistula
    anomalous origin from pulmonary artery
Severe anaemia

Increased myocardial oxygen demand
Left ventricular hypertrophy:
    hypertension
    aortic valve disease
    hypertrophic cardiomyopathy
Tachyarrhythmias

by exertion or lying flat, both of which produce a steep rise in left atrial pressure.

1   Exertional dyspnoea

This is the most troublesome symptom. As left heart failure worsens exercise tolerance deteriorates. In advanced disease the patient is dyspnoeic at rest.

2   Orthopnoea

Dyspnoea on lying flat is very characteristic of left heart failure. To obtain uninterrupted sleep extra pillows are required, and in advanced disease the patient may choose to sleep sitting in a chair.

3   Paroxysmal nocturnal dyspnoea

Frank pulmonary oedema during sleep wakens the patient, with distressing dyspnoea and fear of imminent death. The symptoms are corrected by standing upright, so that gravitational pooling of blood lowers the left atrial pressure.

Fatigue

Exertional fatigue is an important symptom of left and right heart failure and is particularly troublesome towards the end of the day. It is caused by inadequate oxygen delivery to exercising skeletal muscle and reflects an impaired cardiac output.

Palpitation

Awareness of the heart beat is common during exertion or heightened emotion. Under other circumstances it is often symptomatic of cardiac arrhythmia. A description of the rate and rhythm of the palpitation is essential. Rapid irregular palpitation is typical of atrial fibrillation. Rapid regular palpitation occurs in both atrial and ventricular tachyarrhythmias. The pause or the forceful beat that follows an extrasystole may be noticed by introspective individuals but does not necessarily signify important disease.

Dizziness and syncope

Cardiovascular disorders produce dizziness and syncope by transient disturbance of cerebral perfusion. Recovery is usually rapid, unlike with other common causes of syncope (e.g. stroke, epilepsy, overdose).

1   Postural hypotension

Syncope on standing upright reflects inadequate baroreceptor-mediated vasoconstriction. It is common in the elderly. Abrupt reductions in blood pressure and cerebral perfusion cause the patient to fall to the ground, whereupon the condition corrects itself.

2   Vasovagal syncope

Autonomic overactivity in response to emotional or painful stimuli causes vasodilatation and inappropriate slowing of the pulse. These combine to reduce blood pressure and cerebral perfusion. Recovery is rapid if the patient lies down.

3   Carotid sinus syncope

Exaggerated vagal discharge following external stimulation of the carotid sinus (e.g. a tight shirt collar) causes reflex vasodilatation and slowing of the pulse. These combine to reduce blood pressure and cerebral perfusion.

4   Valvar obstruction

Fixed valvar obstruction in aortic stenosis may prevent a normal rise in cardiac output during exertion. Physiological vasodilatation in exercising muscle therefore produces abrupt reductions in blood pressure and cerebral perfusion which lead to syncope. Intermittent obstruction of the mitral valve by left atrial tumors (usually myxoma or ball thrombus) may also cause syncopal episodes.

5   Stokes–Adams attacks

These are caused by self-limiting episodes of asystole or rapid tachyarrhythmias (including ventricular fibrillation). The loss of cardiac output causes syncope and a striking pallor. Following restoration of normal rhythm recovery is rapid and is associated with flushing of the skin as flow through the dilated cutaneous bed is re-established.

Signs of heart disease

Oedema

Oedema which pits on digital pressure occurs in congestive heart failure. It is caused by salt and water retention, which expands the plasma volume and increases the capillary hydrostatic pressure. Hydrostatic forces driving fluid out of the capillary exceed osmotic forces reabsorbing it, so that oedema fluid accumulates in the interstitial space. The effect of gravity on capillary hydrostatic pressure ensures that oedema is most prominent around the ankles in the ambulant patient and over the sacrum in the bed-ridden patient. In advanced heart failure oedema may involve the legs, genitalia and trunk. Transudation into the peritoneal cavity (ascites) and the pleural and pericardial spaces may also occur.

Cyanosis

Cyanosis is a blue discolouration of the skin and mucous membranes caused by increased concentration of reduced haemoglobin in the superficial blood vessels.

1 Peripheral cyanosis

This may result when cutaneous vasoconstriction slows the blood flow and increases oxygen extraction in the skin and the lips. It is physiological during cold exposure. It also occurs in heart failure when reduced cardiac output produces reflex cutaneous vasoconstriction. In mitral stenosis, cyanosis over the malar area produces the characteristic mitral facies.

2 Central cyanosis

This may result from the reduced arterial oxygen saturation caused by cardiac or pulmonary disease. It affects not only the skin and the lips but also the mucous membranes of the mouth. Cardiac causes include pulmonary oedema (which prevents adequate oxygenation of the blood) and congenital heart disease. Congenital defects associated with central cyanosis include those in which desaturated venous blood bypasses the lungs by ('reversed') shunting through septal defects or a patent ductus arteriosus (e.g. Fallot's tetralogy, Eisenmenger's syndrome).

Coldness of the extremities

In patients with heart disease this is an important sign of reduced cardiac output. It is caused by reflex vasoconstriction in the cutaneous bed. Measurement of skin temperature provides a useful indirect means of monitoring cardiac output in patients with heart failure undergoing treatment in the coronary care unit.

Clubbing of the fingers and toes

In congenital cyanotic heart failure clubbing is not present at birth but develops during infancy and may become very marked. Another cardiac cause of clubbing is infective endocarditis.

Arterial pulse and blood pressure

The arterial pulses should be palpated for evaluation of rate, rhythm, character and symmetry.

1 Rate and rhythm

By convention, both are assessed by palpation of the right radial pulse. Rate, expressed in beats per minute, is measured by counting over a timed period of 15 seconds. Normal sinus rhythm is regular but in young patients may show phasic variation in rate during respiration (*sinus arrhythmia*). An irregular rhythm usually indicates atrial fibrillation but may also be caused by frequent premature beats. In patients with atrial fibrillation the rate shoud be measured by auscultation at the cardiac apex because beats that follow very short diastolic intervals may not generate sufficient pressure to be palpable at the radial artery.

2 Character

This is defined by the volume and waveform of the pulse and should be evaluated at the right carotid artery (i.e. the pulse closest to the heart and least subject to damping and distortion in the arterial tree). Pulse volume provides a crude indication of stroke volume, being small in heart failure and large in aortic regurgitation. The waveform of the pulse is of greater diagnostic importance. Aortic stenosis produces a slowly rising carotid pulse; in aortic regurgitation, on the other hand, the large stroke volume vigorously ejected produces a rapidly rising carotid pulse which collapses in early diastole owing to back flow through the aortic valve. In mixed aortic valve disease a *bisferiens pulse* with two systolic peaks is occasionally found. *Pulsus alternans*—alternating high and low systolic peaks—occurs in severe left ventricular failure but the mechanism is unknown. *Pulsus paradoxus*—an inspiratory decline in systolic pressure greater than 10 mmHg—occurs in cardiac tamponade and, less frequently, in constrictive pericarditis and obstructive pulmonary disease. It represents an exaggeration of the normal inspiratory decline in systolic pressure and is not, therefore, truly paradoxical.

3 Symmetry

Symmetry of the radial, brachial, carotid, femoral, popliteal and pedal pulses should be confirmed. An absent pulse indicates an obstruction more proximally in the arterial tree, caused usually by atherosclerosis or thromboembolism. Coarctation of the aorta causes symmetrical reduction and delay of the femoral pulses compared with the radial pulses.

Measurement of blood pressure

Blood pressure is measured indirectly by sphygmomanometry. Supine and erect measurements should be obtained to provide an assessment of baroreceptor function. A cuff (at least 40% the arm circumference) is attached to a mercury or aneroid manometer and inflated around the extended arm. Auscultation over the brachial artery reveals five phases of *Korotkoff sounds* as the cuff is deflated:

Phase 1:	The first appearance of the sounds marking systolic pressure
Phase 2 and 3:	Increasingly loud sounds
Phase 4:	Abrupt muffling of the sounds
Phase 5:	Disappearance of the sounds

Phase 5 provides a better measure of diastolic blood pressure than phase 4, not only because it corresponds more closely with directly measured diastolic pressure, but also because its identification is less subjective. Nevertheless, in those conditions where Korotkoff sounds remain audible despite complete deflation of the cuff (aortic regurgitation, arteriovenous fistula, pregnancy) phase 4 must be used for the diastolic measurement.

Jugular venous pulse

Fluctuations in right atrial pressure during the cardiac cycle generate a pulse which is transmitted backwards into the jugular veins. It is best examined while the patient reclines at 45°. If the right atrial pressure is very low, however, visualization of the jugular venous pulse may require manual pressure over the upper abdomen. This transiently increases venous return to the heart, producing elevation of the jugular venous pulse (hepato-jugular reflux).

1 Jugular venous pressure
The normal upper limit is 4 cm vertically above the sternal angle. This is about 9 cm above the right atrium and corresponds to a pressure of 6 mmHg. Elevation of the jugular venous pressure indicates elevation of the right atrial pressure unless the superior vena cava is obstructed, producing engorgement of the neck veins (Table 2.2). During inspiration the pressure within the chest falls and there is a fall in the jugular venous pressure. In constrictive pericarditis, and less commonly in tamponade, inspiration produces a paradoxical rise in the jugular venous pressure (*Kussmaul's sign*) because the

Table 2.2 Causes of elevated jugular venous pressure

Congestive heart failure
Cor pulmonale
Pulmonary embolism
Right ventricular infarction
Tricuspid valve disease
Tamponade
Constrictive pericarditis
Hypertrophic/restrictive cardiomyopathy
Superior vena cava obstruction
Iatrogenic fluid overload, particularly in
   surgical and renal patients

increased venous return cannot be accommodated within the constricted right side of the heart.

2 Waveform of jugular venous pulse
The jugular venous pulse has a flickering character owing to 'a' and 'v' waves separated by 'x' and 'y' descents. The 'a' wave produced by atrial systole precedes tricuspid valve closure. It is followed by the 'x' descent, marking descent of the tricuspid valve ring. Atrial pressure then rises again, producing the 'v' wave as the atrium fills passively during ventricular systole. The decline in atrial pressure as the tricuspid valve opens to allow ventricular filling produces the 'y' descent. Important abnormalities of the pattern of deflections are shown in Fig. 2.1.

Examination of the heart

Inspection

Chest wall deformities such as pectus excavatum should be noted because these may compress the heart and

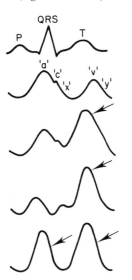

ECG. Electrical events precede mechanical events. Thus the P wave and QRS complex of the ECG precede the "a" and "v" waves, respectively, of the JVP.

NORMAL JVP. The "a" wave is usually the most prominent deflection. The "x" descent is interrupted by the small "c" wave marking tricuspid valve closure.

GIANT "V" WAVE (Arrowed). This is an important sign of tricuspid regurgitation. The regurgitant jet produces pulsatile systolic waves in the JVP.

CANNON "a" WAVE (Arrowed). This is caused by atrial systole against a closed tricuspid valve. It occurs when the atrial and ventricular rhythms are dissociated (e.g. complete heart block) and marks coincident atrial and ventricular systole.

PROMINENT "x" and "y" DESCENTS (Arrowed). These occur in constrictive pericarditis and give the JVP an unusually dynamic appearance. In tamponade only the "x" descent is exaggerated.

Figure 2.1   *Waveform of the jugular venous pulse.*

displace the apex, giving a spurious impression of cardiac enlargement. Large ventricular or aortic aneurysms may cause visible pulsations. Vena caval obstruction is associated with prominent venous collaterals on the chest wall. Prominent venous collaterals around the shoulder occur in axillary or subclavian vein obstruction.

Palpation

The location of the apical impulse inferior or lateral to the fifth intercostal space or the mid-clavicular line, respectively, usually indicates cardiac enlargement. A thrusting impulse occurs in left ventricular hypertrophy associated with vigorous systolic contraction (e.g. aortic valve disease). This must be distinguished from the tapping apex of mitral stenosis produced by the palpable first heart sound. Palpable third and fourth heart sounds give the apical impulse a characteristic double thrust.

Left ventricular aneurysms can usually be palpated medial to the cardiac apex. Right ventricular enlargement produces a systolic thrust in the left parasternal area. The turbulent flow responsible for heart murmurs may produce palpable vibrations ('thrills') on the chest wall, particularly in aortic stenosis and ventricular septal defect.

Auscultation

The diaphragm and bell of the stethoscope permit appreciation of the high- and low-pitched auscultatory events, respectively. The apex, lower left sternal edge, upper left sternal edge and upper right sternal edge should be auscultated in turn. These locations correspond to the mitral, tricuspid, pulmonary and aortic areas, respectively, and loosely identify sites at which sounds and murmurs arising from the four valves are best heard.

1 First sound (S1)
This corresponds to mitral and tricuspid valve closure at the onset of systole. It is accentuated in mitral stenosis because prolonged diastolic filling through the narrowed valve ensures that the leaflets are widely separated at the onset of systole. Thus valve closure generates unusually vigorous vibrations. In advanced mitral stenosis the valve is rigid and immobile and S1 becomes soft again.

2 Second sound (S2)
This corresponds to aortic and pulmonary valve closure following ventricular ejection. S2 is single during expiration. Inspiration, however, causes physiological splitting into aortic followed by pulmonary components because increased venous return to the right side of the heart delays pulmonary valve closure. Important abnormalities of S2 are illustrated in Fig. 2.2.

3 Third and fourth sounds (S3, S4)
These low-frequency sounds occur early and late in diastole, respectively. When present they give a characteristic 'gallop' cadence to the cardiac rhythm. Both sounds are best heard with the bell of the stethoscope at the cardiac apex. They are caused by abrupt tensing of the ventricular walls following rapid diastolic filling. Rapid filling occurs early in diastole (S3) following atrioventricular valve opening and again late in diastole (S4) due to atrial contraction. S3 is physiological in children and young adults but usually disappears after the age of 40. It also occurs in high-output states caused by anaemia, fever, pregnancy and thyrotoxicosis. After the age of 40, S3 is nearly always pathological, usually indicating left ventricular failure or, less commonly, mitral regurgitation or constrictive pericarditis. S4 is sometimes physiological in the elderly. More commonly, however, it is pathological and occurs when vigorous atrial contraction late in diastole is required to augment filling of a hypertrophied, non-compliant ventricle (e.g. hypertension, aortic stenosis, hypertrophic cardiomyopathy).

4 Systolic clicks and opening snaps
Valve opening, unlike valve closure, is normally silent. In

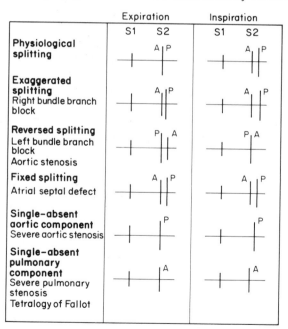

Figure 2.2 *Splitting of the second heart sound. The vertical lines representing S1 and S2 divide the horizontal line into systolic and diastolic intervals. Because auscultation is at the pulmonary area the pulmonary component of S2 is slightly louder that the aortic component; both components are louder than S1. This information is conveyed by the vertical heights of the lines. Additional sounds and murmurs may be superimposed on this basic format, as illustrated in Fig. 2.3.*

aortic stenosis, however, valve opening produces a click in early systole which precedes the ejection murmur. The click is only audible if the valve cusps are pliant and non-calcified and is particularly prominent in the congenitally bicuspid valve. A click later in systole suggests mitral valve prolapse. In mitral stenosis, elevated left atrial pressure causes forceful opening of the thickened valve leaflets. This generates a snap early in diastole which precedes the mid-diastolic murmur.

5 Heart murmurs

These are caused by turbulent flow within the heart and great vessels and may indicate valve disease. Heart murmurs—defined by loudness, quality, location, radiation and timing—may be depicted graphically (Fig. 2.3).

The loudness of a murmur reflects the degree of turbulence. This relates to the volume and velocity of flow and not the severity of the cardiac lesion. Loudness is graded on a scale of 1 (barely audible) to 6 (audible even without application of the stethoscope to the chest wall). The quality of a murmur relates to its frequency and is best described as low-, medium- or high-pitched. The location of a murmur on the chest wall depends on its site of origin and has led to the description of four valve areas (see above). Some murmurs radiate, depending on the velocity and direction of blood flow. The high-velocity systolic flow in aortic stenosis and mitral regurgitation,

for example, is directed towards the neck and the axilla, respectively. The high-velocity diastolic flow in aortic regurgitation is directed towards the left sternal edge. Murmurs are timed according to the phase of systole or diastole during which they are audible (e.g. mid-systolic, pan-systolic, early diastolic).

Murmurs may occur without underlying heart disease. 'Innocent' murmurs of this type usually reflect hyperkinetic circulation in conditions such as anaemia, fever, pregnancy and thyrotoxicosis, which lead to turbulent flow in the aortic or pulmonary outflow tracts. Innocent murmurs are always mid-systolic in timing, are rarely louder than grade 3, may vary with posture and are not associated with other signs of heart disease.

6 Friction rubs and venous hums

A friction rub occurs in pericarditis. It is a high-pitched scratching noise audible during any part of the cardiac cycle and over any part of the left precordium. A continuous venous hum at the base of the heart reflects hyperkinetic jugular venous flow. It is particularly common in infants and usually disappears on lying flat.

Cardiac investigation

The electrocardiogram (ECG)

The ECG records the electrical activity of the heart at the

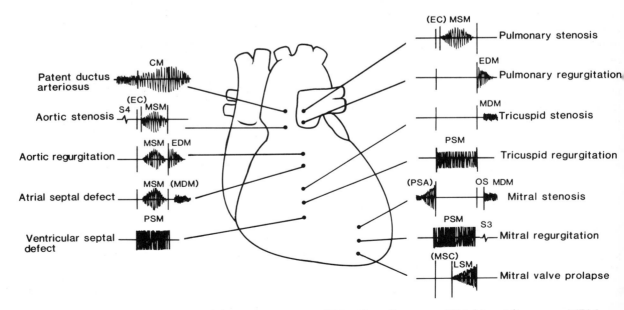

Figure 2.3   *Heart murmurs. EC, ejection click; OS, opening snap; MSM, mid-systolic murmur; LSM, late-systolic murmur; MDM, mid-diastolic murmur; S3, third heart sound; S4, fourth heart sound; MSC, mid-systolic click; CM, continuous murmur; PSM, pansystolic murmur; EDM, early diastolic murmur; PSA, pre-systolic accentuation. Parentheses indicate that the finding is variable and not always present.*

skin surface. A good-quality 12-lead ECG is essential for the evaluation of every cardiac patient.

1 Generation of electrical activity

The wave of depolarization that spreads through the heart during each cardiac cycle has vector properties defined by its direction and magnitude. The net direction of the wave changes continuously during each cardiac cycle and the ECG deflections change accordingly, being positive as the wave approaches the recording electrode and negative as it moves away. Electrodes orientated along the axis of the wave record larger deflections than those orientated at right-angles. Nevertheless the size of the deflections is determined principally by the magnitude of the wave, which is a function of muscle mass. Thus the ECG deflection produced by depolarization of the atria (P wave) is smaller than that produced by the depolarization of the more muscular ventricles (QRS complex). Ventricular repolarization produces the T wave.

2 Inscription of the QRS complex

The ventricular depolarization vector can be resolved into two components:

1 Septal depolarization—spreads from left to right across the septum
2 Ventricular free wall depolarization—spreads from endocardium to epicardium

Left ventricular depolarization dominates the second vector component, the resultant direction of which is from right to left. Thus electrodes orientated to the left ventricle record a small negative deflection (Q wave) as the septal depolarization vector moves away, followed by a large positive deflection (R wave) as the ventricular depolarization vector approaches. The sequence of deflections for electrodes orientated towards the right ventricle is in the opposite direction (Fig. 2.4).

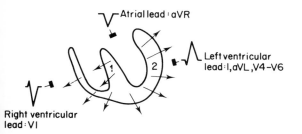

Figure 2.4 *Inscription of the QRS complex. The septal depolarization vector (1) produces the initial deflection of the QRS complex. The ventricular free-wall depolarization vector (2) produces the second deflection which is usually more pronounced. Lead aVR is orientated towards the cavity of the left ventricle and records an entirely negative deflection.*

Any positive deflection is termed an R wave. A negative deflection before the R wave is termed a Q wave (this must be the first deflection of the complex), while a negative deflection following the R wave is termed an S wave.

3 Electrical axis

Because the mean direction of the ventricular depolarization vector (the electrical axis) shows a wide range of normality, there is corresponding variation in QRS patterns consistent with a normal ECG. Thus correct interpretation of the ECG must take account of the electrical axis. The frontal plane axis is determined by identifying the limb lead in which the net QRS deflection (positive and negative) is *least* pronounced. This lead must be at right-angles to the frontal plane electrical axis which is defined using an arbitrary hexaxial reference system (Fig. 2.5).

4 Normal 12-lead ECG

This is illustrated in Fig. 2.6. Leads I to III are the standard bipolar leads, which each measure the potential difference between two limbs:

Lead I: Left arm to right arm
Lead II: Left leg to right arm
Lead III: Left leg to left arm

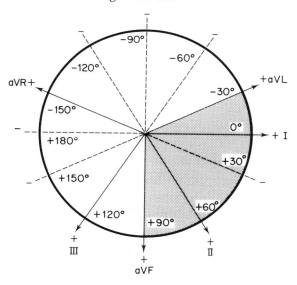

Figure 2.5 *Frontal plane electrical axis. This hexaxial reference system identifies the orientation of each of the standard limb leads to the heart. When the mean frontal QRS axis is directed towards lead I, it is arbitrarily defined as 0°: the maximal positive deflection is in lead I and the equiphasic deflection is in lead aVF. Axis shifts are ascribed, a negative sign if directed leftwards and a positive sign if directed rightwards. Axes between −30° and +90°, within the shaded area of the figure, are normal. Axes less than −30° (left axis deviation) or greater than +90° (right axis deviation) are abnormal.*

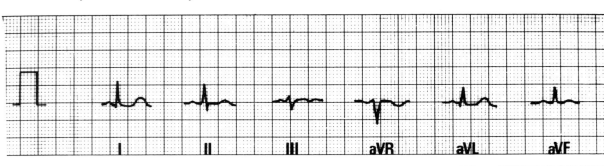

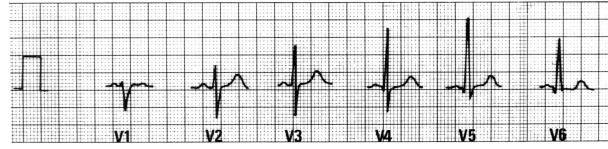

Figure 2.6 *Standard 12-lead ECG. This is a normal recording. The QRS deflections are equiphasic in lead III. This is at right-angles to lead aVR (see Fig. 2.5) which is dominantly negative. The frontal plane QRS axis is, therefore, +30°. The square wave calibration signal is 1 mV.*

The remaining leads are unipolar connected to a limb (aVR to aVF) or to the chest wall (V1 to V6). Because the orientation of each lead to the wave of depolarization is different, the direction and magnitude of ECG deflections is also different in each lead. Nevertheless, the sequence of deflections (P wave, QRS complex, T wave) is identical. In some patients a small U wave can be seen following the T wave. Its orientation (positive or negative) is the same as the T wave but its cause is unknown.

Analysis of the ECG

1 Heart rate
The ECG is usually recorded at a paper speed of 25 mm/s. Thus each large square (5 mm) represents 0.20 seconds. The heart rate (beats/minute) is conveniently calculated by counting the number of large squares between consecutive R waves and dividing this into 300.

2 Rhythm
In normal sinus rhythm, P waves precede each QRS complex and the rhythm is regular. Absence of P waves and an irregular rhythm indicate atrial fibrillation.

3 Electrical axis
Evaluation of the frontal plane QRS axis is described above.

4 P wave morphology
The duration should not exceed 0.10 seconds. Broad-notched P waves (P mitrale) indicate left atrial dilatation caused usually by mitral valve disease or left ventricular failure. Tall-peaked P waves (P pulmonale) indicate right atrial enlargement caused usually by right ventricular failure.

5 PR interval
The normal duration is 0.12 to 0.20 seconds measured from the onset of the P wave to the first deflection of the QRS complex. Prolongation indicates delayed atrioventricular conduction (heart block). Shortening indicates rapid conduction through a tract bypassing the atroventricular node (e.g. Wolff–Parkinson–White syndrome).

6 QRS morphology
The duration should not exceed 0.12 seconds. Prolongation indicates slow ventricular depolarization due to bundle branch block (Fig. 2.7), pre-excitation (Wolff–Parkinson–White syndrome) or electrolyte abnormalities (hypokalaemia).

Exaggerated QRS deflections indicate ventricular hypertrophy (Fig. 2.8). Voltage criteria for left ventricular hypertrophy are fulfilled when the sum of the S and R wave deflections in leads V1 and V6, respectively, exceeds 35 mm (3.5 mv). Right ventricular hypertrophy causes tall R waves in right ventricular leads (V1 and V2). Diminished QRS deflections occur in myxoedema and also when pericardial effusion or obesity insulate the heart. The presence of pathological Q waves (duration greater than 0.04 seconds) should be noted because this usually indicates myocardial infarction.

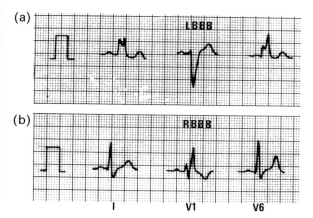

Figure 2.7 *Bundle branch block. (a) Left bundle branch block: the entire sequence of ventricular depolarization is abnormal, resulting in a broad QRS complex with large slurred or notched R waves in I and V6. (b) Right bundle branch block: right ventricular depolarization is delayed, resulting in a broad QRS complex with an rSR' pattern in VI and prominent S waves in I and V6.*

7 ST segment morphology

Minor ST elevation reflecting early repolarization may occur as a normal variant (Fig. 2.9) particularly in negroes. Pathological elevation (> 2.0 mm above the isoelectric line) occurs in acute myocardial infarction, variant angina and pericarditis. Horizontal ST depression indicates myocardial ischaemia. Other important causes of ST depression are digitalis therapy and hypokalaemia.

8 T wave morphology

The orientation of the T wave should be directionally similar to the QRS complex. Thus T wave inversion is normal in leads with dominantly negative QRS complexes (aVR, V1). Pathological T wave inversion occurs as a non-specific response to various stimuli (e.g. viral infection, hypothermia). More important causes of T wave inversion are ventricular hypertrophy, myocardial ischaemia and myocardial infarction. Exaggerated peaking of the T wave is the earliest ECG change in acute myocardial infarction. It also occurs in hyperkalaemia.

The chest X-ray

Good-quality postero-anterior (PA) and lateral chest X-rays are of considerable value in the assessment of the cardiac patient (Fig. 2.10).

1 Cardiac silhouette

Though the PA chest X-ray exhibits a wide range of normality, the transverse diameter of the heart should not exceed 50 per cent that of the chest. Cardiac enlargement is caused either by dilatation of the cardiac chambers or pericardial effusion. Myocardial hypertrophy rarely affects heart size.

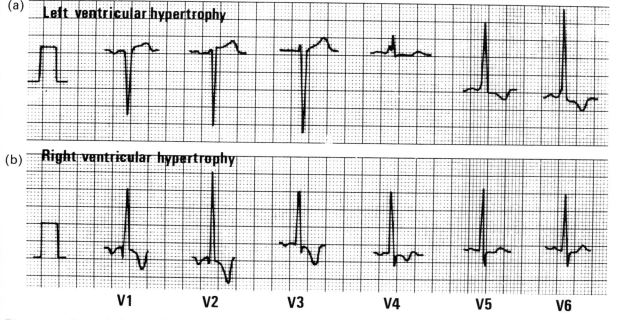

Figure 2.8 *Ventricular hypertrophy. (a) Left ventricular hypertrophy. The QRS voltage deflections are exaggerated such that the sum of S and R waves in VI and V6, respectively, exceeds 35 mm. T wave inversion in V5 and V6 indicates left ventricular 'strain'. (b) Right ventricular hypertrophy. Prominent R waves in VI and V2 associated with T wave inversion ('strain pattern') are shown.*

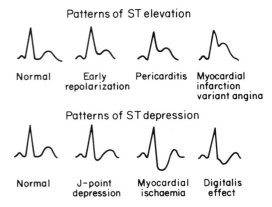

Patterns of ST elevation

Normal   Early repolarization   Pericarditis   Myocardial infarction variant angina

Patterns of ST depression

Normal   J-point depression   Myocardial ischaemia   Digitalis effect

Figure 2.9   *ST segment morphology: common causes of ST segment elevation and depression. Note that depression of the J point (junction between the QRS complex and ST segment) is physiological during exertion and does not signify myocardial ischaemia. Planar depression of the ST segment, on the other hand, is strongly suggestive of myocardial ischaemia.*

Ventricular dilatation. The PA chest X-ray does not reliably distinguish left from right ventricular dilatation. The lateral chest X-ray is more helpful. Thus dilatation of the posteriorly located left ventricle encroaches on the retrocardiac space, while dilatation of the anteriorly located right ventricle encroaches on the retrosternal space.

Atrial dilatation. Right atrial dilatation is usually due to right ventricular failure but occurs as an isolated finding in tricuspid stenosis and Ebstein's anomaly. It produces cardiac enlargement without specific radiographic signs.

Left atrial dilatation occurs in left ventricular failure and mitral valve disease (Fig. 2.11). Radiographic signs are:

1 Flattening and later bulging of the left heart border below the main pulmonary artery
2 Elevation of the left main bronchus, with widening of the carina
3 Appearance of the medial border of the left atrium behind the right side of the heart (double-density sign).

Vascular dilatation. Aortic dilatation caused by aneurysm or dissection may produce widening of the entire upper mediastinum. Localized dilatation of the proximal aorta occurs in aortic valve disease and produces a prominence in the right upper mediastinum. Dilatation of the main pulmonary artery occurs in pulmonary hypertension and pulmonary stenosis and produces a prominence below the aortic knuckle.

Intracardiac calcification. Because the radiodensity of cardiac tissue is similar to that of blood, intracardiac structures can rarely be identified unless they are calcified. Valvar, pericardial or myocardial calcification may occur and usually indicate important disease of these structures. Calcification is best appreciated on the deeply penetrated lateral chest X-ray.

2 Lung fields

Common lung field abnormalities in cardiovascular disease are caused either by altered pulmonary flow or increased left atrial pressure:

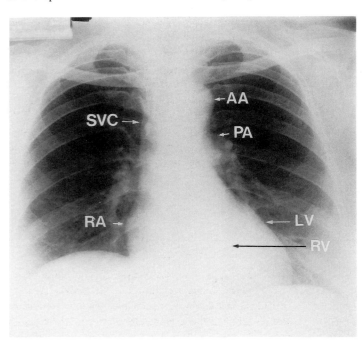

SVC →   ←AA   ← PA   RA →   ← LV   RV

Figure 2.10   *Normal chest X-ray. The standard postero-anterior projection is shown. Note that the heart is not enlarged (cardiothoracic ratio < 50%) and the lung fields are clear. SVC, superior vena cava; RA, right atrium; AA, aortic arch; LV, left ventricle; RA, right atrium; PA, pulmonary artery; RV, right ventricle.*

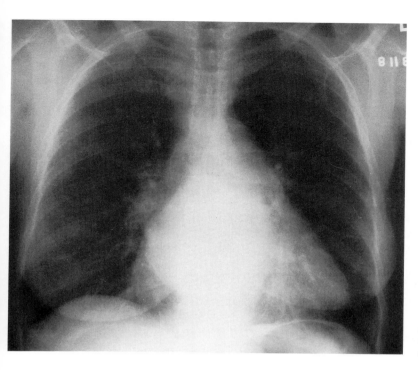

Figure 2.11   *Left atrial dilatation. This is a penetrated PA chest X-ray in a patient with mitral stenosis. The dilated, posteriorly located left atrium is clearly visible. Note flattening of the left heart border, widening of the carina and the double-density sign at the right heart border.*

Altered pulmonary flow. Increments in pulmonary flow sufficient to cause radiographic abnormalities are caused by left-to-right intracardiac shunts (e.g. atrial septal defect, ventricular septal defect, patent ductus arteriosus). Prominence of the vascular markings give the lung fields a plethoric appearance. Reductions in pulmonary flow, on the other hand, cause reduced vascular markings. This may be regional (e.g. pulmonary embolism) or global (e.g. severe pulmonary hypertension).

Increased left atrial pressure. Increased pressure (e.g. mitral stenosis, left ventricular failure) produces corresponding rises in pulmonary venous and pulmonary capillary pressures. Prominence of the upper lobe veins is an early radiographic finding. As the left atrial and pulmonary capillary pressures rise above 18 mmHg, transudation into the lung produces interstitial pulmonary oedema, characterized by prominence of the interlobular septa, particularly at the lung bases (Kerley B lines). Further elevation of pressure leads to alveolar pulmonary oedema characterized by perihilar 'bat's wing' shadowing.

The echocardiogram

Echocardiography is the most versatile and widely applicable imaging technique in clinical cardiology. Reflected ultrasound provides a high-resolution dynamic image of the four cardiac chambers and the myocardial, valvar and pericardial structures. Thus dilatation and hypertrophy of the cardiac chambers can be identified and quantified and ventricular contractile dysfunction is readily appreciated. Echocardiography plays an important role in the diagnosis of valvar heart disease and is the most sensitive technique available for diagnosis of pericardial effusion. Other clinical applications include the detection of intracardiac tumours and thrombus.

Complete echocardiographic examination requires M-mode and two-dimensional studies (Fig. 2.12). The M-mode study provides a unidimensional 'ice-pick' view through the heart, but continuous recording adds a time dimension for appreciation of the dynamic component of the image. The two-dimensional study provides more detailed structural and dynamic information.

Doppler echocardiography

This technique is now widely used for the non-invasive evaluation of valvar regurgitation and valvar stenosis. According to the Doppler principle, when an ultrasound beam is directed towards the blood stream the frequency of the ultrasound reflected from the blood cells is altered.

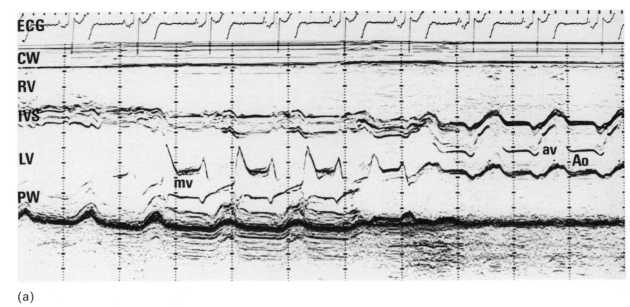

(a)

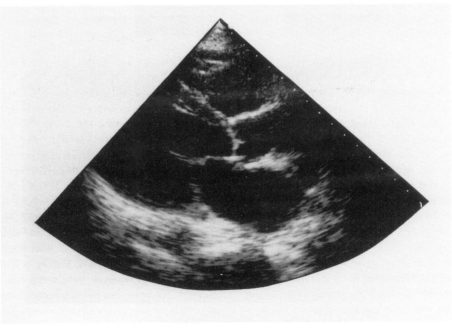

(b)

Figure 2.12 *Normal echocardiograms. (a) M-mode recording: angulation of the ultrasound beam from X to Y (see line drawing in part (c)) permits sequential examination of the right ventricle and the left-side cardiac chambers and heart valves. By convention the anteriorly located ('right-sided') cardiac structures are displayed towards the top of the echocardiogram and the posteriorly located ('left-sided') structures are displayed below. The dense dots are a scale: 1 cm vertically, 1 s horizontally. (b) Two-dimensional recording: interpretation of the echocardiogram is provided by the line drawing, and the dots are a 1 cm scale. (c) Schematic (see opposite): CW, chest wall; IVS, interventricular septum; PW, posterior wall of the left ventricle; RV, right ventricle; LV, left ventricle; Ao, aorta; av, aortic valve; mv, mitral valve.*

The frequency shift—or Doppler effect—is related to the direction and velocity of flow. Thus in valvar regurgitation the retrograde flow that occurs after valve closure is readily detected. In valvar stenosis the velocity of flow across the valve can be measured. Because the peak velocity (as opposed to volume) of flow is directly related to the degree of stenosis, an evaluation of the severity of stenosis can be made.

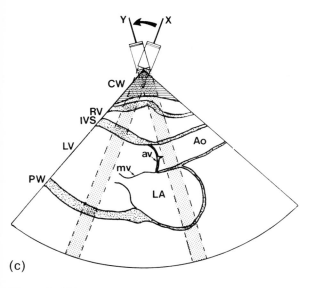

(c)

Figure 2.12(c)

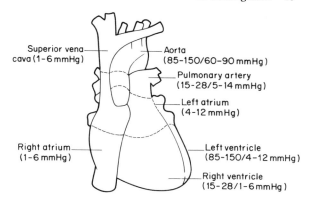

Figure 2.13 *Normal pressure values within the heart and great vessels.*

Radionuclide imaging

1 Radionuclide ventriculography

Red cells labelled with technetium-99m are injected intravenously and allowed to equilibrate within the blood pool. The ventricular chambers are imaged with a gamma camera which records peaks and troughs of radioactivity during diastole and systole, respectively. This permits construction of a dynamic ventriculogram which may be used to examine ventricular wall motion and chamber dimensions.

2 Myocardial perfusion scintigraphy

Thallium-201 injected intravenously is distributed throughout the myocardium according to coronary flow. The distribution is homogeneous, but in coronary artery disease regional impairment of coronary flow produces scintigraphic perfusion defects.

3 Pulmonary scintigraphy (lung scans)

Albumin microspheres labelled with technetium-99m are injected intravenously. These become trapped within the pulmonary capillaries. Imaging with a gamma camera provides a perfusion scintigram. The normal perfusion scintigram shows homogeneous distribution of radioactivity throughout both lung fields, but following thromboembolism regional impairment of pulmonary flow produces a scintigraphic perfusion defect. The appearance, however, is non-specific and occurs in other pulmonary disorders. Simultaneous ventilation scintigraphy enhances specificity. Inhaled xenon-133 is normally distributed homogeneously throughout the alveoli. In pulmonary embolism (unlike other pulmonary disorders) the distribution remains homogeneous. Thus a scintigraphic perfusion defect not 'matched' by a ventilation defect is highly specific for pulmonary embolism.

Cardiac catheterization

Catheters introduced into an artery or vein may be directed into the left or right sides of the heart, respectively. The catheter may be attached to a pressure transducer for measurement of intracardiac pressures. Moreover, catheter delivery of contrast material permits angiographic examination of the internal anatomy of the heart and great vessels.

1 Intracardiac pressure measurement (See Fig. 2.13)

Right-sided pressures are conveniently measured with a Swan Ganz catheter. The catheter has a terminal balloon which may be inflated in a central vein to flow-guide the catheter through the right side of the heart into the pulmonary artery. If the balloon is wedged in a branch of the pulmonary artery the pressure recorded at the tip is an indirect measure of left atrial pressure transmitted retrogradely through the pulmomary veins and capillaries. Pulmonary wedge pressure measurement is widely used in the intensive care unit to monitor left atrial pressure in patients with left ventricular failure. Although right heart catheterization may be performed at the bedside, left heart procedures require the special facilities of a catheterization laboratory. Left ventricular pressure is measured by passing an arterial catheter retrogradely through the aortic valve.

2 Cardiac angiography

This is performed in the catheterization laboratory. Contrast material is injected into the area of interest during radiographic recording on cine-film:

Left ventricular angiography. Contrast injected into the left ventricle demonstrates contractile function and chamber dimensions and also permits evaluation of mitral valve function. The normal mitral valve prevents backflow of contrast, but in mitral regurgitation opacification of the left atrium occurs.

Aortic root angiography—Contrast injected into the aortic root demonstrates the anatomy of the ascending aorta and permits evaluation of aortic valve function. The normal aortic valve prevents backflow of contrast, but in aortic regurgitation opacification of the left ventricle occurs.

Coronary arteriography—This requires selective injection of contrast into the left and right coronary arteries. Intraluminal filling defects or arterial occlusions indicate coronary artery disease, which is nearly always due to atherosclerosis.

Pulmonary angiography—Contrast injection into the main pulmonary artery produces opacification of the arterial branches throughout both lung fields. Intraluminal filling defects and vessel cutoffs usually indicate pulmonary thromboembolism.

Digital subtraction angiography

This recently developed computerized technique may eventually permit high-resolution cardiac angiography using peripheral venous injections of contrast material. Although this will partially avoid the small risk of cardiac catheterization (mortality 0.1–0.2 per cent), it is not yet known to what extent the exciting potential of this new technique will be realized.

Heart failure

Heart failure is a syndrome in which a cardiac disorder produces inadequate cardiac output for the perfusion requirements of metabolizing tissues. It usually implies a disturbance of ventricular function. The major determinants of ventricular function are (Fig. 2.14):

1 Preload—end-diastolic wall tension, conveniently measured by ventricular end-diastolic pressure or atrial pressure (ventricular 'filling pressures')
2 Afterload—systolic wall tension, conveniently measured by arterial pressure
3 Contractility—force and velocity of contraction, independent of loading conditions. Contractility is not amenable to direct measurement.

Aetiology

1 Low-output failure

Cardiac disorders produce low-output failure by restriction of ventricular filling, excessive ventricular loading or impairment of contractile function (Table 2.3).

Restriction of ventricular filling reduces preload, which depresses cardiac output. There is no intrinsic impairment of ventricular contractile function.

Excessive ventricular loading may be caused by either pressure or volume which exert their major influence on afterload and preload, respectively. It is important to distinguish between the effects of acute and chronic loading. In acute pressure loading (e.g. accelerated hypertension, pulmonary embolism) ventricular failure is caused by the abrupt increase in afterload which depresses cardiac output. Acute volume loading (e.g. acute valvar regurgitation) overwhelms the Starling reserve of the ventricle. In chronic pressure or volume loading, however, compensatory mechanisms (see below) protect against heart failure. Nevertheless these compensatory mechanisms are imperfect and ventricular contractile impairment eventually supervenes.

Ventricular contractile impairment is the major cause of low-output failure. It occurs in myocardial infarction, cardiomyopathy and in the end-stage of chronic pressure and volume loading. Once established, ventricular contractile impairment is often irreversible.

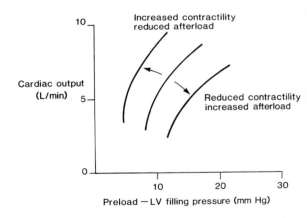

Figure 2.14 *Determinants of left ventricular function. The curvilinear relation between preload (mean left atrial pressure or left ventricular end-diastolic pressure) and cardiac output was described by Starling in 1918. It provides a useful means of evaluating left ventricular function. Changes in contractility and afterload influence ventricular function independently of preload. Thus at a given preload changes in contractility result in changes in cardiac output in the same direction while changes in afterload result in changes in cardiac output in the opposite direction.*

Table 2.3 Causes of heart failure

Ventricular pathophysiology	Clinical examples	Ventricle predominantly affected		
		Left	Right	Both
Restricted filling	Mitral stenosis	×		
	Tricuspid stenosis		×	
	Constrictive pericarditis		×	
	Tamponade		×	
	Restrictive cardiomyopathy			×
	Hypertrophic cardiomyopathy	×		
Pressure loading	Hypertension	×		
	Aortic stenosis	×		
	Coarctation of the aorta	×		
	Pulmonary vascular disease		×	
	Pulmonary embolism		×	
	Pulmonary stenosis		×	
Volume loading	Mitral regurgitation	×		
	Aortic regurgitation	×		
	Pulmonary regurgitation		×	
	Tricuspid regurgitation		×	
	VSD	×		
	Patent ductus arteriosus	×		
Contractile impairment	Coronary artery disease	×		
	Dilated cardiomyopathy			×
	Myocarditis			×
Arrhythmia	Severe bradycardia			×
	Severe tachycardia			×

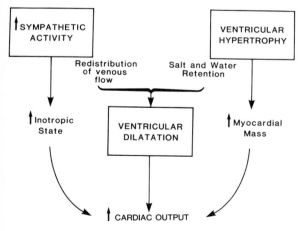

Figure 2.15 *Compensatory physiology in heart failure. If these physiological responses are inadequate, heart failure develops.*

2 High-output failure

Occasionally the perfusion requirements of the body cannot be met despite considerable increments in cardiac output above the normal range. The principal causes of high-output failure are:

1 Increased metabolic rate (e.g. thyrotoxicosis)
2 Reduced oxygen-carrying capacity of the blood (e.g. anaemia) severe lung disease
3 Arteriovenous shunting which reduces the fraction of cardiac output delivered to the metabolizing tissues (e.g. arteriovenous fistula or malformation, beri-beri, Paget's disease)

In all these conditions the volume imposed by chronically elevated cardiac output eventually leads to biventricular failure.

Pathophysiology

1 Compensatory mechanisms

These are directed at maintaining cardiac output despite abnormal loading or contractile impairment (Fig. 2.15).

Increased sympathetic activity helps to maintain cardiac output by increasing the heart rate and contractility. It also constricts the venous capacitance vessels, which redistributes flow centrally and improves cardiac output by increasing preload.

Cardiac dilatation is most marked in the volume-loaded

ventricle. Central redistribution of flow and salt and water retention combine to increase ventricular filling pressures. The heart dilates and the increase in preload helps maintain cardiac output.

Myocardial hypertrophy is most marked in the pressure-loaded ventricle and helps maintain cardiac output by augmenting muscle mass.

Although these compensatory mechanisms can maintain haemodynamic stability for prolonged periods, they are all of limited potential and in the long-term are unable to prevent decompensation from occurring.

2 The kidney in heart failure

The kidney plays an important role in the salt and water retention that characterize heart failure. Reduced renal perfusion and heightened sympathetic activity are major stimuli for renin release from the juxta-glomerular apparatus. This enhances synthesis of angiotensin II which is a potent vasoconstrictor and a stimulus for adrenal secretion of aldosterone. Vasoconstriction helps to maintain blood pressure, but it also increases afterload which may exacerbate left ventricular dysfunction. Aldosterone causes salt and water retention by its effect on the distal nephron. This expands the plasma volume and increases ventricular filling pressures. Although this helps maintain cardiac output, rising atrial pressures eventually lead to pulmonary and systemic oedema.

Clinical features

Most of the clinical features of heart failure are caused by increased sympathetic activity, elevated atrial pressures and reduced cardiac output. Elevated atrial pressures and reduced cardiac output are expressed clinically as congestion (pulmonary and systemic) and peripheral hypoperfusion, respectively. Manifestations of left and right heart failure are conveniently considered separately. Nevertheless, they often occur together, resulting in congestive heart failure.

1 Chronic left heart failure

This is usually the result of left ventricular failure, but in mitral stenosis it occurs without intrinsic impairment of left ventricular contractile function. Symptoms are largely the result of increased left atrial pressure and include exercise-related dyspnoea, orthopnoea and paroxysmal nocturnal dyspnoea (see page 4). Fatigue is usually attributed to inadequate cardiac output. Signs of low cardiac output and reflex sympathetic stimulation include tachycardia, cool skin and peripheral cyanosis. Inspiratory crackles (page 91) are heard at the lung bases. A third

heart sound occurs except in mitral stenosis, where the narrowed valve orifice prevents rapid ventricular filling (see page 7). In severe failure, left ventricular dilatation may stretch the mitral valve ring and papillary muscles, producing 'functional' regurgitation manifested by a pan-systolic apical murmur. Pulsus alternans may also be present in severe failure (see page 5).

2 Acute left heart failure

This is a medical emergency usually caused by myocardial infarction (see page 27). Other causes include acute aortic and mitral regurgitation. Fulminant myocarditis and mitral stenosis may also present acutely. Pulmonary oedema and systemic hypoperfusion are invariable. The patient becomes abruptly dyspnoeic and in severe cases may cough up pink, frothy oedema fluid.

If failure is predominantly 'backward', there will be signs of pulmonary oedema with late inspiratory crackles at the lung bases and sometimes wheezes from associated bronchospasm. There may be cyanosis but the blood pressure and peripheral perfusion are maintained.

If in addition there is 'forward' failure, the blood pressure may fall and peripheral perfusion is poor with cold extremities, mental clouding and a falling urine output (< 20 ml/min).

3 Chronic right heart failure

This is usually the result of chronically elevated pulmonary artery pressure in patients with either left heart failure or obstructive pulmonary disease. In these cases dyspnoea is always prominent. In other cases of right heart failure the effects of low cardiac output, elevated right atrial pressure and salt and water retention dominate the clinical picture. Fatigue, abdominal discomfort and loss of appetite are the principal symptoms. Examination reveals an elevated jugular venous pulse—often with a giant V wave if right ventricular dilatation has stretched the tricuspid valve ring and caused 'functional' tricuspid regurgitation. Peripheral oedema may be severe and commonly involves the abdominal viscera, particularly the liver which is responsible for the abdominal discomfort. In advanced cases hepatic dysfunction results in jaundice and impaired protein synthesis. Hypoalbuminaemia reduces plasma osmolality which exacerbates oedema and contributes to the development of ascites.

4 Acute right heart failure

This is a medical emergency seen in massive pulmonary embolism and, less commonly, in right ventricular infarction. Signs are those of critically reduced cardiac output and include cool skin, systemic hypotension and peripheral cyanosis. Variable elevation of the jugular venous pulse is usually present (see also page 71).

Diagnosis

ECG abnormalities in heart failure are often non-specific and may be limited to T wave changes only. The chest X-ray shows cardiac enlargement, and in left-sided failure this is commonly associated with pulmonary venous dilatation or pulmonary oedema.

The echocardiogram is potentially diagnostic of many of the common causes of heart failure. Left ventricular dilatation and regional contractile impairment indicate ischaemic disease, while four-chamber dilatation and global contractile impairment indicate cardiomyopathy. Heart failure caused by valvar disease is readily apparent.

Cardiac catheterization is rarely necessary for diagnostic purposes, but in patients with surgically correctable lesions (e.g. valvar disease, ventricular aneurysm) the surgeon usually requires precise definition of the lesion with haemodynamic measurements and angiography.

Complications

1 Cardiac arrhythmias

Atrial fibrillation is common in heart failure and often poorly tolerated. Ventricular arrhythmias, however, are more sinister and if sustained cause abrupt clinical deterioration or sudden death.

2 Deep venous thrombosis

This is the result of sluggish flow in the deep veins of the legs and pelvis. Pulmonary thromboembolism is a common cause of death in patients with heart failure.

3 Intracardiac thrombosis

Thrombosis within the dilated cardiac chambers predisposes to systemic and pulmonary thromboembolism.

4 Renal failure

The kidney is particularly sensitive to the effects of hypoperfusion, and worsening renal failure commonly accompanies the progression of heart failure.

5 Hepatic failure

Hepatic congestion causes jaundice and elevation of liver enzymes. This is usually reversible, but in long-standing right heart failure the 'nutmeg' liver of cardiac cirrhosis develops, characterized by centrilobular necrosis and fibrosis.

6 Bronchopneumonia

Chronic pulmonary congestion in left heart failure predisposes to chest infection. Bronchopneumonia is a common cause of death.

Treatment of congestive heart failure

The primary goal of treatment is to identify and correct the underlying cause. In practice this goal cannot always be achieved and once ventricular contractile impairment is established treatment is directed towards controlling symptoms and slowing the progression of disease.

1 Correction of aggravating factors

Cardiac arrhythmias, hypertension and severe anaemia exacerbate heart failure and should be corrected. Salt and water retention in heart failure provides a rationale for limiting salt intake, but the availability of potent diuretics usually makes this unnecessary.

2 Medical therapy (See Table 2.4)

Diuretics are first-line treatment in congestive heart failure. Angiotensin-converting enzyme inhibitors play an important role in patients who fail to respond to diuretics, but other vasodilators and inotropic agents are of less value.

Diuretics promote salt and water excretion. This lowers atrial pressures and corrects pulmonary and systemic congestion. The associated reduction in body weight provides a useful clinical yardstick for assessing the efficacy of treatment. Diuretics do not improve ventricular function. Indeed, by reducing preload they tend to have the reverse effect, and over-diuresis must therefore be avoided.

Thiazides increase sodium excretion in the distal renal tubule. They are mild diuretics, and so in severe heart failure the more potent loop diuretics are necessary. These inhibit sodium reabsorption in the ascending loop of Henle, effectively removing the osmotic gradient in the renal medulla and preventing concentration of the urine.

Angiotensin-converting enzyme inhibitors block the conversion of angiotensin I to angiotensin II. Removal of angiotensin II has two important effects. It produces vasodilatation, which increases cardiac output by reducing blood pressure and afterload. It also removes the major stimulus for aldosterone secretion, enhancing the renal excretion of salt and water. Thus, by increasing cardiac output and promoting salt and water excretion, angiotensin-converting enzyme inhibitors improve both peripheral perfusion and the congestive manifestations of heart failure.

Vasodilators. Drugs with venodilator (e.g. nitrates), arteriolar dilator (e.g. hydralazine) or both properties (e.g. prazosin) have been widely used in the treatment of heart failure. Venodilatation causes pooling of blood in the capacitance vessels, which reduces venous return to the

Table 2.4 Drugs for the treatment of congestive cardiac failure

Drug	How to use	Adverse effects	Interactions
Thiazide diuretics Bendrofluazide Cyclopenthiazide	2.5–10 mg orally daily 250 μg–1.0 mg orally daily	Hypokalaemia; uric acid retention with gout; diminishing glucose tolerance rarely with diabetic-like state	Causes lithium retention; diuresis reduced by NSAIDs
Loop diuretics Frusemide Bumetanide	40–200 mg orally daily 500 μg–5.0 mg orally daily	As for thiazides; high-dose IV frusemide can cause deafness	As for thiazides; also they enhance the nephrotoxicity of aminoglycosides

Both groups of diuretics cause hypokalaemia. Risk factors are high dose, poor diet, concurrent potassium-losing drugs (e.g. steroids) and enhanced toxicity of digitalis which results. At-risk patients should be given either supplementary potassium (25–50 mmol daily as a slow-release preparation) or simultaneously a potassium-sparing diuretic, which is probably more effective.

Potassium-sparing diuretics Amiloride	5–10 mg daily	Hyperkalaemia in poor renal function and diabetes; combined with a thiazide can also cause sodium deficiency	All potassium-sparing diuretics can cause hyperkalaemia if combined with ACE inhibitors or with supplementary potassium
Triamterene	50 mg daily	Hyperkalaemia as above; GI tract upsets	
Spironolactone	50–100 mg daily Takes 2–3 days to work	Hyperkalaemia as above; Gynaecomastia; menstrual upsets; nausea	

A number of fixed-dose preparations containing a thiazide and a potassium-sparing diuretic are available; they are useful if compliance is a problem but do not allow flexibility in dose.

ACE inhibitors Captopril Enalapril	Start with a low dose because of risk of hypotension, especially if the patient is on a diuretic. Captopril: 6.25 mg and increase if necessary to 25 mg three times daily Enalapril: 2.5 mg daily increased to 10–20 mg daily	Hypotension; hyperkalaemia (care in renal failure). Captopril (only in high dose): proteinuria (test urine monthly), leucopenia, patients at risk immunosuppressed, or SLE. Blood counts for first three months. Transient taste disturbances. Cough	Hypotension with other blood-pressure-lowering drugs, especially diuretics; hyperkalaemia with potassium-sparing diuretics
Vasodilators Isosorbide mononitrate	40–80 mg daily	Headache; flushing; hypotension	
Hydralazine	Initially 25 mg daily, increased to 200 mg daily if necessary	Different rates of inactivation; SLE syndrome with higher doses; flushing; headache; GI tract upsets	Action reversed by some NSAIDs

heart and lowers atrial pressures (preload). Arteriolar dilatation improves cardiac output by reducing the blood pressure (afterload). The combination of these effects has the potential to improve both pulmonary congestion and peripheral perfusion, respectively. While there is no doubt about the acute benefits of vasodilator therapy (see below), efficacy is often short-lived so that not all patients experience long-term symptomatic improvement.

Inotropic agents. Of the orally active inotropic agents, digitalis has the time-honoured role in the management of heart failure. Like all other inotropic agents, it increases the availability of intracellular calcium to the myocardial contractile proteins and strengthens the force of contrac-

tion. Despite its mild inotropic properties, digitalis rarely produces appreciable clinical benefit. Moreover, the therapeutic range is narrow and any potential benefit is outweighed by the risk of side-effects. Thus digitalis is no longer recommended for the treatment of heart failure unless the patient is in atrial fibrillation. Digitalis slows the ventricular rate in atrial fibrillation (see page 63) and produces a useful increase in cardiac output. None of the other orally active inotropic agents available for the treatment of congestive heart failure is of proven value. Neither catecholamines nor the more recently introduced non-adrenergic compounds (e.g. amrinone) produce sustained clinical improvement.

Table 2.5 Drugs for treatment of acute left ventricular failure

Drug	How to use	Adverse effects
Opioids		
Morphine	5–10 mg IV bolus	Vomiting (combine with
Diamorphine	2.5–5 mg IV bolus	prochlorperazine 12.5 mg IV); care in obstructive airways disease (use half dose); care in liver disease
Diuretics		
Frusemide	40–80 mg IV	See Table 2.4
Bumetanide	1–2 mg IV	
Vasodilators		
Glyceryl trinitrate	Infusion, starting with 15 μg/minute and increasing as required; max. 200 μg/minute	Headache; flushing; hypotension; tachycardia
Sodium nitroprusside	Infusion, starting with 15 μg/minute and increasing as required; max. 200 μg/minute	5% glucose must be used for infusion solution; protect from light; headaches; nausea; retrosternal pain
Inotropes		
Dopamine	Infusion for renal vasodilatation, 2.5 μg/kg/minute; for inotropic effect, 5–20 μg/kg/minute	Both drugs can cause intense vasoconstriction in overdose; also tachyarrhythmias, nausea, vomiting and headache
Dobutamine	Infusion, 5–20 μg/kg/minute	

Low-dose dopamine may be combined with dobutamine to raise cardiac output and improve renal perfusion.

3 Surgical therapy

Heart failure caused by valve disease, left ventricular aneurysm or certain congenital defects is potentially correctable by surgery, but in the majority of patients with congestive heart failure, heart transplantation is the only surgical option. This is only appropriate in patients with advanced left ventricular contractile impairment resistant to all medical therapy. The risk of perioperative death is small compared with the hazards of organ rejection and immunosuppressive agents. These hazards are greatest during the first year following surgery, but thereafter the threat of accelerated coronary atherosclerosis (the cause of which is unknown) becomes increasingly important. Nevertheless, owing largely to advances in the early recognition and treament of rejection, results of heart transplantation have improved rapidly and there is now an 80 per cent two-year survival.

Treatment of acute left ventricular failure

1 General measures

The patient should be nursed in the head-up position. Correction of cardiac arrhythmias and hypertension is essential. Treatment of hypoxaemia is directed at maintaining an arterial oxygen tension of more than 9 kPa.

2 Medical therapy (Table 2.5)

Opiates and diuretics are first-line agents. Intravenous morphine relieves dyspnoea by a combination of venodilatation, respiratory suppression and relief of anxiety. Intravenous frusemide usually initiates a prompt diuresis. Nevertheless, because diuretic activity depends largely on adequate renal perfusion, frusemide is less helpful in severe low-output states.

Vasodilators and inotropes. If opiates and diuretics are not rapidly effective, vasodilator or inotropic therapy should be started. These drugs should be given by infusion into a central vein with the dual aim of reducing the left atrial pressure and increasing cardiac output. If possible the indirect left atrial pressure (wedge pressure) should be monitored using a Swan Ganz catheter. At a level of 15–20 mmHg pulmonary oedema begins to clear, but further reductions should be avoided because the reduction in preload lowers cardiac output. Cardiac output is best monitored indirectly by measurement of urine flow and skin temperature.

Glyceryl trinitrate and sodium nitroprusside are widely

used vasodilators. Glyceryl trinitrate is predominantly a venodilator, but sodium nitroprusside has a more balanced effect, dilating both veins and arterioles. The venodilator property of both agents reduces the venous return to the heart and lowers the left atrial pressure. The arteriolar-dilator property of sodium nitroprusside, however, ensures that this agent produces greater increments in cardiac output by lowering the blood pressure and afterload. Systolic blood pressure must not be allowed to fall below 90 mmHg because of the risk to vital organ perfusion. Indeed, in patients who are already hypotensive, vasodilators are usually contraindicated.

Dobutamine and dopamine are inotropic agents with sympathomimetic activity. Stimulaton of cardiac beta-1 adrenoceptors enhances contractility and cardiac output. Dopamine (unlike dobutamine) also exhibits important peripheral vascular effects. Low doses (up to 400 μg/minute) selectively dilate the renal arterioles and improve renal perfusion. Higher doses, however, produce widespread alpha adrenoceptor-mediated arteriolar constriction. This improves the blood pressure but further depresses the left ventricular function by increasing afterload. Thus dopamine is best used at low doses for its renal action. Dobutamine, on the other hand, does not share the vascular effects of dopamine and produces dose-related increments in cardiac output. Combination therapy with dobutamine and low-dose dopamine can be particularly beneficial for improving both cardiac output and renal perfusion.

Inotropic agents rarely produce significant reductions in left atrial (pulmonary wedge) pressure. Thus simultaneous treatment with diuretics and vasodilators is often necessary for correction of pulmonary oedema.

3 Surgical therapy

Surgery is potentially life-saving when an acute mechanical lesion produces left ventricular failure without substantial myocardial damage. Thus infective endocarditis complicated by left ventricular failure is usually an indication for urgent valve replacement. Similarly, papillary muscle or septal rupture following myocardial infarction usually requires prompt surgical correction.

Prognosis

Heart failure that is the result of a surgically correctable lesion often has an excellent prognosis following definitive treatment. The majority of patients, however, have irreversible ventricular dysfunction. In these patients prognosis is less good and largely dependent on the degree of ventricular dysfunction. In the most severe cases three-year survival is less than 20 per cent but may be improved by treatment with angiotensin-converting enzyme inhibitors.

Shock

Shock is a syndrome of critically impaired vital organ perfusion which, if not rapidly corrected, leads to irreversible cellular injury with multiple organ failure and death. It is usually caused by severe heart failure (cardiogenic shock), hypovolaemia or septicaemia. The pathogenesis is complex and poorly understood, involving a combination of haemodynamic and toxic factors. Widespread capillary damage characterizes the syndrome and intensifies the perfusion deficit. The myocardial perfusion deficit establishes a vicious cycle of worsening contractile function and end-organ damage. Renal failure occurs early but can be treated by dialysis. Cardiopulmonary failure, on the other hand, is less amenable to treatment. Pulmonary oedema is often 'non-cardiac' in origin and results from pulmonary capillary damage which permits transudation into the lung (*adult respiratory distress syndrome*). Severe hypoxaemia requires mechanical ventilation. Heart failure may respond temporarily to inotropic therapy but the prognosis is very poor with mortality greater than 80 per cent.

Table 2.6 Causes of coronary artery disease

Atherosclerosis
Arteritis:
   systemic lupus erythematosus
   polyarteritis nodosa
   rheumatoid arthritis
   ankylosing spondylitis
   syphilis
   Takayasu disease
Embolism:
   infective endocarditis
   left atrial/ventricular thrombus
   left atrial/ventricular tumour
   prosthetic valve thrombus
   complication of cardiac catheterization
Coronary mural thickening:
   amyloidosis
   radiation therapy
   Hurler's disease
   pseudoxanthoma elasticum
Other causes of coronary luminal narrowing:
   aortic dissection
   coronary spasm
Congenital coronary artery disease:
   anomalous origin from pulmonary artery
   arteriovenous fistula

Coronary artery disease

Aetiology

Coronary artery disease is nearly always caused by atherosclerosis. Indeed the two terms are often used synonymously. Other causes of coronary artery disease are rare (Table 2.6).

Table 2.7 Risk factors for coronary artery disease

Potentially reversible	
Tobacco smoking	Risk rises in proportion to the amount of tobacco smoked
Hypertension	Risk rises in proportion to the level of systolic and diastolic blood pressure
Hyperlipidaemia	Hypercholesterolaemia is the major risk factor, but hypertriglyceridaemia may be important in women. Elevation of low-density lipoproteins (50% cholesterol) increases the risk considerably. High-density lipoproteins (20% cholesterol), however, are protective against the disease
Obesity	The increased risk is due largely to associated hypertension, hypercholesterolaemia and diabetes
Physical inactivity	Evidence is inconclusive. Nevertheless, exercise increases high-density lipoproteins and in some individuals lowers resting blood pressure, both of which might protect against the disease
Diet	Although high-cholesterol diet, and excessive alcohol and coffee consumption, have all been associated with increased risk, the evidence is inconclusive
Irreversible	
Family history	The familial incidence of coronary artery disease is largely the result of genetic predisposition to hypertension, hypercholesterolaemia and diabetes
Advanced age	Risk rises progressively with age
Male sex	Risk is low in young women, but after the menopause it increases and comes to equal that of men
Diabetes mellitus	This increases the risk in both men and women
Personality type	Although the type A personality (chronic sense of time urgency) has been associated with an increased risk compared with the more placid type B personality, the evidence remains inconclusive

The cause of atherosclerotic coronary artery disease is unknown. Epidemiological evidence points to a complex interaction of genetic and environmental influences. Although the cause is unknown a number of risk factors have been identified (Table 2.7). The cumulative effect of multiple risk factors produces an exponential rise in the incidence of future coronary events. Nevertheless it is important to emphasize that risk factors, though associated with coronary artery disease, are not essential for its development. Conversely the presence of risk factors does not necessarily produce atherosclerosis.

Pathology

The disease usually occurs in the proximal 6 cm of the coronary arteries with relative sparing of the smaller distal vessels. It is characterized pathologically by the atherosclerotic plaque, a focal proliferation of smooth muscle cells, collagen and cholesterol esters lying within the intimal and medial layers of the arterial wall. As the plaque increases in size it tends to ulcerate, providing a focus for platelet deposition and thrombosis.

Coronary atherosclerosis is often asymptomatic. The development of symptoms relates to two processes:

1 *Coronary stenosis*—Stenoses in excess of 70 per cent of the coronary luminal diameter may restrict the coronary flow so that myocardial oxygen delivery fails to meet demand. This produces myocardial ischaemia, experienced by the patient as angina.

2 *Thrombotic coronary occlusion*—Total interruption of coronary flow usually produces myocardial infarction in the territory subtended by the occluded artery.

Angina

Clinical features

Angina is experienced as a retrosternal constricting discomfort that may radiate down either arm and into the throat or jaw. Typically, the pain is provoked by exertion and relieved within two to ten minutes by rest. Heightened emotion and sexual intercourse may also provoke angina. Symptoms are usually worse after a heavy meal and in cold weather. Surprisingly the severity of symptoms is not closely related to the extent of coronary artery disease. Indeed extensive disease is sometimes entirely asymptomatic ('silent' myocardial ischaemia), although the risk of myocardial infarction and death remains significant.

The examination is usually normal. Nevertheless, elevated blood pressure and evidence of other major risk factors—including hypercholesterolaemia and diabetes—should be noted. Patients with signs of peripheral vascular disease (absent pulses, arterial bruits) nearly always have associated coronary artery involvement.

Diagnosis

A careful history provides the most useful diagnostic information. Thus in the patient with typical symptoms the probability of coronary artery disease is high, particularly when the patient is male and aged over 40.

1 Exercise testing

Although the resting ECG and thallium-201 perfusion scan are often normal in the patient with angina, exercise-induced myocardial ischaemia may provoke symptoms associated with downward displacement of the ST segment and scintigraphic perfusion defects, respectively. Similarly, exercise-induced abnormalities of left ventricular wall motion may be detected on the radionuclide ventriculogram. These abnormalities reverse during rest and are highly suggestive of coronary artery disease. Nevertheless, exercise testing is imperfect and may give false positive results, particularly in asymptomatic patients and in young women with atypical symptoms. In older patients with more typical symptoms, however, a positive exercise test points strongly to the presence of coronary artery disease.

2 Coronary arteriography

This is the definitive diagnostic test for coronary artery disease (see page 16), although it is not appropriate in every patient suspected of having angina. Coronary arteriography is usually reserved for patients being considered for coronary artery bypass grafting or angioplasty. Other indications are shown in Table 2.8.

Differential diagnosis

1 Neuromuscular disorders

Chest wall pain from the costochrondral junctions or the muscular insertions on to the ribs and sternum is common. The pain is usually sharp and localized and may be provoked by coughing or isometric stess such as pushing or pulling. The affected area is often tender to palpation.

2 Oesophagitis and oesophageal spasm

Oesophageal pain due to acid reflux is retrosternal but may be distinguished from angina by its burning quality and its provocation by stooping or lying flat, particularly after a meal. Antacids often provide effective relief. Oesophageal spasm may be more difficult to distinguish from angina because the pain is retrosternal and may be relieved by glyceryl trinitrate. Nevertheless the pain is often protracted and unrelated to exertion.

3 Psychological disorders

Neurotic anxiety that focuses on the heart is common and disabling. Symptoms, however, are rarely typical of angina. Stabbing pains in the left side of the chest are a common complaint and may be associated with hyperventilation. Time spent discussing the problem with the patient is more productive than extensive investigation, which only serves to reinforce fixed notions of underlying heart disease.

Complications

Angina is a symptom and does not itself produce complications. However, these patients are at risk of all the

Table 2.8 Indications for coronary arteriography

Severe angina unresponsive to medical treatment
Angina in patients aged under 50
Unstable angina
Myocardial infarction in patients aged under 50
Angina or a positive exercise test following myocardial infarction
Cardiac arrhythmias when there is clinical suspicion of underlying coronary artery disease
Preoperatively in patients requiring valve surgery when advanced age (> 50) or angina suggest a high probability of coronary artery disease

Table 2.9 Drugs used to treat angina

Drugs	Dose
Nitrates	
Glyceryl trinitrate:	
sublingual tablet	0.5 mg as required
aerosol spray	0.4–0.8 mg as required
cutaneous patch	25–50 mg daily
	(only 5–10 mg absorbed)
Isosorbide mononitrate	20 mg twice daily
Beta-blockers	
Non-selective:	
propranolol	40–80 mg 3 times daily
slow-release propranolol	160 mg daily
Cardioselective:	
metoprolol	50–100 mg 3 times daily
slow-release metoprolol	200 mg daily
atenolol	50–100 mg once or twice daily
Calcium antagonists	
Nifedipine	5–10 mg 3 times daily
Slow-release nifedipine	20 mg twice daily
Verapamil	40–80 mg 3 times daily
Diltiazem	60–120 mg 3 times daily

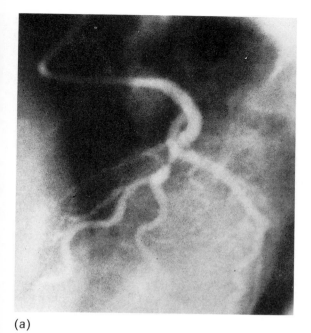

(a)

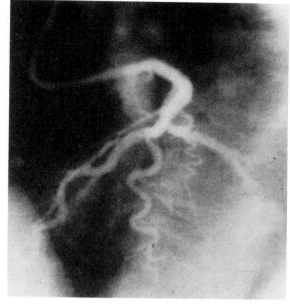

(c)

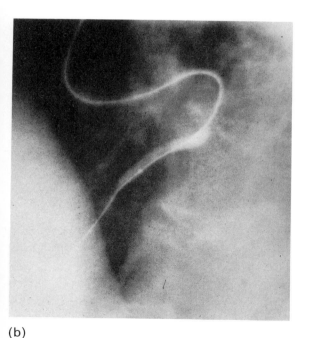

(b)

Figure 2.16 *Coronary angioplasty. (a) Before angioplasty: there is a tight stenosis in the left anterior descending coronary artery. (b) During angioplasty: the angioplasty balloon has been positioned across the stenosis and inflated. (c) After angioplasty: the stenosis has been successfully dilated and the artery is now widely patent.*

other manifestations of coronary artery disease, such as infarction, arrhythmias and heart failure.

Treatment

1 General measures

Severe anaemia, hypertension and thyrotoxicosis exacerbate angina and require treatment. Correction of established risk factors, particularly cigarette smoking, hypertension and hypercholesterolaemia, is usually recommended, but it has been difficult to show that measures other than stopping smoking significantly affect the natural history of the disease.

2 Drug therapy. See Table 2.9

Drugs used to treat angina improve the myocardial oxygen supply-demand imbalance. The only important mechanism for improving oxygen supply is coronary vasodilatation. Reductions in oxygen demand, however, may be achieved by reducing heart rate, contractility or left ventricular wall tension (reflected by blood pressure). Nitrates and beta-blockers are usually used as first-line agents in the treatment of angina, but if symptoms remain troublesome a calcium antagonist can be added.

Nitrates. The vasodilator action of these drugs improves coronary flow and, more importantly, reduces ventricular wall tension by lowering the blood pressure. Sublingual glyceryl trinitrate by tablet or aerosol spray is rapidly absorbed through the buccal mucosa. Relief of angina occurs within about two minutes. The drug can also be used prophylactically to prevent angina during vigorous exertion. A glyceryl trinitrate patch for percutaneous absorption provides a sustained anti-anginal effect in some patients, but responsiveness is variable and the clinical role of this preparation remains uncertain.

Long-term nitrates for regular oral administration are widely used. Isosorbide dinitrate undergoes considerable first-pass metabolism in the liver, but isosorbide mononitrate does not and is the preferred agent in a twice-daily regimen. Side-effects of nitrates relate to vasodilatation and include postural dizziness and headache.

Beta-blockers. These drugs slow the heart rate and reduce contractility and wall tension. A wide variety of different agents are available all with similar anti-anginal efficacy. In general, long-acting drugs such as atenolol are preferred for once- or twice-daily administration. Additional advantages of atenolol are its cardioselectivity and its lipid insolubility, which ensures it does not enter the brain. Beta-blockers, even selective agents, should not be used in patients with a history of asthma because they can precipitate severe attacks of bronchospasm. They should also be avoided in heart failure because of their negative inotropic action.

Calcium antagonists. Like nitrates these drugs are vasodilators and improve the myocardial oxygen balance by their effect on coronary flow and blood pressure. They also cause variable reductions in contractility, particularly verapamil which should be avoided in heart failure. Side-effects include facial flushing, headache and postural dizziness. Mild ankle oedema may also occur but its cause is unclear.

3 Myocardial revascularization procedures

Coronary artery bypass grafting. In patients with proximal coronary artery stenoses or occlusions (demonstrated by arteriography), saphenous vein grafts applied to the ascending aorta may be inserted into the coronary arteries distal to the diseased segments. Alternatively the internal mammary artery can be mobilized and used to bypass the diseased segments. These procedures correct myocardial perfusion and provide significant relief from angina in over 80 per cent of cases. The principal indication for bypass grafting is angina that cannot be controlled by medical therapy. Nevertheless, because surgery improves long-term survival in patients with left main stem or multivessel coronary artery disease, coronary arteriography is now recommended in all symptomatic patients aged under 50 (Table 2.8). This permits identification of those in whom surgery offers prognostic benefit.

Coronary angioplasty (Fig. 2.16) is being used in-creasingly for myocardial revascularization. A catheter with a terminal balloon is introduced percutaneously and positioned across the stenosed coronary arterial segment. Inflation of the balloon dilates the stenosis and restores normal coronary flow. Results are best in patients with a proximal stenosis in only a single major vessel, although multivessel disease may also be treated in this way. Coronary angioplasty provides effective relief of angina, but early recurrence occurs in about 20 per cent of cases. Effects on prognosis are unknown.

Prognosis

Mortality from coronary artery disease has declined in recent years, particularly in the USA. There has probably been a similar decline in the incidence of coronary artery disease. The reasons for this are not known. Nevertheless, the changing natural history of the disease makes prognosis difficult to assess. In the patient with angina, symptoms may remain stable over several years or may even improve as collateral vessels open up. More commonly, however, there is a gradual deterioration with an annual mortality of about 4 per cent.

Unstable angina

Unstable angina may be defined as recurrent episodes of angina occurring on minimal exertion or at rest. Attacks of pain are often associated with reversible ST segment depression on the ECG. The patients usually have critical coronary stenoses, and progression to coronary occlusion with myocardial infarction or death occurs in up to 30 per cent of cases within three months. *Treatment* is with bed-rest and sedation. Glyceryl trinitrate infusion supplemented with oral beta-blockers and calcium antagonists will often control symptoms. The anti-platelet effect of low-dose aspirin (300 mg daily) protects against thrombotic coronary occlusion. In many centres early cardiac catheterization with a view to myocardial revascularization is undertaken. This policy prevents recurrent atttacks of angina but has not been shown to reduce the incidence of myocardial infarction and death.

Variant angina

This relatively unusual anginal syndrome was first described by *Prinzmetal*. It is characterized by unprovoked episodes of chest pain which may be associated with ST segment elevation on the ECG. Coronary artery narrowing is present in 70 per cent of cases, but in the remainder the coronary arteries appear normal at arteriography. An exaggerated increase in coronary arterial tone (spasm) has been demonstrated in these patients during attacks of angina. The spasm is usually focal in distribution, involving the proximal segment of a major coronary artery. Even in the absence of atherosclerosis, spasm can restrict coronary flow sufficiently to produce myocardial ischaemia. These patients are at risk of cardiac arrhythmias, and in prolonged attacks of spasm myocardial infarction may occur. Calcium antagonists prevent spasm and are the treatment of choice. Nitrates are also beneficial, but beta-blockers are of less value and may be detrimental if unopposed alpha-adrenergic stimulation further increases coronary tone.

Myocardial infarction

Myocardial infarction is responsible for 160 000 deaths annually in the UK and for 35 per cent of all deaths in the Western world. Fifty per cent of the deaths occur in the first two hours after the onset of symptoms.

Clinical features

Myocardial infarction usually presents with unprovoked chest pain which is similar in quality to angina but more severe and more prolonged. Autonomic responses produce anxiety, sweating and occasionally vomiting. Examination reveals tachycardia but in other respects may be normal. Nevertheless signs of myocardial damage, including a palpable dyskinetic impulse over the left precordium and the fourth heart sound, are often present. Low-grade fever is common during the first three days. In an estimated 5–10 per cent of cases myocardial infarction is asymptomatic.

Diagnosis

1 Electrocardiogram
Peaking of the T wave followed by ST segment elevation occur during the first hour of pain (Fig. 2.17). Reciprocal ST depression may be seen in the opposite ECG leads. Usually a pathological Q wave (see page 10) occurs during the following 24 hours and thereafter persists indefinitely. The ST segment returns to the isoelectric line within three days and T wave inversion may occur. Occasionally T wave inversion is the only ECG change and is usually attributed to limited subendocardial infarction if other criteria for infarction are fulfilled.

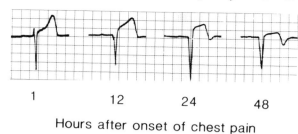

Hours after onset of chest pain

Figure 2.17 *ECG in acute myocardial infarction. This is lead V2 and shows the typical evolution of changes. Peaking of the T wave and elevation of the ST segment occur during the first hour. Thereafter a Q wave develops and usually persists indefinitely. As the ST segment returns to the isoelectric line, T wave inversion may occur.*

The ECG is a valuable indicator of infarct location. Changes in leads II, III and aVF indicate inferior infarction, while changes in leads V1 to V6 indicate anteroseptal (V1 to V3) or anterolateral (V3 to V6) infarction. When the infarct is located posteriorly ECG changes may be difficult to detect, but dominant R waves in leads V1 and V2 often develop.

2 Serum enzymes
Following myocardial infarction enzymes are released into the circulation by the necrosing myocytes (Fig. 2.18).

Creatine phosphokinase is the most useful enzyme for diagnostic purposes. Serum levels peak within 24 hours. The enzyme is also found in skeletal muscle. Thus false positive results may occur following intramuscular injections or external cardiac massage.

Glutamic oxaloacetic transaminase peaks later but remains elevated for about a week. Its diagnostic value is limited by lack of specificity. Thus disease of the liver, kidney and brain may all give false positive results.

Lactic dehydrogenase peaks late but remains elevated for

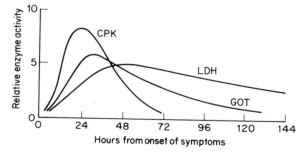

Figure 2.18 *Enzyme release in acute myocardial infarction. These are time activity curves for creatine phosphokinase (CPK), glutamic oxaloacetic transaminase (GOT) and lactic dehydrogenase (LDH). Serum enzyme activity is expressed as multiples of the upper reference limit.*

up to two weeks. It is also found in red cells, and traumatic venesection may give false positive results.

Differential diagnosis

Unstable angina, pericarditis, aortic dissection and pulmonary embolism are important causes of chest pain which may also be associated with ECG changes. All are discussed elsewhere in this chapter.

Complications

1 Cardiac arrhythmias.

Following myocardial infarction, arrhythmia provocation is enhanced by autonomic responses, metabolic abnormalities (particularly hypokalaemia and hypoxaemia), continuing myocardial ischaemia and drug actions. Management of the arrhythmia must include correction of these provocative factors as well as specific anti-arrhythmic therapy.

Atrial arrhythmias. Atrial fibrillation is a common and usually self-limiting arrhythmia in the early hours following myocardial infarction. Paroxysmal attacks may be suppressed with amiodarone or digoxin, but sustained atrial fibrillation may require direct current shock if it produces heart failure or angina.

Ventricular arrhythmias. Ventricular premature beats occur in nearly all patients after myocardial infarction. Certain patterns of ectopy (including very frequent beats or very early 'R on T' beats) have been identified as predictors of ventricular fibrillation. Nevertheless, the logic of treating these 'warning' arrhythmias with lignocaine infusion is now in doubt because there is little evidence that it reduces the incidence of ventricular fibrillation and no evidence that it improves prognosis in patients admitted into the coronary care unit.

Ventricular tachycardia always requires prompt treatment. Paroxysmal attacks may be suppressed with lignocaine bolus followed by infusion (see Table 2.24), but sustained attacks require direct current cardioversion.

Table 2.10 Indications for temporary pacing in acute myocardial infarction

Third-degree (complete) atrioventricular block
    complicating inferior myocardial infarction and any of
    the following:
  (a) rate less than 40 beats per minute, unresponsive
       to atropine
  (b) heart failure
  (c) unreliable escape rhythm
  (d) bradycardia-dependent ventricular arrhythmias
       which require suppression
All cases of third-degree (complete) or Mobitz type II
second-degree atrioventricular block complicating
anterior myocardial infarction
Bifascicular heart block
Underdrive or overdrive suppression of refractory
arrhythmias

Ventricular fibrillation requires urgent direct current cardioversion to prevent death. It usually occurs as a 'primary' electrical phenomenon in the early hours after myocardial infarction, emphasizing the importance of rapid access to resuscitation facilities following the onset of chest pain (Fig. 2.19). Ventricular fibrillation sometimes occurs late after myocardial infarction when it is usually 'secondary' to extensive myocardial damage. If resuscitation is successful, long-term anti-arrhythmic therapy is necessary because secondary ventricular fibrillation predicts a high incidence of sudden death following hospital discharge.

2 Heart block

Myocardial infarction may damage the specialized conducting tissues. If this causes (or threatens to cause) an excessively slow heart rate, temporary pacemaker therapy may be necessary to maintain cardiac output and prevent asystole (Table 2.10). The prognostic implications of heart block in myocardial infarction are shown in Table 2.11.

Atrioventricular block. This is usually a complication of inferior infarction and is caused by inflammation and oedema around the atrioventricular node. In third-degree (complete) atrioventricular block a junctional escape

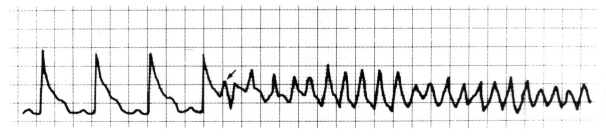

Figure 2.19   *Primary ventricular fibrillation. The ECG shows changes of acute myocardial infarction with sinus tachycardia and ST segment elevation. A very early premature beat (arrowed) triggers ventricular fibrillation.*

Table 2.11 Acute atrioventricular block in myocardial infarction

Conduction defect	Incidence (%)	Risk of progression to third-degree block (%)	Mortality (%)
None	70	6	15
First-degree block	5	6	15
Second-degree block			
Mobitz type I	5	7	15
Mobitz type II	1	70	50
Third-degree block	7	–	25
Left anterior hemiblock	5	3	27
Left posterior hemiblock	1	0	42
Right bundle branch block	2	43	46
Left bundle branch block	5	20	44
Bifascicular block	5	46	45

rhythm usually takes over with a reliable rate of 40 to 60 beats per minute (Fig. 2.20). In most cases this is sufficient to maintain normal cardiac output. Complete recovery of atrioventricular conduction nearly always occurs within two weeks. If the junctional escape rhythm is very slow it will often respond to intravenous atropine (0.6 mg). Indications for pacemaker therapy are shown in Table 2.10. When atrioventricular block complicates anterior myocardial infarction, this usually implies extensive left ventricular injury with damage to both left and right bundle branches. Ventricular escape rhythms are always slow and unreliable, and whether the block is complete or intermittent (Mobitz type II) pacemaker therapy is indicated.

Bundle branch block. Isolated left or right bundle branch block is an adverse prognostic sign but requires no specific treatment. Left or right axis deviation (hemiblock) in myocardial infarction often indicates damage to the anterior or posterior fascicle of the left bundle, respectively. When hemiblock is associated with right bundle branch block ('bifascicular block'), atrioventricular conduction is dependent upon the remaining fascicle of the left bundle. The risk of complete heart block developing is considerable and prophylactic pacing should be undertaken.

3 Left ventricular failure

This affects up to half of all patients with myocardial infarction and is the principal cause of death following admission to the coronary care unit. Because right ventricular damage is rarely severe, left ventricular failure usually dominates the clinical picture. The severity of failure is closely related to infarct size; when about 40 per cent of the left ventricle is damaged cardiogenic shock occurs (see page 22). The principal clinical manifestations of left ventricular failure are pulmonary oedema and peripheral hypoperfusion, caused by elevated left atrial pressure and reduced cardiac output, respectively. Four subsets of patients have been identified based on these clinical manifestations and defined by a cardiac output of 3.5 litres per minute and a left atrial (pulmonary artery wedge) pressure of 18 mmHg (Fig. 2.21):

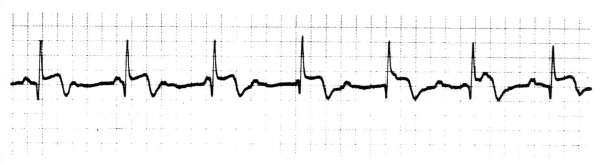

Figure 2.20 *Third-degree (complete) heart block in inferior myocardial infarction. Block is at the atrioventricular node and has caused dissociation of the atrial and ventricular rhythms. Thus the P waves and the QRS complexes are completely independent of one another. Because the 'escape' rhythm is junctional in origin, the QRS complexes are narrow and the rate is well maintained. The monitoring lead is III and shows a Q wave with ST segment elevation.*

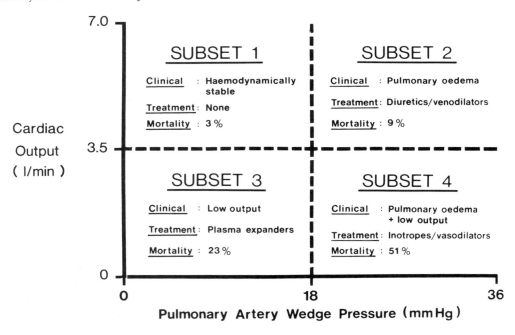

Figure 2.21 *Haemodynamic subsets in acute myocardial infarction. The subset divisions are defined by the intersection of a pulmonary artery wedge pressure of 18 mmHg and a cardiac output of 3.5 l/minute. The clinical, therapeutic and prognostic correlates of subset classification are illustrated.*

Subset 1: Well-preserved left ventricular function requiring no specific therapy.

Subset 2: Dominantly 'backwards' failure with pulmonary oedema but well-maintained cardiac output. Treatment with morphine and diuretics is usually effective.

Subset 3: Dominantly 'forwards' failure without pulmonary oedema. Oliguria and hypotension are corrected by infusion of a plasma volume expander (e.g. plasma, blood) which increases cardiac output by the Starling mechanism. Careful monitoring of pulmonary artery wedge pressure is essential to prevent overloading the circulation. Pulmonary oedema develops if the wedge pressure rises above 18 mmHg.

Subset 4: Low cardiac output and pulmonary oedema occur together. Treatment must be directed towards improving left ventricular function with vasodilators or inotropes. These drugs should be given by controlled intravenous infusion to reduce pulmonary artery wedge pressure and improve cardiac output. Responses are best monitored with a Swan Ganz catheter.

Subset classification provides not only a useful basis for therapeutic decision making but also a means of predicting prognosis. Thus mortality rises from less than 5 per cent in subset 1 to greater than 50 per cent in subset 4.

4 Right ventricular failure

Occasionally, inferior myocardial infarction is associated with extensive right ventricular damage and leads to right ventricular failure with elevation of the right atrial and jugular venous pressures.

From the clinical point of view, low cardiac output is the principal problem, and a useful improvement can often be achieved by further increasing the right atrial pressure with infusions of plasma volume expander. This increases the right ventricular output by the Starling mechanism. Monitoring of pulmonary capillary wedge pressure is a sensible precaution during the infusion in order to guard against pulmonary oedema.

5 Myocardial rupture

This usually occurs during the first ten days following myocardial infarction. When it involves the free wall of the ventricle it causes severe tamponade, which is usually fatal. Rupture of a papillary muscle or the interventricular distinguish. In most cases urgent cardiac catheterization is required to define the lesion and to assess the potential for surgical correction.

6 Pericarditis and Dressler's syndrome

Pericarditis during the first three days after myocardial infarction is a direct consequence of the underlying muscle damage and usually resolves rapidly. Pericarditis which presents later may indicate Dressler's syndrome, particularly when associated with fever, pleurisy and an elevated erythrocyte sedimentation rate. Dressler's syndrome is probably an autoimmune phenomenon. It is self-limiting, but anti-inflammatory analgesics (e.g. aspirin) provide effective symptomatic relief. Occasionally corticosteroids are necessary. Relapses up to two years after myocardial infarction may occur.

7 Thromboembolism

Deep venous thrombosis and intracardiac mural thrombosis (overlying the infarcted ventricular myocardium) are potential sources of pulmonary and systemic thromboembolism, respectively. Heparin therapy reduces the risk of these complications.

8 Ventricular aneurysm

If scar formation is inadequate following myocardial infarction, a thin-walled left ventricular aneurysm may develop. This is often associated with persistent ST segment elevation on the ECG. Ventricular aneurysm predisposes to arrhythmias, heart failure and thromboembolism and may require surgical excision.

Treatment

1 Home versus hospital care

In acute myocardial infarction the need for early medical supervision has already been emphasized. Only the presence of personnel with appropriate skills and equipment can prevent death from ventricualr fibrillation. In certain cases, however, the familiar environment afforded by home care may compensate for lack of resuscitation facilities. The patient whose symptoms are of more than six hours standing has survived beyond the period of maximum risk and, in the absence of complications, the added anxiety of hosptial referral may confer no prognostic advantage. The full weight of hospital intensive care is also inappropriate in the very elderly.

2 General measures

The patient should be admitted to the coronary care unit and attached to an ECG monitor. An intravenous line should be established. If the early course is uncomplicated the patient may be transferred to the general ward after 24 hours. Mobilization is started after three days with a view to discharge after seven to ten days.

3 Specific therapy

Pain relief and sedation are of overriding importance. Intravenous diamorphine (2.5–5.0 mg) is the drug of choice for both purposes, and should be repeated as necessary. Drug-induced nausea and vomiting are reduced by intravenous cyclizine (50 mg). All patients should be treated with subcutaneous heparin, 5000 units three times daily, to guard against deep venous and mural thrombosis.

Thrombolytic agents (e.g. streptokinase) can recanalize a recently occluded coronary artery by lysing the thrombus (Fig. 2.22). This permits reperfusion of the jeopardized myocardium. Because the full extent of myocardial damage takes up to six hours to develop, reperfusion within this time may limit the extent of myocardial damage and thereby improve prognosis. Recent information suggests that the use of fibrinolytic agents following myocardial infarction reduces early mortality. Streptokinase (1.5 mega units) is infused over one hour, but it only apears to be effective if given within six hours of the onset of pain. This excludes many patients admitted to hospital. Contraindications to streptokinase include recent peptic ulceration or stroke.

It may well be that in the future tissue plasminogen activators or a plasminogen streptokinase actived complex will be found to be more effective with less risk.

Intravenous beta-blockers given early after myocardial infarction also improve the prognosis, though the mechanism is obscure. It may relate to limitation of the infarct size owing to reductions in myocardial ischaemia, but anti-arrhythmic effects may also be important. Atenolol 5–10 mg IV is recommended in the absence of contraindications (bronchial asthma, heart failure).

4 Rehabilitation

Most patients require considerable reassurance. On return home they should make a graded return to activity within the limits of their exercise tolerance.

They should be strongly advised to stop smoking and to reduce their weight (if overweight) to the ideal level for their height and age. They should not drive for two months. Normal sexual activity can be resumed after a month provided exercise tolerance is satisfactory.

Patients may require advice about their future occupation. They should usually be able to return to work in 8–12 weeks and questions of retirement, etc. will need individual discussion; but patients should be encouraged to lead as full and as normal a life as possible.

5 Secondary prevention

In the year that follows myocardial infarction there is a significant risk of recurrent infarction or suddden death. The only measures of proven value for reducing that risk

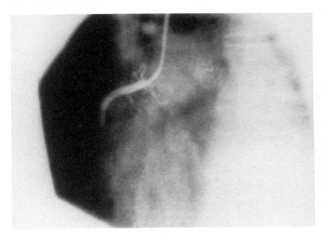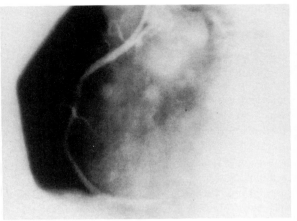

Figure 2.22   *Thrombolytic therapy in acute myocardial infarction. The panel on the left shows the right coronary arteriogram in a patient with inferior myocardial infarction. The artery is occluded near its origin. The panel on the right shows the arteriogram following strep-tokinase therapy. The artery is now recanalized but there is a tight residual stenosis. Further management must include measures to prevent re-occlusion, such as anticoagulant therapy or revascularization (angioplasty, bypass surgery).*

are stopping cigarette smoking and treatment with beta-blockers.

Although patients with left ventricular failure have a poor prognosis following myocardial infarction, attempts to identify other high-risk subgroups have been disappointing. Evidence that residual myocardial ischaemia is portentous of early reinfarction and death has led to a policy of early exercise stress-testing for patients recovering from myocardial infarction. Patients who develop ST segment depression suggestive of ischaemia (see page 11) or ventricular arrhythmias undergo cardiac catheterization with a view to revascularization by coronary bypass surgery or angioplasty. Despite continuing enthusiasm for this relatively simple method of selecting and treating 'high-risk' patients, convincing evidence for its efficacy in terms of improving long-term prognosis has not been forthcoming.

Prognosis

Myocardial infarction is fatal in about 50 per cent of cases. Of these, 65 per cent die within six hours of the attack before hospital admission. The remainder of deaths occur in hospital (15 per cent) or during the first year after discharge (20 per cent). The pre-hospital mortality is due to primary ventricular fibrillation in the majority of cases. Primary ventricular fibrillation, however, does not necessarily reflect extensive myocardial damage, and prognosis following resuscitation is similar to that of other early survivors.

Hospital mortality is closely related to infarct size. When infarction is sufficiently extensive to cause severe

Table 2.12 Adverse prognostic factors in myocardial infarction

Advanced age
Anterior transmural infarction
Bundle branch block and advanced atrioventricular block
Heart failure
Systolic hypotension
Complex ventricular arrhythmias occurring greater than
  24 hours after the onset of symptoms
History of previous myocardial infarction
Diabetes mellitus

heart failure, mortality exceeds 50 per cent. Other factors, apart from overt heart failure, are also predictive of a poor prognosis (Table 2.12). With the exception of advanced age, however, these are all variably related to extensive myocardial damage, emphasizing the important relation between infarct size and prognosis.

Cardiomyopathy

The cardiomyopathies are a group of chronic heart muscle disorders of unknown cause. This definition excludes those specific heart muscle disorders that are secondary to coronary artery disease, valvar disease, hypertension and other systemic disorders.

Dilated cardiomyopathy

Aetiology

The cause of dilated cardiomyopathy is by definition

a)

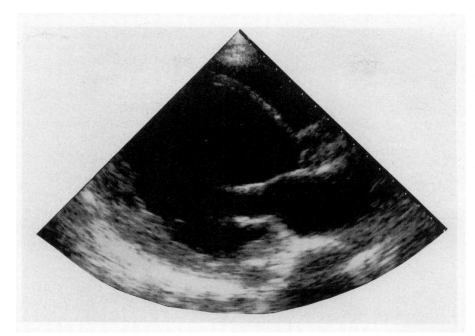

b)

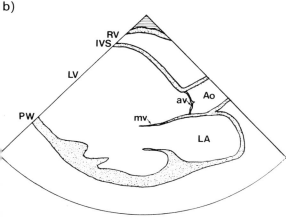

Figure 2.23 *Echocardiogram in dilated cardiomyopathy. Two-dimensional recorded showing enormous dilatation of the left ventricle (compare with Fig. 2.12(b)).*

the atrioventricular valve rings can lead to functional mitral and tricuspid incompetence. These complications produce additional impairment of ventricular function.

Clinical features

Dilated cardiomyopathy often remains asymptomatic in its early stages, but with progression of disease symptoms and signs of congestive heart failure develop (see page 18).

Diagnosis

The chest X-ray shows cardiac enlargement with dilated upper lobe veins and, in advanced cases, pulmonary oedema. The echocardiogram shows four-chamber dilatation and global left ventricular contractile impairment (Fig. 2.23). Doppler studies often reveal mitral and tricuspid regurgitation even if these are not evident clinically.

Differential diagnosis

This includes all those conditions listed in Table 2.13 that cause specific heart muscle disease. Coronary artery disease is suggested by a history of angina or myocardial infarction associated with pathological Q waves on the ECG. Valvar disease is confirmed by echocardiography.

unknown. There is some evidence for an infectious–autoimmune aetiology related to viral myocarditis, but this is unproven.

Pathology and pathophysiology

Dilated cardiomyopathy is characterized by progressive dilatation, hypertrophy and fibrosis of all the cardiac chambers. Contractile function is severely impaired. Atrial fibrillation commonly supervenes and stretching of

Table 2.13 Common causes of specific heart muscle disease

Cardiovascular
Coronary artery disease
Chronic valvar disease
Hypertension

Infective
Viral (e.g. Coxsackie A & B)
Influenza, Varicella, Mumps
Herpes simplex
Protozoal (e.g. Trypanosomiasis-Chagas' disease)

Metabolic
Thiamine deficiency (beriberi)
Kwashiorkor

Endocrine
Thyrotoxicosis
Myxoedema
Diabetes mellitus

Toxic
Alcohol
Doxorubicin
Cobalt

Connective tissue disease
Polyarteritis nodosa
Systemic lupus erythematosus

Neuromuscular disease
Muscular dystrophy
Friedreich's ataxia

Infiltrative
Amyloidosis
Haemochromatosis
Sarcoidosis
Neoplastic

Miscellaneous
Post-partum cardiomyopathy
Obesity

septum produces abrupt left ventricular failure associated with a pan-systolic murmur. Clincially they are difficult to Hypertensive and alcoholic heart disease are sometimes impossible to distinguish from dilated cardiomyopathy. Nevertheless a careful history often provides the aetiological diagnosis, and the examination may reveal non-cardiac manifestations of hypertensive or alcoholic end-organ damage. Viral myocarditis is usually a subclinical complication of upper respiratory infection, but occasionally it causes severe heart failure and mimics dilated cardiomyopathy. Complete recovery, however, can be expected in most cases of viral myocarditis. Doxorubicin, a widely used anti-neoplastic agent, causes dose-related myocardial toxicity. The risk is particularly high once a cumulative dose of $550\,mg/m^2$ has been exceeded. Once heart failure is established the condition is similar to dilated cardiomyopathy but progresses more rapidly.

Complications

Cardiac arrhythmias are common in dilated cardiomyopathy, particularly atrial fibrillation and ventricular extrasystoles. More complex ventricular arrhythmias (ventricular tachycardia and fibrillation) are a cause of sudden death.

Intracardiac mural thrombosis—the result of haemostasis within the dilated heart—predisposes to systemic and pulmonary thromboembolism.

Treatment

No specific treatment affects disease progression in dilated cardiomyopathy. It should be managed in the same way as other causes of heart failure.

Prognosis

This depends on the severity of left ventricular dysfunction. Once symptoms of heart failure develop the average five-year survival is less than 50 per cent. In patients with end-stage disease, heart transplantation improves the prognosis (see page 21).

Hypertrophic cardiomyopathy

Aetiology

Hypertrophic cardiomyopathy shows an autosomal dominant pattern of inheritance but it occurs sporadically in about half of all cases.

Pathology

Hypertrophic cardiomyopathy is characterized anatomically by ventricular hypertrophy usually with disproportionate involvement of the interventricular septum. Histologically there is disarray and disorganization of the cardiac myocytes.

The physiological disorder is one of impaired diastolic relaxation. Systolic contraction is normal and often hyperdynamic. The hypertrophied ventricle is stiff (non-compliant) and adequate filling demands high end-diastolic pressure. Atrial contraction provides an important boost to ventricular filling, and the development of atrial fibrillation results in abrupt clinical deterioration.

In the past considerable importance has been attached to the pressure gradient which can often be demonstrated in the left ventricular outflow tract beneath the aortic valve. It is now clear, however, that the pressure gradient does not reflect significant obstruction to flow and, im-

(a)

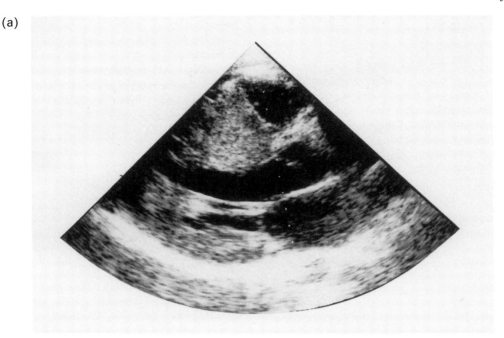

(b)

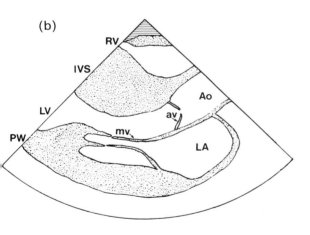

Figure 2.24 *Echocardiogram in hypertrophic cardiomyopathy. Two-dimensional recording showing massive left ventricular hyper-trophy predominantly affecting the interventricular septum (compare with Fig. 2.12(b)).*

portantly, its presence influences neither symptoms nor prognosis in patients with hypertrophic cardiomyopathy.

Clinical features

Hypertrophic cardiomyopathy is often asymptomatic. The most common complaint is exercise-related dyspnoea which is due to the elevated left atrial pressure required to fill the stiff, non-compliant ventricle. In advanced cases frank congestive heart failure occasionally develops. Angina, due to the excessive oxygen demand of the hypertrophied ventricle, may also be troublesome.

Examination reveals a 'jerky' carotid pulse owing to vigorous left ventricular ejection in early systole. The apical impulse is prominent and often has a double thrust owing to a palpable fourth heart sound. Auscultatory features include the fourth heart sound and a mid-systolic ejection murmur at the aortic area owing to turbulent flow in the left ventricular outflow tract. Mitral regurgitation affects nearly half of all cases and when present produces an apical pan-systolic murmur.

Diagnosis

The ECG shows left ventricular hypertrophy. This is confirmed by the echocardiogram which usually shows disproportionate involvement of the interventricular septum (Fig. 2.24). Other echocardiographic findings are systolic anterior motion of the mitral valve and early closure of the aortic valve. When the diagnosis remains unclear, cardiac catheterization can be performed for measurement of the pressure gradient in the left ventricular outflow tract and angiographic demonstration of the abnormal left ventricular contraction pattern.

Differential diagnosis

Hypertension and aortic stenosis both produce left ventricular hypertrophy and share many of the clinical and ECG features of hypertrophic cardiomyopathy. Nevertheless, the elevated blood pressure and slow rising pulse which, respectively, characterize these conditions help in making the correct differential diagnosis. Moreover, in both conditions the echocardiogram shows concentric left ventricular hypertrophy without other features of hypertrophic cardiomyopathy; the valvar abnormality in aortic stenosis is readily apparent.

Hypertrophic cardiomyopathy must also be differentiated from coronary artery disease. This may required coronary arteriography in patients with angina.

Complications

Cardiac arrhythmias are the major complication. Atrial fibrillation causes abrupt clinical deterioration (see page 57). Paroxysmal ventricular arrhythmias produce dizziness and syncope (Stokes–Adams attacks) and are portentous of sudden death.

Treatment

No drugs affect the progression of disease in hypertrophic cardiomyopathy. Treatment is aimed at correcting symptoms and preventing sudden death. Beta-blockers and verapamil control angina and also produce a variable improvement in ventricular diastolic relaxation. This reduces the left atrial pressure and improves dyspnoea. All patients should undergo ambulatory ECG monitoring (see page 57). If ventricular arrhythmias are detected amiodarone is the drug of choice because it may prevent sudden death. Screening of family members and genetic counselling should be undertaken, as with other inherited disorders.

Restrictive cardiomyopathy

Restrictive cardiomyopathy is characterized by endomyocardial fibrosis with progressive obliteration of the ventricular cavities. Systolic function is normal but diastolic relaxation is restricted. Restrictive cardiomyopathy is rare in this country and nearly always associated with cryptogenic hypereosinophilia. Presentation is with congestive heart failure. Steroids or cytotoxic agents lower the eosinophil count and may halt the progression of disease.

Primary amyloidosis commonly involves the heart and may produce a syndrome clinically and physiologically indistinguishable from restrictive cardiomyopathy, although hypereosinophilia is not present. There is no effective treatment and death occurs within two years of presentation.

Pericardial disease

Acute pericarditis

Aetiology

Causes of pericarditis are listed in Table 2.14. Viral infection probably accounts for the majority of cases including many of those idiopathic cases in which a specific cause cannot be positively identified.

Pathology

Pathological features are those of any acute inflammatory process. An inflammatory exudate commonly occurs resulting in pericardial effusion.

Clinical features

Central chest pain is the predominant symptom and may be associated with fever. The pain is typically sharp in quality and is aggravated by deep inspiration, coughing

Table 2.14 Causes of acute pericarditis

Idiopathic
Infective:
    viral (Coxsackie B, influenza, *Herpes simplex*)
    bacterial (*Staphylococcus aureus, Mycobacterium tuberculosis*)
Connective tissue disease:
    systemic lupus erythematosus
    rheumatoid arthritis
    polyarteritis nodosa
Uraemia
Malignancy (e.g. breast, lung, lymphoma, leukaemia)
Radiation therapy
Acute myocardial infarction
Post myocardial infarction/cardiotomy (Dressler's syndrome)

and changes in posture. Auscultation usually reveals a pericardial friction rub (see page 8). If pericardial effusion develops the heart sounds diminish in intensity but the friction rub does not necessarily disappear.

Diagnosis

The ECG shows widespread ST segment elevation. The ST segments are concave upwards (unlike myocardial infarction) and return towards baseline as the pericardial inflammation subsides.

The aetiological diagnosis in viral pericarditis requires demonstration of elevated serum viral antibody titres with return towards normal during convalescence. In connective tissue disorders there is usually evidence of multisystem disease, and specific serology, including rheumatoid or anti-nuclear factors, may be positive. When the aetiological diagnosis is obscure pericardial fluid (if present) should be aspirated for bacterological, cytological and serological examination.

Differential diagnosis

Important differential diagnoses are myocardial infarction and pleurisy, though it should be appreciated that both conditions may themselves be associated with pericarditis. The quality of pericarditic pain, the failure of Q waves to develop on the ECG and the absence of significant serum enzyme changes effectively exclude myocardial infarction. Pleuritic pain is similar to pericarditic pain but its location is different, and a pleural rub is usually audible over the painful area.

Complications

The major complication of pericarditis is pericardial effusion which may cause tamponade. Pericarditis can also progress to pericardial constriction. The reputed association between pericarditis and atrial arrhythmias has not been confirmed in prospective studies.

Treatment

Anti-inflammatory analgesics (e.g. aspirin) are effective for controlling chest pain. In viral pericarditis no other treatment is necessary. Bacterial pericarditis requires vigorous antibiotic therapy.

Pericarditis may be a recurrent illness particularly in Dressler's syndrome, connective tissue disorders and idiopathic disease. When recurrence is frequent, low-dose corticosteroid therapy (prednisolone 5 to 10 mg daily) offers effective prophylaxis.

Prognosis

Pericarditis is usually a benign disorder and the prognosis depends on the underlying cause. Nevertheless, the development of tamponade or pericardial constriction may be fatal if not corrected.

Cardiac tamponade

Aetiology

In this country the principal causes of cardiac tamponade are haemopericardium following heart surgery and pericardial effusion complicating neoplastic disease. Nevertheless, almost any other cause of pericardial haemorrhage or effusion may cause tamponade, depending principally on the rate of fluid accumulation within the pericardial sac.

Pathophysiology

Gradual accumulation of fluid permits progressive stretching of the pericardial sac such that a substantial effusion may develop without significant elevation of intrapericardial pressure. Rapid accumulations, on the other hand, cause elevation of pressure within the pericardial sac, which leads to tamponade. This tends to constrict the heart and impede diastolic relaxation. Adequate ventricular filling depends on the diastolic pressures in both ventricles rising to equilibrate with the intrapericardial pressure. As tamponade worsens, progressive increments in ventricular filling pressures become inadequate to maintain cardiac output.

Clinical features

Presentation is abrupt following pericardial haemorrhage but is usually more gradual in patients with pericardial effusion. Shortness of breath and fatigue are the principal complaints. Examination reveals tachycardia, elevated jugular venous pressure, hypotension and signs of reduced cardiac output or cardiogenic shock. Pulsus paradoxus is invariable, and in some patients Kussmaul's sign is also present. The heart sounds are faint and a pericardial friction rub may be audible.

Diagnosis

The chest X-ray shows globular cardiac enlargement. The ECG shows diminished voltage deflections which may be associated with electrical alternans (Fig. 2.25). Echocardiography confirms pericardial effusion.

Differential diagnosis

Tamponade must be differentiated from other causes of low cardiac output and shock, including myocardial infarction, pulmonary embolism and septicaemia. The differential diagnosis is not difficult if pulsus paradoxus and pericardial effusion can be demonstrated.

Treatment

Tamponade requires urgent pericardiocentesis in order to decompress the heart. A needle is introduced into the angle between the xiphisternum and the left costal margin and advanced beneath the costal margin towards the left shoulder. Following entry into the pericardial sac, the effusion is aspirated. Further treatment is directed at the underlying cause.

Prognosis

Cardiac tamponade is potentially fatal, but following pericardiocentesis the prognosis depends on the underlying cause of the fluid accumulation.

Constrictive pericarditis

Aetiology

Constrictive pericarditis is no longer common in this country owing largely to the declining incidence of tuberculosis. Most cases are now idiopathic in origin.

Pathophysiology

Fibrosis and shrinkage of the pericardial sac impedes diastolic relaxation of the ventricles and prevents adequate filling. Thus constrictive physiology is very similar to that seen in tamponade (see page 37).

Clinical features

Constrictive pericarditis is a chronic wasting illness. Although symptoms and signs of low cardiac output are usually present, the consequences of elevated right atrial pressure and salt and water retention dominate the clinical picture. The appearances are those of severe right heart failure with elevation of the jugular venous pressure, hepatomegaly, ascites and peripheral oedema. Kussmaul's sign is always positive, but pulsus paradoxus

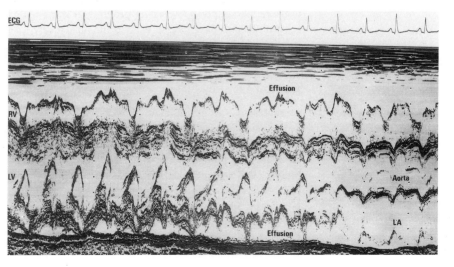

Figure 2.25   *ECG and echocardiogram in pericardial effusion. This M-mode echocardiogram shows a pericardial effusion evidenced by the echo-free space in front of and behind the heart (compare with Figure 2.12(a)). The movement of the heart within the effusion is unrestricted resulting in beat-to-beat variation in the electrical axis of the ECG (electrical alternans).*

is seen less commonly. Auscultation reveals an early third heart sound (pericardial 'knock').

Diagnosis

The ECG shows diminished voltage deflections. The chest X-ray is often normal but may show pericardial calcification, particularly in tuberculous disease. Cardiac catheterization confirms elevation of the left and right atrial pressures, which equalize with loss of the normal differential. The ventricular diastolic pressure signal shows a characteristic dip and plateau configuration (the 'square-root' sign).

Differential diagnosis

This includes all other causes of right heart failure. Cirrhosis of the liver must also enter the differential diagnosis. In most cases of right heart failure the heart is enlarged and right ventricular dilatation can be demonstrated by echocardiography. Moreover, in the majority of cases associated pulmonary disease or left heart failure is evident. Cirrhosis of the liver produces ascites and debilitation but does not share the cardiovascular manifestations of constrictive pericarditis.

Treatment

Diuretics control salt and water overload, but pericardiectomy is the treatment of choice. The procedure is technically demanding but if successful the results are excellent.

Rheumatic fever

Aetiology

A small proportion (less than 1 per cent) of patients with group A haemolytic streptococcal pharyngitis develop rheumatic fever two to three weeks later. The disease occurs most commonly between the ages of five and fifteen years. The precise pathogenic role of the streptococcus is unknown but a number of features suggest an autoimmune process. These include the characteristic latency period between throat infection and development of rheumatic fever and the immunological cross-reaction between streptococcal antigens and myocardial sarcolemma.

The tendency for rheumatic fever to be familial and the high incidence of recurrence after an initial attack indicate heightened susceptibility in certain individuals, possibly due to genetic predisposition. Nevertheless, the major factors predisposing to the disease are crowding and social deprivation which encourage spread of the streptococcus. Improvements in housing and welfare have undoubtedly played the major role in reducing the incidence of rheumatic fever throughout the developed world. Other contributory factors have been the availability of penicillin and the changing virulence of the streptococcus itself.

Pathology

Myocarditis and a transient pericarditis occur commonly but are rarely severe. Endocarditis is the major cardiac lesion. Inflammation of the valve cusps is associated with verrucous nodules along the lines of valve closure. This may cause severe valve damage acutely, but more commonly valve function is little affected in this phase of the illness. During healing, however, progressive scarring of the valve may lead to chronic rheumatic heart disease (see below).

Clinical features

Fever and arthralgia are often the only symptoms. These may be attributed to a simple viral infection which is soon forgotten by the patient.

1 Carditis

This affects about 50 per cent of cases. It may cause severe heart failure and death, although usually it produces no symptoms at all. Tachycardia, gallop rhythm and a soft ejection murmur at the aortic area are typically present, but in children these findings are non-specific manifestations of any feverish illness. Thus a diagnosis of rheumatic carditis should not be made unless there is clear evidence of valvar involvement. The apical pan-systolic murmur of mitral regurgitation is the most constant finding. A mid-diastolic murmur at the same location also indicates mitral disease. The early diastolic murmur of aortic regurgitation occurs less commonly.

2 Non-cardiac disease

Polyarthritis usually affects the large joints of the extremities. A migratory pattern is characteristic and as one joint recovers another becomes involved. Cutaneous involvement is characterized by small painless nodules and erythema marginatum—an evanescent rash which occurs on the trunk but never on the face. *Chorea (Sydenham's chorea, St Vitus' dance)* often occurs several months after the initiating streptococcal pharyngitis. Severity is variable, ranging from occasional involuntary movements to violent jerking movements of the entire body.

Diagnosis

If recent streptococcal throat infection can be confirmed by demonstration of elevated serum antistreptolysin O titre, Jones' criteria may be used for diagnosis of rheumatic fever (Table 2.15). The presence of two major criteria, or one major and two minor criteria, indicates a high probability of rheumatic fever.

Differential diagnosis

Differential diagnoses include other causes of childhood arthritis, bacterial endocarditis and viral pericarditis. Still's disease—the major cause of childhood arthritis—runs a chronic course and other criteria for rheumatic fever are not present. Bacterial endocarditis, though associated with fever and heart murmurs, causes relentless clinical deterioration. Positive blood cultures and other stigmata of the condition should be sought. Simple viral pericarditis is never associated with valvar disease, unlike rheumatic pericarditis in which valvar involvement and heart murmurs are always present.

Treatment

In patients with a streptococcal throat infection, amoxycillin 250 mg three times daily (or if vomiting, benzylpenicillin 600 mg 12-hourly IM) is effective in preventing rheumatic fever.

In established rheumatic fever no specific treatment affects the course of the illness. Bed-rest is usually recommended and a course of penicillin should be given to eradicate residual streptococcal infection. Aspirin, starting at 100 mg/kg/day, is highly effective for treating fever and arthritis. Steroids are equally effective and are sometimes preferred in patients with carditis, though there is no evidence that they prevent chronic valvar damage. Following rheumatic fever, phenoxymethylpenicillin 125 mg orally twice daily should be given to guard against recurrent attacks and continued up to the age of 25.

Table 2.15 Jones' criteria for the diagnosis of rheumatic fever

Major criteria	Minor criteria
Carditis	Fever
Polyarthritis	Arthralgia
Erythema marginatum	Previous rheumatic fever
Chorea	Elevated ESR
Subcutaneous nodules	Prolonged P–R interval

Prognosis

Acute rheumatic fever usually subsides within six weeks but intractable carditis or chorea may last up to six months. Recurrent attacks are common, and in patients with carditis these exacerbate cardiac damage and increase susceptibility to heart failure and death. In most cases, however, heart failure is delayed until the development of chronic rheumatic heart disease several years later. Chorea and arthritis rarely produce chronic sequelae.

Chronic rheumatic heart disease. Following an attack (or recurrent attacks) of rheumatic fever, cardiac function usually returns to normal. During healing of the inflamed valves, however, progressive scarring may lead to chronic rheumatic heart disease 15 to 20 years later. Adhesion of the valve commissures and shrinkage of the cusps and subvalvar apparatus produce variable stenosis and regurgitation. Valvar calcification exacerbates the process. By the age of 30 many patients have had their first attack of congestive heart failure, which is often precipitated by the onset of atrial fibrillation or by the stress of pregnancy. The percentage incidence of involvement of the various valves is approximately as follows:

Mitral valve	80
Aortic valve	45
Tricuspid valve	10
Pulmonary valve	1
Mitral valve alone	50
Mitral and aortic valves together	20

Infective endocarditis

Infective endocarditis usually involves the heart valves but may also affect other congenital or acquired cardiac defects. Infection of the endothelial lining of arterial aneurysms or arteriovenous fistulae produces a similar illness.

Aetiology

Endocarditis is now seen increasingly in the elderly, unlike 50 years ago when it was more common in young adults. *Streptococcus viridans* is the most common infecting organism. It is a normal commensal of the upper respiratory tract and produces a chronic, subacute illness. Other more virulent organisms, notably *Staphylococcus aureus*, produce a rapidly progressive acute illness (Table 2.16).

Endocarditis may affect healthy patients with entirely

Table 2.16 Organisms implicated in endocarditis

Organism	Typical source of infection	First-choice antibiotics (pending sensitivity studies)
Streptococcus viridans	Upper respiratory tract	Benzylpenicillin; gentamicin
Streptococcus faecalis	Bowel and urogenital tract	Ampicillin; gentamicin
Anaerobic streptococcus	Bowel	Ampicillin; gentamicin
Staphylococcus epidermidis	Skin	Flucloxacillin; gentamicin
Fungi: Candida, Histoplasmosis	Skin and mucous membranes	Amphotericin B*; 5-fluoro-cytosine*
Coxiella Burnetti	Complication of Q fever	Chloramphenicol*; tetracycline*
Chlamydia psittaci	Contact with infected birds	Tetracycline* and erythromycin
Acute disease		
Staphylococcus aureus	Skin	Flucloxacillin; gentamicin
Streptococcus pneumoniae	Complication of pneumonia	Benzylpenicillin; gentamicin
Neisseria gonorrhoeae	Venereal	Benzylpenicillin; gentamicin

*These drugs are not cidal and valve replacement is nearly always necessary to eradicate infection.

normal hearts. Nevertheless patients at greater risk are those with pre-existing valvar disease. Other high-risk groups are shown in Table 2.17. The left-sided heart valves, ventricular septal defects, and patent ductus arteriosus are the most common sites of infection. Right-sided endocarditis is rare, usually affecting main-lining drug addicts.

The source of infection cannot usually be identified. *Streptococcus viridans* bacteraemia is almost invariable during dental surgery, but fewer than 15 per cent of patients with endocarditis give a history of recent dental treatment. Instrumentation of the genitourinary and gastrointestinal tracts also causes bacteraemia but is not often implicated in the development of endocarditis.

Pathology

Endocarditis leads to aggregation of fibrin, platelets and

Table 2.17 Groups at increased risk of endocarditis

The elderly (> 60 years)
Patients with intrinsic cardiovascular disease; high-risk
    lesions are:
        ventricular septal defect
        aortic regurgitation
        mitral regurgitation
        aortic stenosis
        patent ductus arteriosus
        coarctation of the aorta
Patients with valve prostheses, tissue grafts and other
    intracardiac foreign material
Mainlining drug addicts (right-sided valvar endocarditis
    occurs relatively commonly in this group)
Immunosuppressed patients
    acquired immunodeficiency syndrome
    immunosuppressive drugs

other blood products at the site of infection. This produces a vegetation which is relatively avascular and tends to isolate the infective organism from host defences and antimicrobial agents. Valve destruction produces worsening regurgitation and commonly leads to heart failure. In endocarditis caused by *Staphylococcus aureus*, valve destruction is rapid and local abscess formation commonly occurs. In less aggressive infections (e.g. from *Streptococcus viridans*) the progression of disease is slower and large craggy vegetations develop which are prone to embolism. The chronic infection may lead to immune complex disease with vasculitic involvement of kidneys, joints and skin.

Clinical features

In subacute disease the onset is insidious, with influenza-like symptoms including fever, night-sweats, arthralgia and fatigue. Petechial haemorrhages in the skin and under the nails ('splinter' haemorrhages) are a common but non-specific finding. Valvar endocarditis causes regurgitant murmurs (typically aortic or mitral) owing to destruction of the valve leaflets. Other 'classical' manifestations of endocarditis, including Osler's nodes (tender erythematous nodules in the pulps of the fingers), Roth's spots in the retina, clubbing of the fingers and splenomegaly are now rarely seen.

Diagnosis

Endocarditis should be considered in every patient with fever and a heart murmur. Laboratory findings include leucocytosis, normochromic, normocytic anaemia and elevation of the erythrocyte sedimentation rate. Analysis of the urine commonly reveals haematuria. Blood cultures are usually positive and should always be obtained before antibiotic treatment is started: up to six specimens should be collected over 24–48 hours. Culture-negative endocarditis is caused by pretreatment with antibiotics, inadequate blood sampling or infection with unusual micro-organisms. The echocardiogram identifies underlying valvar disease and vegetations may also be seen if large enough.

Differential diagnosis

Infective endocarditis must be distinguished from other causes of fever and heart murmurs (e.g. rheumatic fever). Particular difficulty arises in patients with pre-existing valvar disease who develop an associated trivial infection (e.g. viral pharyngitis). Nevertheless, if recovery is not rapid investigation to exclude endocarditis is essential.

Complications

1 Heart failure
This is the major complication of endocarditis and the usual cause of death.

2 Immune complex disease
Vasculitic rash and arthritis with red, tender joints occasionlly occur. More important, however, is glomerulonephritis which may progress to intractable renal failure.

3 Embolism
Vegetations may embolize peripherally, threatening limbs or major organs. Metastatic abscesses are not uncommon, particularly in the spleen or brain. Coronary embolism with myocardial infarction is seen occasionally.

4 Heart block
Abscess formation in the aortic valve ring may cause heart block by damaging the conducting tissue in the interventricular septum.

5 Mycotic aneurysm
Aneurysm may develop locally in the sinuses of Valsalva or elsewhere in the circulation. They result from embolic occlusion of the vasa vasorum and may be infected or sterile. Rupture can occur during the acute phase of the illness or at any time following its eradication.

Treatment

This must not be delayed beyond the time necessary to obtain up to six blood specimens for culture. Bactericidal antibiotic therapy should then be started and continued for at least four weeks. For the first two weeks combination therapy with two antibiotics is recommended. These should be given intravenously using a central line. Thereafter the course may be completed using a single antibiotic given orally. Because streptococcal infection accounts for over 70 per cent of cases, initial treatment should be with benzylpenicillin, 6.0 g daily, and low-dose gentamicin which enhances penicillin activity. When the results of blood cultures become available different antibiotics may be necessary depending on the organism grown.

Valve replacement may be necessary in endocarditis, but ideally this should be delayed until antibiotic therapy has resolved the infection. Nevertheless urgent surgical intervention during the acute phase of the illness is necessary if heart failure develops; any delay often results in the death of the patient. Other relative indications for early surgery are conduction defects, recurrent embolism, fungal endocarditis and resistant infection, particularly in prosthetic valve endocarditis.

Prophylaxis. Antibiotic prophylaxis—to prevent bacteraemia during dental surgery and other non-sterile invasive procedures—is required in all patients with valve disease and other cardiac defects. A single 3 g oral dose of amoxycillin should be given one hour before dental work (scaling, filling, extraction). Erythromycin can be used in penicillin-sensitive patients.

Ampicillin (1 g IM) with gentamicin (120 mg IM) immediately before the procedure, followed after six hours by amoxycillin (500 mg orally), is appropriate prophylaxis during instrumentation of the gastrointestinal or genitourinary tracts.

Prognosis

With the introduction of penicillin nearly 50 years ago, mortality in endocarditis fell from 100 per cent to about 30 per cent. It has remained at that level since that time. The continuing high mortality is the result of multiple factors, including the emergence of antibiotic-resistant organisms, the introduction of prosthetic heart valves, the widespread use of immunosuppressive therapy, the worsening problem of intravenous drug abuse, and the older more debilitated age group now at risk. The major impediment to effective treatment, however, is delayed diagnosis. The insidious onset of endocarditis often causes it to be overlooked until it is too late to save the patient.

Valvar heart disease

The heart valves direct the cardiac output forwards into the pulmonary and systemic circulations without impeding the flow. Valvar dysfunction is the result of incompetence or stenosis which produce backward flow (regurgitation) or impeded flow, respectively. Regurgitant valve lesions volume-load the ventricles, while stenotic lesions of the ventricular outflow valves (aortic and pulmonary) pressure-load the ventricles. Stenotic lesions of the ventricular in-flow valves (mitral and tricuspid), on the other hand, impede filling and reduce preload. Abnormal loading has the potential to cause heart failure, but this may be delayed by the effects of compensatory mechanisms (see page 17), particularly in chronic valve disease.

The important role of echocardiography in the diagnosis of valve disease has already been emphasized. Used in conjunction with Doppler studies the pressure gradient across the stenosed valve and the regurgitant flow through an incompetent valve can be quantitated. Indeed, in patients with valve disease, cardiac catheterization is rarely necessary for diagnostic purposes. Despite this, cardiac catheterization is usually performed before proceeding to valve replacement, particularly in elderly patients who are at risk of coronary artery disease. This not only documents the valve lesion but also permits angiographic examination of the coronary arteries. In patients with coronary disease, bypass grafting can be performed at the same time as valve replacement.

Surgery has revolutionized the management of valvar heart disease and can produce complete haemodynamic correction. The timing of valve surgery is important because if it is delayed until ventricular dysfunction or pulmonary hypertension have become irreversible the risks are greater and the results less satisfactory. In mitral stenosis dilatation of the valve (valvotomy) is effective if the valve is competent and not calcified. Regurgitant lesions of the mitral and tricuspid valves can sometimes be corrected by repair procedures. In most cases of valve disease, however, surgical correction requires replacement of the valve with a tissue graft or prosthesis. Porcine xenografts are widely used because, unlike prostheses, they are not thrombogenic and do not expose the patient to the inconvenience and risk of long-term anticoagulant therapy. Nevertheless tissue grafts are prone to calcification and failure within seven years and for this reason prostheses are often preferred. Prostheses are usually ball and cage or tilting disc mechanisms. Both types are reliable but tilting discs present less obstruction to flow. Long-term anticoagulant therapy is essential following insertion of a prosthetic valve.

It is convenient to consider each of the important valve lesions separately. It must be recognized, however, that an individual valve may be both regurgitant and stenosed. Moreover, disease involving more than one valve is not uncommon, particularly in rheumatic disease and endocarditis. Multivalvar disease increases the haemodynamic burden on the heart and often leads to heart failure earlier than disease affecting a single valve.

Mitral stenosis

Aetiology

Mitral stenosis is nearly always rheumatic in origin. Rarely it occurs as a congenital defect.

Pathology and pathophysiology

In mitral stenosis the valve commisures are fused and the leaflets are thickened and often calcified. Adequate filling of the left ventricle is impaired, and the left atrial pressure rises producing a diastolic pressure gradient across the valve (Fig. 2.26). Left ventricular contraction is unaffected, but because filling is impeded adequate cardiac output cannot be maintained, particularly during exercise. As the pressure rises in the left atrium it dilates and is prone to fibrillate. This compromises left ventricular filling still further, partly because of the rapid heart rate which reduces diastolic filling time, and partly because of the loss of atrial asystole.

The elevated left atrial pressure produces pulmonary congestion and pulmonary hypertension which in turn leads to right ventricular failure. In advanced mitral stenosis, irreversible pulmonary hypertension may develop.

Clinical features

Mitral stenosis produces orthopnoea and exertional fatigue and dyspnoea in the same way as other causes of left heart failure. In advanced disease life-threatening attacks of acute pulmonary oedema occur. Chronic pulmonary congestion may produce cough and haemoptysis and predisposes to winter bronchitis. The onset of atrial fibrillation is often associated with abrupt clinical deterioration. A similar deterioration may occur during pregnancy owing to the increase in circulating volume and increased cardiac output.

Cyanotic discolouration of the cheeks produces the typical mitral facies. Atrial fibrillation results in an

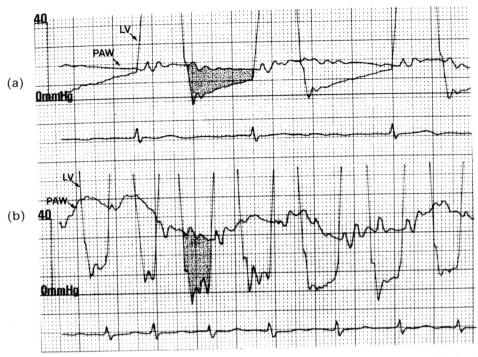

Figure 2.26   *Cardiac catheterization in mitral stenosis. (a) Recording made at rest. The heart rate is slow and the diastolic pressure gradient (shaded area) is trivial. (b) Recording made during exertion. This produced tachycardia and a steep rise in left atrial pressure. The diastolic pressure gradient (shaded area) is now substantial. The ECG shows atrial fibrillation. LV, left ventricular pressure signal; PAW, pulmonary artery wedge pressure signal.*

irregular pulse. The apical impulse has a tapping quality but is not usually displaced. Auscultation at the cardiac apex reveals a loud first sound and an opening snap in early diastole followed by a low-pitched mid-diastolic murmur. Pre-systolic accentuation of the murmur occurs only in sinus rhythm. In advanced mitral stenosis the loud first sound and the opening snap become less prominent, and the opening snap and the start of the murmur move closer to the second heart sound as the left atrial pressure rises.

The development of right ventricular failure produces elevation of the jugular venous pulse and peripheral oedema. The dilated right ventricle displaces the apical impulse towards the left axilla and causes a left parasternal systolic thrust. Prominence of the pulmonary component of the second heart sound reflects pulmonary hypertension.

Diagnosis

The ECG shows P mitrale when the patient is in sinus rhythm. Atrial fibrillation, however, is more common. Signs of right ventricular hypertrophy may be present in advanced disease. The chest X-ray shows left atrial en-

largement often with a normal heart size. Prominence of the upper lobe veins is almost invariable; pulmonary oedema may also occur. Calcification of the mitral valve or left atrial wall is sometimes seen on penetrated lateral films.

The echocardiogram is diagnostic and shows thickening and rigidity of the mitral valve leaflets associated with dilatation of the left atrium (Fig. 2.27). The right-sided cardiac chambers may also be dilated. Doppler studies permit quantification of the pressure gradient across the valve. This may be confirmed by cardiac catheterization (see Fig. 2.26).

Differential diagnosis

Mitral stenosis must be differentiated from other conditions in which dyspnoea is associated with added diastolic sounds. Left ventricular failure produces similar symptoms and the unwary may mistake the third heart sound for an opening snap or a mid-diastolic murmur. A mid-diastolic apical murmur also occurs in severe aortic regurgitation owing to preclosure of the mitral valve (Austin-Flint murmur). Perhaps the most important differential diagnosis is left atrial myxoma. This is difficult

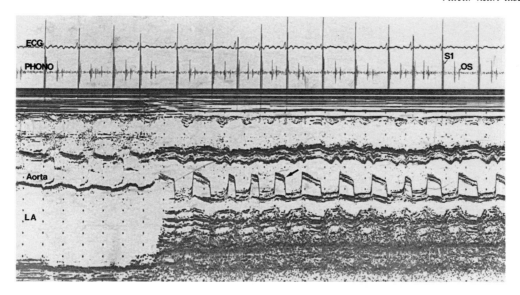

Figure 2.27 *Echocardiogram in mitral stenosis. This M-mode recording shows thickening and rigidity of the mitral valve (arrowed). The left ventricle is normal but the left atrium (LAS) is considerably dilated (compare with Fig. 2.12(a)). The phonocardiogram shows a loud first heart sound (S1) followed by a normal second heart sound. The opening snap (OS) in early diastole has also been recorded. The ECG shows atrial fibrillation.*

to distinguish from mitral stenosis on clinical grounds but the echocardiogram is diagnostic.

Complications

1 Atrial arrhythmias
Atrial fibrillation nearly always develops in long-standing mitral stenosis.

2 Thromboembolism
Haemostasis in the dilated left atrium predisposes to thrombosis, particularly following the onset of atrial fibrillation. The risks of systemic embolism to the brain or elsewhere are reduced by prophylactic anticoagulation with warfarin.

3 Pulmonary vascular disease
Pulmonary hypertension is an inevitable consequence of elevated left atrial pressure and may become irreversible because of obliterative pulmonary vascular disease in the presence of severe right ventricular failure. The process is irreversible so mitral valve replacement does not produce clinical improvement.

4 Endocarditis
This rarely occurs in pure mitral stenosis unassociated with mitral regurgitation. Nevertheless, antibiotic prophylaxis prior to dental surgery and other non-sterile invasive procedures should always be given.

5 Chest infection
Chronic pulmonary congestion predisposes to chest infections which are a common cause of death in mitral stenosis.

Treatment

Diuretics produce effective symptomatic relief by correcting pulmonary and systemic congestion. Following the onset of atrial fibrillation, digitalis should be prescribed to control the ventricular rate, and anticoagulation with warfarin is mandatory to protect against thromboembolism.

Indications for surgery are dyspnoea unresponsive to medical treatment and right ventricular failure. Valvotomy is the procedure of choice, but if the valve is calcified or regurgitant it must be replaced with a tissue graft or prosthesis.

Prognosis

Following rheumatic carditis in childhood, symptomatic mitral stenosis may take up to 20 years to develop, though pregnancy or the development of atrial fibrillation may prompt an earlier presentation. Once symptoms are established progressive deterioration often leads to death within five to ten years unless surgery is performed. Death may be the result of pulmonary oedema, chest infection, endocarditis or thromboembolism.

Mitral regurgitation

Aetiology

Mitral regurgitation has many causes, the majority of which relate to acquired disease of the valve leaflets or the subvalvar apparatus (Table 2.18).

1 Mitral valve prolapse

This is a common and usually asymptomatic condition in which one or both of the mitral valve leaflets bulge backwards into the left atrium during systole. This produces mitral regurgitation in some but not all cases. Only rarely is the mitral regurgitation severe. Mitral valve prolapse affects about 5 per cent of the population and is particularly common in young women. Most cases are idiopathic but it may also be associated with a variety of cardiac and systemic disorders, including rheumatic and ischaemic heart disease and Marfan's syndrome. Chest pain and cardiac arrhythmias may occur, particularly ventricular extrasystoles and supraventricular tachycardias. Auscultation typically reveals a mid-systolic click followed by a murmur. Definitive diagnosis requires echocardiography which identifies the prolapsing leaflet.

2 Chordal rupture

This is usually idiopathic in origin but may also occur in endocarditis or rheumatic disease. It usually produces acute mitral regurgitation and may present abruptly with pulmonary oedema.

3 Papillary muscle disease

Myocardial ischaemia can cause dysfunction of the papillary muscles with variable mitral regurgitation. Papillary muscle rupture complicating myocardial infarction always produces torrential mitral regurgitation and pulmonary oedema requiring urgent valve replacement.

Table 2.18 Causes of mitral regurgitation

*Valve leaflet diease**
Mitral valve prolapse
Rheumatic disease
Infective endcarditis†

*Subvalvar disease**
Chordal rupture†
Papillary muscle dysfunction
Papillary muscle rupture†

Dilating left ventricular disease
'Functional' mitral regurgitation

* Note that the subclassification into valve leaflet and subvalvar disease is to some extent artificial because all the causes of valve leaflet disease are usually associated with subvalvar dysfunction.
† These disorders produce acute mitral regurgitation.

Pathophysiology

Mitral regurgitation volume-loads the left ventricle leading to compensatory dilatation and hypertrophy. The increase in left atrial pressure and volume causes pulmonary congestion. The dilated left atrium is prone to fibrillate.

Clinical features

Mitral regurgitation is usually asymptomatic until the left ventricle begins to fail. In acute mitral regurgitation this occurs abruptly but in chronic disease it may take several years. Symptoms including orthopnoea and exercise-related fatigue and dyspnoea are the same as occur in other causes of left heart failure. Severe pulmonary hypertension is unusual in mitral regurgitation and for this reason features of right ventricular failure are rarely prominent.

The pulse is often irregular owing to atrial fibrillation. The cardiac apex is displaced, reflecting cardiac enlargement. Auscultation at the apex reveals a pan-systolic murmur which radiates into the left axilla. The third heart sound is often present owing to rapid filling from the volume-loaded left atrium.

Diagnosis

The ECG shows P mitrale if the patient is in sinus rhythm. The chest X-ray shows cardiac enlargement, left atrial dilatation and prominence of the upper lobe veins. The echocardiogram confirms dilatation of the left sided chambers which is associated with worsening contractile impairment as the left ventricle fails. Diagnostic abnormalities of the valve itself occur when the leaflets are diseased. In subvalvar disease, however, the echocardiogram may show an apparently normal valve. Doppler studies identify the regurgitant jet in the left atrium. The diagnosis is confirmed by left ventricular angiography which documents the severity of mitral regurgitation and left ventricular contractile impairment.

Differential diagnosis

Mitral regurgitation must be distinguished from other causes of a pan-systolic murmur, particularly tricuspid regurgitation and ventricular septal defect. In both conditions, however, the murmur is loudest at the left sternal edge and does not radiate into the axilla.

Complications

Patients with mitral regurgitation are prone to thrombo-embolism from the dilated left atrium, particularly following the development of atrial fibrillation. The risk of endocarditis is considerable and antibiotic prophylaxis is required prior to dental surgery and other non-sterile invasive procedures. Nevertheless, the major complication of mitral regurgitation relates to left ventricular volume overload which may lead eventually to irreversible impairment of contractile function.

Treatment

Diuretics are often sufficient to control dyspnoea in mitral regurgitation. The development of atrial fibrillation requires digitalis to control the ventricular rate and anticoagulation with warfarin. Vasodilators such as prazosin or hydralazine act by lowering peripheral vascular resistance; forward flow into the aorta increases, reducing the volume of blood that regurgitates backwards through the mitral valve.

If symptoms cannot be controlled by medical measures, mitral valve replacement should be considered. If surgery is delayed unnecessarily, irreversible deterioration in left ventricular contractile function occurs. In acute mitral regurgitation diuretics and vasodilators are helpful, but early valve replacement is usually necessary.

Prognosis

Chronic mitral regurgitation is only slowly progressive and is compatible with a normal life-span. Nevertheless, if the volume-loaded left ventricle develops contractile failure the prognosis is considerably worse and death usually occurs within five to ten years.

Aortic stenosis

Aetiology

In the UK aortic stenosis is usually caused by calcification of the valve leaflets. This is a slowly progresive, degenerative process. When it affects a previously normal valve it rarely presents before the age of 60. When it affects a congenitally bicusid valve, on the other hand, presentation in middle-age is more common. Rheumatic aortic stenosis is relatively unusual and rarely occurs without associated mitral disease. All the important causes of aortic stenosis are also causes of aortic regurgitation. Thus a combination of both defects commonly occurs in the same patient.

Pathophysiology

Aortic stenosis obstructs left ventricular outflow. A systolic pressure gradient is produced across the valve, and this increased load leads to left ventricle hypertrophy. The hypertrophied ventricle is stiff and non-compliant so that adequate filling depends on a high diastolic pressure. Atrial contraction provides an important boost to ventricular filling, and the development of atrial fibrillation often produces clinical deterioration. As aortic stenosis worsens, irreversible impairment of left ventricular contractile function eventually occurs. Forward flow across the valve can no longer be maintained and the heart dilates, leading to frank left ventricular failure.

Clinical features

Elevation of the left atrial pressure produces exertional dyspnoea, which is particularly severe following the onset of left ventricular failure. Other major symptoms include angina (caused by the exaggerated oxygen demands of the hypertrophied left ventricle) and syncope. Syncope typically occurs during exertion because flow through the stenosed aortic valve cannot increase sufficiently to maintain blood pressure in the face of vasodilation in exercising skeletal muscle (see page 4). Vasodilator drugs can produce hypotension and syncope by the same mechanisim and should be avoided in aortic stenosis. Syncope may also result from paroxysmal ventricular arrhythmias (Stokes–Adams attacks).

The carotid pulse has a slow upstroke. Left ventricular hypertrophy does not displace the apex beat, which is thrusting in character and may have a double impulse owing to a palpable fourth heart sound. A systolic thrill is often palpable over the aortic area and the carotid arteries. Auscultation reveals a medium-pitched mid-systolic murmur which is loudest at the aortic area and radiates into the neck. It is preceded by an ejection click if the valve cusps are pliant and not heavily calcified. A fourth heart sound and reversed splitting of the second heart sound are usually present.

Diagnosis

The ECG shows left ventricular hypertrophy. The chest X-ray shows a normal heart size unless there is left ventricular failure or associated aortic regurgitation. Post-stenotic dilatation of the ascending aorta is usually evident (Fig. 2.28) and the penetrated lateral film may reveal valvar calcification. The echocardiogram shows a

(a)

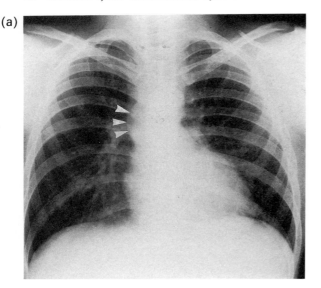

(b)

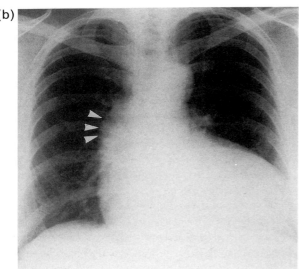

Figure 2.28   *Chest X-ray in aortic valve disease. Aortic valve disease produces dilatation of the ascending aorta (arrowed). (a) In aortic stenosis, the heart size is normal because the pressure-loaded left ventricle hypertrophies but does not dilate until failure supervenes. (b) In aortic regurgitation, volume loading produces a variable degree of left ventricular dilatation.*

thickened, rigid aortic valve and symmetrical ventricular hypertrophy. Doppler studies may be used to quantify the valve gradient.

Cardiac catheterization permits direct measurement of the pressure gradient across the aortic valve (Fig. 2.29). Angiographic assessment of left ventricular contractile function can also be obtained. Because angina is common in aortic stenosis, coronary arteriography is essential before valve replacement to rule out associated coronary artery disease.

Differential diagnosis

Hypertrophic cardiomyopathy and hypertension are both associated with left ventricular hypertrophy and have many of the clinical features of aortic stenosis. These include angina, mid-systolic murmur and the fourth heart sound. Moreover, ECG abnormalities in both conditions are similar to those in aortic stenosis. Nevertheless, in neither hypertrophic cardiomyopathy nor hypertension is the carotid pulse slow-rising, nor does the echocardiogram show a thickened aortic valve.

Innocent mid-systolic murmurs should not be confused with aortic stenosis. They may occur in healthy individuals but are more common in conditions such as anaemia, fever, thyrotoxicosis and pregnancy. The hyperdynamic circulation characteristic of these conditions increases the velocity of ejection sufficiently to produce turbulence across the aortic and pulmonary valves. Innocent murmurs are usually soft, are always mid-systolic in timing and are never associated with a slow-rising carotid pulse.

Complications

1 Left ventricular failure
The chronic pressure load may eventually lead to irreversible left ventricular contractile impairment.
2 Endocarditis
This is an ever-present risk in aortic stenosis. Antibiotic prophylaxis prior to dental surgery and other non-sterile invasive procedures is essential.
3 Arrhythmias
Atrial fibrillation is not uncommon in aortic stenosis and often produces clinical deterioration. More important are ventricular arrhythmias which are a cause of syncope and sudden death.
4 Heart block
This is an occasional complication of calcific aortic stenosis and results from calcific destruction of the conducting tissue in the adjacent part of the interventricular septum.

Treatment

Aortic stenosis that is subcritical requires no specific treatment while it remains asymptomatic. The development of symptoms, however, is an indication for valve replacement. Other indications for valve replacement are

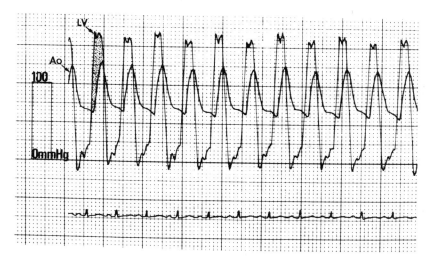

Figure 2.29 *Cardiac catheterization in aortic stenosis. Aortic stenosis causes a systolic pressure gradient across the aortic valve (shaded area) such that left ventricular pressure is higher than aortic pressure. LV, left ventricular pressure signal; Ao, aortic pressure signal.*

left ventricular contractile impairment and critical aortic stenosis (peak systolic pressure gradient above 50 mmHg) even in the absence of symptoms. Balloon valvuloplasty may be possible in patients unfit for surgery.

Prognosis

Aortic stenosis is well-tolerated and most patients are over 60 before they die. Nevertheless, following the development of symptoms death usually occurs within three to five years. The outlook is worse in patients with left ventricular failure. Valve replacement improves both symptoms and prognosis in patients with aortic stenosis.

Aortic regurgitation

Aetiology

Aortic regurgitation may be caused either by disease of the valve cusps or by aortic root disease which leads to dilatation of the valve ring (Table 2.19).

Pathophysiology

Aortic regurgitation volume-loads the left ventricle. When this occurs acutely it may cause severe decompensation by overwhelming the Starling reserve of the ventricle. In chronic aortic regurgitation, however, left ventricular dilatation and hypertrophy compensate for the volume load. The regurgitation of blood through the aortic valve increases diastolic filling and produces vigorous ventricular contraction by the Starling mechanism. This maintains forward cardiac output despite regurgitation through the aortic valve. These compensatory mechanisms, however, have limited potential and contractile function may eventually deteriorate, leading to left ventricular failure.

Clinical features

Acute aortic regurgitation may present dramatically with pulmonary oedema and low-output failure. Chronic aortic regurgitation, however, often remains asymptomatic for several years until the development of exertional fatigue and dyspnoea marks the onset of left ventricular failure. Angina may also occur owing to the increased oxygen requirements of the dilated, hypertrophied ventricle. The

Table 2.19 Causes of aortic regurgitation

Valve leaflet disease
Congenital bicuspid valve
Calcific disease
Rheumatic disease
Infective endocarditis*

Aortic root dilating disease
Marfan's syndrome
Ankylosing spondylitis
Syphilis
Hypertension
Aortic dissection*
Aortic root aneurysm
Deceleration injury*

* These disorders produce acute AR. In the remainder the course is chronic.

carotid pulse is visible in the neck (Corrigan's pulse). It has a rapid upstroke and collapses in early diastole owing to regurgitation of blood into the left ventricle. The pulse pressure is widened, with exaggeration of the systolic peak and the diastolic nadir. The apex beat is displaced towards the left axilla and has a prominent impulse. Auscultation reveals a high-pitched early diastolic murmur which is often louder at the left sternal edge than the aortic area. A mid-systolic ejection murmur is commonly present: it reflects the increased volume and velocity of flow across the aortic valve and does not necessarily indicate associated aortic stenosis. In severe disease the regurgitant jet causes preclosure of the anterior leaflet of the mitral valve and results in an apical mid-diastolic (Austin Flint) murmur.

Diagnosis

The ECG shows evidence of left ventricular hypertrophy. The chest X-ray shows an enlarged heart and dilatation of the ascending aorta (Fig. 2.28). Penetrated lateral films may reveal calcification of the aortic valve. The echocardiogram shows an abnormal aortic valve only if the cusps are diseased. In aortic root disease the valve itself appears normal though the aorta is dilated. The regurgitant jet produces fine vibrations on the anterior leaflet of the mitral valve which are often visible on the M-mode recording. The left ventricle shows variable dilatation and vigorous contractile function until this deteriorates in end-stage disease. Doppler studies identify the regurgitant jet. Left ventricular and aortic root angiography permit direct assessment of contractile function and the severity of aortic regurgitation, respectively.

Differential diagnosis

Aortic regurgitation must be distinguished from other conditions with an early diastolic murmur. Pulmonary regurgitation is relatively unusual and is nearly always associated with evidence of severe pulmonary hypertension (see page 72). In patent ductus arteriosus the murmur is continuous, but loudest at end-systole/early diastole. The pulse pressure is usually widened and confusion with aortic regurgitation, therefore, is not uncommon.

Complications

Irreversible left ventricular contractile impairment and endocarditis are the major complications of aortic regur-

gitation. Antibiotic prophylaxis prior to dental surgery and other invasive non-sterile procedures is essential.

Treatment

In acute aortic regurgitation associated with left ventricular failure, valve replacement should not be delayed. In chronic aortic regurgitation symptoms are rarely obtrusive until the onset of left ventricular failure. Mild shortness of breath may respond to diuretic therapy. Vasodilators (e.g. hydralazine, prazosin) are often useful, because reductions in peripheral vascular resistance increase forward flow and reduce regurgitation through the valve.

When aortic regurgitation becomes significantly symptomatic valve replacement is usually indicated, particularly when symptoms are associated with echocardiographic evidence of left ventricular contractile impairment. If surgery is delayed contractile impairment becomes irreversible and the results of valve replacement are less satisfactory.

Prognosis

Mild aortic regurgitation is compatible with a normal life-span. In more severe cases left ventricular failure develops, and thereafter prognosis is poor and similar to that of other causes of left ventricular failure. Timely valve replacement that anticipates deterioration in ventricular function improves the prognosis considerably.

Tricuspid valve disease

Tricuspid stenosis

Tricuspid stenosis is almost invariably rheumatic and is usually associated with mitral valve disease. Indeed, symptoms of mitral valve disease usually dominate the clinical picture. Severe tricuspid stenosis, however, may produce right heart failure characterized by fatigue, elevation of jugular venous pulse and peripheral oedema. A low-pitched mid-diastolic murmur, augmented during inspiration, is audible at the lower left sternal edge. These findings, associated with echocardiographic evidence of tricuspid valve thickening and right atrial dilatation, are diagnostic. Surgery is indicated only when right heart failure is severe.

Tricuspid regurgitation

Tricuspid regurgitation is the most common right-sided

valve lesion. It is usually 'functional', caused by stretching of the tricuspid valve ring in patients with advanced right ventricular failure. Other causes, including rheumatic disease, infective endocarditis, Ebstein's anomaly and carcinoid syndrome, are rare.

Tricuspid regurgitation volume-loads the right ventricle and may lead to (or, more commonly, exacerbate) right heart failure. The regurgitant jet produces systolic waves in the jugular veins, called giant V waves. Sometimes systolic expansion of an enlarged liver can also be detected. Auscultation reveals a pansystolic murmur at the lower left sternal edge. Confirmation of tricuspid regurgitation is provided by Doppler echocardiography which demonstrates the regurgitant jet in the right atrium.

Tricuspid regurgitation is often well-tolerated. Diuretics control peripheral oedema and reduce right ventricular volume, which improves functional regurgitation. Tricuspid valve surgery is only rarely necessary.

Pulmonary valve disease

Rheumatic disease of the pulmonary valve is rare. Endocarditis occurs occasionally, usually in main-lining drug addicts. The most common pulmonary valve defects are congenital stenosis (see page 82) and regurgitation secondary to pulmonary hypertension. Pulmonary regurgitation produces a high-pitched early diastolic murmur at the upper left sternal edge (Graham Steell murmur) very similar to that of aortic regurgitation. Nevertheless, signs of pulmonary hypertension are usually prominent (see page 72) and the carotid pulse is normal. Pulmonary regurgitation is well-tolerated and produces negligible haemodynamic embarrassment. The prognosis is determined by the severity of the associated pulmonary hypertension.

Conducting tissue disease

Synchronized contraction of the four cardiac chambers is dependent upon the organized spread of a wave of depolarization through the heart. All cardiac cells will depolarize in response to a stimulus of sufficient magnitude. Only the specialized conducting tissues, however, will depolarize spontaneously. This property —called automaticity—is essential to the pacemaker function of the sinus node, the conducting tissue with the highest intrinsic firing rate. The impulse generated by the sinus node first triggers atrial depolarization and then spreads through the atrioventricular node into the His–Purkinje tissue, triggering ventricular depolarization. The atrioventricular node provides the only pathway connecting the atria and the ventricles. The remainder of the atrioventricular ring tissue is electrically inert. Impulse conduction through the atrioventricular node is slow; this ensures that ventricular filling is complete before the onset of systole and that the ventricles will not respond to excessively rapid atrial rates.

Sinoatrial disease

Aetiology

Causes of sinoatrial disease are shown in Table 2.20. The most common cause is idiopathic fibrosis, a disease of the elderly which may affect the conducting tissue anywhere in the heart.

Pathology

The spontaneous discharge of the normal sinus node is influenced by a variety of neurohumoral factors, particularly vagal and sympathetic activity which slow and quicken the heart rate, respectively. A rate of 35–40 beats per minute is normal during sleep, but this may rise to 200 beats per minute during exertion. The rate of sinus node discharge is also influenced by age and slows progressively after the age of 50.

Sinus node discharge is not itself visible on the surface ECG, but the atrial depolarization it triggers produces the P wave. Sinus node discharge may be suppressed by drugs and disease or it may be blocked and fail to activate atrial depolarization. Under these circumstances the pacemaker function can be assumed by foci lower in the atrium, the atrioventricular node or the His–Purkinje conducting tissue in the ventricles. The intrinsic rate of these 'escape' pacemaker foci is slower than the normal sinus rate.

Table 2.20 Causes of sinoatrial disease

Acute
Myocardial infarction
Drugs (e.g. beta-blockers, digitalis)
Hypothermia
Atrial surgery

Chronic
Idiopathic fibrotic disease
Congenital heart disease
Ischaemic heart disease
Amyloid

Clinical features

Sinoatrial disease is commonly asymptomatic. Dizzy attacks or blackouts may occur, caused by extreme brady-cardia or prolonged sinus pauses without an adequate escape rhythm. Generally speaking pauses of greater than four seconds are necessary to produce symptoms. Additional complaints may include exertional fatigue or dyspnoea due to failure of physiological increments in heart rate. Palpitations also occur caused by premature beats or paroxysmal tachyarrhythmias (see below).

Diagnosis

In common with all other cardiac arrhythmias, electro-cardiographic documentation of sinoatrial disease is a prerequisite of accurate diagnosis. Although the resting ECG may be helpful, the disorder often occurs intermit-tently, in which case continuous in-hospital or ambulatory ECG monitoring is necessary (see page 57).

1 Sinus bradycardia (less than 50 beats per minute)

This is physiological during sleep and in trained athletes but in other circumstances often reflects sinoatrial disease, particularly when the heart rate fails to increase normally with exercise.

2 Sinoatrial block

If the sinus impulse is blocked and fails to trigger atrial depolarization, a pause occurs on the ECG. No P wave is seen during the pause owing to the absence of atrial depolarization. The electrically 'silent' sinus discharge, however, continues uninterrupted. Thus the pause is always a precise multiple of preceding P–P intervals. Sinoatrial block that cannot be abolished by atropine-induced vagal inhibition usually indicates sinoatrial disease, particularly with pauses longer than two seconds.

3 Sinus arrest (Fig. 2.30)

Failure of sinus node discharge produces a pause on the ECG that bears no relation to the preceding P–P interval. Pauses longer than two seconds are usually pathological.

Prolonged pauses are often terminated by an escape beat from a 'junctional' focus in the bundle of His.

4 Bradycardia–Tachycardia syndrome

In this syndrome atrial bradycardias are interspersed by paroxysmal tachyarrhythmias (e.g. atrial flutter or fibrilla-tion). Nevertheless, it is the bradycardias that usually cause symptoms, particularly dizzy attacks and blackouts.

Differential diagnosis

Sinoatrial disease must be distinguished from other cardiac and non-cardiac causes of dizzy attacks and syncope (see page 4).

Complications

1 Tachyarrhythmias

Paroxysmal atrial arrhythmias occur in the bradycardia–tachycardia syndrome (see above). Ventricular arrhyth-mias may also occur owing to associated His–Purkinje disease.

2 Thromboembolism

Systemic emboli from the left atrium occasionally occur in the bradycardia–tachycardia syndrome.

Treatment

Asymptomatic patients require no treatment, although drugs such as beta-blockers which suppress the sinus node should be avoided. In patients with symptomatic bradycardias and sinus pauses, however, pacemaker therapy is indicated (see page 55). This maintains the heart rate, preventing syncopal episodes and improving exercise tolerance.

Troublesome tachycardias in the bradycardia–tachy-cardia syndrome require anti-arrhythmic drug therapy. Drugs of this type often exacerbate sinus node dysfun-ction, and a pacemaker is usually necessary to protect against severe bradycardia. Anticoagulation with

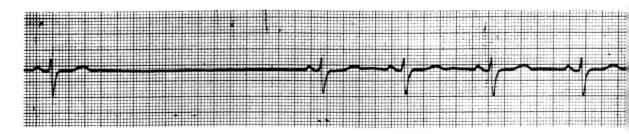

Figure 2.30   *Sinus arrest. After the first sinus beat there is a long pause before sinus rhythm re-establishes itself.*

warfarin is sometimes recommended in the bradycardia–tachycardia syndrome in order to protect against thromboembolism.

Prognosis

Sinoatrial disease caused by idiopathic fibrosis of conducting tissue has a good prognosis. Dizzy attacks and syncopal episodes are inconvenient but not directly life-threatening and do not appear to influence the prognosis; when sinoatrial disease is ischaemic in origin, however, the prognosis is less good.

Heart block

Aetiology

Myocardial infarction is the commonest cause of acute heart block (Table 2.21). Chronic heart block in the UK is usually due to idiopathic fibrosis of the bundle branches, particularly in the elderly, though ischaemic disease is more common in middle-aged patients. Chagas' disease in Central and South America, however, is the commonest cause of heart block world-wide.

Pathology

Heart block delays or completely interrupts atrioventricular conduction, either in the atrioventricular node itself or in the bundle branches. When conduction is merely delayed (e.g. first-degree atrioventricular block, bundle branch block) the heart rate is unaffected. When conduction is completely interrupted, however, the heart rate may slow sufficiently to produce symptoms. In second-degree atrioventricular block failure of conduction is, by definition, intermittent, and if sufficient sinus impulses are conducted to maintain an adequate ventricular rate symptoms may be avoided. In third-degree atrioventricular block there is complete failure of conduction and continuing ventricular activity depends on the emergence of an escape rhythm. If the block is within the atrioventricular node the escape rhythm usually arises from a focus just below the node in the bundle of His (junctional escape) and is often fast enough to prevent symptoms. If both bundle branches are blocked, however, the escape rhythm must arise from a focus lower in the ventricles. Ventricular escape rhythms of this type are nearly always associated with symptoms because they are not only very slow but are also unreliable, and may stop altogether producing prolonged asystole.

Clinical features

1 First-degree atrioventricular block
This is an electrocardiographic diagnosis and produces no symptoms or signs.
2 Second-degree atrioventricular block
Intermittent failure of atrioventricular conduction rarely produces symptoms unless the heart rate is very slow. On examination, occasional dropped beats may be detected, but diagnosis is effectively impossible without an ECG.
3 Third-degree (complete) atrioventricular block
The ventricular escape rhythm is often slow and does not speed up significantly during exercise. Exertional fatigue is always troublesome, and frank congestive heart failure may occur if the rate is very slow, particularly when there is associated valvar or myocardial disease. Moreover, if the escape rhythm is unreliable, intermittent periods of asystole produce dizzy attacks or syncope.

Examination reveals a slow regular pulse, usually about 40 beats per minute. The atrial and ventricular rhythms are 'dissociated'. Signs of dissociation include intermittent cannon 'a' waves in the jugular venous pulse (see Fig. 2.1), and beat-to-beat variation in the intensity of the first heart sound. These signs, however, are not present if the atria are fibrillating.

Diagnosis

Definitive diagnosis of heart block depends upon electrocardiographic documentation of the rhythm. If the disorder is intermittent this may require in-hospital or ambulatory ECG monitoring (see page 57).
1 First-degree atrioventricular block
Delayed atrioventricular conduction causes prolongation of the PR interval (> 0.20 seconds). Ventricular depolarization occurs rapidly by normal His–Purkinje pathways and the QRS complex is usually narrow.

Table 2.21 Causes of atrioventricular heart block

Acute
Myocardial infarction
Drugs (e.g. beta-blockers, verapamil, digitalis)
Surgical or catheter ablation of the His bundle

Chronic
Idiopathic bilateral bundle branch fibrosis
Ischaemic heart disease
Congenital heart block
Calcific aortic valve disease
Chagas' disease
Infiltrative disease (amyloid, haemochromatosis)
Granulomatous disease (sarcoid, tuberculosis)

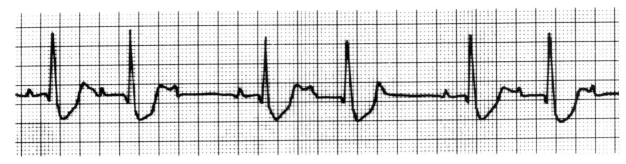

Figure 2.31   *Mobitz type I second-degree atrioventricular block. Three Wenckebach cycles are shown, during each of which gradual prolongation of the PR interval culminates in a non-conducted impulse (2:1 block).*

2   Second-degree atrioventricular block

Mobitz type I (Wenckebach). See Fig. 2.31. This occurs commonly in inferior myocardial infarction. Successive sinus beats find the atrioventricular node increasingly refractory until failure of conduction occurs. The delay permits recovery of nodal function and the process may then repeat itself. The ECG shows progressive prolongation of the PR interval, culminating in a dropped beat. Block is within the atrioventricular node itself and ventricular depolarization occurs rapidly by normal pathways. Thus the QRS complex is usually narrow.

Mobitz type II. See Fig. 2.32. This always indicates advanced conducting tissue disease and is commonly seen in idiopathic fibrosis. Intermittent failure of atrioventricular conduction produces dropped beats. The PR interval is constant. Block is nearly always within the bundle branches, and ventricular depolarization is commonly prolonged, occurring by abnormal pathways to produce a broad QRS complex.

3   Third-degree (complete) atrioventricular block

The atrial and ventricular rhythms are 'dissociated' because none of the atrial impulses is conducted. Thus the ECG shows regular P waves (unless the atrium is fibrillating) and regular QRS complexes occurring independently of each other. When block is within the atrioventricular node (e.g. inferior myocardial infarction, congenital atrioventricular block) a junctional escape rhythm with a reliable rate (40–60 beats per minute) takes over (see Fig. 2.20). Ventricular depolarization occurs rapidly by normal pathways, producing a narrow QRS complex. However, when block is within the bundle branches (e.g. idiopathic fibrosis) there is always extensive conducting tissue disease. The ventricular escape rhythm is slow and unreliable, with a broad QRS complex (Fig. 2.33).

4   Right bundle branch block (See Fig. 2.7)

This may be a congenital defect but is more commonly the result of organic conducting tissue disease. Right ventricular depolarization is delayed, resulting in a broad QRS complex with an rSR pattern in lead VI and prominent S waves in leads I and V6.

5   Left bundle branch block (See Fig. 2.7)

This always indicates organic conducting tissue disease. The entire sequence of ventricular depolarization is abnormal, resulting in a broad QRS complex with large slurred or notched R waves in leads I and V6.

Treatment

The treatment of acute atrioventricular block complicating myocardial infarction has already been discussed (see page 28). In chronic atrioventricular block, treatment is necessary only in Mobitz type II second-degree block and

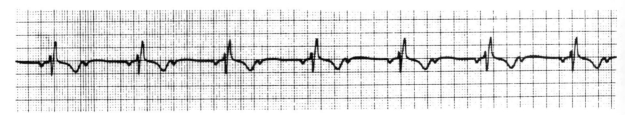

Figure 2.32   *Mobitz type II second degree block. Alternate P waves are not conducted (2:1 block). Note that the PR interval of the conducted beats is normal and that the QRS complex is broad with c bundle branch block pattern—both typical features of Mobitz type II block.*

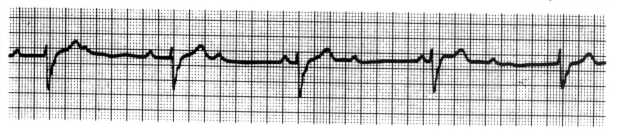

Figure 2.33 *Third-degree (complete) atrioventricular block. The patient had idiopathic fibrosis of both bundle branches. Note the dissociated atrial and ventricular rhythms and the slow ventricular escape rhythms with a broad QRS complex (compare with Fig. 2.20).*

third-degree (complete) block. In both conditions there is always the risk of prolonged asystole and sudden death. Thus pacemaker therapy is mandatory.

Pacemaker therapy. A pacemaker wire with a terminal electrode is introduced into a central vein and directed into the apex of the right ventricle. The wire is attached to a power source for delivery of electrical pulses which depolarize the ventricles and stimulate systolic contraction. Temporary pacing using an external power source is appropriate when the need for rate control is likely to be short-lived (e.g. heart block in inferior myocardial infarction) or as a prelude to permanent pacing in patients with severe bradycardias. Permanent pacing is required for chronic Mobitz type II block, complete atrioventricular block and also for patients with symptomatic sinoatrial disease (see page 52). The generator powered by lithium batteries (life 7–10 years) is implanted subcutaneously, usually in the infraclavicular pectoral position.

Ventricular inhibited-demand units are used most commonly. These deliver electrical pulses at a preselected rate which can be programmed into the power source. Spontaneous ventricular beats inhibit the power source. This prevents 'competitive' pacing in which the delivery of electrical pulses during the vulnerable period of the cardiac cycle (the T wave) may initiate ventricular fibrillation. Thus ventricular inhibited-demand units are only activated when the spontaneous ventricular rate falls below the preselected pacemaker rate.

The pacing rate that is selected depends on the indication for pacing. If the pacemaker is prophylactic against occasional sinus pauses, a rate of 50 per minute is sufficient to guard against syncopal attacks. In complete block associated with a slow and unreliable ventricular escape rhythm, however, a faster pacing rate is necessary to maintain adequate cardiac output.

Ventricular pacing does not, of course, restore synchronous atrial activity in patients with heart block, nor does it permit physiological increments in heart rate during exertion. Pacing systems are now available which re-establish the normal atrioventricular relationship by delivering electrical pulses first to the right atrium and then to the ventricle. Alternatively, if normal atrial activity is intact the power source will sense atrial depolarization and then stimulate the ventricle. Systems of this type not only produce a more favourable haemodynamic result by recruiting atrial systole but, if normal atrial activity is intact, they allow the sinus node to control the heart rate such that a normal tachycardia occurs during exertion.

Prognosis

First-degree and Mobitz type I second-degree atrioventicular block pose no direct threat to the patient, and the prognosis is therefore determined by the cause of the underlying conducting tissue disorder. The same is true of isolated left or right bundle branch block. Mobitz type II second-degree block and third-degree atrioventricular block always carry the risk of prolonged asystole and sudden death. Nevertheless, following pacemaker insertion this risk is effectively abolished and prognosis then relates to the underlying conducting tissue disorder. In idiopathic fibrosis of the conducting system, for example, the prognosis is excellent. In ischaemic disease, on the other hand, the prognosis is much worse.

Tachyarrhythmias

Aetiology

Many factors may predispose to the development of tachyarrhythmias. These include both cardiac and noncardiac disorders and the effects of drug toxicity (Table 2.22).

Table 2.22 Causes of atrial (A) and ventricular (V) arrhythmias

Cardiac disorders	
Coronary artery disease	A and V
Pericardial disease	A
Cardiomyopathy	A and V
Mitral valve prolapse	A and V
Mitral stenosis/regurgitation	A
Aortic stenosis/regurgitation	V
Pre-excitation syndromes	A
Concealed bypass tracts	A
Long QT syndrome	V
Chagas' disease	V
Cardiac trauma	A and V
Non-cardiac disorders	
Thyrotoxicosis	A
Phaeochromocytoma	V
Dystrophia myotonica	A and V
Hypothermia	A and V
Hypokalaemia	A and V
Hypomagnesaemia	A and V
Hyperkalaemia	V
Hypoxaemia	A and V
Acidosis	A and V
Drug toxicity	
Caffeine	A and V
Alcohol	A
Aminophylline	A and V
Tricyclic antidepressants	A and V
Sympathomimetic amines	A and V
Anaesthetic agents	A and V
Digitalis	A and V

Pathology

The principal mechanisms involved in the pathogenesis of tachyarrhythmias are enhanced automaticity and re-entry.

1 Enhanced automaticity

Automaticity—spontaneous depolarization—is a property common to all the specialized conducting tissues within the heart (see page 51). The automatic discharge of the sinus node, however, normally proceeds at a faster rate than the remainder of the conducting tissue which is, therefore, continuously suppressed. Neverthe-less, a variety of stimuli (e.g. trauma, ischaemia, drug toxicity) can enhance the automaticity of an ectopic atrial or ventricular focus, allowing it to depolarize more rapidly than the sinus node. This produces a premature beat. Repeated automatic discharge from an ectopic focus of this type at a rate in excess of the sinus node can take over the pacemaker function and result in sustained atrial or ventricular tachyarrhythmias.

2 Re-entry

The basic requirements for re-entry are the coexistence of unidirectional block to impulse traffic in one part of the conducting system and retrograde conduction over an alternative pathway. A typical re-entry circuit involving the atrioventricular node and a fast conducting bypass tract is shown in Fig. 2.34. A premature impulse A is blocked at point B in the fast pathway but conducts through the atrioventricular node. Rapid ventricular de-polarization occurs by His–Purkinje pathways, and cells immediately distal to the block are activated. By now, the bypass tract is no longer refractory and conducts the impulse retrogradely into the atria, thereby completing the re-entry circuit and initiating self-sustaining tachycar-dia.

Clinical features

Both atrial and ventricular tachyarrhythmias may be entirely asymptomatic. Generally speaking symptoms are determined by the ventricular rate and the presence and severity of underlying heart disease.

Palpitation is the most common symptom caused by tachyarrhythmias. Nevertheless, isolated premature beats usually pass unnoticed, although the patient is occasion-ally aware of the pause or the forceful beat that follows. Paroxysmal tachycardias may also pass unnoticed, par-ticularly if the attacks are short. More commonly, however, the patient will notice the abrupt onset and termination of the attack. Sustained tachyarrhythmias usually produce rapid palpitation which is irregular in atrial fibrillation.

Angina may occur if the rapid ventricular rate causes myocardial oxygen demand to exceed supply. Although angina is particularly troublesome in patients with

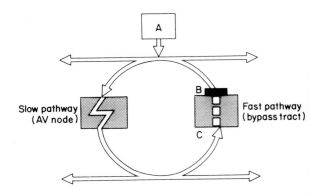

Figure 2.34 *A model of re-entry involving the atrioventricular (AV) node and a fasty-conducting nodal bypass tract (see text for discussion).*

coronary artery disease, it may also occur in the presence of normal coronary arteries.

Tachyarrhythmias may present with dyspnoea due to heart failure particularly in patients with associated left ventricular or valvar disease. Tachyarrhythmias are an important treatable cause of heart failure.

Syncopal episodes (Stokes–Adams attacks) occur when paroxysmal tachyarrhythmias produce abrupt reductions in cardiac output and cerebral perfusion. Paroxysmal ventricular arrhythmias are usually responsible and if sustained may cause death. Sudden death is an inevitable consequence of sustained ventricular fibrillation.

Diagnosis

1 Arrhythmia detection

Electrocardiographic documentation of the arrhythmia should be obtained prior to instituting treatment. In patients with sustained arrhythmias a recording at rest provides the necessary information. Nevertheless many patients have paroxysmal arrhythmias and special techniques may be required to obtain electrocardiographic documentation.

In-hospital ECG monitoring. Patients who have had out-of-hospital cardiac arrest or severe, arrhythmia-induced heart failure should undergo ECG monitoring in hospital under the continuous surveillance of trained staff.

Ambulatory ECG monitoring. Patients with intermittent palpitation or dizzy attacks should have a continuous 24-hour ECG recording while engaging in normal day-to-day activities. Portable cassette recorders are available for this purpose. Analysis of the tape often identifies the cardiac arrhythmias, particularly if symptoms were experienced during the recording.

Patient-activated ECG recording. For patients with very infrequent symptoms, the detection rate with 24-hour ambulatory monitoring is low and patient-activated recorders are therefore more useful. When symptoms occur the patient applies the recorder to the chest wall and may then transmit the ECG by telephone to the hospital for scrutiny by the physician.

Exercise testing. ECG recording during exercise may be helpful when there is a history of exertional palpitation. Arrhythmias provoked by ischaemia or increased sympathetic activity are more likely to be detected during exercise.

Programmed cardiac stimulation. This technique requires cardiac catheterization with electrode catheters. Premature stimuli are introduced into the atria or ventricles with a view to stimulating re-entry arrhythmias such as supraventricular tachycardia, ventricular tachycardia or ventricular fibrillation. In the normal heart sustained arrhythmias of this type are rarely provoked by premature stimuli. Thus arrhythmia provocation during programmed stimulation is usually diagnostic, particularly when the arrhythmia reproduces symptoms.

2 Electrocardiographic diagnosis

Careful analysis of the ECG permits diagnosis of the large majority of cardiac arrhythmias. If possible, a standard 12-lead recording should be obtained as well as a long continuous recording of the lead showing the clearest P wave (if present). In this chapter the term 'supraventricular tachycardia' describes all tachyarrhythmias originating from the atria or atrioventricular junction, not just AV nodal re-entry tachycardia (see page 58).

Atrial premature beats. These rarely indicate heart disease. They often occur spontaneously but may be provoked by toxic stimuli such as caffeine, alcohol and cigarette smoking. They are caused by the premature discharge of an atrial ectopic focus and an early and often bizarre P wave is essential for the diagnosis. The premature impulse enters and depolarizes the sinus node such that a partially compensatory pause occurs before the next sinus beat during re-setting of the sinus node. No treatment is necessary.

Atrial fibrillation. See Fig. 2.27. This is common in ischaemic heart disease, mitral valve disease, thyrotoxicosis and left ventricular failure. It also occurs after major surgery and in response to various toxic stimuli, particularly alcohol. Atrial activity is chaotic and mechanically ineffective. P waves are therefore absent and are replaced by irregular fibrillatory waves (rate 300–600 per minute). The long refractory period of the atrioventricular node ensures that only some of the atrial impulses are conducted to produce an irregular ventricular rate of 130–200 beats per minute. If the atrioventricular node is diseased the ventricular rate is slower, but in the presence of a fast-conducting nodal bypass tract (e.g. Wolff–Parkinson–White syndrome) dangerous ventricular rates above 300 beats per minute may occur. Treatment is directed at either converting the arrhythmia to sinus rhythm (direct current shock, amiodarone) or controlling the ventricular response with drugs that slow conduction through the atrioventricular node (digitalis, beta-blockers, verapamil).

Atrial flutter. See Fig. 2.35. This is less common than atrial fibrillation but occurs under exactly similar circumstances. Re-entry mechanisms produce an atrial rate close to 300 beats per minute. The normal atrioventricular node conducts with 2:1 block giving a ventricular rate of 150 beats per minute. Higher degrees of block may reflect intrinsic disease of the atrioventricular node, but the

(a)

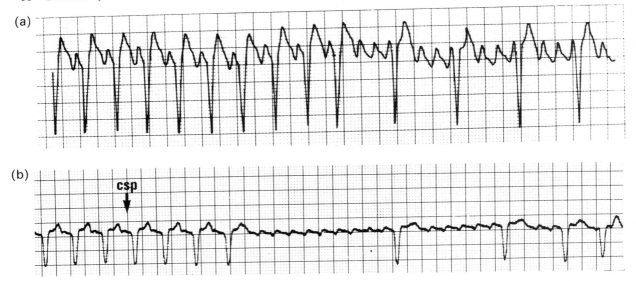

(b)

Figure 2.35 *Atrial flutter. (a) Typical sawtooth flutter waves are seen. AV conduction is initially with 2:1 block but later changes spontaneously to 4:1 block. (b) Flutter wave are less obvious until the application of carotid sinus pressure (csp) exacerbates AV block and reveals the underlying atrial rhythm.*

conduction ratio is nearly always multiples of two (i.e. 4:1 or 6:1). The ECG characteristically shows saw-tooth flutter waves which are most cleary seen when block is increased by carotid sinus pressure. Atrial flutter is an unstable rhythm which usually converts spontaneously to sinus rhythm or atrial fibrillation. Specific treatment to restore sinus rhythm requires either atrial pacing or direct current shock (see below). Satisfactory control of the ventricular rate can usually be achieved with drugs that slow conduction through the atrioventricular node (e.g. digoxin).

Nodal re-entry tachycardia. Commonly called supraventricular tachycardia, this arrhythmia is usually paroxysmal without obvious cardiac or extrinsic causes. It is caused by re-entry within the atrioventricular node. The rate is

usually 150–200 beats per minute. Ventricular depolarization usually occurs rapidly by normal His–Purkinje pathways, producing a narrow QRS complex which confirms the supraventricular origin of the arrhythmia. Aberrant intraventricular conduction or pre-existing bundle branch block, on the other hand, produce broad ventricular complexes difficult to distinguish from ventricular tachycardia (Fig. 2.36). The arrhythmia is usually self-limiting but will sometimes respond to carotid sinus pressure. If this fails intravenous verapamil is usually effective by blocking the re-entry circuit within the atrioventricular node.

Ventricular premature beats. These may occur in normal individuals in response to toxic stimuli such as caffeine or sympathomimetic drugs. When ventricular premature

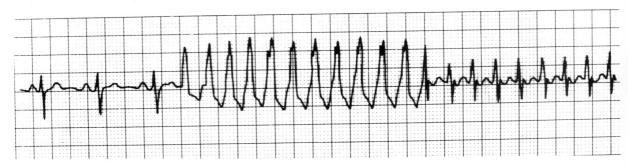

Figure 2.36 *Supraventricular tachycardia. Sinus rhythm is terminated by the onset of a broad-complex tachycardia. Although this resembles ventricular tachycardia, the QRS complexes become abruptly narrow confirming the supraventricular origin on the arrhythmia. Thus the broad QRS complexes must have been caused by aberrant intraventricular conduction.*

beats are frequent or complex (i.e. multifocal or occurring in couplets) they usually indicate heart disease. They are caused by the premature discharge of a ventricular ectopic focus which produces an early and broad QRS complex. The premature impulse may be conducted backwards into the atria, producing a retrograde P wave, but penetration of the sinus node is rare. Thus resetting of the sinus node does not usually occur and there is a fully compensatory pause before the next sinus beat. Ventricular premature beats may be suppressed by a variety of anti-arrhythmic drugs, but this does not necessarily affect the natural history of the underlying disorder (see page 28).

Accelerated idioventricular rhythm. (Fig. 2.37). This is a ventricular rhythm with a rate of 60–120 beats per minute. It usually occurs as a complication of acute myocardial infarction. The slow ventricular ectopic focus is in continuous competition with the sinus node such that the broad complex ventricular rhythm is often interspersed with episodes of sinus rhythm. The slow ventricular rhythm rarely produces haemodynamic disturbance and treatment is not necessary.

Ventricular tachycardia. This is always pathological. It is defined as three or more consecutive ventricular beats at a rate above 120 per minute. Ventricular depolarization

inevitably occurs slowly by abnormal pathways; the QRS complex is therefore broad and bizarre. Supraventricular tachycardia with aberrant intraventricular conduction or pre-existing bundle branch block can also produce a broad complex tachycardia (see Fig. 2.36) which may be difficult to distinguish from ventricular tachycardia. Any one of the following ECG findings, however, confirms the diagnosis of ventricular tachycardia:

1. Atrioventricular dissociation (Fig. 2.38)—During ventricular tachycardia, atrial depolarization often continues uninterrupted though at a slower rate. This produces P waves which can be seen 'marching through' the broad-complex ventricular tachycardia.
2. Ventricular capture or fusion beats (Fig. 2.39)— Because atrial depolarization often continues uninterrupted during ventricular tachycardia, it may penetrate the ventricle by conduction through the atrioventricular node. This produces either a normal ventricular complex (capture) or a broad hybrid complex representing fusion of the atrial and the ventricular beats.
3. Torsades de pointes (Fig. 2.40)—Changing wavefronts in broad-complex tachycardias occur only in ventricular tachycardia and are particularly characteristic of the long QT syndrome.

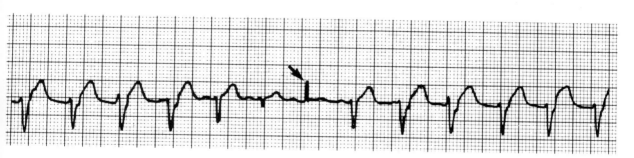

Figure 2.37 *Accelerated idioventricular rhythm. The broad-complex idioventricular rhythm is interrupted by 'fusion' beats (part sinus and part ventricular in origin) and a single sinus beat (arrowed).*

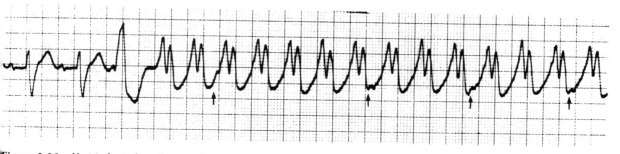

Figure 2.38 *Ventricular tachycardia: AV dissociation. P waves (arrowed) are seen 'marching' through the broad-complex tachycardia. AV dissociation confirms the ventricular origin of the arrhythmia.*

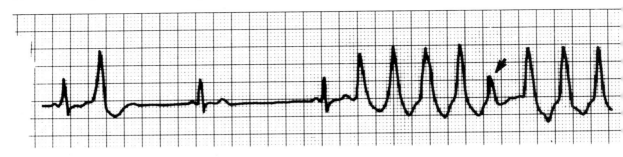

Figure 2.39   *Ventricular tachycardia: fusion beats. The second complex is an early ventricular premature beat. This recurs after the fourth complex and initiates a broad-complex tachycardia. The tachycardia is interrupted by a fusion beat (arrowed) which is part sinus and part ventricular in origin. The fusion beat confirms the ventricular origin of the arrhythimia.*

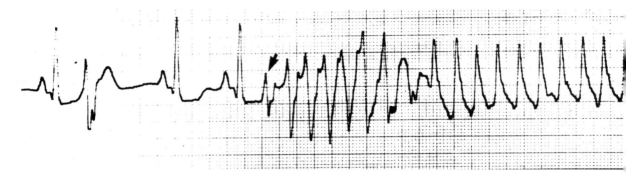

Figure 2.40   *Ventricular tachycardia: torsades de pointes. The second complex is an early ventricular premature beat. This recurs (arrowed) after the fourth complex and initiates a broad-complex tachycardia. The changing wavefronts (torsades de pointes) of the arrhythmia confirm its ventricular origin.*

Other ECG findings suggestive of ventricular tachycardia in patients with broad-complex tachyarrhythmias include extreme left axis deviation and concordant QRS deflections in leads V1 to V6 (all positive or all negative).

Ventricular tachycardia always requires treatment, either by direct current shock or by ventricular pacing. In patients with paroxysmal attacks, appropriate suppressive therapy must be instituted.

Ventricular fibrillation. See Fig. 2.19. This occurs most commonly in severe myocardial ischaemia either with or without frank infarction. It is a completely disorganized arrhythmia characterized by irregular fibrillatory waves with no discernible QRS complexes. There is no effective cardiac output and death is inevitable unless resuscitation is instituted rapidly.

Complications

Myocardial ischaemia, heart failure and death are the major complications of cardiac arrhythmias (see page 56). Pulmonary and systemic thromboembolism may occur, particularly in atrial fibrillation when prophylactic anticoagulation with warfarin is often recommended.

Treatment

The usual aims of treatment are to suppress paroxysmal arrhythmias and to convert established arrhythmias to sinus rhythm. In patients with atrial arrhythmias (particularly atrial fibrillation) in whom these aims cannot be fulfilled, treatment is directed at controlling the rate of the ventricular response.

1 General measures
A number of factors are known to predispose to cardiac arrhythmias (see Table 2.22) and where possible these should receive specific treatment.

2 Non-pharmacological therapy
Carotid sinus pressure/Valsalva. The reflex vagotonic response to these manoeuvres causes slowing of conduction through the atrioventricular node. This can interrupt re-entry circuits and convert nodal re-entry tachycardia to sinus rhythm.

Pacemaker therapy. Arrhythmias caused by re-entry mechanisms are amenable to treatment of this type. Either underdrive or overdrive pacing may be used—in which the heart is paced at a rate slower or faster, respectively, than the arrhythmia rate. Because the pacing rate is different from the arrhythmia rate, pacing stimuli are delivered randomly throughout the cardiac cycle and may penetrate and break the re-entry circuit. Withdrawal of pacing permits re-establishment of sinus rhythm.

Implantable anti-tachycardia pacemakers are now being used increasingly in the management of paroxysmal atrial and ventricular re-entry arrhythmias. The pacemaker senses the abrupt increase in heart rate at the onset of the arrhythmia and delivers strategically timed electrical stimuli in order to block the re-entry circuit and permit return to normal conduction.

Electrode ablation. Electrode ablation catheters placed strategically within the heart may be used to deliver low-energy electrical shocks in order to cause selective damage to the conducting system. The technique is particularly useful for atrial arrhythmias resistant to conventional drug therapy. Electrode ablation of the atrioventricular node or bundle of His produces complete heart block and prevents conduction of the arrhythmia to the ventricles. This abolishes troublesome palpitation and other consequences of a rapid ventricular response (see page 56). Following the procedure permanent ventricular pacing is required.

Surgery. Left ventricular aneurysmectomy often corrects intractable cardiac arrhythmias. In patients with myopathic disease, surgical excision of the irritable focus is occasionally beneficial. The supraventricular arrhythmias associated with Wolff–Parkinson–White syndrome are abolished by surgical interruption of the bundle of Kent (see page 64).

Direct current shock. Electrode paddles placed against the chest wall permit delivery of a high-energy direct current shock across the heart. General anaesthesia is necessary if the patient is conscious. This technique corrects the majority of acute-onset atrial and ventricular tachyarrhythmias by depolarizing the heart and allowing the sinus node to re-establish itself. The rapid, almost instantaneous response makes this the treatment of choice in emergency management.

3 Drug therapy

Table 2.23 shows the Vaughan Williams classification of antiarrhythmic drugs. Because all these drugs may themselves exacerbate cardiac arrhythmias, a cautious and rational approach to treatment must be adopted. Electrocardiographic documentation of the arrhythmia is essential before starting treatment in order that the appropriate agent may be selected. The therapeutic range for most drugs is very narrow and regular measurements of plasma concentrations should be made if possible in order to avoid toxic side-effects. Careful electrocardiographic monitoring of the response to treatment is important, and if the arrhythmia persists despite therapeutic plasma concentrations an alternative and appropriate drug should be substituted. A partial response might justify combination with a second agent, but regimens of this type should if possible be avoided because of the risk of drug interactions and exaggerated side-effects. Class 3 and class IA drugs, for example, both prolong the QT interval and their combination can induce the long QT syndrome which is associated with severe ventricular arrhythmias. Class 2 and class 4 drugs both slow conduction through the atrioventricular node. The combination is usually safe for oral administration, but by the intravenous route it can cause complete heart block and asystole.

(a) *Class I drugs*. These drugs stabilize irritable foci within the conducting tissue by depressing the rapid influx of sodium ion that initiates the action potential. Effects on repolarization are variable and provide the basis for a subclassification into groups A, B and C which prolong, shorten and have little effect on the QT interval, respectively.

Disopyramide is the most widely used class IA drug. It can be given intravenously to terminate both ventricular and supraventricular arrhythmias. It should not, however, be given in supraventricular arrhythmias with a narrow QRS complex (e.g. atrial flutter) as this can cause a dangerous rise in ventricular rate.

It is also used orally in the prevention of both ventricular and supraventricular arrhythmias.

Disopyramide has marked negative inotropic properties and must be used with caution in heart failure. Its anti-cholinergic properties help to maintain the sinus rate (by blocking vagal activity) but may lead to a dry mouth and to urinary retention in the elderly.

Lignocaine is the most widely used class IB drug. It suppresses ventricular arrhythmias and is particularly useful in myocardial infarction (see page 28). It is ineffective against atrial arrhythmias. Parenteral administration is always necessary because of gastrointestinal side-effects and first-pass metabolism in the liver. It can be given as an initial bolus of 50–100 mg followed by an infusion of 4.0 mg/minute which is gradually reduced and should not normally be continued for more than 48 hours. In patients with liver disease or poor hepatic perfusion (e.g. heart failure) the perfusion rate should not exceed 1.0 mg/minute.

Lignocaine is negatively inotropic, but less so than disopyramide. More important side-effects include bradycardia, hypotension, drowsiness and convulsions.

Mexiletine is in all respects similar to lignocaine except that it may be given orally and is suitable therefore for

Table 2.23

Vaughan-Williams classification	Acute intravenous therapy		Chronic oral therapy daily dose (mg)	Therapeutic blood levels (mg/l)
	Bolus* (mg)	Infusion (mg/min)		
Class 1A				
Quinidine	†	†	1000	2.0–5.0
Disopyramide	100–150	0.5	300–800	2.0–5.0
Class 1B				
Lignocaine	50–200	1.0–4.0	†	2.0–5.0
Mexiletine	125–250	0.5–1.0	600–1000	0.75–2.0
Class 1C				
Flecainide	100–150	0.25	200–400‡	0.4–1.0
Class II				
Practolol	5–10	†	†	–
Atenolol	5–10	†	50–100	0.1–1.0
Class III				
Amiodarone	300–900	0.5–1.0	200–400	0.6–2.5
Bretylium	500–1000	0.5–2.0	†	–
Class IV				
Verapamil	5–10	0.05–0.1	120–240	0.1–0.2

* Bolus injections should always be given slowly over at least five minutes. The injection may be repeated after 15 minutes if the desired effects is not achieved.
† Not available.
‡ Half the dose for the elderly.

outpatient use (although nausea may be a problem).

Flecainide is the only class IC drug available for clinical use. It is a potent anti-arrhythmic agent effective against both atrial and ventricular arrhythmias. Oral and parenteral preparations are available. Flecainide is less negatively inotropic than other class I drugs but nevertheless should be used with caution in heart failure. It also prolongs the PR and QRS intervals on the ECG. Other side-effects including dizziness are rarely troublesome.

(b) *Class 2 drugs.* These are all beta-blockers which protect the heart against catecholamine stimulation. They are particularly effective for suppressing atrial and ventricular premature beats, and are of value in arrhythmias due to thyrotoxicosis and anaesthetic agents. Beta-blockers slow conduction through the atrioventricular node and may be used to treat nodal re-entry tachycardias. Moreover, when adequate control of the ventricular rate in atrial flutter or fibrillation cannot be achieved with digitalis alone, the addition of a beta-blocker is usually effective.

Practolol, a cardioselective beta-blocker, is the drug of choice for intravenous use, but it cannot be used orally because of long-term toxic side-effects. Thus other cardioselective beta-blockers such as atenolol or metoprolol should be used for maintenance therapy.

Side-effects of beta-blockers are described on page 68.

(c) *Class 3 drugs.* Amiodarone is the most important drug in this class, although sotalol, a beta-blocker, also has mild class 3 activity. Amiodarone prolongs the duration of the action potential, increasing the effective refractory period of the conducting tissues. The drug is available for oral and parenteral use and is effective against a wide range of atrial and ventricular arrhythmias. Therapeutic plasma concentrations may take a week or more to achieve during oral administration; and because the half-life is very long activity persists for up to four weeks following discontinuation of the drug. It is usual, therefore, to start treatment with 200 mg three times daily orally for one week, then reduce the dose to the minimum necessary. The drug is more rapidly effective following intravenous loading, but occasionally causes profound hypotension and bradycardia and should be given via a central line over 30 minutes. Chronic therapy has been associated with a variety of side-effects, including photosensitivity rashes, skin discolouration, pulmonary infiltrates and hepatic and thyroid dysfunction. Thyroid function tests should be performed 6-monthly.

(d) *Class 4 drugs.* Verapamil is the most important drug in this class, though diltiazem, another calcium antagonist, also has class 4 activity. Selective blockade of the calcium slow channel decreases the rate of depolarization and slows conduction through the atrioventricular node. Given intravenously it is the drug of choice in nodal re-entry tachycardia when conversion to sinus rhythm is often achieved. Verapamil may also be used to control the ventricular rate in atrial flutter and fibrillation, particularly when digitalis alone is ineffective. It is negatively inotropic and should be used with caution in heart failure. Intravenous verapamil is contraindicated in patients taking beta-blockers.

(e) *Digitalis.* Digitalis, a cardiac glycoside, defies classification by Vaughan Williams' criteria. In addition to its mild positive inotropic effect (see page 20) this drug slows conduction through the atrioventricular node by a direct effect on depolarization and vagal stimulation. It is the drug of choice for slowing the ventricular rate in atrial flutter and fibrillation. Nodal re-entry tachycardia will often respond to digitalis, and in paroxysmal attacks maintenance therapy often reduces the frequency of recurrence.

Digoxin is the most widely used cardiac glycoside. In an emergency it may be given intravenously, the usual dose being 500 μg followed after an hour by a further 250 μg. Intravenous digoxin should not be used if the patient has had digitalis in the previous six weeks. The usual oral dose is 500 μg initially followed by 250 μg 8-hourly for three doses. The maintenance dose is 125–500 μg, depending on clinical response. Reduced dosage (usually half or less) is required in the elderly and—because digoxin is excreted largely by the kidney—in patients with impaired renal function. The risk of toxicity is also increased in hypokalaemia (often induced by diuretics), hypomagnesaemia, hypercalcaemia and hypothyroidism.

The therapeutic plasma concentration range for digoxin is narrow (0.9–2.0 μg/litre). There is, however, some variation in the therapeutic range between patients and some overlap between therapeutic and toxic concentrations. Estimations of plasma levels is often not helpful in controlling dosage unless the problem is one of overdose or compliance.

Important toxic manifestations are loss of appetite, nausea, vomiting and bradycardias. Digitalis may also cause tachyarrhythmias by enhancing the automaticity of atrial and ventricular ectopic foci.

Digitalis therapy produces important ECG abnormalities, including prolongation of the PR interval and sagging of the ST segment. These abnormalities, however, do not necessarily indicate digitalis toxicity.

Cardiac arrest

Aetiology

Cardiac arrest is usually caused by ventricular fibrillation or asystole. It may also be caused by rapid ventricular tachycardia. These arrhythmias are usually the result of severe myocardial ischaemia or infarction but may also complicate hypoxia, electrolyte imbalance and a variety of drug interventions. Autonomic reflexes in response to endotracheal intubation or urethral catheterization may occasionally cause cardiac arrest.

Clinical features

In cardiac arrest there is no effective cardiac output. The diagnosis is made clinically by loss of the arterial pulse followed rapidly by unconsciousness, apnoea and dilatation of the pupils. Irreversible brain damage usually occurs if the circulation is not re-established within four minutes, though factors such as hypothermia may prolong this time.

Treatment

A firm thump over the sternum occasionally converts ventricular tachycardia or fibrillation to sinus rhythm. If this fails, full cardiopulmonary resuscitation should be instituted. The patient is placed supine on a firm surface with the neck extended. The airway is cleared and positive pressure ventilation and external cardiac massage are started. These should be continued uninterrupted until adequate spontaneous circulatory and respiratory function are restored. Acidosis develops rapidly after cardiac arrest and should be corrected with sodium bicarbonate which, like all drugs during resuscitation, is given into a central vein. Between 25 and 50 ml of an 8.4% solution usually suffices.

1 Positive pressure ventilation
The lungs should be inflated between 10 and 12 times per minute. Adequate oxygenation of the blood can usually be achieved by hand ventilation, using a face mask, or by mouth-to-mouth techniques. Endotracheal intubation, however, should not be delayed because this not only improves alveolar ventilation but also protects the airway against regurgitated gastric contents.

2 External cardiac massage
This is applied by sharp compression of the lower end of the sternum about 60 times per minute. As soon as possible the patient should be attached to an ECG monitor in order to determine the cardiac rhythm. Further

management is directed at restoring an effective spontaneous cardiac output.

3 Ventricular fibrillation

This is treated with direct current shock (see page 61) using between 200 and 400 joules. If the fibrillatory waves are very fine, adrenaline (1 mg) may increase their amplitude, producing a coarser pattern which is often more susceptible to cardioversion. Anti-arrhythmic drugs such as lignocaine (100 mg, given slowly intravenously) make resistant ventricular fibrillation more responsive to direct current cardioversion.

4 Asystole

Treatment is difficult. Atropine (600 μg) disinhibits the sinus node. Inotropic drive is provided by adrenaline (1 mg) and calcium chloride (5 ml) in 10% solution, and an isoprenaline infusion of 1 to 5 μg per minute. If a pacemaker catheter can be introduced into the right ventricle a paced rhythm can be established, but electromechanical dissociation often prevents restoration of effective cardiac output.

If these measures succeed in restoring spontaneous circulatory function, further management is directed towards maintaining stable cardiac rhythm and oxygenation of the blood. Prophylactic anti-arrhythmic drugs are usually necessary, and many patients require mechanical ventilation.

Prognosis

Following resuscitation, the prognosis depends on the cause of the cardiac arrest and the presence of ischaemic cerebral damage. Prompt resuscitation prevents neurological sequelae, and in those cases caused by drugs and other toxic insults, life expectancy may be normal. In the majority of cases, however, cardiac arrest reflects severe underlying heart disease and the prognosis is usually poor. An important exception is primary ventricular fibrillation in acute myocardial infarction, when prognosis following resuscitation is often no worse than that of other survivors of myocardial infarction (see page 28).

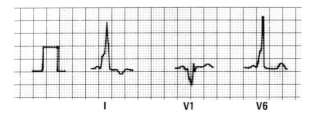

I   V1   V6

Figure 2.41 *Wolff–Parkinson–White syndrome: ECG. The short PR interval and the slurred initial defection (delta wave) of the QRS complex are clearly seen.*

Wolff–Parkinson–White (WPW) syndrome

Aetiology

This is a congenital disorder in which there is an anomalous conduction pathway (bundle of Kent) between the atria and the ventricles.

Pathophysiology

Atrial impulses conduct more rapidly through the bundle of Kent than through the atrioventricular node. Thus the initial phase of ventricular depolarization occurs early (pre-excitation) and spreads slowly by abnormal pathways. The PR interval is therefore short and the initial deflection of the QRS complex is slurred, producing a 'delta wave'. The remainder of ventricular depolarization is rapid because the delayed arrival of the impulse conducted through the atrioventricular node completes ventricular depolarization by normal His–Purkinje pathways.

Patients with WPW syndrome are prone to paroxysmal re-entry tachycardia. The re-entry circuit employs the atrioventricular node and the bundle of Kent (see Fig. 2.34). These patients are also prone to atrial fibrillation, which is potentially lethal if the rapid atrial discharge is conducted without block through the bundle of Kent producing an uncontrolled ventricular response. This may degenerate into ventricular fibrillation and cause sudden death.

Clinical features

The WPW syndrome is often asymptomatic. The most common complaint is paroxysmal palpitation due to re-entry tachycardia. Other clinical features of tachyarrhythmias may also occur (see page 56).

Diagnosis

A short (less than 0.12 seconds) PR interval and a delta wave on the ECG confirm the diagnosis (Fig. 2.41). The abnormality may be intermittent and multiple recordings are sometimes necessary for its demonstration. The delta wave is absent during episodes of tachycardia. Similar conditions may occur in which the PR interval is short but there is no delta wave (Lown–Ganong–Levine syndrome).

Complications

Sudden death is the major complication of the WPW syndrome but only occurs in those patients in whom the bundle of Kent will conduct at very fast rates (more than 300 beats per minute) during atrial fibrillation.

Treatment

Patients with Wolff–Parkinson–White syndrome should undergo an atrial stimulation study in which the right atrium is paced at rates in excess of 300 beats per minute. This often causes atrial fibrillation. In most cases the bundle of Kent is unable to conduct at this rapid rate and such patients, therefore, are not at risk of sudden death.

Drugs such as amiodarone and disopyramide are usually effective in the WPW syndrome. They slow conduction in the bundle of Kent so that re-entry tachycardia and a rapid ventricular response to atrial fibrillation are both prevented. Nevertheless, atrial stimulation studies should be repeated on treatment. Those patients who can still conduct at very rapid rates may require surgical excision of the bundle of Kent.

Digitalis should not be used in the WPW syndrome. Although it prevents re-entry tachycardia by slowing conduction through the atrioventricular node, conduction through the bundle of Kent may be facilitated, increasing the risk of sudden death in atrial fibrillation.

Prognosis

Life expectancy is normal in those patients without cardiac arrhythmias. Those patients with atrial fibrillation and a rapid ventricular response, on the other hand, are at high risk of sudden death if not adequately treated.

Hypertension

Hypertension is abnormal elevation of the arterial blood pressure. It is an important and potentially treatable cause of cardiovascular disease and death. Abnormal elevation of blood pressure implies a level above which the risk of morbid complications rises substantially. This level, however, is impossible to define because the risk of complications rises in approximately linear relation to both systolic and diastolic measurements. Moreover, the influence of blood pressure on morbid cardiovascular events is modified importantly by other factors such as age, race and sex, with young black males being at greatest risk. Attempts to define limits of normality are further confounded by the diurnal variability of blood pressure, with peak levels occurring early in the day and trough levels at night. Superimposed on this diurnal rhythm are the effects of exertion and anxiety, both of which increase blood pressure substantially. Blood pressure also shows long-term variability and in Western societies rises progressively with age, men on average having higher levels than women.

For all these reasons any definition of hypertension must inevitably be arbitrary. For practical purposes, however, hypertension in adults may be defined as follows (the diastolic level representing disappearance of sounds; see page 5):

Mild	140/90 to 160/100 mmHg
Moderate	160/100 to 180/120 mmHg
Severe	> 180/120 mmHg

Aetiology

Blood pressure is determined by cardiac output and systemic vascular resistance. Hypertension is nearly always the result of increased systemic vascular resistance caused by arteriolar constriction. In the majority of patients no specific aetiological factor can be identified. Essential hypertension of this type must be distinguished from secondary hypertension in which a specific cause can be identified.

1 Essential hypertension

This accounts for 95 per cent of all cases. The cause is by definition unknown, but evidence points to an interaction between hereditary and environmental factors. A hereditary influence must account in part for the familial incidence of essential hypertension. Abnormal membrane handling of sodium has often been demonstrated but its aetiological significance is unclear. Increases in circulating catecholamines and activation of the renin–angiotensin system occur in individual cases but are often not present. Environmental factors that have been associated with hypertension include obesity, alcohol consumption and urban living. The role (if any) of a high salt intake has yet to be defined. Cigarette smoking appears to be of aetiological importance only in accelerated hypertension (see page 69).

2 Secondary hypertension

In most cases, secondary hypertension is the result of renal disease or hormonal disorders (Table 2.24). Renal causes include both vascular and parenchymal disease, and in both cases activation of the renin–angiotensin system accounts at least in part for the elevation of blood pressure (see page 300). Hormonal disorders are responsible for hypertension in primary aldosteronism and Cushing's syndrome, owing to excessive mineralocorticoid activity, and in phaeochromocytoma owing to the

Table 2.24 Causes of secondary hypertension

Renal parenchymal disease
Glomerulonephritis
Pyelonephritis
Polycystic disease
Diabetic nephropathy
Connective tissue disease
Hydronephrosis

Renal artery stenosis
Atherosclerosis
Fibromuscular hyperplasia
Congenital

Endocrine disease
Adrenal cortex (Cushing's syndrome, Conn's syndrome)
Adrenal medulla (phaeochromocytoma)
Acromegaly
Iatrogenic (contraceptive pill, corticosteroids,
    sympathomimetic agents)

Miscellaneous
Coarctation of the aorta
Pregnancy (pre-eclampsia, eclampsia)
Acute porphyria
Increased intracranial pressure

effects of adrenal catecholamines (see page 303). The most common hormonal cause of hypertension, however, is the oral contraceptive which almost invariably produces an increase in blood pressure. Nevertheless, the increase is usually small and reverses promptly on stopping the drug. Activation of the renin–angiotensin system is probably responsible.

Pathology

Hypertension is usually the result of peripheral arteriolar constriction. In the early stages this is reversible, but in the long-term irreversible fibrinoid necrosis develops in the arteriolar wall. Hypertension is an important risk factor for atherosclerosis and accelerates the disease, particularly in the coronary, cerebral and renal circulations.

1 The heart
Hypertension is a major risk factor for coronary artery disease and predisposes to myocardial ischaemia and sudden death. Left ventricular hypertrophy occurs to compensate for the increase in afterload (see page 16). In long-standing disease, however, irreversible deterioration in left-ventricular contractile function may develop, leading to heart failure. The reduction in cardiac output often normalizes the blood pressure and the condition may be clinically indistinguishable from dilated car-

diomyopathy.
2 The brain
Accelerated atherosclerosis and microaneurysms are the principal cerebral consequence of hypertension. Both predispose to stroke by causing cerebral infarction and cerebral haemorrhage, respectively.
3 The kidney
Vascular changes in the renal arterioles and glomerular tufts decrease the glomerular filtration rate and produce tubular dysfunction. Proteinuria and haematuria occur and a vicious cycle of worsening renal function and increasing hypertension may develop.

Clinical features

Uncomplicated hypertension is usually asymptomatic. Contrary to popular belief the incidence of headache and epistaxis is not significantly increased and the onset of symptoms usually signals the development of major complications. Angina due to coronary atherosclerosis, left ventricular hypertrophy or a combination of the two is common, and in end-stage disease symptoms of heart failure occur. Retinal haemorrhage and exudates produce blurring of vision, while cerebrovascular disease may lead to transient ischaemic episodes or major stroke.

Examination confirms elevated blood pressure. The cardiac apex is not usually displaced, but it may have a thrusting quality and a double impulse due to a palpable fourth heart sound. Auscultation confirms the fourth sound and reveals accentuation of the aortic component of the second sound. An innocent mid-systolic murmur at the aortic area is not uncommon owing to forceful ejection by the hypertrophied left ventricle. Occasionally the early diastolic murmur of aortic regurgitation is also present.

Examination of the optic fundus permits direct inspection of the small blood vessels. Four grades of hypertensive retinopathy are recognized:

Grade I: Narrowing and increased tortuosity of the retinal arteries
Grade II: Accentuation of the arterial changes and apparent narrowing (nipping) of the retinal veins at arteriovenous crossings
Grade III: Vascular changes associated with haemorrhages and exudates
Grade IV: Previous grades with papilloedema

Grades I and II are not specific for hypertension, but grades III and IV are pathognomonic of hypertensive retinal damage.

Diagnosis

Hypertension is diagnosed by sphygmomanometry (see page 5). Blood pressure may show considerable variation in an individual; if it is found to be elevated, further measurements should be taken after a brief rest period and again at a subsequent clinic visit before committing the patient to life-long anti-hypertensive treatment. If the diagnosis is confirmed further investigation is directed at determining the aetiological diagnosis and assessing end-organ damage.

1 Aetiological diagnosis

Because the large majority of patients have essential hypertension, a routine search for unusual causes is unnecessary. Thus special investigations to screen for secondary hypertension (e.g. renal angiography or urography, urinary VMA, dexamethasone suppression test) are only indicated when the clinical findings are suggestive of a treatable underlying cause. Nevertheless, the threshold for undertaking special investigations of this type should be low for hypertensives under 35 years old, particularly when there is no family history of hypertension because in this group the incidence of secondary hypertension is relatively high.

2 Assessment of end-organ damage

Routine cardiac investigations should include an ECG and chest X-ray for assessment of left ventricular hypertrophy and failure. Renal status is evaluated by analysis of the urine for blood and protein and measurement of blood levels of urea and creatinine. A serum potassium level is needed as a baseline prior to starting diuretic therapy. This also provides a simple screen for primary aldosteronism.

Complications

The major complications of hypertension are heart disease, stroke, retinal damage and renal failure.

Treatment

Only a small minority of patients have hypertension that is amenable to surgical correction. This includes those with adrenal disease, unilateral renal disease and coarctation. The remainder require medical management.

1 Aims of treatment

Treatment is aimed at lowering the blood pressure with a view to reducing the incidence of major complications. The efficacy of treatment for preventing stroke is well-established, but reductions in the incidence of myocardial infarction have been more difficult to demonstrate.

Nevertheless, the overall mortality of treated hypertensives is lower than for those who receive no treatment.

2 Who to treat?

Patients with mild hypertension (up to 160/100 mmHg) do not require treatment because it produces no appreciable benefit in terms of long-term morbidity and mortality. The benefit of treating moderate and severe hypertension is, however, well-established.

There is no evidence that treatment differs radically in particular age or sex groups, but there is a strong impression that black patients respond poorly to beta-blockers and better to vasodilators. In addition, the very elderly (> 70 years) are often less able to tolerate anti-hypertensive drugs and it is reasonable to pursue a less aggressive policy in this subgroup since the aim of treatment is not only to prolong life but also to preserve its quality.

3 General measures

In certain patients dietary control is important. Thus the obese patient should be encouraged to lose weight because this often produces a significant reduction in blood pressure. Moderation of alcohol consumption is beneficial in the heavy drinker. Dietary sodium restriction is of unproven benefit, although it may potentiate the efficacy of anti-hypertensive drugs.

Relief of stress, though difficult to achieve, is beneficial in some patients. Thus relaxation techniques such as meditation have been shown to lower blood pressure, at least in the short-term.

Undoubtedly the most important general measure in the treatment of hypertension is the avoidance of other risk factors for arterial disease. In the majority of clinical trials smoking has emerged as a more important predictor of both myocardial infarction and stroke than a moderate increase in blood pressure.

4 Drug therapy

See Table 2.25. In hypertension, treatment must usually continue indefinitely, Thus the acceptability of treatment in terms of dosage frequency and side-effects must always be a major consideration. Indeed, poor compliance to the treatment regimen is the usual reason for inadequate control of blood pressure. From the wide range of drugs available, four groups of agents come closest to fulfilling the combined requirement for anti-hypertensive efficacy and patient acceptability.

Diuretics. These are useful in mild or moderate hypertension. Salt and water excretion reduces plasma volume and cardiac output. Nevertheless, these changes are short-lived and the mechanisms responsible for the long-term anti-hypertensive efficacy of diuretics are unknown.

Though thiazide and loop diuretics are equally

Table 2.25 Drugs used to treat hypertension

Drug	How to use	Adverse effects	Interactions
Thiazide diuretics Bendrofluazide	2.5 mg orally once daily	See Table 2.4	See Table 2.4
Beta-blockers Atenolol	Start with 50 mg once daily; increase if necessary to 100 mg daily	Avoid in asthma, cardiac failure and care in diabetics. Lack of energy; cold hands; bradycardia; depression and nightmares (especially propranolol) and impotence	Don't combine with IV verapamil Action increased by cimetidine (metoprolol) Action decreased by some NSAIDs Antagonizes the effects of theophylline
Metoprolol	Start with 100 mg once daily; increase to 100 mg twice daily if necessary		
Oxprenolol (slow release)	160–320 mg once daily		
ACE inhibitors Captopril	12.5 mg twice daily; increase if necessary to 50 mg twice daily	See Table 2.4	See Table 2.4
Enalapril	5.0 mg once daily and increase if necessary		
Calcium antagonists Nifedipine	20 mg twice daily (may be too much for the elderly)	Headaches; flushing; dyspepsia; 'hot legs'; ankle swelling	
Verapamil	120–160 mg twice daily	Constipation; flushing; headaches; is a negative inotrope	
Other vasodilators Prazosin	Initial dose 0.5 mg before retiring because of postural hypotension on first dose; thereafter 1.0 mg three times daily, increased as necessary	Drowsiness; headache; constipation; postural hypotension	Action reversed by some NSAIDs
Hydralazine	25–50 mg twice daily with a beta-blocker to prevent tachycardia; max 200 mg daily	See Table 2.4	See Table 2.4

beneficial in hypertension, thiazides are usually preferred because they produce a less vigorous diuresis, except in patients with impaired renal function. They should be used in low dose as the dose response curve is almost flat, but the incidence of adverse effects (especially hypokalaemia) is dose-related.

Plasma potassium should be measured one month after starting treatment, and if it is below 3.0 mmol/litre, which is unusual, a potassium-sparing diuretic should be added to the regimen.

Thiazides cause modest elevation of blood sugar and triglycerides, but there is no evidence that these metabolic side-effects increase long-term cardiovascular morbidity.

Beta-blockers. These drugs are effective in all degrees of hypertension. Although beta-blockers inhibit renin release from the kidney and also reduce cardiac output, it seems that these mechanisms are not necessarily involved in their hypotensive action, which remains undecided.

Beta-blockers may be used alone or may be combined

with diuretics or vasodilators. The choice of beta-blockers depends principally on patient acceptability (see page 67). Atenolol is often preferred because it is long-acting, cardioselective and does not cross the blood–brain barrier. Occasionally a beta-blocker with some intrinsic sympathetic action, such as oxprenolol, is used if bradycardia is a problem.

Calcium antagonists. These drugs relax vascular smooth muscle, producing arteriolar dilatation and reductions in systemic vascular resistance. They are effective in all degrees of hypertension, and have the advantage of increasing peripheral blood flow, which may be important in the older patient.

Angiotensin-converting enzyme inhibitors. These drugs block the synthesis of angiotensin II, producing arteriolar dilatation and reductions in systemic vascular resistance. They are effective in all degrees of hypertension but are usually reserved for the more resistant cases. Nevertheless, their use is increasing because their side-effects are rarely troublesome and the quality of life is often better preserved than with other anti-hypertensive drugs.

Other drugs. Prazosin, a post-synaptic alpha adrenergic blocker, continues to be widely used in moderate or severe hypertension. As with other vasodilators, postural hypotension may be troublesome. Hydralazine is also a vasodilator, acting directly on vascular smooth muscle.

Choice of drugs

There is still no universal agreement as to the best drug or combination of drugs to use in hypertension. At present it is usual to start with a single drug. For patients under 60 a beta-blocker is commonly used. In the elderly a diuretic is popular because of its lack of immediate side-effects and its ease of use. One or other of these drugs should control the blood pressure in 40–50 per cent of hypertensives.

If the resulting control of blood pressure is inadequate, the diuretic and beta-blockers should be combined and the success rate will rise to around 80 per cent. For those still poorly controlled, a vasodilator may be added to the regimen.

This stepwise approach is not always satisfactory. The side-effects of both beta-blockers and some vasodilators can be unacceptable to certain patients, and the long-term metabolic disturbances with thiazides may be a problem.

Other combinations which are used include a beta-blocker with a vasodilator such as nifedipine, or an ACE inhibitor can be used alone or combined with a diuretic.

It seems likely that in the future, quality of life as well as control of blood pressure will decide the drugs that are chosen.

Prognosis

The prognosis is determined by the extent of associated cardiac, cerebral and renal disease. It relates principally to the duration of hypertension and its severity. Thus by detecting hypertension at an early stage and treating it effectively the prognosis can be improved (principally by reducing the incidence of stroke). Prognosis is also affected by the age, race and sex of the patient, with young black men being at greatest risk of premature death. The interaction of other cardiovascular risk factors, particularly cigarette smoking, increase the risk considerably.

Accelerated hypertension

This affects about 1 per cent of all hypertensive patients and occurs in both essential and secondary hypertension. Cigarette smoking is a predisposing factor. Severe elevation of the blood pressure (often above 200/140 mmHg) may be associated with encephalopathy characterized by headache, nausea, clouding of consciousness and convulsions. The marked increase in afterload commonly causes left ventricular failure and pulmonary oedema. Grade IV retinopathy is invariable. Impairment of renal function usually occurs and if treatment is not instituted rapidly oliguric renal failure develops.

Accelerated hypertension is a medical emergency. Treatment is aimed at reducing the diastolic blood pressure to between 90 and 110 mmHg. Blood pressure reduction should be smooth and controlled because there is risk of cerebral infarction if it drops abruptly to very low levels. For this reason bolus injections of diazoxide or hydralazine are no longer recommended because the blood pressure response is unpredictable and difficult to control. A graded reduction in blood pressure can be achieved by intravenous infusions of nitroprusside or labetalol. Nitroprusside infusion should start at 25 μg per minute with small increments every 15 minutes until the desired response is achieved. Labetalol infusion should start at 1 mg per minute with increments every 30 minutes. Because labetalol is a beta-blocker as well as an alpha-blocker, it should be used cautiously in severe left ventricular failure. Following control of the blood pressure oral treatment should be prescribed to prevent recurrence of the hypertensive crisis.

Cardiac tumours

Primary tumours

Primary cardiac tumours are rare. The histologically

benign *myxoma* accounts for at least half of all cases. Myxomas usually arise in the left atrium but may also be found in the other cardiac chambers. Typically the tumour is pedunculated and attached to the interatrial septum such that it prolapses into the mitral valve orifice during diastole. This impedes diastolic filling of the left ventricle and produces symptoms similar to those of mitral stenosis. Dyspnoea, however, is often episodic and provoked by changes in posture which encourage gravitational prolapse of the tumour into the mitral valve. On examination there is a low-pitched noise in mid-diastole (tumour 'plop') probably caused by the myxoma striking the left ventricular wall. This may be mistaken for the mid-diastolic murmur of mitral stenosis. Other symptoms and signs of myxoma include fever, weight loss and clubbing but these are unusual. The erythrocyte sedimentation rate may be raised and systemic thromboembolism is common. Sudden death may occur if the tumour causes unrelieved obstruction of the mitral valve. In the past left atrial myxoma was usually misdiagnosed as mitral stenosis, but the echocardiogram now permits visualization of the tumour and rules out mitral valve disease. Treatment is by surgical excision of the tumour.

Metastatic tumours

Metastases account for the majority of cardiac tumours and usually originate from the breast or lung. The pericardium is most commonly affected but any other part of the heart may also be involved. Most cases are clinically silent. Pericardial effusion and tamponade is the most common clinical presentation. Invasion of the conducting tissue may produce heart block. Occasionally extensive myocardial involvement or valvar obstruction leads to heart failure.

Carcinoid syndrome

Carcinoid tumours in the appendix and other parts of the small bowel secrete kinin peptides and serotonin which are largely inactivated in the liver. Following metastasis to the liver, however, the systemic cirulation is no longer protected from these substances which are responsible for the characteristic clinical features of carcinoid syndrome. These include diarrhoea, bronchospasm, flushing attacks and telangiectasia. Cardiac manifestations are the result of toxic damage to the tricuspid or pulmonary valves. Variable regurgitation or stenosis often develops. Left-sided valvar disease is rare but is occasionally seen in patients with pulmonary metastases.

Pregnancy

The requirements of pregnancy cause an increase in plasma volume which by the third trimester may be 50 per cent greater than pre-pregnancy levels. This is associated with a fall in plasma osmotic pressure which predisposes to oedema even in the absence of pre-eclampsia. Oedema is usually mild and tends to affect the lower limbs where venous pressure is high owing to compression of the pelvic veins by the uterus. Elevated venous pressure is also an important factor in the development of varicose veins and haemorrhoids, which are commonly seen during pregnancy.

In pregnancy the skin is warm and often flushed owing to peripheral vasodilatation. The pulse rate is increased and may have a collapsing quality. During the third trimester the pregnant uterus may cause upward displacement of the diaphragm. This compresses the heart such that the apex beat becomes palpable in the fourth intercostal space in the anterior axillary line. Auscultation during this period commonly reveals an 'innocent' ejection murmur at the base of the heart and a third heart sound—both manifestations of the hyperdynamic circulation.

The ECG and chest X-ray are usually normal, but late in pregnancy may show changes reflecting cardiac compression. These include a degree of left axis deviation and apparent radiological cardiac enlargement. Atrial and ventricular premature beats are frequently found.

Heart disease in pregnancy

Flow murmurs, added heart sounds, peripheral oedema and minor ECG and chest X-ray abnormalities often give rise to a spurious impression of heart disease in the pregnant woman. In such cases the echocardiogram provides a safe and useful means of ruling out valvar and myocardial disorders.

Valvar and myocardial disease typically present during the third trimester or at the time of delivery when increments in plasma volume and cardiac output are at their peak. Mitral stenosis in particular is poorly tolerated and there is a considerable risk of pulmonary oedema. It is best treated by valvotomy before the onset of labour, but if valvar calcification or regurgitation contraindicate this procedure, medical management is preferable to valve replacement. Although mild bacteraemia is common during vaginal delivery, the risk of endocarditis in women with valvar disease is negligible and antibiotic prophylaxis (intravenous gentamicin and amoxycillin) is required only for complicated instrumented deliveries.

Dilated cardiomyopathy that presents three months before or after labour has been named *peripartum cardiomyopathy*. This appears to be a specific entity related to pregnancy and is particularly common in women of West African origin. Nevertheless, it remains unclear whether peripartum cardiomyopathy represents the direct effects of pregnancy on a previously normal heart or merely a deterioration in a pre-existing cardiomyopathy.

The pulmonary circulation

Acute pulmonary embolism

Aetiology

In the large majority of cases pulmonary embolism is caused by thrombus which usually derives from the iliofemoral veins or, less commonly, from the right-sided cardiac chambers. Other causes include air, tumour, amniotic fluid and fat and are seen less commonly.

Pathology

Generally speaking, the severity of pulmonary embolism is determined by the extent of pulmonary vascular obstruction and the associated increase in pulmonary artery pressure. If this is severe the abrupt rise in afterload may cause acute right ventricular failure. Occasionally, however, the degree of pulmonary hypertension is out of proportion to the extent of pulmonary vascular obstruction. It has been proposed, therefore, that pulmonary arteriolar constriction caused by ill-defined neurohumoral mechanisms may contribute to the pathophysiology of pulmonary embolism.

Arterial hypoxaemia occurs in severe pulmonary embolism. It is caused principally by ventilation—perfusion mismatch (see page 94), though right ventricular failure and low cardiac output may also contribute.

Pulmonary infarction occurs in fewer than 10 per cent of cases since the lung is protected by the bronchial arterial supply arising from the thoracic aorta, and it also obtains oxygen directly from the alveoli.

Clinical features

Pulmonary embolism is clinically silent in many cases. When symptoms occur they are variable and usually non-diagnostic. Nevertheless, patients commonly complain of the acute onset of dyspnoea and chest pain. The chest pain is usually retrosternal and is not necessarily pleuritic in nature. Cough, haemotysis, sweating and syncope occur less frequently. The most consistent clinical signs are tachypnoea, tachycardia and accentuation of the pulmonary component of the second heart sound. Elevation of the jugular venous pressure, a third heart sound and cyanosis are more variable. In the most severe cases the patient is shocked with severe hypotension and other signs of critically impaired cardiac output (see page 18).

Diagnosis

The chest X-ray is often normal, though loss of lung volume (elevated hemidiaphragm) and regional oligaemia are sometimes seen. When pulmonary infarction occurs the development of a radiographic density takes 12 to 24 hours to develop and does not contribute to early diagnosis. The ECG changes are as variable as the clinical features. Tachycardia may be the only abnormality, but in some cases features of acute right heart strain are seen. These include P pulmonale, an S wave in lead I and a narrow Q wave in lead III associated with T wave inversion (SI, Q3, T3). Right bundle branch block and atrial fibrillation may also occur.

In severe pulmonary embolism, arterial gas analysis shows hypoxaemia associated with hypocapnia and respiratory alkalosis.

More definitive diagnostic information is obtained by the radionuclide lung scan, particularly when ventilation and perfusion scans are performed (see page 15). Perfusion defects not matched by ventilation defects are highly specific for pulmonary embolism (Fig. 2.42). Pulmonary angiography is usually diagnostic if arterial filling defects and vessel cutoffs are seen. These occur only in pulmonary embolism, although other abnormalities including regional oligaemia are less specific.

Differential diagnosis

This includes other causes of acute-onset chest pain and dyspnoea, the most important of which is myocardial infarction. Pneumonia and pneumothorax are differentiated by inspection of the chest X-ray.

Complications

Non-fatal pulmonary embolism usually resolves without complications. In a minority of cases recurrent (often subclinical) attacks result in worsening pulmonary hypertension and right ventricular failure (see below).

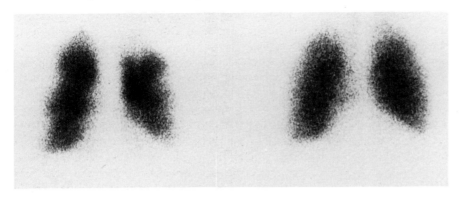

Figure 2.42 *Pulmonary embolism: ventilation–perfusion scintigraphy. The perfusion scintigram on the left shows multiple defects involving both lungs. The ventilation scintigram on the right, however, is normal showing homogenous distribution of the isotope. Ventilation–perfusion 'mismatch' of this type is highly specific for pulmonary embolism.*

Treatment

In most cases the degree of pulmonary artery blockage is mild. The initial pulmonary embolus will break up and the symptoms resolve. The main aim of treatment is to prevent further emboli.

Oxygen and heparin should be given immediately without waiting for the results of diagnostic tests. Heparin prevents extension of thrombosis within the lungs and allows endogenous fibrinolysis to proceed uninterrupted. It also reduces the risk of recurrent thromboembolism. After seven days oral anticoagulation with warfarin should be substituted and continued for three to six months (see page 390).

In severe pulmonary embolism the degree of pulmonary artery obstruction may lead to low-output cardiac failure, and this requires haemodynamic support with inotropic agents (see page 21). Thrombolytic therapy with streptokinase should be considered in these circumstances. Streptokinase is best given through a catheter positioned in the pulmonary artery.

In the shocked patient who fails to respond rapidly to these measures pulmonary embolectomy must be considered, though the mortality is high.

Prognosis

Pulmonary thromboembolism often goes unnoticed or causes only transient haemodynamic disturbance. Only a minority of embolic events are fatal. Trivial pulmonary embolism should not be ignored, however, because it may presage a more severe recurrence.

The prognosis in non-thrombotic pulmonary embolism is often less favourable. Thus amniotic fluid embolism in labour leads to shock and death in many cases. Fat embolism following surgical or accidental bony injury typically presents after a latent period of up to 36 hours with severe cardiopulmonary embarrassment. Mortality is high.

Chronic pulmonary embolism

Repeated, often subclinical, episodes of pulmonary embolism may lead to progressive obliteration of the pulmonary vascular tree. This is a chronic process associated with slowly rising pulmonary artery pressure providing time for the development of compensatory right ventricular hypertrophy. The clinical presentation is usually with severe pulmonary hypertension and right ventricular failure. The patient may be cyanosed. Signs of *pulmonary hypertension* include a left parasternal systolic thrust due to right ventricular hypertrophy and a loud pulmonary component of the second heart sound, often associated with the early diastolic murmur of pulmonary regurgitation. The development of right ventricular failure produces elevation of the jugular venous pulse, hepatomegaly and peripheral oedema. Functional tricuspid regurgitation is almost invariable in advanced cases. At this stage the pulmonary vascular disease is usually irreversible and treatment must be directed at preventing futher embolic events. Life-long anticoagulation with warfarin is essential, and in some cases a filter in the inferior vena cava may be used to prevent further embolism from the iliofemoral veins. The prognosis, however, is poor and few patients survive beyond five years.

Pulmonary heart disease

Aetiology

Pulmonary heart disease is sometimes called cor pulmonale. In this country chronic obstructive pulmonary disease is the leading cause. Other causes are shown in Table 2.26.

Pathology

Pulmonary heart disease is the result of chronic pulmonary hypertension caused by obliteration of the pulmonary vascular bed and hypoxic pulmonary arteriolar constriction. The right ventricle compensates by progressive hypertrophy but dilatation and contractile failure eventually supervene.

Clincial features and treatment

These are described on page 119.

Peripheral vascular disease

Aortic aneurysm

Aetiology

Aortic aneurysm is nearly always the result of atherosclerosis. Other causes include syphilis, Marfan's syndrome and idiopathic cystic medial necrosis.

Pathology

The wall tension in a blood vessel is determined by the product of intravascular pressure and diameter (Law of Laplace). The aorta is the largest artery in the body and its walls, therefore, are under considerable tension. Disease of the aortic wall causes destruction of the elastic fibres in the media which allows the vessel to dilate. The dilatation itself increases wall tension and a vicious cycle of worsening dilatation and increasing wall tension becomes established.

Most aortic aneurysms are fusiform, involving the total circumference of a segment of the vessel wall. Ocassionally they are saccular and consist of an outpouching of the vessel wall. Aneurysms occur most commonly in the abdominal aorta below the renal arteries, although any other part of the aorta may be affected.

Clinical features

Aortic aneurysms are usually asymptomatic. Local pressure may cause pain in the lumbar or thoracic spine depending on the location of the aneurysm. Rupture causes more severe pain and commonly leads to hypovolaemic shock and death.

Abdominal aortic aneurysms produce a pulsatile mass in the abdomen. A bruit is often audible owing to turbulent flow through the aneurysm. Thoracic aneurysms usually produce no physical signs unless they involve the aortic root, when the early diastolic murmur of aortic regurgitation may be audible.

Diagnosis

A plain chest or abdominal X-ray is often diagnostic, particularly when the aneurysm is calcified. Ultrasound studies are also useful, but computed tomography provides definitive diagnostic information. Angiography is usually required before surgery but is not necessary for diagnostic purposes.

Differential diagnosis

Abdominal aneurysms must be distinguished from other abdominal masses, particularly those which overlie the aorta and transmit pulsation. Nevertheless, only aortic aneurysms are expansile. Thoracic aneurysms must be distinguished from other causes of a mediastinal mass, particularly carcinoma.

Complications

1 Thromboembolism

Thrombosis within the aneurysm predisposes to thromboembolism.

Table 2.26 Causes of pulmonary heart disease

Obstructive airways disease
Bronchitis
Emphysema
Asthma

Parenchymal lung disease
Sarcoidosis
Pneumoconiosis
Bronchiectasis

Neuromuscular and chest wall disease
Poliomyelitis
Kyphoscoliosis

Impaired respiratory drive
Respiratory centre abnormalities
Sleep apnoea syndrome

Pulmonary vascular disease
Primary pulmonary hypertension
Chronic pulmonary embolism
Eisenmenger's syndrome

2 Infection
Aortic aneurysms may become infected and produce a syndrome almost identical to endocarditis, though heart murmurs are not present.

3 Aortic regurgitation
Aneurysmal involvement of the aortic valve ring is not uncommon in Marfan's syndrome and causes aortic regurgitation.

4 Rupture
Aneurysmal rupture is a surgical emergency which is often fatal.

Treatment

Blood pressure control is important and beta blockade delays the progress of aneurysm formation. Surgical resection is indicated when symptoms or complications (e.g. aortic regurgitaiton) cannot be controlled, or when rupture threatens. Aneurysms of the abdominal aorta are most prone to rupture and when greater than 6 cm in diameter require prompt surgical resection.

Prognosis

Atherosclerotic aortic aneurysms are nearly always associated with advanced coronary artery disease. Indeed, myocardial infarction is the usual cause of death. Five-year survival is less than 50 per cent.

Aortic dissection

Aetiology

Like aortic aneurysm, dissection is caused by disease of the aortic media, usually atherosclerosis. The majority of patients are hypertensive, particularly when the dissection arises in the aortic arch.

Pathology

The development of a tear in the aortic intima causes the high-pressure aortic blood to create a false lumen for a variable distance through the diseased media. The tear is usually proximal just above the sinus of Valsalva, but in about 25% of cases it is distal and located within the aortic arch. The dissection can partially or completely occlude any of the branch arteries arising from the aorta and, if proximal, may disrupt the aortic valve ring producing aortic regurgitation. The false lumen may rupture externally (particularly into the pericardial or left pleural spaces) or may re-enter the true lumen of the aorta more distally.

Clinical features

Presentation is with the abrupt onset of severe tearing pain in the front or the back of the chest. Examination may reveal absent pulses caused by side branch occlusions. The blood pressure is often elevated but in the event of rupture may be very low owing to hypovolaemia or tamponade. The early diastolic murmur of aortic regurgitation is commonly present in proximal dissections.

Diagnosis

ECG changes are non-specific but may show acute infarction if the dissection occludes the coronary ostium. The chest X-ray shows dilatation of the aorta, often with widening of the entire mediastinum. External rupture into the pericardial or pleural spaces causes cardiac enlargement or left pleural effusion, respectively. The echocardiogram often demonstrates the false lumen in proximal dissections and may also show pericardial haematoma and signs of aortic regurgitation. More useful information is provided by computed tomography which reliably demonstrates the true and false aortic lumens separated by an intimal flap. When the diagnosis is in doubt urgent aortic root angiography is required to define the origin and the extent of the false lumen (Fig. 2.43).

Differential diagnosis

Differential diagnosis is from other causes of acute chest pain, including myocardial infarction, pericarditis, pulmonary embolism and pneumothorax.

Complications

1 Branch artery occlusion
This may cause myocardial infarction, stroke, intestinal infarction, renal failure or limb ischaemia. If both vertebral arteries are occluded paraplegia occurs.

2 Aortic regurgitation
Disruption of the aortic valve ring may demand valve replacement during surgical repair of the dissection.

3 Rupture
Rupture into the pericardial sac causes severe tamponade. Rupture into the pleural or peritoneal spaces may lead to hypovolaemic shock.

Treatment

The first step is to relieve pain, which will usually require

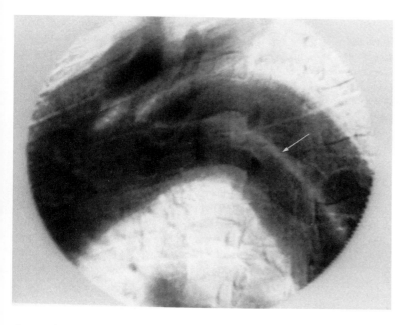

Figure 2.43 *Aortic dissection: angiography. This digital subtraction angiogram of the aortic arch shows abrupt widening of the aorta after the left subclavian branch. The intimal flap (arrowed) dividing the true and the false lumens is clearly seen.*

diamorphine (2.5–5 mg IV) with prochlorperazine (12.5 mg IV) as an anti-emetic.

In proximal dissection, expeditious surgical repair improves the prognosis and is the treatment of choice. In uncomplicated distal dissection, surgery has not been shown to affect the prognosis, but strict control of the blood pressure is essential. Beta-blockers are drugs of first choice because they reduce the pulse pressure as well as lowering the blood pressure.

Prognosis

Untreated proximal dissection is usually fatal within three weeks of presentation. Patients with distal dissection fare little better, though lowering the blood pressure helps prevent rupture and may permit longer survival.

Acute limb ischaemia

Aetiology

Acute limb ischaemia is usually caused by embolic, thrombotic or traumatic arterial occlusion. Emboli usually originate from the left side of the heart in conditions such as mitral valve disease, cardiomyopathy, myocardial infarction and endocarditis. Thrombosis is usually the result of advanced atherosclerosis or local trauma.

Pathology

Acute arterial occlusion provides no time for the develop-ment of collateral supply to the threatened limb. Profound ischaemia is therefore inevitable. This causes severe cell swelling and leads to irreversible damage within six hours. Muscle swelling in the anterior compartment of the leg may exacerbate tissue damage by compressing muscular arterioles. Decompression by fasciotomy may prevent ongoing tissue damage following surgical revascularization of the leg.

Clinical features

Acute arterial occlusion causes the abrupt onset of pain in the distal part of the limb, which thereafter becomes pale and cold. No pulses are palpable beyond the occlusion. Later the pain becomes less severe, but within six hours irreversible ischaemic damage develops.

Diagnosis

Diagnosis is by clinical criteria. Arteriography is unnecessary and needlessly delays definitive treatment.

Treatment

Urgent surgery is necessary if the limb is to be salvaged. Embolectomy may be performed under local anaesthesia. In the patient with thrombotic occlusion of diffusely atherosclerotic vessels, emergency bypass surgery may be necessary. Fasciotomy to relieve compression in the anterior compartment of the leg is sometimes helpful (see above).

If embolectomy fails, treatment is directed at preserving flow to the limb, which should be elevated to prevent swelling. Vasodilators such as nifedipine are usually prescribed, though their efficacy is unproven. Heparin and dextran infusions prevent extension of thrombosis within the limb. Infusion of streptokinase directly into the femoral artery may stimulate thrombolysis and restore flow.

Prognosis

Acute arterial occlusion in the lower limb nearly always progresses to gangrene and amputation if flow is not restored soon enough. In the arm, gangrene is rare but ischaemic contracture (Volkmann's) renders the limb useless.

Chronic limb ischaemia

Aetiology

Chronic limb ischaemia is nearly always the result of atherosclerosis. Risk factors are the same as for coronary artery disease. Thus men over 50 are most frequently affected, particularly if there is associated cigarette smoking, hyperlipidaemia or hypertension. Diabetic patients are also at increased risk.

Pathology

The atherosclerotic plaque which characterizes the condition enlarges and causes arterial stenosis which may proceed to thrombotic occlusion. This impairs distal perfusion of the limb. The lesions are found mainly in the large and medium-sized arteries, particularly the aorta and iliofemoral vessels. The upper limb is rarely affected. Diabetics are prone to more extensive disease, often with small vessel involvement.

Clinical features

Clincial features are largely dependent on the site of the obstruction. Two syndromes can be defined.

1 Femoro-popliteal obstruction

This is the more common syndrome. The femoro-popliteal disease results in intermittent claudication—a cramp-like pain felt in the calf which is brought on by walking and relieved by rest. As the disease advances, exercise capacity becomes progressively more limited until eventually rest pain occurs. Rest pain is usually felt in the feet and is most troublesome at night when it prevents sleep. Some relief is obtained by hanging the legs over the edge of the bed. On examination popliteal and pedal pulses are either reduced or absent. Arterial bruits may be audible over the femoral pulses. The skin of the legs is typically shiny and hairless. In severe ischaemia, areas of gangrene may develop. This often follows trauma, particularly around the nail bed and over the heels. In the most advanced cases, gangrene may extend to involve the whole foot and the leg.

2 Aorto-iliac obstruction

The main obstruction is in the lower aorta at its bifurcation and in the iliac arteries. Calf claudication is an early symptom but the pain spreads to the thighs and buttocks. This may be associated with impotence (Leriche syndrome). On examination the femoral pulses are reduced or absent, often with wasting of the buttock and thigh muscles. Auscultation over the lower abdomen and femoral pulses may reveal arterial bruits.

Diagnosis

The diagnosis is usually clear on the basis of the history and examination, particularly when there are absent pulses in the leg. Doppler studies permit flow measurements in the leg at rest and during exercise. This quantitates the perfusion deficit. If surgical treatment is contemplated arteriography is essential to define the location and the extent of disease.

Differential diagnosis

The chronically ischaemic limb must be distinguished from other causes of exercise-related pain in the legs, particularly musculoskeletal disorders and nerve root irritation in the lumbosacral spine.

Complications

Ischaemic ulcers and gangrene are the major complications. Ulcers often develop in response to minor trauma. Healing is always slow. Gangrene is the result of severe ischaemia and may require amputation of the limb. Diabetic patients are particularly at risk of these serious complications.

Treatment

1 General measures

Exercise is helpful because it encourages collateral flow and may improve symptoms. Trauma to the feet (e.g. ill-fitting shoes) should be avoided and a chiropodist should be enlisted to help with care of the toe-nails. The bed at night should not be excessively warm because cutaneous vasodilatation diverts flow away from muscle and exacerbates rest pain. Cigarette smoking must be strongly discouraged: it accelerates disease progression and produces vasoconstriction, which further reduces blood flow.

2 Specific therapy

Vasodilator drugs are of no value. Improved blood flow to the ischaemic limb can only be achieved by sympathectomy, angioplasty or bypass surgery. Most patients with intermittent claudication, however, never need surgical therapy.

Lumbar sympathectomy causes arteriolar dilatation and improves perfusion of the ischaemic limb. It is not helpful in intermittent claudication but relieves rest pain in about 50 per cent of cases. Nevertheless, early recurrence of symptoms is common. Angioplasty is only feasible in patients with isolated iliofemoral stenoses. The role of lasers in iliofemoral occlusions is under investigation. Bypass surgery corrects peripheral ischaemia in most cases. Results are better in patients with aorto-iliac disease than those with more distal disease. In patients with severe rest pain or gangrene, amputation may be necessary.

Prognosis

Prognosis is poor in patients with symptomatic peripheral vascular disease, with a five-year survival of less than 50 per cent. Myocardial infarction is the usual cause of death because nearly all these patients have associated coronary artery disease.

Buerger's disease

This is a rare condition occurring almost exclusively in men aged between 20 and 40. It is always associated with heavy cigarette smoking. The lesions occur principally in the small arteries of the feet (less commonly the hands) and lead to progressive arterial obliteration. Severe claudication often involving the instep is characteristic. Examination reveals absent foot pulses with normal femoral and popliteal pulses. Effective treatment is difficult. Abstinence from smoking is essential. Lumbar sympathectomy may help, but amputation is often necessary.

Raynaud's syndrome

Raynaud's syndrome is caused by spasm of the digital arteries in response to cold exposure. It is usually idiopathic and develops during adolescence, more commonly in women. Occasionally the syndrome is secondary to some other disorder (Table 2.27). This should be suspected when the onset is later in life, particularly in men, and when the digital involvement is either unilateral or asymmetrical.

Cold exposure typically causes a triphasic colour response. Profound blanching of the fingers and hands (the hallmark of Raynaud's) is followed by cyanotic mottling. During recovery the hands become pink and warm. The toes and even the nose may also be affected. In long-standing disease trophic changes in the finger-tips occur, sometimes progressing to frank gangrene.

Treatment is by avoiding cold exposure. Underlying causes, if present, should be corrected. Vasodilator drugs such as nifedipine may be helpful. Sympathectomy is beneficial in some cases but early relapse is common.

Deep venous thrombosis

Aetiology

Prolonged immobility in bed is the usual cause of thrombosis in the deep veins of the legs and pelvis. This affects up to 35 per cent of patients following major surgery—particularly abdominal and hip operations. Other risk factors for deep venous thrombosis are shown in Table 2.28. Upper limb venous thrombosis is less common but may occur after trauma to the axillary vein or in association with indwelling catheters, pacemaker wires or external compression.

Pathology

Thrombosis is usually in the iliac, femoral or calf veins. In about 10 per cent of cases a portion of thrombus may break off and cause pulmonary embolism (see page 71). This is unlikely if thrombosis is confined to the calf veins but becomes more likely with extension to the iliofemoral veins.

Table 2.27 Causes of Raynaud's sydrome

Idiopathic
Connective tissue disease (scleroderma, systemic lupus erythematosus)
Thoracic outlet syndrome (cervical rib)
Occupational (use of vibrating tools)
Drugs (beta-blockers)
Malignant disease

Table 2.28 Risk factors for deep venous thrombosis

Immobility, particularly following hip and abdominal
surgery
Venous stasis in legs (varicose veins, vena caval
compression (e.g. gravid uterus), bony fractures of legs)
Heart disease (myocardial infarction, heart failure)
Endocrine/metabolic factors (diabetes, obesity,
contraceptive pill, post-partum period)
Malignant disease, particularly pancreatic and bronchial
carcinoma
Miscellaneous (polycythaemia, Behçet's disease)

Clinical features

Symptoms and signs of deep venous thrombosis in the
legs are variable and non-diagnostic. Pain and swelling of
the calf occur, but many cases are clinically silent. Confirmation of the diagnosis requires special investigations.

Diagnosis

1 I¹²⁵-labelled fibrinogen test

1 I^{125}-labelled fibrinogen test

Radiolabelled fibrinogen is given intravenously, becomes
incorporated during the thrombotic process and may be
detected by imaging under a gamma camera. The
fibrinogen, however, is not taken up by thrombus that
has already formed and this limits the sensitivity of the
test.

2 Doppler ultrasound

This detects reductions in blood flow velocity caused by
thrombosis in the iliofemoral veins. It is of no value for
detecting thrombosis in the smaller veins of the calf.

3 Venography

This provides definitive evidence of deep venous
thrombosis. Following injection of contrast medium into
a vein in the foot, radiographic imaging of the leg and
pelvis identifies venous filling defects caused by
thrombosis.

Differential diagnosis

Deep venous thrombosis is usually unilateral and must be
distinguished from other causes of a swollen leg,
including trauma and infection. In patients with arthritis
of the knee, rupture of a Baker's cyst into the calf is
commonly mistaken for deep venous thrombosis.
Bilateral deep venous thromboses must be distinguished
from cardiac oedema, dependent oedema of the elderly
and lymphoedema.

Complications

Pulmonary embolism is the most important complication
of deep venous thrombosis and is a major cause of
in-hospital morbidity and mortality. Embolism is less
common with upper limb thrombosis. Thrombotic
damage to the veins and their valves may compromise
venous drainage and lead to chronic elevation of venous
pressure around the ankles. This produces the post-
thrombotic syndrome characterized by varicose veins and
trophic skin changes, including pigmentation (haemo-
siderosis) and ulceration of the skin around the ankles.

Treatment

1 Prophylaxis

Patients at risk of deep venous thrombosis may be given
prophylactic heparin. This is now regular practice
following ·myocardial infarction and also in patients
undergoing major surgery. Subcutaneous heparin, 5000
units eight-hourly, is effective and in surgical patients
should start preoperatively.

2 Specific therapy

In established deep venous thrombosis, anticoagulation
should begin with intravenous heparin followed by oral
anticoagulation with warfarin (see page 390). In patients
with recurrent pulmonary embolism, life-long anticoagulation is sometimes necessary.

Thrombolytic agents (e.g. streptokinase) effectively
lyse fresh venous thromboses but their role, if any, in the
management of this condition is not yet defined.

Prognosis

Complete resolution of deep venous thrombosis usually
occurs following anticoagulation and mobilization. In the
absence of pulmonary embolism, therefore, the prognosis
is good unless there is underlying malignant disease or
other serious systemic disorders.

Superficial thrombophlebitis

This is an acute inflammatory process involving superficial veins in the arms or legs. The aetiology is often
obscure, although it may occur as a complication of
varicose veins. In hospital practice it is commonly
associated with indwelling venous cannulae when
infection or local irritation by parenterally administered
drugs are the likely causes. The thrombosed vein may be
palpated as a cord. It is tender and the overlying skin is
erythematous. The risk of pulmonary embolism is

negligible. Treatment is directed at reducing inflammation by elevating the limb and prescribing anti-inflammatory analgesics.

Lymphoedema

Inadequate drainage of lymph from the extremities leads to its accumulation in the interstitium. This produces lymphoedema. Lymphoedema may be congenital but more commonly it is the result of lymphatic obstruction by organisms (e.g *Wuchereria bancrofti*), trauma (e.g. burns, irradiation, surgery) or malignancy. Essential lymphoedema of unknown cause (*Milroy's disease*) appears at puberty and mainly affects women. The *yellow-nail syndrome* is an unusual association of thick yellow nails, lymphoedema, pleural effusions and bronchiectasis.

The affected limb becomes progressively more oedematous and in chronic cases the skin becomes coarse and discoloured. The oedema is characteristically non-pitting, in contrast to cardiac oedema. Response to diuretics is poor. Surgical excision of oedematous tissue is reserved for the most severe, disfiguring cases.

Congenital heart disease

Cardiac defects are the most common of all serious congenital abnormalities. About 0.8 per cent of babies born alive have congenital heart disease, a figure that excludes non-stenotic bicuspid aortic valve and mitral valve prolapse. Untreated, the mortality is high, and by the age of five 70 per cent of affected children are dead. Those who survive have less severe cardiac lesions but few live beyond the age of 40. Congenital defects in which survival to adulthood is common are shown in Table 2.29.

Aetiology

Genetic factors can be identified in less than 1 per cent of cases (Table 2.30). These include cardiac disorders which occur in congenital syndromes, those associated with

Table 2.29 Congenital heart defects in which survival to adulthood is common

Bicuspid aortic valve
Pulmonary stenosis
Coarctation of the aorta
Atrial septal defect (secundum)
Patent ductus arteriosus
Tetralogy of Fallot
Complete heart block

recognizable chromosomal abnormalities (e.g. Down's syndrome, Turner's syndrome) and single-gene disorders which account for the familial incidence of certain defects. In most cases, however, the relatives of patients with congenital heart disease have only a slightly increased risk of being affected. Indeed, concordance for congenital cardiac defects is unusual in monozygotic twins. Thus environmental factors are likely to play an important role either directly or through interaction with genetic predisposition. Environmental factors known to influence the development of the heart during early pregnancy include maternal rubella and certain drugs.

Intracardiac shunts

(a) Atrial septal defect

Pathology

Communications between the atria may be caused by sinus venosus defects high in the septum or 'primum' defects low in the septum. These are commonly associated with anomalous pulmonary venous drainage and mitral valve abnormalities, respectively. However, the most common atrial septal defect is the 'secundum' defect of the oval fossa. Blood shunts preferentially from the left atrium through the right side of the heart into the low-resistance pulmonary circulation. The chronic increase in pulmonary flow may cause irreversible obliterative disease of the pulmonary arterioles during adulthood. Rising pulmonary vascular resistance causes pulmonary hypertension and right ventricular hypertrophy. This leads to progressive reductions in both cardiac output and left-to-right shunting. Eventually the pressures in the pulmonary and systematic circulations equilibrate and shunting becomes negligible or reverses (*Eisenmenger's syndrome*).

Clinical features

Atrial septal defect is usually asymptomatic until the chronic increase in pulmonary flow leads to pulmonary hypertension during adulthood. This causes fatigue and dyspnoea owing to reductions in cardiac output. Symptoms are exacerbated by atrial fibrillation, which may precipitate right ventricular failure. Physical signs are fixed splitting of the second heart sound and a mid-systolic murmur at the pulmonary area owing to increased flow through the valve. When the shunt is large a mid-diastolic tricuspid flow murmur may also be present. The primum type of defect is often associated

Table 2.30 Aetiology of congenital heart disease

Genetic factors		
(a)	Chromosomal abnormalities:	
	Trisomy 21 (Down's syndrome)	ASD, VSD, Fallot's tetralogy
	XO (Turner's syndrome)	VSD, PDA, Pulmonary stenosis
	XXXY	PDA, ASD
(b)	Single-gene disorders:	
	Autosomal dominant	ASD (secundum), hypertrophic cardiomyopathy, mitral valve prolapse
	Autosomal recessive	ASD (primum)
(c)	Congenital syndromes:	
	Autosomal dominant	
	Marfan	Aortic and mitral regurgitation
	Leopard	Pulmonary stenosis, hypertrophic cardiomyopathy
	Holt–Oram	ASD, VSD
	Romano–Ward	Prolonged QT interval
	Autosomal recessive	
	Osteogenesis imperfecta	Aortic regurgitation
	Pseudoxanthoma elasticum	Mitral regurgitation
	Laurence–Moon–Biedl	VSD
Environmental factors		
(a)	Viral infection:	
	Rubella	PDA, pulmonary stenosis, ASD
(b)	Drugs:	
	Alcohol	ASD, PDA
	Trimethadone	Complete transposition, Fallot's tetralogy
	Lithium	Ebstein's anomaly, ASD
	Amphetamines	VSD, PDA, complete transposition

ASD—Atrial septal defect, PDA—patent ductus arteriosus, VSD—ventricular septal defect.

with an apical pan-systolic murmur and other signs of mitral regurgitation.

In those patients who develop severe pulmonary hypertension and shunt reversal (Eisenmenger's syndrome), central cyanosis occurs owing to mixing of venous and arterial blood in the left atrium. This is associated with digital clubbing, polycythaemia and signs of pulmonary hypertension (see page 72).

Infective endocarditis is rare in atrial septal defect, though patients with a primum defect are prone to infection of the mitral valve.

Diagnosis

The ECG shows left axis deviation in primum atrial septal defect, but in the more common secundum defect the axis is normal or to the right. The chest X-ray shows cardiac enlargement with dilatation of the proximal pulmonary artery and plethoric lung fields reflecting increased pulmonary flow. The echocardiogram shows dilatation of the right-sided cardiac chambers and is potentially diagnostic if the defect can be imaged. Cardiac catheterization confirms the diagnosis. Serial measurements of oxygen saturation in the vena cava, right atrium, right ventricle and pulmonary artery shows an abrupt 'step-up' at right atrial level owing to shunting of oxygenated blood through the defect. The catheter can be directed across the defect into the left atrium. Measurements of pulmonary and systemic flow using the Fick principle permit quantification of the shunt ratio. When a high oxygen saturation is found in the superior vena cava, or when the catheter enters a pulmonary vein directly from the right atrium, a sinus venosus defect with anomalous pulmonary drainage is likely.

Treatment

Surgical correction of atrial septal defect is recommended

in all patients with a pulmonary-to-systemic flow ratio in excess of 2:1. This policy protects against the development of Eisenmenger's syndrome. In established Eisenmenger's syndrome, pulmonary hypertension is irreversible and closure of the defect is, therefore, unhelpful. Total heart and lung transplantation is the only surgical option.

Prognosis

Untreated, atrial septal defect rarely permits survival beyond the age of 60.

(b) Ventricular septal defect

Pathology

Ventricular septal defect is the most common congenital cardiac anomaly. It usually occurs in the perimembranous part of the septum. Blood shunts preferentially from left to right into the low-resistance pulmonary circulation. About 40 per cent of defects close spontaneously in early childhood, but in those that remain patent the chronic increase in pulmonary flow predisposes to obliterative pulmonary vascular disease and Eisenmenger's syndrome.

Clinical features

If the shunt is large, heart failure occurs in infancy. Smaller shunts often remain asymptomatic until adulthood when fatigue and shortness of breath are common. These symptoms are accentuated by the development of obliterative pulmonary vascular disease. Examination reveals cardiac enlargement with a prominent left ventricular impulse. A systolic thrill over the lower left sternal edge can often be felt in association with a pan-systolic murmur at the same location.

Patients with ventricular septal defect are always at risk of endocarditis, and antibiotic prophylaxis is essential.

Diagnosis

The ECG and chest X-ray may be normal if the defect is small. Larger defects produce left ventricular hypertrophy and cardiomegaly with pulmonary plethora caused by increased pulmonary flow. The echocardiogram is diagnostic if the defect can be imaged. Cardiac catheterization confirms the diagnosis. There is a step-up in oxygen saturation at right ventricular level (see page 80), and left ventricular angiography produces prompt opacification of the right ventricle through the defect.

Differential diagnosis

Differential diagnosis is from other causes of a pan-systolic murmur. In mitral regurgitation the murmur is apical and radiates into the axilla. In tricuspid regurgitation the location of the murmur at the lower left sternal edge is similar to ventricular septal defect, but the murmur is accentuated by inspiration and giant V waves are visible in the jugular venous pulse (see page 6).

Treatment

Ventricular septal defect requires urgent repair if it causes heart failure in infancy. In asymptomatic cases conservative management is usually appropriate; but if signs of pulmonary hypertension develop during follow-up, cardiac catheterization is required with a view to closure of the defect. In established Eisenmenger's syndrome closure of the defect is unhelpful and total heart and lung transplantation is the only surgical option.

Prognosis

When spontaneous closure of ventricular septal defect occurs in childhood, life expectancy is normal. Persistent small defects (Maladie de Roger) are consistent with a normal life-span. Larger defects may produce heart failure and death in infancy or lead to Eisenmenger's syndrome in later life.

(c) Patent ductus arteriosus

Pathology

The ductus arteriosus joins the main pulmonary trunk to the aorta. In the fetus gas exchange takes place at the placenta. Saturated vena cava blood from the placenta passes through the right side of the heart and shunts through the ductus arteriosus into the low-resistance systemic circulation, bypassing the high-resistance pulmonary bed. At birth the lungs take over the role of gas exchange. Systemic resistance rises with loss of the placental circuit and pulmonary resistance falls owing to inflation of the lungs. Flow through the ductus arteriosus therefore diminishes and the effects of local prostaglandins stimulate its closure.

In the premature infant persistent patency of the ductus arteriosus is common because normal mechanisms for its closure are not developed. At full-term relative hypoxaemia (high-altitude, pulmonary disease, cyanotic heart disease) delays normal closure. In other cases a patent ductus arteriosus is properly regarded as a congenital defect which occurs more commonly in females. Blood shunts from left to right across the patent ductus arteriosus into the low-resistance pulmonary bed. This increases the pulmonary flow and volume-loads the left side of the heart. If the shunt is large, obliterative pulmonary vascular disease and Eisenmenger's syndrome may develop.

Clinical features

The chronic volume-load may lead to left ventricular failure which, in the premature infant, exacerbates respiratory distress caused by hyaline membrane disease. In the full-term infant, left ventricular failure may also occur, but in many cases the condition remains asymptomatic. Examination reveals a collapsing carotid pulse owing to diastolic shunting through the ductus. The cardinal physical sign, however, is a continuous 'machinery' murmur at the upper left sternal edge caused by turbulent flow through the ductus which occurs throughout the cardiac cycle. The murmur is loudest at end-systole and early diastole.

Diagnosis

The chest X-ray is usually normal but may show cardiac enlargement and pulmonary plethora if the shunt is large. In adults, calcification of the ductus arteriosus may be visible. Cardiac catheterization is necessary to confirm the diagnosis.

Complications

When the shunt is large, a patent ductus arteriosus may cause left ventricular failure or obliterative pulmonary vascular disease, leading to Eisenmenger's syndrome. The risk of endocarditis is considerable.

Treatment

Patent ductus arteriosus always requires closure regardless of the size of the shunt. It is a low-risk procedure and guards against the development of complications, particularly endocarditis. In the premature infant cyclo-oxygenase inhibitors (e.g. indomethacin) may be effective, but in older children surgical closure is required. Recently catheterization techniques have been developed which permit closure of the ductus by a synthetic obstructor. This avoids the small risk of surgery.

Prognosis

The natural history of patent ductus arteriosus is variable. If the shunt is large the risk of life-threatening complications is considerable. Endocarditis is an ever-present risk regardless of the size of the shunt. Nevertheless, patients with a very small defect may have a normal life-span.

Obstructive valvar and vascular lesions

(a) Aortic stenosis

Congenital aortic stenosis is caused by commissural fusion which results most commonly in a bicuspid valve. Associated anomalies may include patent ductus arteriosus and coarctation of the aorta. Bicuspid aortic valve may present in infancy with left ventricular failure due to outflow obstruction. More commonly, however, significant valvar stenosis does not occur until adulthood, when the cusps calcify (see page 47). On examination the carotid pulse may be slow-rising, depending on the degree of valvar stenosis. An ejection click followed by a mid-systolic murmur is audible at the aortic area. Heart failure in infancy requires surgery (usually valvotomy), but asymptomatic cases without significant valvar stenosis require no specific treatment apart from antibiotic prophylaxis to protect against endocarditis.

In a minority of cases the obstruction is subvalvar caused by a muscular band or diaphragm. Clinical manifestations are very similar to valvar stenosis. Supravalvar aortic stenosis occurs at the superior margin of the sinuses of Valsalva above the coronary arteries. It is commonly associated with idiopathic hypercalcaemia, mental retardation and characteristic elfin-like facies.

(b) Pulmonary stenosis

This is one of the most common congenital cardiac anomalies. The right ventricular outflow obstruction produces a pressure gradient across the valve and variable right ventricular hypertrophy. Auscultation reveals an ejection click at the pulmonary area followed by a mid-systolic murmur. Mild-to-moderate pulmonary stenosis (peak systolic valve gradient less than 70 mmHg) is only rarely symptomatic and is consistent with a normal life-span. In more severe cases, right ventricular failure may occur and valvotomy is required to relieve the outflow obstruction. Effective relief of outflow obstruction may also be achieved by balloon dilatation of the pulmonary valve during cardiac catheterization, which avoids the risks of surgery.

(c) Tetralogy of Fallot

Pathology

The tetralogy consists of subvalvar pulmonary outflow obstruction, ventricular septal defect, overriding of the aorta and right ventricular hypertrophy. Depending largely on the severity of the right ventricular outflow obstruction, desaturated blood shunts from right to left across the ventricular septal defect. In severe outflow obstruction the shunt is large and cyanosis severe. In mild outflow obstruction, on the other hand, pulmonary flow may be close to normal and shunting is negligible— 'acyanotic Fallot's'. Nevertheless, even in acyanotic Fallot's, the outflow obstruction is often progressive and cyanosis usually develops during early childhood.

Clinical features

Tetralogy of Fallot is the most common cardiac cause of central cyanosis after the first year of life. When pulmonary outflow obstruction is very severe and shunting considerable, the volume-loaded left ventricle fails in infancy. Unprovoked attacks of intense cyanosis may occur leading to syncope, convulsions or death. In less severe cases important symptoms do not occur until later, when the child is troubled by exertional dyspnoea and may squat to relieve symptoms. Squatting improves arterial oxygen saturation by increasing systemic vascular resistance, thereby reducing the shunt through the ventricular septal defect. Examination reveals central cyanosis and clubbing. Physical development is often impaired, though mental development is usually normal. A midsystolic ejection murmur is audible at the pulmonary area, but the pulmonary component of the second heart sound is absent. A left parasternal systolic thrust due to right ventricular hypertrophy is usually present.

Diagnosis

The ECG shows variable right ventricular hypertrophy depending on the degree of outflow obstruction. The chest X-ray shows a boot-shaped heart with a deep concavity of the left heart border due to a diminutive pulmonary artery. The echocardiogram is diagnostic if the ventricular septal defect and overriding aorta are imaged. The diagnosis is confirmed by cardiac catheterization.

Differential diagnosis

Tetralogy of Fallot can usually be distinguished from other cardiac causes of central cyanosis (Table 2.31) on the basis of the echocardiographic findings. In the adult, Eisenmenger's syndrome is the major differential diagnosis. Both conditions are associated with central cyanosis, clubbing and heart murmurs. Nevertheless, the pulmonary component of the second heart sound which is loud in Eisenmenger's syndrome is absent in tetralogy of Fallot.

Complications

In severe cases the right-to-left shunt can cause left ventricular failure in infancy. In children and adults, on the other hand, right ventricular failure is more common owing to chronic outflow obstruction. Other complications include cardiac arrhythmias and endocarditis.

Treatment

Treatment is by total correction of the abnormality, which involves closure of the ventricular septal defect and relief of pulmonary outflow obstruction. In infants, however, palliative procedures are usually performed pending total correction later in life. These procedures are directed at improving the pulmonary flow by creating an anastomosis between the ascending aorta and the pulmonary artery (Waterston shunt) or the subclavian artery and the pulmonary artery (Blalock shunt).

Prognosis

Death in infancy may occur if right ventricular outflow obstruction is very severe. Less severe disease permits survival into adulthood but few patients live beyond the age of 40. In infants cyanotic attacks are the major cause of death, but in children and adults right ventricular failure, arrhythmias and endocarditis are more important.

Table 2.31 Causes of central cyanosis in congenital heart disease

Plethoric lung fields	Oligaemic lung fields
Transposition of great arteries	Tricuspid atresia
Total anomalous pulmonary drainage	Severe pulmonary stenosis
Common atrium	Severe Fallot's tetralogy
Hypoplastic left heart syndrome	Eisenmenger's syndrome
Common arterial trunk	

(d) Coarctation of the aorta

Pathology

Coarctation is a localized fibrotic narrowing of the aorta which arises in association with the ductus arteriosus just beyond the origin of the left subclavin artery. It occurs more commonly in males and may be associated with bicuspid aortic valve, Berry aneurysm or gonadal dysgenesis (Turner's syndrome).

If coarctation is severe and obstruction to aortic flow complete, left ventricular failure occurs in infancy. More commonly, however, the obstruction is partial and heart failure is avoided by the development of compensatory left ventricular hypertrophy and collateral flow around the coarctation.

Clinical features

Coarctation is usually asymptomatic if heart failure in infancy does not occur. On examination the femoral pulses are delayed and diminished compared with the radial pulses (radiofemoral delay). The blood pressure in the arms is elevated but in the legs it is normal or low. Left ventricular hypertrophy produces a prominent apical impulse and a fourth heart sound. A systolic murmur is almost invariable from turbulent flow through the coarctation and collateral vessels. The murmur is often louder over the back of the chest and may be continuous if the collateral circulation is extensive. In adults with coarctation the shoulders and arms are often noticably better developed than the lower extremities.

Diagnosis

The ECG shows left ventricular hypertrophy depending on the severity of hypertension. The chest X-ray characteristically shows notching on the underside of the ribs owing to erosion by dilated interocostal collateral arteries (Fig. 2.44). Angiography confirms the diagnosis.

Differential diagnosis

Other obstructive lesions of the aorta also cause diminished or absent femoral pulses. The most important of these is advanced atherosclerosis. Nevertheless patients with atherosclerosis are usually elderly and complain of intermittent claudication, which is not a feature of coarctation.

Complications

The principal complications are those of sustained hypertension in the upper half of the body. This produces left ventricular failure and predisposes to stroke and aortic

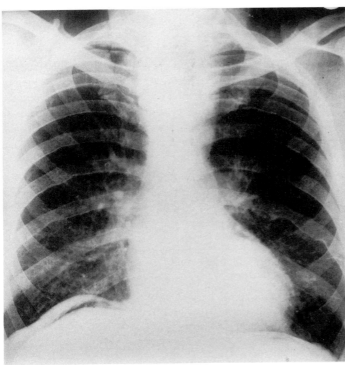

Figure 2.44   *Coarctation: PA chest X-ray. Notching of the inferior margins of the ribs is shown. The air under the diaphragm was the result of recent abdominal surgery.*

dissection. Patients with coarctation are also prone to subarachnoid haemorrhage (due to ruptured berry aneurysm), endocarditis and arrhythmias.

Treatment

Treatment is by resection of the coarctation and end-to-end anastomosis of the aorta. This should be performed electively in childhood when relief of aortic obstruction corrects hypertension and removes the risk of left ventricular failure and stroke. Later in life hypertension may become irreversible.

Complications

Complications of coarctation rarely permit survival beyond the age of 40 unless surgical correction is undertaken.

Congenital heart block

Congenital complete heart block may not present until adolescence or early adult life. Treatment is by implantation of a permanent pacemaker.

Further reading

Braunwald, E. (1988) *Heart Disease*, 3rd edn. W.B. Saunders, Philadelphia.

Timmis, A.D. (1988) *Essentials of Cardiology* Blackwell Scientific Publications. Oxford.

Julian, D.G. (1988) *Cardiology*, 5th edn. Baillière Tindall, London.

3
Disorders of the Respiratory System

Introduction

The lungs and respiratory tract are constantly exposed to infecting and noxious agents in the air we breathe. Antibiotics have altered the outlook for bacterial infections, but as yet there is no specific treatment for viral infections of the respiratory tract which are amongst the most common types of infection seen in man. The importance of industrial lung diseases such as occupational asthma and that occurring in miners and those exposed to asbestos has received much prominence and has modified manufacturing processes. The hazards of cigarette smoking have received world-wide recognition; apart from the morbidity and mortality associated with progressive impairment of lung function in smokers, cancer of the lung is the commonest form of cancer in the Western world and a major cause of death. Much research into asthma has given a better understanding of the mechanisms involved in its causation and of its treatment.

Defence mechanisms

The air passages are lined with ciliated epithelium down as far as the respiratory bronchioles, and the rich blood supply of the lining membrane enables it to warm and moisten the inspired air. A thin film of mucus is secreted by the submucosal glands in the larger bronchi and by the goblet cells extending throughout the respiratory tract. It is kept continuously moving away from the lungs by the sweeping action of the cilia—the so called ciliary escalator—and this is a most effective filter in removing particulate matter from the air before it reaches the lungs. Another local defence mechanism is the cough reflex, whereby foreign matter is expelled explosively (see page 88). Further, the synthesis of immunoglobulin (secretory

IgA) by plasma cells in the submucosa and its passage through the epithelium, together with the presence of alveolar macrophages, provide mechanisms for destruction and phagocytosis of infecting agents and particulate matter.

Disease states occur when any of these defence mechanisms are deficient. For example, patients with the immotile cilia syndrome (*Kartagener's syndrome*, see page 114) invariably suffer from rhinitis, sinusitis and chronic bronchitis, recurrent respiratory infections occur in patients with IgA deficiency, and opportunist lung infections with unusual organisms occur in patients with impaired immune response due to disease and/or treatment (page 112).

Anatomy

The bronchi to the separate lobes of each lung arise from the main bronchi on their respective sides. The primary subdivision of the lobar bronchi, together with the segments of lung which they supply, form the bronchopulmonary segments. The segmental bronchi are regarded as the first generation of the subdivisions of the intrapulmonary bronchi, which continue to divide and subdivide to produce some 15–20 generations. By definition, once cartilage is lost from the wall, the airway becomes a bronchiole. The terminal bronchiole is the last airway proximal to the respiratory bronchioles, which in turn open directly into the alveoli. The alveoli are lined by type I and type II pneumocytes, the latter probably being responsible for the production of surfactant which is of importance in lowering the surface tension of the alveoli and terminal airways.

The pulmonary and the bronchial arteries follow the pattern of the branching airways, the former supplying the alveoli and the latter the bronchi and bronchioles. Blood from lung tissue and the airways drains into the pulmonary veins which enter directly into the left atrium. The bronchial veins drain blood form the proximal bronchi only, as well as the hilar structures, and enter the azygos veins. Thus, an anastomosis between systemic and pulmonary circulations occurs in the lungs.

Lymphatics exist in the connective tissue of the lung, in the pleura and in the interlobular septa which occur at the lung edges. Oedema or prominence of the lymphatics of the septa (such as occurs, for example, in mitral stenosis, left ventricular failure, pneumoconiosis and lymphangitis carcinomatosa) produces Kerley B (septal) lines on the chest X-ray; they are short (less than 2 cm), horizontal lines extending from the pleural surface and are most marked at the lung bases. Lymphatic drainage of the lungs mostly follows the bronchovascular pattern, but some lymphatic vessels course irregularly through the lungs, and when prominent from distension or infiltration produce Kerley A lines; these are more central, not connected to the pleura and are some 2–4 cm in length.

The fissures

The upper and lower lobes of the left lung are separated by the oblique fissure. The right lung is composed of three lobes and the right oblique fissure separates the lower lobe from the upper and middle lobes. On each side the oblique fissure extends from the anterior end of the 6th rib and runs upwards and backwards round the chest wall, usually along the line of the 5th or 6th rib to the vertebral column. Its surface marking roughly corresponds to the position of the medial border of the scapula when the hand is placed on top of the head. The horizontal fissure separates the right upper lobe from the middle lobe. Its surface marking starts at the fourth right costal cartilage and runs horizontally around the chest to join the oblique fissure in the mid-axillary line. The segment of the left lung which occupies the position corresponding to the middle lobe is called the lingula, and it is part of the left upper lobe.

The bronchopulmonary segments

A proper knowledge of the anatomy of the bronchopulmonary segments (Fig. 3.1) is essential to an understanding of the localization and spread of many diseases of the lung. Many lung infections spread via the bronchi and the distribution of the infection is determined by the segments which these bronchi supply. The segments of each lobe are named after their corresponding bronchi as follows.

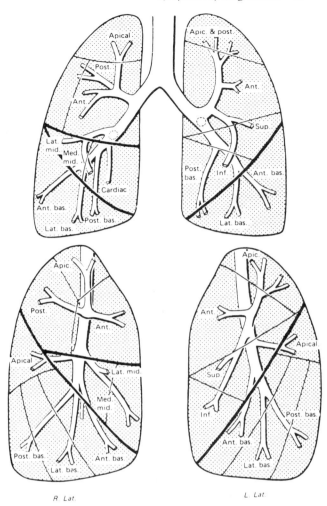

Figure 3.1 *The bronchopulmonary segments.*

1 The upper lobes
The right upper lobe bronchus divides almost immediately into anterior, apical and posterior branches. The anterior and posterior bronchi have axillary branches which supply the lateral part of the upper lobe.

The left upper lobe bronchus quickly gives origin to the lingula bronchus which runs downwards and forwards, subdividing into superior and inferior branches. It then gives off branches to the anterior, apical and posterior segments of the lobe, but differs from the right side in having a common apicoposterior bronchus.

2 The middle lobe
This is only present on the right side and runs downwards and forwards dividing into lateral and medial divisions.

3 The lower lobes

The right lower lobe bronchus gives off an apical branch which arises opposite the middle lobe bronchus and runs backwards to the apical segment of the lower lobe. The basal bronchi consist of anterior, lateral, and posterior branches and, in addition, a medial basal (or cardiac) bronchus supplies a small segment in the medial aspect of the lower lobe.

On the left side the arrangement is similar, but the medial basal is usually insignificant or absent.

Symptoms of lung disease

Types of cough and sputum

A forced expiration against a closed glottis produces a high pressure in the trachea and bronchi, and the sudden opening of the glottis is followed by the explosive discharge of air, producing the characteristic barking noise of a cough. This removes secretions and foreign material from the air passages. The cough reflex is stimulated by irritation of nerve endings in the larynx, trachea, bronchi, and even the pleura.

1 Respiratory tract infections

In the early stages, inflammatory swelling of the mucous membrane causes the cough to be dry and unproductive. With the later development of inflammatory exudate, the cough produces clear or whitish, and later yellow, sputum.

2 Whooping cough

The exudate here is particularly tenacious. The patient gives a series of quickly repeated coughs during one expiratory movement and this is followed by an inspiratory 'whoop', through a partially closed glottis. The cough typically occurs in paroxysms and is not always associated with a 'whoop', but may be accompanied by vomiting.

3 Purulent sputum

This is yellow or greenish in colour and occurs with secondary pyogenic infection during respiratory tract infections, in pneumonia, lung abscess and bronchiectasis. Purulent sputum tends to be more fluid as enzymes from the pus cells liquefy the mucus.

4 Bronchiectasis

The patient coughs up the infected sputum which has collected in the dilated bronchi during the night with change of posture on waking in the morning. The quantity of sputum depends on the degree of infection and extent of the disease. It may amount to several ounces per day and is sometimes very offensive in smell owing to the action of putrefactive bacteria.

5 Bronchial carcinoma

The cough is at first persistent and unproductive owing to invasion of the mucous membrane. When partial bronchial obstruction develops, distal infection produces mucopurulent sputum which may be blood-stained.

6 Pulmonary tuberculosis

There may be no sputum in the earlier stages of the disease. If sputum is produced it is clear or white and very sticky, so that it remains in separate lumps in the sputum pot (nummular sputum). Later it becomes frankly purulent.

7 Pneumococcal pneumonia

In the early stages the patient may cough up very viscid sputum tinged with blood which gives it a rusty colour.

8 Pulmonary oedema

In severe cases fluid exudes into the alveoli and the attack is associated with the expectoration of a large quantity of clear, frothy sputum, which is sometimes pinkish in colour owing to the presence of red cells.

9 Bronchial asthma

The sputum consists of firm, whitish pellets, which can sometimes be unravelled in water into spiral ribbons (Curschmann's spirals). These represent casts of the bronchial tubes in which they have formed. At times the sputum is yellow owing to the presence of eosinophils.

Haemoptysis

The coughing up of blood must be distinguished from haematemesis, the vomiting of blood. Blood from the lungs is usually bright red, frothy and mixed with sputum, while that from the stomach is usually dark in colour, having been altered to acid-haematin by hydrochloric acid, and often mixed with food particles. Many patients can state definitely whether the blood has been coughed up or vomited, and often there will be symptoms or signs which point to disease of the lungs or the alimentary tract.

The common causes of haemoptysis are either respiratory or cardiovascular. Among the former conditions are carcinoma of the bronchus, pulmonary tuberculosis, acute or chronic bronchitis, bronchiectasis and lung abscess. Cardiovascular conditions include pulmonary infarct, mitral stenosis and acute left ventricular failure.

1 In *carcinoma of the bronchus*, although there may be an isolated haemoptysis, the ulcerated area leads to repeated daily blood-streaking of sputum.

2 In *pulmonary tuberculosis*, an early lesion sometimes presents with an haemoptysis of an ounce or more of bright-red blood, not associated with sputum.

3 *Fungal colonization* with *Aspergillus fumigatus* of a cyst,

often an old tuberculous cavity, to form a mycetoma may produce persistent or profuse haemoptysis.

4 *Infection* of the respiratory tract or lung commonly leads to blood-streaking of sputum from inflamed mucosa.

5 In *bronchiectasis*, it is sometimes severe from ulceration of bronchial arteries.

6 *Pulmonary embolism* may cause haemoptysis and may be the first sign in a woman who is pregnant or taking the contraceptive pill.

Every patient presenting with haemoptysis should be fully examined and have a chest X-ray, particularly to exclude bronchial carcinoma and pulmonary tuberculosis. A normal chest X-ray does not exclude bronchial carcinoma, and so bronchoscopy should be performed if this possibility exists. However, unless there are good clinical grounds for suspecting a bronchial carcinoma, bronchoscopy is often not justified at this stage and it is sufficient for the patient to be followed up carefully with fairly frequent chest X-rays. The majority of such patients do not develop any serious disease, and in nearly half of all patients presenting with a small haemoptysis, no definite cause is found.

Pain in the chest

Acute pleuritic pain from pleurisy is sharp and stabbing in character and aggravated by coughing or deep breathing. The pain is usually localized to the site of the pleurisy, but it may be referred to the abdominal wall and be confused with an acute abdominal condition. With diaphragmatic pleurisy the pain is referred to the tip of the shoulder, as the skin in this situation has the same sensory nerve supply (C3, 4 and 5).

Lesions of the chest wall, such as fractures or malignant disease involving the chest wall or the ribs, may cause severe local pain and tenderness. The aetiology of *Tietze's syndrome* is uncertain, but it is a painful condition, usually involving one of the upper costochondral junctions. Chest pain may also be referred from the thoracic spine. The seventh cervical nerve supplies the pectoralis major, and pain referred from this root may be felt in that muscle as well as in the arm. Intrathoracic structures, other than the lungs, can produce pain in the chest, common examples being pain from ischaemic heart disease and from oesophageal spasm and hiatus hernia.

Respiration types and abnormalities

Respiration in men is mainly diaphragmatic in type, women have a greater costal input. Inspiration is a more powerful muscular movement than expiration, the latter depending on elastic recoil of the lungs and relaxation of the diaphragm and intercostal muscles. Obstruction to the large air passages outside the thoracic cage produces a prolonged inspiratory phase with stridor. The bronchi and bronchioles normally dilate on inspiration and narrow on expiration, so that obstruction of the airways, as in asthma, leads to prolonged, wheezy and difficult expiration.

Respirations in *pneumonia* and *pleurisy* are rapid and shallow, the inspirations being abruptly stopped, often with an audible grunt, as soon as the pleuritic pain is felt. Normally, expiration immediately follows inspiration and there is then a pause before the next breath. In pneumonia this rhythm is sometimes reversed, the pause taking place between inspiration and expiration.

The acidosis which occurs with uraemia, aspirin poisoning and diabetic ketosis causes very deep breathing, known as *air hunger*, or *Kussmaul's breathing*, owing to marked stimulation of the respiratory centre.

Cheyne–Stokes breathing is a characteristic respiratory arrhythmia occurring when the respiratory centre has a diminished sensitivity to carbon dioxide in the blood. The amplitude of respiration progressively deepens until a maximum is reached and then diminishes until there is a period of apnoea. During the period of apnoea, the carbon dioxide in the blood rises to a level high enough to stimulate the respiratory centre. There is then an exaggerated response producing the period of hyperventilation, which washes the carbon dioxide out of the blood until the stimulus to respiration is removed and apnoea occurs. The whole cycle lasts two or three minutes and is then repeated. This type of breathing occurs with left ventricular failure and respiratory centre depression and often during sleep in normal subjects.

Hyperventilation syndrome may be associated with excessive panting or with compulsive sighing, and hypocarbia may result. The patient may complain of chest pain, breathlessness, faintness and paraesthesia in the extremities. It is usually a feature of anxiety.

Clubbing of the fingers

The earliest change is a filling in of the angle between the skin at the base of the nail and the base of the nail itself, the skin becoming swollen and shiny. The base of the nail may be fluctuant. Later increased curvature of the nails occurs, and finally the pulps of the fingers become enlarged.

Clubbing has many unrelated causes. Cardiovascular causes include infective endocarditis, cyanotic congenital heart disease and arteriovenous communications in the arm. Respiratory causes include carcinoma of the bronchus, chronic suppuration in the chest—such as bronchiectasis, lung abscess and empyema and fibrosing alveolitis.

At times clubbing is familial and there is no underlying disease. More rarely it is associated with cirrhosis of the liver, steatorrhoea or polyposis of the colon.

Inspection of the chest

The general contours

1 Kyphosis and kyphoscoliosis

These may be developmental in origin. If gross, they may in later years give rise to severe impairment of lung function and heart failure. Abnormalities of spinal curvature also occur secondary to intrathoracic disease.

2 Funnel-shape depression of the sternum (pectus excavatum)

This may occur in varying degrees. Deep depression may displace the heart to the left and lead to the erroneous diagnosis of cardiac enlargement.

3 Over-inflation of the lungs

Over-inflation, such as occurs with asthma and emphysema, leads to an increase in the anteroposterior diameter of the chest, and so the shoulders are held high.

4 Unilateral flattening

Long-standing pulmonary or pleural fibrosis can cause flattening of the chest.

Respiratory movements

The respiratory rate is increased in many conditions, including acute and chronic lung disease, cardiac failure and anxiety. It is decreased with depression of the respiratory centre, as in narcotic poisoning and with various cerebral lesions.

The accessory muscles of respiration may be used if there is severe respiratory distress, as in an asthmatic attack.

Decreased movement on one side of the chest indicates disease of the lung or pleura of that side.

The respiration may have a special character (see page 89).

Table 3.1 Examination of the chest

Condition	Inspection	Palpation	Percussion	Auscultation
Consolidation*	Respiration rate increased; movement decreased on affected side	Mediastinum central; TVF increased over consolidation	Dullness over consolidation	Bronchial breathing Bronchophony WP Late crackles } Over consolidation
Absorption collapse	Movement diminished on affected side	Mediastinum shifted to affected side; absent TVF over collapsed segment	Dullness over collapsed area	Breath sounds diminished or absent; voice sounds diminished or absent
Fibrosis	Flattening of the chest and diminished movement on affected side	Mediastinum shifted to affected side; increased TVF over fibrosis.	Dullness over fibrosis	Bronchial breathing Bronchophony WP } Over fibrosis Early coarse crackles due to concomitant bronchiectasis
Fluid	Movement diminished on affected side	If large, mediastinum shifted to opposite side; TVF absent over fluid	Stony dullness over fluid, the line tending to rise in the axilla with moderate effusions	Absent breath sounds and voice sounds over fluid; sometimes bronchial breathing, WP, and aegophony above upper level of fluid
Pneumothorax	Movement diminished on affected side	If large, mediastinum shifted to opposite side	Normal or hyper-resonant; diminished cardiac dullness of the left and liver dullness on right	Breath sounds and voice sounds diminished or absent; sometimes if large, bronchial breathing, WP, and positive coin sound

*These signs are only heard over a considerable area of consolidation. With small patches of pneumonia, or when the pneumonic process has not reached the surface of the lung, signs may be scanty and are often confined to a small area of inspiratory crackles.

Palpation

The position of the mediastinum is assessed by determining the position of the apex beat and the trachea. Shift of the mediastinum towards the side of the lesion indicates shrinkage of the lung due to collapse or fibrosis. Displacement away from the lesion occurs with fluid or air in the pleural cavity. Displacement of the trachea alone is more likely with contraction of an upper lobe and shift of the apex beat alone in a lesion of a lower lobe.

Tactile vocal fremitus (TVF) is decreased with air or fluid in the pleural cavity and with pulmonary collapse. Increased TVF occurs with conditions that also produce bronchial breathing.

Percussion

Normally the lungs are resonant to percussion and there are areas of dullness over the heart and liver. In emphysema and pneumothorax, hyper-resonance is sometimes found and cardiac and liver dullness are either diminished or absent. Impaired resonance is found over consolidated, collapsed or fibroid lung, or with pleural thickening. A flat, dull note is found over pleural fluid.

Auscultation

The breath sounds

The breath sounds heard over the chest wall are in part the result of turbulence of airflow in the more peripheral airways, together with a component of filtered and attenuated sound transmitted from the central airways.

The normal breath sounds are rustling, with a long inspiratory phase followed by a short expiratory phase. Over the lung roots the normal breath sounds take on a bronchial character. The breath sounds are diminished or absent with fluid or air in the pleural cavity and with impaired inflation of the lung, as in emphysema and collapse. In *bronchial breathing*, the breath sounds have a harsher quality and the expiratory phase is longer than the inspiratory, with a short gap between the two.

When bronchial breathing is heard over the lungs, this indicates a pathological process which is enhancing the transmission of the tracheal sound to the chest wall. It occurs with pneumonic consolidation, with fibroid lung (fibrosis plus bronchiectasis), and over a large cavity. It also sometimes occurs above the upper level of a pleural effusion and over a large pneumothorax, which acts as a resonating chamber. Bronchial breathing is always accompanied by whispering pectoriloquy and by increased TVF and bronchophony.

The voice sounds

Normally, when the stethoscope is placed over a peripheral part of the lungs the spoken voice comes through in a modified form so that the consonants are blurred and indistinct; the whispered voice (a pharyngeal sound) cannot be heard at all. Transmission of the spoken and whispered voice in an unmodified bronchial form (such as can be heard in the normal subject by listening over the trachea, though it is not necessarily as loud as this) are called respectively *bronchophony* and *whispering pectoriloquy* (WP). They occur under the same circumstances as bronchial breathing.

Aegophony is the peculiar nasal quality to the voice sounds heard above the upper level of an effusion.

Wheezes (rhonchi)

A wheeze is a musical squeak produced by air passing through an airway on the point of closure; vibrations of the wall act like the reed of a toy trumpet. *Polyphonic* wheezing occurs in obstructive airways disease when expiration produces dynamic compression and sequential narrowing of the larger airways. Also in bronchitis and asthma, wheezing occurs from narrowing of the airways from spasm, mucosal swelling or exudate; and it is more marked on expiration. Narrowing of a single bronchus from stricture or bronchial neoplasm may produce a persistent *monophonic* wheeze, either in inspiration or expiration or both.

Crackles (Râles)

Crackles are popping noises caused by explosive equalizations in air pressure which occur with the sudden opening of airways; they are most marked on inspiration. When associated with bronchitis or bronchiectasis they start early in the inspiration, with regular spacing between the crackles owing to boluses of air passing through at regular intervals. With pulmonary oedema, pneumonia and fibrosing alveolitis the crackles are high-pitched and start later in inspiration, as sequential opening of abnormal alveoli begins at this phase of respiration. Late crackles are heard best in the most dependant parts of the lungs at the lung bases and vary in intensity with alterations in posture.

Investigations

Radiology

The chest X-ray

A chest X-ray is an integral part of the examination of a patient suspected of lung disease, and indeed in many conditions radiological abnormalities are present long before the development of physical signs.

The film should be examined in a systematic, rather than haphazard, manner. First it should be ensured that the film has been taken straight by observing that the medial ends of the clavicles are equidistant from the centre of the spine. Undue rotation can produce abnormal looking appearances of the mediastinum and the hilar shadows, as well as gross differences in the opaqueness of the two lungs.

The trachea should be central; displacement may be due to rotation, shift of the mediastinum (see palpation, page 91) or to a superior mediastinal swelling (page 132). The diaphragms should be examined next; flattening of the diaphragms occurs with over-inflated lungs, and undue elevation of a diaphragm may be due to diminished lung volume on that side, to diaphragmatic paralysis or to pathology below the diaphragm. The right diaphragm is normally higher than the left and the costophrenic angle should be clear and at an acute angle, filling-in being due to fluid or pleural thickening.

The lung fields are then examined by comparing one side with another; the apices of the lungs above the clavicles are first compared, then coming down the chest using the anterior ends of the ribs as markers one interspace is compared with the other on the opposite side. In this way small focal lesions can be detected. In addition, the pulmonary vascular markings should be examined and an assessment made as to whether there is any diffuse shadowing in addition to the normal markings. The position of the horizontal fissure should be noted. The hilar regions should be examined; enlargement may be due to a prominent pulmonary artery, pathological enlargement of the pulmonary artery, enlarged lymph glands or hilar mass.

Starting with the first ribs, and comparing one side with another, both the posterior and anterior parts of the ribs should be examined for abnormalities. A lateral chest X-ray will be necessary for full interpretation of a lesion and for correct anatomical localization (see page 87), and in addition a lateral film is essential for a suspected lesion in the left lower lobe as it may be obscured in the straight X-ray by the heart shadow.

Tomograms

Tomograms may give additional information by defining lesions and cavitation more exactly and by demonstrating narrowing of major bronchi. Both anteroposterior and lateral tomograms may be undertaken.

Computerized tomograms

A CT scan, when available, is of particular value in demonstrating abnormalities in the mediastinum (see page 132), and is used for assessment of mediastinal lymphadenopathy prior to operation for lung carcinoma. It is more likely to pick up small intrapulmonary and intrapleural lesions (such as secondary deposits) not shown by conventional radiology; to define questionable lesions seen on a chest X-ray; to reveal lung lesions in the presence of a pleural effusion; and to demonstrate bullae and bronchiectasis.

Isotope lung scanning

Isotope scanning of the lung is of value in the diagnosis of pulmonary embolism. A perfusion scan is performed after the intravenous injection of macroaggregates of albumin labelled with radioactive technetium, and a ventilation scan after the inhalation of a radioactive gas such as krypton. With pulmonary embolism and a normal chest X-ray there are segmental defects of perfusion with a normal ventilation scan. With lung disease defects of perfusion and ventilation are matched in the areas involved, but may make the diagnosis of a pulmonary embolus with its unmatched defect more difficult.

Ultrasound

Ultrasound examination is used to distinguish fluid from other pleural or lung disease. Demonstration of the precise localization of the fluid within the chest enables satisfactory aspiration to be carried out.

Respiratory function tests

Tests of respiratory function aid the clinical assessment of a patient, for they provide a quantitative method of estimating the respiratory ability. They may be helpful, for example, when thoracic surgery is being considered, and serial recordings are of value, both in assessing the effectiveness of a form of treatment and in following the progress of a disease. In addition, they may indicate the nature of the underlying respiratory disease as a cause of breathlessness, either an *obstructive ventilatory defect*, as in asthma, chronic bronchitis and emphysema, or a *restrictive ventilatory defect*, as in fibrosing alveolitis and kyphoscoliosis.

Some tests are easy to perform and others require skill and complicated apparatus. Each has its limitations and it may be necessary to test several aspects of function

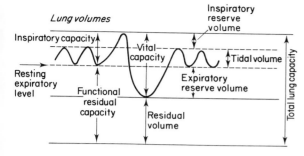

Lung volumes

Figure 3.2 *Tests of pulmonary ventilation.*

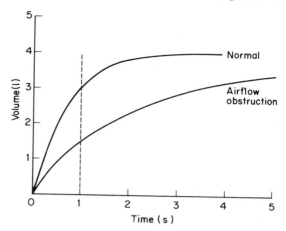

Figure 3.3 *Timed volume study.*

before reaching a satisfactory conclusion. It is proposed to discuss the principles involved, rather than the technical aspects.

Tests of ventilation

Figure 3.2, which is self-explanatory, illustrates the various subdivisions of the lung volume. The *tidal volume* is the volume of air breathed in or out at rest. The *functional residual capacity* (FRC) is the volume of the lung at the end of expiration and the *total lung capacity* (TLC) is the maximum volume of gas in the lungs after a full inhalation. A full unhurried exhalation from TLC gives the *vital capacity* (VC). A reduction in all of these volumes indicates a *restrictive ventilatory defect*, and is a feature of many disorders of the lung, pleura and thoracic cage where there is stiffness, deformity or weakness.

The *residual volume* (RV) is the volume of gas remaining in the lungs after a full unhurried exhalation and its proportion of the TLC is fairly constant. Up to the age of 30 years it forms 20–25 per cent of the TLC but it then increases with age. The RV/TLC ratio is abnormally increased in those diseases where there is airflow obstruction, and consequently over-inflation of the lungs, as in asthma and emphysema. However, neither RV nor TLC can be measured by normal spirometry—they require body plethysmography or helium dilution techniques for their estimation.

Airflow obstruction is best measured when the vital capacity is determined with reference to time. For this, the robust and portable 'Vitalograph' can be used. The *forced vital capacity* (FVC) is the volume of a maximal exhalation carried out as rapidly as possible following a maximal inhalation to TLC. The volume expired during the first second of the FVC is termed the *forced expiratory volume in one second* ($FEV_{1.0}$). The percentage of the FVC expired during this first second is termed the *forced expiratory ratio* (FER) and is normally 70 per cent or more. A reduction in both the $FEV_{1.0}$ and FER occurs in those

disorders with an *obstructive ventilatory defect* (see Fig. 3.3). Improvement of the $FEV_{1.0}$ occurring fifteen minutes after an inhalation of a bronchodilator, such as salbutamol, helps to distinguish reversible airflow obstruction (asthma) from irreversible airflow obstruction (as in emphysema or chronic bronchitis). Alternatively, in a patient with normal spirometry but suspected of having asthma, an exercise test can be performed to demonstrate the development of airways obstruction.

The *peak expiratory flow rate* (PEFR) is the maximal expiratory flow rate achieved during a maximal forced exhalation. It is measured with a Wright's peak flow meter, which is small, portable and easy to operate. Although measuring rather different aspects of airflow, both the *peak flow* and $FEV_{1.0}$ are reduced in the diseases causing airflow obstruction.

All the measurements described are determined by the patient's race, sex, age and size, being larger in males than in females, increasing until adulthood, and then declining with age. The predicted values for any individual have a large normal range. For example, for a man of 39 years, who is 1.79 m (5 ft 11 in) tall, the normal ranges are:

$FEV_{1.0}$	2.9–4.7 litres
FVC	4.0–6.0 litres
FER	63–92 per cent
PEFR	482–722 litres/minute

Blood gas analysis

Measurements of the oxygen and the carbon dioxide tensions in arterial blood can be used to assess the efficiency of alveolar ventilation as well as the matching between ventilation and perfusion of the lung. Normally the arterial partial pressure for CO_2 ($PaCO_2$) is 40 mmHg

(5.3 kPa) with a range of 36–44 mmHg (4.8–5.9 kPa); and for O_2 (PaO_2) is 90 mmHg (12 kPa) with a range of 70–110 mmHg (9.3–14.6 kPa).

Alveolar hypoventilation leads to arterial oxygen desaturation and retention of carbon dioxide in the blood, with a consequent rise in its arterial partial pressure ($PaCO_2$) and the development of a respiratory acidosis. This state of affairs may be *precipitated* by any complication producing severe impairment of ventilation, such as poliomyelitis or respiratory depression from drugs, or it may be *persistent* in patients with chronic chest disease.

'Mismatching' between ventilation and perfusion occurs when there is filling of the air space (as in pulmonary oedema or pneumonia), with infiltration of the lung, with emphysema and with widespread airway narrowing. In these conditions there are areas of the lung in which perfusion continues but ventilation is prevented. This effectively results in venous blood passing straight through the lung without being oxygenated, as in intracardiac right-to-left shunts. There is a resulting reduction in the partial pressure of arterial oxygen (PaO_2), but unless the mismatch is very severe there is no increase in the partial pressure of carbon dioxide ($PaCO_2$). Indeed, hyperventilation is often present at rest, which may produce an increased excretion of carbon dioxide by the lungs with a reduction in the $PaCO_2$, and the development of a respiratory alkalosis. At rest, the reduction of the partial pressure of arterial oxygen depends on the severity of the condition, and the compensatory hyperventilation, but on exertion PaO_2 may fall more with a further reduction in $PaCO_2$.

In chronic carbon dioxide retention the respiratory centre depends on the hypoxia for its stimulation. Relief of severe hypoxia by oxygen therapy is an important part of the treatment of cor pulmonale, but this may release the respiratory centre from its 'hypoxic drive' and depress ventilation. The patient may thus be relieved from hypoxia, but the additional reduction in alveolar ventilation leads to further retention of carbon dioxide and respiratory acidosis. Mental disturbance usually occurs when the arterial pH is less than 7.2 or the $PaCO_2$ higher than 100 mmHg (13.3 kPa), and coma usually supervenes with arterial levels of pH below 7.1 or the $PaCO_2$ above 120 mmHg (16.0 kPa). The serial estimation of the $PaCO_2$ from arterial puncture is thus an essential part of the proper control of oxygen administration in such patients.

Gas transfer

In certain conditions the predominant physiological defect is the impairment of transfer of gases between the pulmonary capillaries and the alveoli. This occurs in such diseases as fibrosing alveolitis, asbestosis, infiltration of the lungs with sarcoid granulomata, lymphangitis carcinomatosa, and pulmonary oedema.

The abnormality can be determined by measuring the *transfer factor* of the lung for carbon monoxide (TLCO). There are various methods for its measurement, but the most usual is to measure the uptake of carbon monoxide from the lung after a single full inhalation to TLC of a gas mixture containing a low concentration of carbon monoxide and helium. The TLCO is recorded as the uptake (mmol) per minute of CO per partial pressure gradient of CO. The inert gas helium is not absorbed and is used to calculate the volume of alveolar gas (Va). The TLCO per litre of alveolar gas is known as the *transfer coefficient* or *diffusion coefficient* (KCO). In the above conditions, hyperventilation may be present even at rest, and the impaired gas transfer may be reflected in a lowered PaO_2, and a normal or low $PaCO_2$, these changes becoming more marked after exertion (see 'mismatching' between ventilation/perfusion, above). In the conditions described, in addition to the blood gas changes and reduced TLCO, if the pathological changes are sufficiently advanced, then there will be a restrictive ventilatory defect with reduction in FVC and $FEV_{1.0}$, but the FER and the PEFR are usually normal. In contrast, although the TLCO is lowered in emphysema, because of ventilation–perfusion mismatch and reduction in the area of the alveoli available for gas transfer, the FER and the PEFR are also reduced by the associated airflow obstruction.

Flow–volume curves

Decreases in flow rates at different lung volumes are easily seen when flow is displayed against volume in a maximal expiratory flow–volume loop; this is constructed by use of a spirometer or an integrated pneumotachograph. From a point soon after peak flow the configuration is relatively independent of effort. Flow rates at low lung volumes may reflect particularly the function of smaller airways, and it has been suggested that they may be used to detect early chronic bronchitis. With the addition of a maximal inspiratory phase the shape of the flow–volume loop is useful in evaluating obstruction in large airways. Any fixed obstruction cuts off peak inspiratory and expiratory flows; a variable obstruction in an extrathoracic airway predominantly affects inspiratory flow while in an intrathoracic airway it predominantly affects expiratory flow.

Bronchoscopy

1 Fibreoptic bronchoscopy

This is carried out under local anaesthesia, when the bronchial tree can be examined and material obtained for histological and/or bacteriological examination. In addition, transbronchial biopsies, brushings and *bronchoalveolar lavage* (BAL) can be undertaken for more peripheral lesions or for diffuse lung disease.

2 Rigid bronchoscopy

This technique requires general anaesthesia and is usually carried out by a thoracic surgeon particularly for preoperative assessment. It is also required when foreign bodies have to be removed, to assess major haemoptysis, and when a general anaesthetic is preferred. Fibreoptic examination can also be carried out at the same time.

Bronchography

The introduction of contrast material to outline the bronchial tree can be performed at the time of fibreoptic branchoscopy (see above) or as a separate procedure by a radiologist. It is an investigation that is done infrequently now, its use being confined to the assessment of bronchiectasis.

Biopsy procedures

Tissue can be obtained from the bronchi or lungs at the time of bronchoscopy (see above), or tissue from the mediastinum obtained at mediastinoscopy or mediastinotomy. For peripheral lung lesions, aspiration or biopsy may be carried out by transcutaneous needle biopsy under radiological screening. Open lung biopsy can be undertaken by a thoracic surgeon. Pleural biopsy can be performed with an Abram's needle at the time of pleural aspiration, or it can be carried out by a thoracic surgeon at thoracoscopy or as an open procedure.

Hay fever and perennial rhinitis

These are allergic disorders characterized by bouts of sneezing, profuse watery nasal discharge, smarting and watering of the eyes. Hay fever is due to sensitivity to grass and tree pollens and occurs during the months of April to August; a type I (IgE mediated) hypersensitivity reaction occurs. Perennial (vasomotor) rhinitis is due to sensitivity to a variety of allergens, such as house dust mite, and may occur throughout the year. The conditions may be associated with nasal polyps.

Treatment

Antihistamines are of considerable value during an attack of hay fever. Usually one preparation can be found to suit the patient. Among the most valuable are chlorpheniramine (4 mg twice daily) or non-sedating drugs such as terfenadine (60 mg once or twice daily). Sodium cromoglycate or beclomethasone inhaled into the nose are both valuable in the prophylactic treatment of hay fever. Occasionally in severe cases where there is great disability, monthly injections of a depot corticosteroid, such as methyl prednisolone, may be justified.

Desensitization vaccines are occasionally given if skin testing confirms pollen sensitivity. This is done by giving subcutaneous injections at weekly or fortnightly intervals of a suitable preparation of allergen extract in progressively increasing concentrations over a 7–10 week period, starting in January and finishing before the pollen season starts. Anaphylactic reactions can occur—which may be severe or even fatal—and suitable precautions must be taken (see under asthma, page 96). The effectiveness of such regimens is disputed.

In *perennial rhinitis*, known precipitants such as house dust, pets or feathers should be avoided. Skin testing is seldom helpful as the patient is often sensitive to many allergens. Antihistamines may be tried, but are not usually as successful as in hay fever. Good symptomatic relief may be obtained with local steroid sprays.

Asthma

Asthma is widespread airflow obstruction which is partly or completely reversible with time or treatment. Patients with bronchial asthma suffer attacks of wheezing and difficulty in breathing owing to bronchospasm, mucosal swelling and sticky secretions; at times these symptoms may be persistent with intermittent acute exacerbations. Asthma can be divided broadly into extrinsic and intrinsic forms, although there is some overlap between them.

1 Extrinsic asthma

This is most likely to start in childhood or early adult life. It is often associated with hay fever and a previous history of eczema as well as a family history of allergic disorders. An atopic individual is prone to develop increased amounts of reaginic antibody (IgE) which becomes attached to mast cells in the bronchial mucosa. Inhaled allergen combines with IgE and damage to mast cells releases inflammatory agents and spasmogens such as histamine, bradykinin and slow-reacting substance of anaphylaxis SRS-A, which is now identified as the leucotrienes C_4, D_4 and E_4 derived from arachidonic acid by the lipoxygenase pathway. This is a *type I hypersensitivity reaction.*

There are a large number of substances to which the asthmatic may be allergic. They are most often inhaled, common examples being pollens (grasses and trees), spores from moulds (*Aspergillus fumigatus* and dry rot), dusts of various kinds (house dust, which contains the mite *Dermatophagoides pteronyssinus* which lives on the scales of human skin), and animal danders. Ingested allergens are less often to blame and less easy to identify.

Eosinophilia suggests that allergy is important but may also be present with intrinsic asthma. The history is the best guide to the part that allergy plays. If attacks occur in the spring and early summer it is reasonable to suspect that pollens are responsible; attacks in the winter months may be related to infection or to bronchopulmonary aspergillosis (see page 113); or attacks may be induced by proximity to a domestic animal such as a cat or a horse.

Skin sensitivity tests can be performed. Drops of specially prepared solutions of a range of suspected allergens are placed on the skin of the forearm and superficial pricks made through the drops. The result is positive if a raised wheal appears within 15 minutes. A positive skin test does not necessarily imply that the asthma is related to that particular antigen, and is only of significance if it coincides with the history. Skin tests are not affected by sodium cromoglycate or corticosteroids, but they are by antihistamines. Specific IgE may also be detected in the blood by radio-allergosorbent tests (RAST).

In addition to allergy, the following may play a part in the aetiology:

1 Infections of the respiratory tract commonly precipitate asthma, and in some patients they may be the main cause.
2 Various stimuli may induce attacks by a *reflex* vagal mechanism. Examples are sudden exposure to cold, laughing and physical exertion (see below).
3 Psychological factors play some part in a large number of asthmatics, and anxiety or depression may have a role if not in starting the asthma, at least in maintaining it.
4 There may be pharmacological causes. Beta-blockers, given for angina or hypertension, may precipitate asthma. Aspirin-induced asthma, which occurs in a small number of patients, is the result of inhibition of prostaglandin synthetase activity. It may also be induced by other non-steroidal anti-inflammatory agents. It is usually associated with nasal polyps and occurs most often in patients with intrinsic asthma (see below).

2 Intrinsic asthma

This form usually occurs for the first time in later life. Although mast-cell instability may be present, allergic factors are not evident in the history or demonstrable by skin testing or by increased IgE production. It is more often associated with bronchitis and psychological factors. It may occur for the first time after a respiratory infection, and persistent cough and wheezing may be misinterpreted as chronic bronchitis. It tends to be more intractable and response to bronchodilators may be disappointing.

3 Special types of asthma

There are various special types, which may give rise to diagnostic difficulties.

Exercise-induced asthma. Although exercise may induce asthma in most asthmatics, in some patients asthma is produced almost exclusively by exertion. Hyperventilation producing cooling and drying of the airways seems to be the trigger mechanism; mast-cell degranulation is probably involved and the asthma can be prevented by prophylactic use of sodium cromoglycate, as well as by salbutamol inhalation.

Paroxysmal cough and early-morning asthma. There may be no abnormal signs at the time the patient presents. Typical features which should suggest the diagnosis of asthma are a paroxysmal cough and cough or wheezing occurring in the early hours of the morning (at the time of the early-morning 'dip' in peak flow).

Late-onset asthma superimposed on chronic bronchitis and/ or emphysema is likely to be misinterpreted as a progressive worsening of the chronic condition. Furthermore, reversibility of the airways obstruction to inhalation of a bronchodilator may not be present, as quite often there is poor response to bronchodilators in this type of asthma; reversal of the airways obstruction may, however, be achieved by a therapeutic/diagnostic course of corticosteroids. Clinical clues to the existence of this state of affairs are marked fluctuations in the degree of wheezing and disability; response to inhalation of a bronchodilator when it occurs; a family history of asthma; eosinophilia or eosinophils in the sputum. Terminology becomes confused in such patients but the important point is to test the effect of bronchodilators and corticosteroids.

Allergic bronchopulmonary aspergillosis is associated with marked blood eosinophilia (see pulmonary eosinophilia, page 99).

Occupational asthma. The inhalation of organic dusts, fumes or vapours may induce an *immediate* (type I) attack of asthma in atopic subjects. The immediate asthmatic reaction can also occur in non-atopic individuals if the concentration of the inhalant is high and the exposure is prolonged.

The relationship of asthma to an occupational cause may be overlooked when there is 'late' asthma occurring some 4–6 hours after exposure. It is probably associated with a *type III immune response*, and extrinsic allergic alveolitis may also be present with precipitins to the specific allergen in the blood.

Some inhalants may produce both immediate and late asthma; for instance, isocyanates used in the production of polyurethanes, and enzymes produced by *Bacillus subtilis* used in 'biological' soap powders.

Clinical features

There may be no abnormal signs at the time a patient is seen and the diagnosis then depends on the history of attacks. During a typical attack the patient complains of tightness in the chest, difficulty in breathing and wheeziness. There is often cough—dry at first but towards the end of an attack strings of clear mucus may be produced. The sputum is yellow when infection is present or when it contains large numbers of eosinophils. If examined at the time of an attack the chest is over-inflated and there are widespread wheezes, most marked on expiration. Tests of respiratory function such as peak flow rate and $FEV_{1.0}$ show airways obstruction.

It is important to assess the severity of an attack of asthma using a combination of the clinical signs and objective measurements. Features of a severe attack are shown in Table 3.2.

Treatment

1 The mild attack

Most patients can abort or cut short an attack by using a pressurized aerosol containing a B_2 agonist, such as salbutamol. The patient must be carefully instructed in its use; after breathing out fully, release of the metered dose should be timed with the start of a deep slow inspiration, followed by breath holding for up to ten seconds. Other inhalation devices are available for those unable to use metered dose inhalers. With more severe or prolonged

Table 3.2 Features of a severe attack of asthma

Pulse rate greater than 110/minute
Respiratory rate greater than 30/minute
Inability to speak in sentences
Pulsus paradoxus
Absence of wheezing in the chest through severe reduction
   in air entry
Cyanosis
Hypercapnia
Peak flow rate less than 100/minute

attacks, salbutamol can also be given by inhalation from a nebulizer of 1 ml (5 mg) of 0.5% solution diluted to 4 ml with saline. In some cases asthmatics can be provided with this for use in the home. However, this carries the danger that the patient may stay at home too long rather than seek alternative further help. Tachycardia and tremor (owing to stimulation of B_2 receptors in striated muscle) are unwanted side effects of salbutamol therapy, and are dose-related. They are more likely to occur with oral therapy than when given by inhalation.

2 Severe acute asthma

Adequate therapy for severe attacks is essential, because the great majority of asthma deaths are associated with poor assessment of attacks and under-treatment. Features of severe attacks are shown in Table 3.2. Patients known to have severe attacks must have easy access to medical help and to hospital, and be sure of the way to manage any exacerbations.

Bronchodilators. B_2 stimulants are the mainstay of bronchodilator treatment. In most cases they can be given by nebulizer in a dose of 5 mg of salbutamol initially (reduced to 2.5 mg in the presence of ischaemic heart disease). This can be repeated at intervals of one to four hours according to the response. In some cases subcutaneous B_2 stimulant injections may be more convenient. Occasionally acute asthma fails to respond to nebulized therapy and intravenous B_2 stimulants are necessary.

Nebulized ipratropium bromide (250–500 µg) occasionally provides an additional effect and can be used as an alternative if there are adverse effects of B_2 stimulants.

Intravenous aminophylline is often used in an acute attack of asthma. It is associated with more side effects than nebulized bronchodilators and is unnecessary in the majority of cases. An initial loading dose of 5 mg/kg should be given intravenously by a slow infusion over 20 minutes. If the patient has been taking oral theophyllines this initial dose should be reduced by 50 per cent. The loading dose can be followed by an infusion, up to 500 µg/kg/hour. Blood levels must be measured if the infusion is continued for more than 24 hours. Therapeutic levels lie in the range 10–20 mg/l, and toxic effects consist of nausea, vomiting, cardiac arrhythmias and fits.

It is important to assess the response regularly and to keep the patient under close observation until it is certain that a satisfactory response is maintained.

Corticosteroids. These play an important part in the treatment of deteriorating asthma control and acute severe attacks. They can usually be given as oral prednisolone in a dose of 40 mg daily; but severe attacks dictate intravenous hydrocortisone, 300 mg initially, then

Table 3.3 Adverse effects of short courses of corticosteroids

Indigestion
Glucose intolerance
Hypertension
Fluid retention
Hypokalaemia
Proximal myopathy

200 mg 6-hourly. There are few serious side effects of a short course of corticosteroids (Table 3.3).

Oxygen. In exacerbations of chronic airflow obstruction oxygen must be given in carefully controlled concentrations; but in asthma it can be given freely. Nebulizations should be driven by oxygen.

Fluid and potassium. There is often a degree of fluid depletion in acute asthma and intravenous rehydration may be necessary. Hypokalaemia can be exacerbated by hyperventilation, corticosteroids, B_2 stimulants and aminophylline.

Antibiotics. These are not necessary for the majority of asthma attacks since precipitating organisms are likely to be viruses. However, if there is a suggestion of bacterial infection, such as purulent sputum or leucocytosis, then amoxycillin (250 mg 8-hourly) should be given.

Ventilation. If deterioration occurs, as judged by exhaustion of the patient and hypercapnia, mechanical ventilation may be necessary.

3 General management

Attacks of asthma need treatment as they arise, but the main aim of management should be to prevent asthma occurring. The patient must be educated to take prophylactic treatment regularly to suppress a wheezy state; and once this is fully established in a good phase for a reasonable period of time, the treatment can be gradually tailed down. Recurrence of symptoms as treatment is reduced means that the patient should continue with the minimal dosage required to keep free of asthma for a longer period. In patients with chronic asthma, self-monitoring of the peak flow can be extremely helpful, both in detecting sudden deterioration and in aiding adjustment of treatment.

Allergic subjects should avoid contact with known allergens as far as possible. When there is sensitivity to house dust the bedroom should be kept clean and furnishings which harbour dust and the dust mite *Dermatophagoides pteronyssinus* should be avoided. Feather quilts should not be used and non-allergic substitutes should replace feather pillows and hair mattresses.

There is little if any convincing evidence for the effectiveness of hyposensitization in the treatment of asthma.

4 Suppressive therapy

The main adrenergic receptors in the lung are principally B_2; and so apart from their immediate bronchodilator effect, regular use of the more specific B_2 *agonists* may have a suppressive effect, possibly by an anti-inflammatory action. They are best given by inhalation rather than orally as the same therapeutic effect is achieved by a much smaller dose, and side effects of tachycardia and tremor are less likely to occur. Salbutamol, for example, can be administered by pressurized aerosol, as a dry powder or as a nebulized solution.

Sodium cromoglycate has been thought to act as a mast-cell 'stabilizer' although this mechanism has been doubted. Its regular use may be of great value in the prevention of allergic asthma. It is usually ineffective in intrinsic asthma. It is administered by inhalation, either as a powder using a Spinhaler (up to one capsule 20 mg q.d.s.) or by the use of a pressurized inhaler (Intal 5 inhaler, 2 puffs (10 mg) q.d.s.); if effective the frequency of administration can be progressively reduced to the minimum required to keep the patient free of asthma. The newer *nedocromil sodium* may have a wider action in older patients.

Corticosteroids by inhalation have revolutionized the management of asthma, particularly persistent asthma. They are effective in suppressing both intrinsic and extrinsic asthma, and may avoid the use of systemic steroids or produce a systemic steroid-saving effect. Corticosteroids have an anti-inflammatory effect on bronchial mucosa, and as preparations such as beclomethasone dipropionate are poorly absorbed systemic side effects do not occur at normal doses. Beclomethasone dipropionate can be administered by pressurized aerosol, or as a dry powder, and budesonide is available as an aerosol. Corticosteroids should be taken regularly (usually twice daily) and once the asthma is suppressed the dose can be gradually reduced to the minimum necessary to keep the patient free of symptoms. Above 2 mg daily, inhaled corticosteroids may start to produce adrenal suppression but at normal doses they are very safe. Oropharyngeal candidiasis may occur, and can be treated with nystatin or amphotericin. The incidence is reduced by spacer devices on the inhalor.

Theophylline and aminophylline. Regular administration of oral slow-release preparations may complement the effect of B_2 agonists, particularly for nocturnal symptoms. Hepatic metabolism of theophylline may show individual variations and be affected by drugs, smoking or other factors. It is advisable to check blood levels after a week's treatment to ensure that the therapeutic range of 10–20 mg/l is achieved.

Oral corticosteroids are extremely effective in the treatment of asthma. Serious side-effects, such as those experienced in patients with Cushing's syndrome (see page 296), are only likely to occur when used in high dosage for long-term therapy. Short courses are an essential part of the treatment of exacerbation of asthma. Side effects are unlikely provided that there is a gap of several weeks between courses. In patients with chronic asthma, which is most likely to be intrinsic, often the only effective treatment is some form of corticosteroid therapy. In a good number of patients the asthma can be suppressed with corticosteroids by inhalation (see above). Those who continue to have disabling symptoms can be greatly helped by adding oral prednisolone on a long-term basis. In such patients the benefits of treatment outweigh the dangers, which can be minimized by keeping the dose as small as possible, preferably on alternate days.

Pulmonary eosinophilia

There is a group of conditions characterized by a varying degree of constitutional upset, cough, fluctuating infiltration of the lung and eosinophilla in the blood.

Worm and parasite infiltration

Pulmonary infiltration and eosinophilia may result from the migration through the lungs of the larvae of *Ascaris lumbricoides* (see page 444).

Asthma

Some patients develop pulmonary eosinophilia at the time of an attack of asthma, perhaps associated with an infection, or with some other allergic response.

Allergic bronchopulmonary aspergillosis occurs in patients with extrinsic asthma (page 95) and is more likely to arise during the autumn and winter when high spore counts are prevalent. It produces asthma, changing shadows on the chest X-ray and a high eosinophil count in the blood and sputum. Precipitins are often present in the blood, and the skin prick test to aspergillus antigen is positive. The patient may cough up plugs of yellow sputum in which the mycelia may be detected. The radiographic appearances are those of fluctuating areas of consolidation or collapse, or the proximal bronchi, distended with tenacious sputum, may be seen as band-like shadows or their inflamed walls visible as tramline shadows. Chronic changes may develop with proximal

bronchiectasis visible as tubular or ring shadows, and fibrosis of the upper lobes may develop, mimicking tuberculosis.

Treatment with oral prednisolone usually resolves the asthma and clears the X-ray changes rapidly, and a small suppressive dose may be required to prevent relapse. A course of oral di-iodohydroxy quinoline (1500–1800 mg a day) has been reported to produce worthwhile remission in a proportion of cases.

Tropical eosinophilia

This is a well-defined clinical entity, occurring in tropical countries, particularly India and Pakistan, and due to microfilarial infestation. The symptoms may be acute or chronic, with fever, cough, malaise and attacks of dyspnoea. Radiography may show miliary mottling and there is always a marked eosinophilia.

The condition usually responds to diethylcarbamazine in oral doses of 4 mg/kg t.d.s. for four days.

Cryptogenic pulmonary eosinophilia

General symptoms of malaise and fever are associated with radiographic changes of diffuse shadowing around the periphery of the lungs—a 'reversed bat's wing', but the appearances may change rapidly from day to day. There is marked eosinophilia and a high ESR, and eosinophils are present in the sputum.

The condition rapidly resolves with prednisolone, and after a prolonged remission it may be possible to tail off the treatment completely without relapse.

Allergic granulomatosis

Churg Strauss syndrome (allergic granulomatosis), a variant of polyarteritis nodosa, may produce asthma and transient infiltration in the lung with eosinophilia. Unlike polyarteritis renal involvement is unusual and cardiac or pericardial involvement is common.

Drug reactions

Some drugs, in particular nitrofurantoin but rarely others such as antituberculous drugs and sulphonamides, may produce pulmonary infiltration and blood eosinophilia.

Wegener's granulomatosis

This is a vasculitic condition with necrotizing granulomas involving the upper respiratory tract, lungs and kidneys (see page 274). Local involvement of one system may

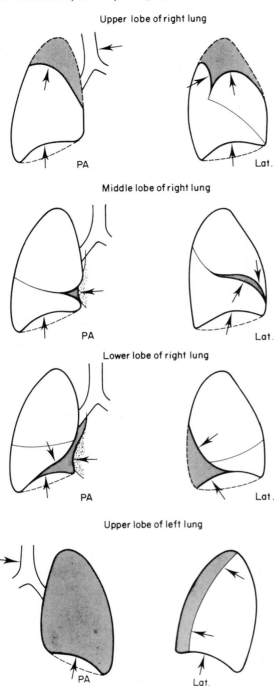

Upper lobe of right lung

PA   Lat.

Middle lobe of right lung

PA   Lat.

Lower lobe of right lung

PA   Lat.

Upper lobe of left lung

PA   Lat.

Figure 3.4 *Diagrams of radiographic appearances of lobar absorption collapse.*

occur. Treatment is with corticosteroids and cyclophosphomide.

Goodpasture's syndrome (see page 274)

Pulmonary collapse

1 Absorption collapse (atelectasis)

If a bronchus either to a whole lung or to a segment of lung becomes completely blocked, then the air in that portion of lung is absorbed into the blood stream and it becomes airless and collapses to a smaller size (see Fig. 3.4). The space formerly occupied by the collapsed lung is then filled by any combination of the following:

(a) elevation of the diaphragm;

(b) the mediastinum moving towards the side of the collapsed lung (see palpation, page 91);

(c) the remaining lung becoming hyperinflated, a condition known as 'compensatory emphysema'.

Bronchial obstruction may be due to several causes; the more important are:

1 Bronchial carcinoma, or more rarely bronchial adenoma (see page 120).

2 Foreign material in the bronchial tree. Mucus or inflammatory exudate may collect following an operation, but also occurs in asthma, bronchitis, bronchiectasis, measles and whooping cough. Sometimes foreign material may be inhaled—for instance a blood clot from the mouth following dental extraction, or foreign bodies such as beads, peanuts or pieces of bone.

3 Compression of the bronchus from outside may occur from enlarged lymph nodes in tuberculosis, sarcoidosis or lymphoma, or occasionally may be due to aortic aneurysm.

Collapse of major segments of the lungs occurs with bronchial carcinoma, external compression of the bronchus and with mucus.

With *viral respiratory tract infections*, segmental areas of collapse/consolidation (Fig. 5.4) due to blockage of a bronchus with infected sputum is the commonest form of pneumonia. With collapse, if the lung does not return to normal within a few weeks, then permanent residual lung changes are likely to occur.

2 Pneumothorax and hydrothorax

If air or fluid is introduced into the pleural space then the lung will be compressed to a smaller size, the degree of collapse depending on the volume of air or fluid in the pleural cavity. The mediastinum may be displaced to the opposite side if the pneumothorax or effusion is large.

Symptoms and signs

The symptoms of collapse depend on the extent of lung involved. They may also be overshadowed by the symptoms of the underlying lung disease. Obstruction of a large bronchus usually gives rise to dyspnoea and to a feeling of tightness across the chest, but at times the symptoms may be minimal. If obstructive pneumonitis occurs, there may be fever and constitutional upset.

There may be increase in the pulse and respiratory rate and at times cyanosis. Examination of the chest will show a shift of the mediastinum towards the side of the lesion, with dullness to percussion and absent breath sounds over the collapsed area. Smaller segments of collapse may give rise to little in the way of symptoms and signs and are diagnosed by radiography (Fig. 3.4). The interpretation of chest X-rays in this conditions depends on a knowledge of the anatomy of the bronchopulmonary segments (see page 87); both anteroposterior and lateral films are required for exact localization.

Treatment

In those cases where bronchial obstruction is due to plugging with mucus or inflammatory exudate, postural drainage should be carried out with percussion of the chest wall and 'assisted' coughing. Respiratory infection and asthma should receive appropriate treatment; with postoperative collapse adequate analgesia should be given as the pain caused by coughing, particularly with abdominal and chest operations, is the major cause of this complication. Using these methods the plug is usually dislodged, but at times aspiration through a bronchoscope is required.

Table 3.4 The most frequent causes of pneumonia

Bacteria
  H. influenzae
  Strep. pneumoniae
  Staph. aureus
  Klebsiella pneumoniae
  Legionella pneumophila
  Mycobacterium tuberculosis

Viruses
  Influenza
  Para-influenza
  Adenovirus
  Respiratory syncytial virus
  Cytomegalovirus

Other organisms
  Mycoplasma pneumoniae
  Chlamydiae
  Coxiella burnetti

Protozoa
  Pneumocystis carinii

Fungi
  Aspergillus fumigatus

Identification of respiratory infections

The pneumonias

Classification can be based both on the nature of the *infecting organism* and on the *anatomical distribution* of the pneumonia.

Infecting organisms which may produce pneumonia are shown in Table 3.4. In general, leucocytosis above 15 000 per millimetre strongly suggests a bacterial infection. Identification of the organism should be attempted by direct examination of the sputum with Gram staining, and if necessary by Ziehl–Neelsen stain. Culture of the sputum and antibiotic sensitivities should be performed. Blood cultures are of value in severe pneumonias.

Blood for serological tests can be taken if Legionnaire's pneumonia, psittacosis, Q fever, viral or mycoplasma pneumonia are suspected. A fourfold rise in antibody titre over a two-week period is significant, but suffers the disadvantage that it is by then a retrospective diagnosis.

Not infrequently there is a failure to identify the infecting organism in spite of every attempt to do so, in which case antibiotic therapy is directed at the infection most likely to be present in a given clinical setting.

The chest X-ray will demonstrate the anatomical distribution of the pneumonia. There are, however, no absolute diagnostic radiological appearances which will reveal the nature of the infecting organism upon which treatment should be based.

1 Bronchopneumonia
This is consolidation occurring in patches around infected terminal bronchi. It may be confined to a small segment of lung or it may be widespread throughout both lungs, tending to be more marked at the bases. It is often the result of secondary bacterial infection following an acute viral bronchitis; organisms such as *Strep. pneumoniae* or *Haemophilus influenzae*, can spread down the air passages to infect terminal bronchi. It has a greater tendency to occur in the very young, the elderly, in those with established heart and lung disease, and the debilitated. It is often the terminal event in a seriously ill patient.

Influenza may at times cause a fulminating bronchopneumonia with super-added bacterial infection usually with *Staph. aureus*.

Tuberculosis by bronchogenic spread throughout the lung may produce a widespread bronchopneumonia.

2 Segmental pneumonia
The aspiration of infected material into the lungs may give rise to pneumonia. The distribution of the consolida-

tion depends on the quantity of material inhaled and its nature. If large amounts of highly infected or irritating material are inhaled, as when an anaesthetized patient inhales vomit, a widely distributed and severe bronchopneumonia involving both lungs may result. If a smaller amount of highly infected material is inhaled into a segment of lung this will result in pneumonic consolidation of the segment, and unless aspirated material is coughed up or sucked out and the infection controlled, the consolidation may proceed to abscess formation.

The commonest type of pneumonia seen in general practice follows a respiratory tract infection. It is due to bronchial obstruction by mucus, with subsequent infected lobular or segmental collapse. The mucus is aspirate from the upper respiratory tract at the time of a cold or sinus infection, or it may have a bronchial origin at the time of bronchitis. *Aspiration pneumonitis* may also occur owing to the inhalation of anaerobic organisms from the oropharynx. The clinical picture varies considerably depending on the nature of the accompanying bacterial infection. At one extreme the pneumonitis may be discovered by chance on radiography at the time of a cold, there being no localized or constitutional symptoms. With virulent organisms, however, the clinical picture resembles that of the specific bacterial pneumonias. Most commonly, a few days after a cold or bronchitis, the patient's general condition becomes a little worse and there is malaise, cough, continuing fever and sometimes pleuritic pain. Usually the only physical sign is a patch of crackles over the affected area. Radiography of the chest shows an opacity owing to an area of segmental collapse and consolidation.

3 Lobar pneumonia

Lobar consolidation bounded by the fissures and with the normal size of the lobe maintained is characteristic of infection with virulent strains of *Strep. pneumoniae*. It diffusely involves one or at times more lobes of the lung. It also occurs with *Klebsiella pneumoniae* (Friedlander's pneumonia), when lung sloughing and cavitation may occur. Cavitation also occurs with infections with *Staph. aureus* and *M. tuberculosis* which may also produce lobar or lobular pneumonia.

It should be remembered that segmental or lobar pneumonia with collapse/consolidation may be due to an obstructive lesion such as carcinoma of the bronchus.

Viral and *mycoplasma* infections produce hazy lobular or lobar shadowing, which may be extensive.

Virus infections

The following are some of the viruses that affect the respiratory tract:

Rhinovirus
Adenovirus
Influenza virus
Parainfluenza virus
Respiratory syncytial virus
Coxsackie (an enterovirus)
ECHO (an enterovirus)

All these viruses have a nucleic acid content of RNA, with the exception of the adenovirus which contains DNA. An increasing number of serotypes are being identified with some of the above viruses; for example, there are more than 90 serotypes of the rhinovirus and 33 of the adenovirus. The enteroviruses, ECHO and Coxsackie A and B, also produce respiratory infections as well as other illnesses such as pericarditis and meningitis (see pages 36 and 425). The influenza virus consists of types A, B and C; influenza A virus is the cause of pandemics and major epidemics, B virus causes smaller epidemics and is a less virulent type of infection, and influenza C is principally endemic producing a fairly trivial respiratory infection. Major changes in the antigenic nature of influenza A virus occur about every ten to fifteen years, but minor changes may occur during the intervening years—the so-called, 'antigenic drift'. For this reason effective vaccines against influenza should contain type B virus and the latest strain of type A. The development of effective vaccines against the other respiratory viruses has not been possible because of the large number of viruses involved and because there would be no crossprotection between the different serotypes in the same group.

Generally speaking each type of acute respiratory illness can be produced by a number of different viruses. A cold, for example, can be caused by the rhinovirus and the adenovirus, and the latter virus may also be responsible for a sore throat, an influenza-like illness or pneumonia.

Acute tracheitis and bronchitis

Acute tracheitis and bronchitis may complicate colds, influenza, measles and other virus infections, and are particularly liable to occur in cold, damp and foggy weather. Laryngitis may also be present. After the first few days, secondary bacterial invasion commonly occurs. Bronchiolitis in infants is often due to the respiratory syncytial virus.

Acute tracheitis causes a dry, painful cough with soreness behind the sternum. Spread of infection to the bronchi produces tightness of the chest, with wheezing and difficulty in breathing. At first there is a little sticky, mucoid sputum, but secondary bacterial infection soon makes it yellow and more profuse. The severity and duration of the fever and of the general malaise are very variable; usually the illness is a mild one, lasting a few days. It may be serious and lead to pneumonia in young children, in the elderly or debilitated, or in patients with chronic bronchitis.

The signs of *acute bronchitis* are moderate fever, raised respiratory rate, particularly in children or in those with underlying lung disease, widespread wheezes and often crackles.

The patient should be kept in bed with severe attacks. The room should be warm and the atmosphere not too dry. Steam inhalations reduce the soreness and aid expectoration. A dry, troublesome cough is helped by linctus codeine (5–10 ml t.d.s.) or elixir diphenhydramine (10–20 ml); the latter also aids sleep.

After a few days the fever settles and the cough disappears. Convalescence is advisable after an attack of acute bronchitis, as early return to work with exposure to cold and a smoky atmosphere may delay complete recovery. Antibiotics are not required in mild, uncomplicated acute bronchitis. They are required where the risks of bronchopneumonia are greater:

    (a) in a patient with severe bronchitis;

    (b) in children and in the elderly and infirm;

    (c) in the presence of complicating disease, such as heart disease;

    (d) in patients with chronic bronchitis or bronchiectasis.

In these circumstances amoxycillin (250 mg three times daily) or tetracycline (250 mg four times daily), or co-trimoxazole (two tablets twice a day) are usually effective.

Bacterial pneumonias

Pneumococcal pneumonia

Pneumococcal lobar pneumonia may occur at any age; it is quite a common terminal event in the lives of the elderly or infirm, but it may equally attack people in the prime of life. It is more common in the winter months, and usually occurs sporadically. It is due to infection with virulent strains of pneumococci.

Clinical features

The onset is usually sudden with shivering or even a rigor and sometimes vomiting. The temperature rises abruptly and fever remains continuous. The face is typically hot and flushed and cyanosis may be marked. The respiration rate rises out of proportion to the temperature. An acute dry pleurisy develops over the affected lobe, leading to severe pain on respiration, so that the breathing becomes rapid, shallow and sometimes grunting. The development of herpes on the lips completes the classical picture. A painful cough is common at this stage of the disease and the sputum may have a 'rusty' tinge.

Examination of the chest at the onset usually shows little except diminished movement on the affected side together with reduced breath sounds, and perhaps some crackles or a pleural rub. After the first 24–48 hours, the signs of consolidation appear—dullness, bronchial breathing, whispering pectoriloquy, and bronchophony over the consolidated lobe. There is a polymorphonuclear leucocytosis. Chest radiography confirms the presence of lobar consolidation.

Prognosis

In the days before antibiotics were available recovery occurred by crisis at about the seventh day, the temperature falling quite rapidly and the patient's general condition taking a sudden turn for the better. Antibiotic treatment modifies the course of the disease and the patient's condition usually begins to improve within 48 hours of starting treatment. As the signs of consolidation disappear they are replaced by coarse crackles owing to the liquefying inflammatory exudate.

In the elderly, lobar pneumonia may not produce the dramatic picture outlined above. There may be little fever and the diagnosis depends on finding signs of consolidation.

Complications

1 Delayed resolution

The time taken for the lung to return to normal, with disappearance of physical signs and radiological clearing, varies a good deal in different patients. If resolution is delayed for more than two or three weeks the possibility of some underlying condition such as carcinoma or bronchiectasis must be investigated. Alternatively the pneumonia may be due to organisms resistant to the antibiotic in use, such as the tubercle bacillus. This will require careful and perhaps repeated examination of the sputum. Bronchoscopy and bronchography may be required. Pneumonia responds slowly to treatment in patients with diabetes, cirrhosis, chronic alcoholism or nephritis.

There remains a small group of patients in whom the pneumonia, instead of resolving, proceeds to fibrosis and chronic suppuration. Postural drainage and inhalations should be used, but the affected lobe may require surgical resection.

2 Effusions

Since the advent of chemotherapy, empyemata have become uncommon, but serous pleural effusions appearing about one to two weeks after the onset of the pneumonia continue to occur.

The pleural fluid should be aspirated and cultured for organisms and systemic antibiotics should be continued. The site of the aspiration is determined by the position of the physical signs and by radiography. The majority of serous effusions subside within a week or so of treatment.

3 Empyema

In a small proportion of patients the effusion becomes purulent and the patient's condition deteriorates. Fever recurs and becomes remittent in type. The patient looks ill and suffers from anorexia, malaise, and drenching sweats. Examination of the chest reveals signs of fluid (see page 90). A white count shows considerable polymorph leucocytosis. The diagnosis is confirmed by aspirating pus from the pleural cavity. Empyema is considered further on page 130.

4 Heart failure

Cardiac failure complicated perhaps by cardiac arrhythmia, particularly atrial fibrillation, may occur in elderly patients. For treatment see page 19.

5 Other complications

These include pericarditis, endocarditis and meningitis. Certain patients have severe headache and some neck stiffness in the early stages of pneumonia, although the cerebrospinal fluid is normal. The syndrome is called *meningism*.

Staphylococcal pneumonia

Staphylococcal pneumonia may occur at any age. It can occur as a primary infection but more commonly as a complication of influenza. It can be part of a staphylococcal septicaemia and there may be a history of a recent boil or some other staphylococcal infection. Pulmonary infarcts may be secondarily infected with staphylococci.

Clinical features

The onset is often acute with malaise, vomiting, anorexia and rigors. Pleurisy may occur. The sputum is purulent and may be blood-stained. Fever is characteristically remittent.

Signs are variable and often inconspicuous. They are often bilateral with patches of impaired resonance, reduced breath sounds and crackles. Bronchial breathing may be present.

Diagnosis

Radiography of the chest confirms the presence of consolidation which often cavitates to form an abscess. Alternatively thin-walled abscesses may occur which are distension cysts typical of staphylococcal pneumonia, particularly when part of a septicaemia. Empyema and spontaneous pneumothorax may also occur. The diagnosis is confirmed by sputum culture or by direct examination of the sputum with Gram staining. The sensitivity of the organism to various antibiotics should be determined, as it may be widely resistant.

Prognosis

It is often striking that a lung riddled with pneumonia and abscesses can resolve completely with antibiotic treatment, but residual areas of fibrosis and cyst formation are not uncommon. The lung abscesses and pleural infection rarely require surgical treatment.

At times staphylococcal pneumonia complicating influenza becomes a fulminating infection (see page 106).

Klebsiella pneumonia

Pneumonia due to Friedlander's bacillus (*Klebsiella pneumoniae*) is not uncommon. It usually presents acutely as lobar consolidation, in which case the lobe may be so distended with inflammatory exudate that there is bulging of the fissure—the so-called 'heavy' lobe. At times it may have an insidious onset when it may mimic tuberculosis or carcinoma. Friedlander's pneumonia has a tendency to progress to lung sloughing with abscess formation and fibrosis. The mortality rate is considerable. The diagnosis is confirmed by culturing the organism in the sputum, or more immediately by identification of the Gram-negative bacilli on direct examination.

Treatment of specific bacterial pneumonias

1 General

Severe pleuritic pain is best treated with oral co-codaprin or subcutaneous morphine (10–15 mg). The beneficial effects of these drugs in promoting rest far outweigh the dangers of respiratory depression. A persistent unproductive cough may be relieved by codeine linctus (10 ml).

If the patient becomes cyanosed, oxygen should be given. An oxygen mask may frighten or distress the patient and so careful explanation and reassurance are important. Care should be taken on administering oxygen to patients with chronic lung disease because of the danger of CO_2 retention (see page 119).

Patients severely ill with pneumonia are not infrequently dehydrated and need adequate fluid intake, either orally or intravenously.

Most patients can be allowed up five to seven days after the temperature has become normal, but this will be influenced by the patient's age and the severity of the illness. Breathing exercises should begin when the temperature falls and should be continued through convalescence, the length of which depends on the occupation and the home environment.

2 Specific treatment

In practice it is not always possible to be sure of the causative organism. Culture of sputum and blood takes time to produce results and in fact may not be helpful. Initial antibacterial treatment is therefore on the 'best bet' principle based on the clinical picture and on the prevailing pattern of pathogens in the area. Further modification of antibacterial treatment may be required in the light of the patient's response and the results of cultures.

Pneumococcal lobar pneumonia responds satisfactorily to treatment with ampicillin (500 mg 6-hourly, IV initially).

The patient usually responds within 48 hours, but treatment should be continued for one to two weeks. If clinical response is satisfactory the dosage can be reduced to 250 mg of amoxycillin 8-hourly.

Other antibiotics are occasionally required when the patient is sensitive to ampicillin or when the organisms are resistant. Penicillin resistance is a problem in some countries and in pneumonia complicating chronic bronchitis or bronchiectasis. In these patients it is often advisable to use an alternative antibiotic, such as erythromycin (500 mg four times daily).

In *staphylococcal pneumonia*, quite frequently infection is due to penicillin-resistant organisms, and if the patient is severely ill there is no time to await the result of sputum culture or the clinical response to benzylpenicillin. Under these circumstances flucloxacillin (500 mg IV 6-hourly) with sodium fusidate (500 mg orally or IV, three times daily) should be given. Subsequent antibiotic treatment will depend on the response of the patient and the result of sensitivity tests, and it is advisable to continue treatment for several weeks because of the liability to relapse. If clinical response is satisfactory, flucloxacillin can be continued orally.

Recovery is usual in these severe cases, but when staphylococcal infection is associated with *fulminating influenzal pneumonia* the outlook is grave (see below).

Friedlander's pneumonia is resistant to penicillin but responds to gentamicin (60–120 mg 8-hourly). Blood levels of gentamicin should be monitored. Many strains of *K. pneumoniae* are also sensitive to co-trimoxazole and cefotaxime. The sensitivity of the organism to antibiotics should be determined whenever possible. If abscess formation or fibrosis ensues, surgical treatment may be required.

Legionnaires' disease

This type of pneumonia occurs sporadically or in outbreaks. It is due to a Gram-negative aerobic organism (*Legionella pneumophila*) which can be grown on blood agar with additives. The reservoir for the organism is probably in humid and wet situations. In the early stages malaise, myalgia, headache and fever, with rigors, predominate. Respiratory symptoms of dry cough and pleuritic pain may then be overshadowed by gastrointestinal and central nervous system symptoms —namely vomiting and diarrhoea and mental confusion. Laboratory findings include moderate leucocytosis (usually less than 15×10^9/litre); proteinuria and haematuria; hyponatraemia (serum Na less than 130 mmol/litre); and abnormal liver function tests. Examination of the chest reveals crackles only. The chest X-ray shows segmental or lobar pneumonia which may be widespread and which is slow to clear. Pleural effusions may be present. Diagnosis can be confirmed by detection of antibodies by an indirect fluorescent antibody test or by identification or culture of the organism. The illness varies from a mild pneumonia to a severe illness with respiratory failure and a generalized disorder involving the central nervous, renal and gastrointestinal systems, and fatalities occur.

Treatment

This is with erythromycin (up to 1 g 6-hourly IV for the first 48 hours and then orally) combined with rifampicin (600 mg b.d.).

Tuberculous pneumonia

Tuberculosis may at times present with lobar pneumonia or more commonly widespread bronchopneumonia, associated with severe constitutional symptoms. It will fail to respond to penicillin. The sputum of every patient with pneumonia which does not respond to ordinary antibiotic treatment must be examined, and the diagnosis of tuberculous pneumonia will be established by finding the organism.

Treatment is along the usual lines for tuberculosis (see page 111).

Pneumonia complicating influenza

Influenza is sometimes complicated by pneumonia; this is rare when influenza is sporadic, but may become common during epidemics and accounts for the majority of deaths that occur.

Any type of pneumonia may complicate influenza. The most common is a localized aspiration pneumonia (see page 102) and staphylococcal pneumonia is common. Of particular importance is the severe infection called *fulminating influenzal pneumonia*. There is overwhelming toxaemia often caused by a combination of infection with the influenzal virus and *Staph. aureus*.

Clinical features

The onset of severe pneumonia complicating influenza is rapid, often alarmingly so. The patient has a simple attack of influenza which appears to be progressing in the usual way when over a few hours the condition deteriorates rapidly. The respiration rate becomes rapid, cyanosis appears, sometimes with a typical greyish blue colour (heliotrope cyanosis). There may be evidence of circulatory collapse with rising pulse rate and falling blood pressure. Pleuritic pain is uncommon. Examination of the chest shows evidence of patchy consolidation with scattered crackles and perhaps an occasional area of bronchial breathing. Leucopenia is common.

Treatment

In fulminating influenzal pneumonia treatment must be started before the results of sputum culture are available. Antibiotics are therefore used which are active against both the staphylococcus and other unknown organisms. Flucloxacillin (500 mg 6-hourly, IV) should be used because of the possibility of penicilllin-resistant organisms. There is also a good case for giving a broad-spectrum antibiotic in addition until the nature of the infecting organism has been established—for example, gentamicin or one of the newer cephalosporins such as cefuroxime. Once staphylococcal infection has been identified, sodium fusidate (500 mg 8-hourly, IV) may be given as a second antistaphylococcal agent in severely ill patients. Erythromycin should be used in any case in patients known to be allergic to penicillin.

Oxygen therapy may be indicated and circulatory collapse with a falling blood pressure can be treated with hydrocortisone (200 mg 4-hourly, IV) until improvement occurs.

Virus pneumonias

Most cases of so-called virus pneumonia have, in fact, an area of collapse/consolidation occurring at the time of a viral respiratory tract infection. This is the result of blockage of a bronchus with sputum with superimposed secondary bacterial infection (see segmental pneumonia, page 101). Infections with viruses, such as the adenovirus and influenza, can affect the lungs producing pneumonia, but the roles of primary virus infection and bacterial infection are often in doubt. In these cirumstances it is reasonable to give antibiotic treatment as for bacterial infection. Respiratory syncytial virus causes bronchiolitis in infants and cytomegalovirus produces pneumonia in immunosuppressed patients (see page 107).

Other pneumonias

Mycoplasma pneumonia

The organism *Mycoplasma pneumoniae* has features of both a virus and a bacterium. Although it is small and has no cell wall, at the same time it does not require a living organism for culture and is sensitive to the tetracycline group of drugs and to erythromycin. It is not sensitive to the penicillins as these depend on their action on the bacterial cell membrane for their antibiotic effect.

Clinical features

The disease starts with the general symptoms of a virus infection—namely malaise, anorexia, headache, backache, and sometimes depression, followed within a day or two by cough and sometimes pleurisy. Venous thromboses may occur and severe cases may develop haemolytic anaemia, myocarditis, pericarditis and pleural effusions.

Examination of the chest usually shows only a patch of crackles or perhaps an area of impaired resonance and bronchial breathing. The chest X-ray will show areas of consolidation having a rather ground glass appearance, and which may be bilateral. Pleural effusion may occur occasionally.

Diagnosis and treatment

Leucocytosis is not a feature but cold agglutinins develop in the blood in about 50 per cent of patients. Serological tests will show a fourfold increase or more in the mycoplasma antibody titre over a 2–3 week period.

Erythromycin should be given in a dosage of 500 mg 6-hourly.

Anaerobic infections

Anaerobic infections of the lung usually follow the inhalation of mixed organisms form the oropharynx. In most cases there is infection of the gums, but the absence of teeth does not exclude the diagnosis. Other predisposing factors include alcoholism and epilepsy, and loss of consciousness from coma, drug overdose or general anaesthesia. Defective cough due to neurological disease and dysphagia from any cause may also predispose to inhalation. The types of infection include aspiration pneumonitis (see page 102), a necrotising pneumonia (to be distinguished from tuberculosis and from staphylococcal or klebsiella pneumonia), lung abscess and empyema. The infection is likely to be sited in the most dependent parts of the lung at the time of inhalation (see lung abscess, below). In addition, anaerobic organisms may secondarily darily infect bronchiectasis and devitalized lung, as with pneumoconiosis and emphysematous bullae, and obstructive pneumonitis from carcinoma. The sputum and the breath are characteristically extremely foul (putrid or fetid) with anaerobic infections, owing to the presence of short-chain fatty acids produced by the organisms.

Treatment

The infection responds to treatment with benzylpenicillin and metronidazole. The most effective cephalosporin against anaerobes is latamoxef but it is expensive and the above treatment is usually satisfactory.

Psittacosis (ornithosis)

The organism *Chlamydia psittaci* occurs widely among many species of birds. Human infection is caught mainly from parrots, budgerigars, canaries, poultry and pigeons. It is an influenza-like illness and the patient may develop patchy consolidation in the lungs. Splenomegaly is common and rose spots resembling those seen in typhoid fever may be found. At times a severe fulminating pneumonia with considerable mortality may develop.

In the early stages the organism can be cultured from the blood or sputum and at a later stage a rising titre of serum antibodies can be demonstrated.

Treatment

The organism responds to tetracycline which should be given in full doses of 500 mg four times daily.

Q fever (see page 447)

This Rickettsial disease is caused by the organism *Coxiella burneti*. It is known to infect domestic animals such as sheep, cows and goats. Human infection probably occurs from inhaling dust from excreta of infected animals or ticks, or from drinking raw infected milk. It is characterized by fever, toxaemia, headache, cough and 'atypical' pneumonia, with a ground-glass appearance on chest X-ray similar to mycoplasma pneumonia. Q fever endocarditis may also occur, particularly on diseased aortic valves. Serological tests will show a rising titre to phase II antigens in acute infections, and to phase I antigens in chronic infection, such as endocarditis.

Treatment

Tetracycline in full doses is effective but response is slow. Treatment may have to be prolonged, particularly with endocarditis when it may have to be continued for six months to a year.

Opportunist lung infection

Lung infection is a not-infrequent complication when immune responses are impaired. This may result from disease, such as reticulosis, leukaemia or AIDS, or because of drug treatment, such as cytotoxic therapy, immunosuppressant drugs or corticosteroids. Infection with the usual bacteria or tuberculosis often occurs, but at times infection may be with organisms not commonly pathogenic to the lungs; these include protozoa (*Pneumocystis carinii*), viruses (*Cytomegalovirus*), yeasts (*Cryptococcus neoformans* and *Candida albicans*) and fungi (*Aspergillus fumigatus*). Fibreoptic bronchoscopy with transbronchial biopsy and lung lavage may be required to establish the nature of the infecting organism. Abnormalities on the chest X-ray may be caused by drug reactions, haemorrhage or infiltration by an underlying leukaemic or lymphomatous process in such patients.

Pneumocystis infection responds to co-trimoxazole in large doses. Invasive aspergillosis (see page 113) can be treated with intravenous amphotericin B, often in combination with flucytosine, and possibly ketoconazole in addition. Cryptococcal and candidal infections are discussed on page 113.

Lung abscess

Lung abscess is not a definitive diagnosis for it has many different causes, and the symptoms often depend on the underlying cause. In a small proportion of patients with lung abscess, no cause can be found.

1 Inhalation of infected material

Inhalation into the bronchial tree from the upper respiratory tract, particularly gross periodontal infection, is liable to occur when the cough reflex is suppressed during sleep, or when the patient is in a coma or under anaesthesia. Infected pus and blood clots may also be inhaled at the time of dental extractions. The material is inhaled into a dependent bronchopulmonary segment, and this leads to segmental pneumonia which breaks down to form an abscess. The contents are coughed up, leaving a chronic abscess cavity usually infected with a mixed group of organisms. If they include anaerobic organisms the pus becomes foul-smelling (*putrid lung abscess*). The breakdown of lung tissue may be very rapid and this state is sometimes called *gangrene of the lung*. Inhalation of foreign bodies, food or vomit may also cause lung infection leading to abscess formation.

With 'putrid' lung abscess, the onset of symptoms is usually acute. There may be a history of coma or an anaesthetic in the presence of periodontal infection, or of recent dental extraction or some other operation on the upper respiratory tract. The patient complains of fever, shivering, night sweats, malaise and anorexia. Pleurisy is quite common. There is usually a cough with mucoid sputum; after some days the abscess discharges into a bronchus and the patient coughs up foul purulent sputum. This may be preceded by a foul smell to the breath and is pathognomonic of this type of lung abscess. When the abscess has discharged, the patient's general condition may improve but he continues to cough up purulent sputum sometimes mixed with blood. There is the risk of cerebral abscess, of blocking of the abscess cavity with rapid deterioration in the patient's condition and of spread of infection into the pleural cavity, leading to an empyema.

Clubbing of the fingers develops. The signs over a lung abscess are variable. Usually there is impairment to percussion together with crackles and sometimes bronchial breathing; a pleural rub may also be heard. Both posteroanterior and lateral chest X-rays must be taken; the exact segment of lung involved will then be apparent. In the early stages the affected segment is opaque, but when discharge of the abscess has occurred a cavity can be seen containing a fluid level and sometimes a slough. The site of inhalation lung abscess is influenced by gravity. As the unconscious patient usually lies on his side or back the most dependent segments in these positions are the segments supplied by the axillary branches of the upper lobe bronchi, the posterior segment

of the upper lobe and the apex of the lower lobe. Anaerobic organisms can be identified in the sputum and the white count shows a polymorphonuclear leucocytosis.

2 Carcinoma of the lung

A peripheral tumour may undergo central necrosis, producing an abscess cavity lined with malignant tissue; the chest X-ray characteristically shows a cavity with thick and irregular walls. Alternatively there may be breakdown of a suppurative pneumonitis distal to an obstructing carcinoma.

3 Specific infections

Abscesses may develop in the course of certain specific infections, such as staphylococcal pneumonia, Friedlander's pneumonia and tuberculosis. The infecting organism can be identified by bacteriological examination of the sputum.

4 Granulomas

An abscess cavity may result from the breakdown of an arteritic granuloma, such as Wegener's granulomatosis.

5 Rarer infections

These include extension of an amoebic abscess of the liver through the diaphragm, actinomycosis, infected hydatid cyst, and abscesses developing during the course of a pyaemia. Pulmonary emboli may produce pulmonary infarction and cavity formation. This may lead to a lung abscess if the embolus itself comes from a septic source or if there is secondary infection in the lung.

Pulmonary tuberculosis

Infection with the tubercle bacillus in a subject who has never previously experienced contact with the organism is called *primary tuberculosis*; reinfection after the primary lesion is called *post-primary tuberculosis*. The disease follows different courses in the two instances, the difference being attributed to the acquisition of a delayed cell-mediated hypersensitivity reaction (type IV) by sensitized T cells and macrophages in response to the primary lesion.

In Great Britain and the USA, and in most countries in the West, infection is almost entirely with the human bacillus. In less economically developed countries milk may still serve as a vehicle for infection with the bovine organism, although this is becoming increasingly uncommon.

The human bacillus is spread almost exclusively by droplet infection and lesions are most often limited to the lungs. Susceptibility to the disease has a wide range and may depend on inborn, racial and environmental factors.

For example, dwellers in isolated communities have little natural resistance and when exposed to the infection for the first time are prone to develop florid disease. Resistance may also be conditioned by such factors as alcoholism, diabetes, malnutrition and general debility. The risks of infection are much increased by proximity, either from overcrowding of housing, or individual exposure, for example in dentists, doctors or nurses working with tuberculous patients.

Deaths from tuberculosis of all forms fell steadily in all civilized communities from the turn of the century. The rate of decline was so regular (with the exception of the war years) in the British Isles that it may be concluded that it was little influenced by any passing fancy in therapy and that the improvement was more likely to be due to public health measures. Since the introduction of effective chemotherapy death rates have declined precipitously.

Primary tuberculosis

Characteristically the initial lesion is small and the local lymph nodes bear the brunt of the infection.

A small pneumonic lesion (Ghon focus) may be situated in any part of the lungs. Lymphatic spread soon occurs and the local lymph nodes become enlarged. The radiographic appearance of a small shadow in the lung associated with hilar lymphadenopathy is known as the *primary complex*. It is accompanied by a change in the tuberculin reaction to positive (see page 111). There is usually little upset in health and the natural tendency is to heal by fibrosis and calcification. In the past, primary tuberculosis commonly occurred in young people and up to 1950 over 95 per cent of urban dwellers had unknowingly healed such lesions before reaching adult life. Not all primary lesions heal spontaneously and without complications. As tuberculosis is now less common, an increasing proportion of children reach adult life without infection and it is these for whom protection is sought by vaccination with BCG (see page 112).

Complications

Sometimes the lung lesion progresses, and rarely it may cavitate. This is more liable to occur in young adults, who are also prone to develop primary *tuberculous pleural effusions* (see page 128).

In infants and young children particularly, the enlarged hilar lymph nodes may cause compression of a bronchus with segmental collapse, producing the radiographic appearance known as *epituberculosis*. This may lead to permanent bronchiectasis, such as the *middle lobe syndrome* (see page 114). An infected lymph node may also rupture through the wall of a bronchus, the caseous material being discharged into the bronchial tree and causing a widespread *tuberculous bronchopneumonia* (page 105). Alternatively, the nodes may erode blood vessels to produce miliary tuberculosis and blood-borne tuberculosis may occur in such sites as bone, joints, kidney, epididymus, Fallopian tubes, brain or meninges. Tuberculous pericarditis may develop as a result of direct spread of infection from mediastinal glands.

Miliary tuberculosis

Miliary tuberculosis is due to widespread haematogenous dissemination. In primary tuberculosis it usually results from a caseous lymph node eroding a bronchial vessel, but it also occurs with infection spreading into the blood stream with post-primary lesions and in the elderly.

Clinical features

The onset is usually insidious with general malaise, pyrexia, loss of weight and sweats. Children often become listless and lose interest in their toys. Evidence of miliary spread through the lungs is not obvious early in the disease but later cough develops, with little sputum or dyspnoea. In some cases meningeal involvement is the most prominent feature and the patient presents with a tuberculous meningitis (see page 220).

Chest signs are either absent or confined to scattered fine crackles. The spleen is often just palpable and careful examination of the retina may show choroidal tubercles. They are greyish-white lesions about one-third the size of the optic disc. A chest radiograph shows the typical fine mottling of miliary tubercles throughout the lungs.

Treatment is along the usual lines with chemotherapy (see page 111). The prognosis is good provided meningeal involvement is not too advanced.

Tuberculous cervical lymphadenitis

The initial infection occurs in the tonsillar crypts and spreads to the cervical lymph nodes. These may become chronically enlarged and heal by fibrosis and calcification. They may undergo caseous necrosis, the pus tracking through the fascial planes to form a superficial cold abscess at some distance from the nodes ('collar stud' abscess). This type of infection is now uncommon in the UK, except in immigrants.

Post-primary tuberculosis

The infection is almost invariably pulmonary and usually occurs in the upper lobes or the apical segment of the lower lobes, where the lung is relatively over-ventilated and under-perfused. It is due to reinfection or the reactivation of a primary lesion. The early lesion of an area of tuberculous bronchopneumonia which radiographically appears as soft shadowing. Spread is initially by direct extension to adjacent lung. Later *caseation* occurs and the necrotic centre of the lesion is discharged into a bronchus, producing a cavity in the lung, and cough with sputum. The infected sputum may be inhaled into other parts of either lung, producing new tuberculous lesions by *bronchogenic spread*. The expectoration of infected sputum may cause *tuberculous tracheitis, laryngitis,* or *tuberculous ulcers on the tongue.* Peripheral lesions may cause *pleurisy,* which may progress to tuberculous *effusions* or empyema (see page 128). *Haemoptysis* occurs with erosion of blood vessels. *Endobronchial tuberculosis* may produce a valvular obstruction to the bronchi draining a cavity, so that it distends to form a *tension cavity.* A *tuberculoma* is a blocked cavity with thick walls and full of inspissated material. It shows on the chest radiograph as a rounded opacity with clear-cut edges and may show areas of calcification.

The rate of progress of the disease is variable. It is rapid at times, but more commonly it is slow, the early lesion taking some years to develop into widespread tuberculosis. It depends on the extent and severity of the original infection and on the patient's resistance. The disease may become arrested at any stage, either permanently or temporarily, owing to spontaneous healing by resolution, fibrosis and calcification, or as the result of treatment. Alternatively widespread tuberculous bronchopneumonia, miliary tuberculosis or metastatic tuberculosis may supervene. As opposed to *acute tuberculosis,* with infiltration and cavitation, a state of *chronic fibrocaseous* or *fibroid tuberculosis* may develop with gross fibrous contraction of the upper lobes and over-inflation of the lower lobes. Respiratory reserve is then diminished and dyspnoea becomes a prominent symptom.

In patients with longstanding extensive disease, secondary amyloidosis may develop (see page 342).

Clinical features

Most patients with early tuberculosis of the lungs are free of symptoms but some present with haemoptysis.

The disease is usually well advanced by the time symptoms have developed. Classically they are chronic ill health, cough with mucoid sputum, low-grade fever, anorexia, tiredness, progressive weight loss, and night sweats. In advanced cases the patient appears ill, sweating and has lost weight, and the continual coughing up of infected sputum may spread infection and lead to further symptoms. Tracheitis causes retrosternal soreness, and laryngitis, hoarseness and dysphagia. Tuberculous ulcers in the mouth, usually around the edge of the tongue, are extremely painful.

There are no abnormal signs from an early lesion. The first physical sign to appear is usually a small area of persistent crackles at one or other apex, but by this time lung involvement is considerable. With more extensive disease there will be impairment to percussion, more widespread crackles and sometimes areas of bronchial breathing if consolidation or cavities are near the chest wall. Fibrosis of an upper lobe leads to shift of the trachea towards the lesion, flattening of the upper chest with diminished movement and impaired percussion note, bronchial breathing, and crackles.

Signs of fluid will be present if there is an associated pleural effusion or empyema.

Abdominal tuberculosis

The swallowing of large quantities of infected sputum may lead to *gastritis* with dyspepsia and more rarely to *tuberculous ileitis* with diarrhoea, fever and weight loss. *Fistula-in-ano* may occur with sero-sanguinous perianal discharge.

Tuberculous peritonitis may arise from direct spread from infected mesenteric glands (*tabes mesenterica*) or by haematogenous spread. It presents with fever, weight loss, abdominal pain and bowel disturbance. Ascites or subacute intestinal obstruction may develop. The ascitic fluid is lymphocytic and the diagnosis is confirmed by histological and bacteriological examination of peritoneal tubercles seen on laparatomy. The diagnosis should always be suspected when such symptoms occur, particularly in Asian or African immigrants.

Tuberculous pericarditis (see also page 38)

The infection nearly always arises as a result of direct spread from mediastinal lymph nodes. It is usually associated with a large pericardial effusion and signs of tamponade may be present (pulsus paradoxus, raised jugular venous pulse with rapid Y descent, increase in the venous pulse on inspiration, and a third heart sound). A late manifestation is calcific constrictive pericarditis.

Investigations

1 Radiography

Chest X-ray is essential for diagnosis and is required to assess the extent and nature of the disease, to detect cavities and to follow progress. Tomograms may be helpful to demonstrate cavities and delineate the extent of the lesion.

It is difficult to judge the activity of a lesion from a single X-ray. Cavitation means activity and soft fluffy opacities are usually of recent onset. Hard and calcified shadows suggest healing and inactivity. Serial films provide the best way of judging both the activity and progress of the disease.

There is no radiological appearance which is diagnostic of tuberculosis, although cavitating disease involving the upper lobes is extremely suggestive of it. Often the diagnosis depends on exclusion of other diseases or the confirmation of tuberculosis by sputum examination. Relatives and close contacts must be X-rayed, and may require follow-up examinations.

2 Sputum

Sputum examination is essential in a patient suspected of having pulmonary tuberculosis. The finding of tubercle bacilli confirms the diagnosis and indicates that the disease is active.

The auramine fluorescence technique is preferable to the traditional *Ziehl–Neelsen technique.* Culture on *Lowenstein's* medium takes 6–8 weeks but increases the chance of finding tubercle bacilli, and sensitivity tests to chemotherapeutic agents may be made. When acid-fast bacilli are seen on microscopy cultures are positive in 98 per cent of cases, but only 85 per cent of those with positive cultures will be positive on microscopy. Lung washouts on fibreoptic bronchoscopy, and pleural fluid, may be similarly examined. In general, the ease of finding the organism and the number found are indications of the activity of the disease, except in miliary tuberculosis where, such sputum as there is, is often negative.

3 Sedimentation rate

A normal ESR does not exclude an active lesion. A raised ESR, although a non-specific test, may be additional evidence of activity, and serial measurements are useful in following the progress of the disease.

4 Tuberculin test

A delayed cell-mediated hypersensitivity reaction (type IV), initiated by T cells in the tissues, develops in response to infection with the tubercle bacillus, and this hypersensitivity state to the tubercle bacillus antigen persists after the infection has become inactive. There are rare exceptions to this; for instance, in some cases of overwhelming miliary tuberculosis. The delayed hyper-sensitivity can be demonstrated by injecting intradermally an antigen prepared from dead tubercle bacilli (tuberculin). A local reaction occurs in the skin, producing an area of redness and swelling and rarely ulceration. A *positive result* is judged as a papule larger than 5 mm which appears within 2–4 days of injection. False positive results appear in the first 48 hours and last only a day or two. The test may be carried out by using a Tine test or a Heaf multipuncture test. In the Mantoux test, 0.1 ml of a solution of PPD (purified protein derivative) containing 1 TU (tuberculin unit) is injected intradermally. If negative, increasing concentrations containing 10 TU or 100 TU can be injected. A positive result simply indicates previous exposure; it is not a measure of activity. A negative result would indicate that a radiographic pulmonary opacity is not tuberculous.

Treatment

Active disease requires treatment, whereas healed disease only requires observation. Disease must be regarded as active in any of the following circumstances:

    (a) there is clinical evidence of disease (e.g. fever and weight loss);

    (b) there are tubercle bacilli in the sputum;

    (c) there is radiological evidence of spread of the disease (comparison with the past chest X-rays is invaluable in this respect);

    (d) there are cavities.

1 General measures

With effective chemotherapy hospital treatment or prolonged bed-rest is no longer required, but the patient should be kept in bed if he is ill with fever or toxaemia. The patient can be regarded as not infectious to others after taking chemotherapy for two weeks. Good food is essential. This means adequate, but not excessive calories, plenty of protein, with sufficient vitamin and mineral content. The aim should be to regain, but not exceed, the normal body weight.

2 Chemotherapy

Some general principles governing drug therapy may be stated:

    (a) Chemotherapy is indicated if the disease is active.

    (b) It should be continued for a prolonged period.

    (c) No drug should be given alone. Combinations of the drugs should be used to avoid the emergence of drug-resistant strains of tubercle bacilli.

Treatment is started with three or four drugs to obtain a maximum therapeutic effect and to cover the possibility that the organism is resistant to one of the drugs. Sputum culture and tests of the organism's sensitivity to the drugs will subsequently determine this.

The standard treatment used in the UK at the present time is:

ethambutol 15 mg/kg body weight daily
rifampicin 450–600 mg (10 mg/kg body weight) daily
isoniazid 300 mg daily

All three drugs can be given together in a single dose before breakfast, as rifampicin is best absorbed on an empty stomach. Rifampicin and isoniazid are best taken combined in a single tablet. It is usual to add pyridoxine (10 mg daily) to prevent neuropathy developing in patients in long-term isoniazid.

All three drugs are given for the first two months of treatment; ethambutol is then stopped when the sensitivity of the cultured organism should be available. Rifampicin and isoniazid are continued as long-term therapy. A course of nine months is satisfactory, but if pyrazinamide is added to the regimen for two months the length of treatment can be shortened to six months.

Rifampicin is relatively free from side-effects. It may cause a transient disturbance of liver function tests, which can be disregarded; but hepatitis with jaundice, which is more likely to occur with intermittent high-dose therapy and those whose liver function is already impaired, is an indication for stopping the drug. Patients should be warned that rifampicin produces a reddish colour in the urine and reduces the efficacy of the contraceptive pill.

Isoniazid causes peripheral neuropathy in high doses, particularly in those who inactivate the drug slowly.

Ethambutol can cause optic neuritis, so that patients taking it as long-term therapy should have their visual acuity tested before treatment and thereafter at regular intervals. Patients must be warned to report any impairment in vision and to stop taking the drug.

Pyrazinamide is being used increasingly and can be added to the regimen for one or two months. It is bactericidal for tubercle bacilli. Used in the recommended doses it rarely causes liver damage but liver function should be measured regularly whilst on treatment urate may be increased. It is particularly useful in tuberculous meningitis and tuberculous lymphadenopathy. It is given as follows:

Body weight	Dose
< 50 kg	1.5 g daily
50–74 kg	2.0 g daily
> 75 kg	2.5 g daily

Corticosteroids are safe in the treatment of tuberculosis provided that effective chemotherapy is given at the same time. They are of value in acute tuberculosis with severe toxaemia, and with tuberculous pleural (page 128) or pericardial (page 38) effusions which are not resolving quickly enough to chemotherapy alone.

Prophylaxis

There should be measures to raise standards of hygiene and to improve nutrition and living conditions, and the detection of both early and infectious cases of pulmonary tuberculosis by sputum examination and by routine radiography in countries where tuberculosis is still common.

Efforts have been made to increase individual resistance by vaccinating susceptible (tuberculin negative) subjects with an attenuated strain of the tubercle bacillus (*Bacille Calmette–Guerin*; BCG). Freeze-dried BCG is the most reliable preparation. An intradermal injection of 0.1 ml of the vaccine is made and the appearance of a papule at the site of the injection within 10–14 days indicates a successful vaccination. Conversion of the tuberculin test to positive should occur between the sixth and eighth week after vaccination. Complications include abscesses and persistent ulceration at the site of injection, and enlargement of the axillary lymph glands; they may require treatment with rifampicin and isoniazid.

The World Health Organization have used BCG vaccination on an enormous scale in India, Africa and some parts of Asia with few ill effects and benefits that are variable. It is part of the routine vaccination programme in the UK (see page 414), but the declining incidence of tuberculosis has reduced its value. In the future it may be best reserved for those exposed to tuberculous infection and contacts.

Opportunist mycobacterial infection

Acid-fast bacilli distinct from *M. tuberculosis* may at times produce a lung infection which mimics an indolent form of tuberculosis. These different 'atypical' mycobacteria can be distinguished on cultures by their rate of growth and ability to produce pigment. *M. kansasii*, the commonest variety seen in the UK, produces a yellow pigment when cultures grown in the dark are exposed to light. *M. xenopi* and *M. avium intracellulare* are also prone to infect emphysematous lungs.

Treatment

The organisms often show resistance to many of the drugs on *in vitro* sensitivity tests. Response to treatment is slow and it may have to be continued for up to two ears. *M. kansasii* is usually sensitive to rifampicin and thambutol and partially sensitive to pyrazinamide. *M. enopi* infection usually responds to treatment with rifampicin, isoniazid and streptomycin. *M. avium intracell-dare* is usually resistant to most of the anti-tubercular rugs, but clinical response to rifampicin, isoniazid, thambutol and pyrazinamide may occur in spite of drug resistance being demonstrated by *in vitro* tests.

Fungus infections

Histoplasmosis, *coccidiodomycosis* and *blastomycosis* are fungus diseases of the lungs occurring in the USA, but hey are not endemic in the UK.

Sporadic cases of *torulosis* occur and it may arise as an opportunist lung infection (see page 107). It is due to infection with the yeast *Cryptococcus neoformans*. Pulmonary lesions may develop into cavitating granulomas, or into tumour-like masses. Infection may spread by the blood stream to the meninges mimicking tuberculous meningitis, even when the pulmonary lesions are small. Treatment consists of surgical resection, where feasible, combined with intravenous amphotericin B. Cryptococcal meningitis has also been successfully treated with flucytosine.

The fungus *Aspergillus fumigatus* is not normally pathogenic to the normal respiratory tract. However, it may infect pulmonary infarcts, and cysts or cavities which have resulted from such diseases as tuberculosis, sarcoidosis, staphylococcal pneumonia or ankylosing spondylitis. A solid ball of fungus (*mycetoma*) grows free in the cavity. On tomography a crescent of air may be seen above the opacity, which can be seen to move its position when the patient is tipped. Precipitins to aspergillus can be detected in the blood. Recurrent haemoptyses may occur and the sputum may be thick and purulent.

An invasive necrotizing pneumonia may occur as part of an opportunist lung infection (see page 107), and haematogenous spread to the brain, meninges and other organs may occur.

Allergic bronchopulmonary aspergillosis is a distinct syndrome resulting from hypersensitivity to aspergillus in atopic subjects. It produces asthma, radiographic changes and eosinophils in the blood and sputum (see pulmonary eosinophilia, page 99). Aspergillus skin tests are positive and precipitins may be present.

Invasive aspergillus pneumonia can be treated with intravenous amphotericin B, but treatment has to be prolonged and there is a risk of nephrotoxicity. It can be combined with flucytosine and possibly ketoconazole in addition.

A mycetoma responds poorly to this treatment. Ideally it is best removed surgically, but this is rarely possible because associated severe lung disease precludes operation.

Candida albicans

The yeast *Candida albicans* is a normal saprophyte found in the respiratory tract and in the intestines. The administration of antibiotics and corticosteroids may encourage its growth so that it may be abundant in the sputum but not necessarily pathogenic. It may, however, invade the mucosa, causing *thrush* in the mouth and pharynx, and at times in the oesophagus and in the trachea and bronchi; it may also cause diarrhoea and anogenital pruritus. Oral candidiasis may be a complication of treatment with inhaled corticosteroids. Rarely, in debilitated patients and in patients on treatment with antibiotics, steroids and cytotoxic drugs (with such diseases as leukaemia and reticuloses), blood stream infection and meningitis may occur.

Oral thrush is treated by nystatin or amphotericin. Neither drug is absorbed in significant amounts. In the rare systemic infections intravenous amphotericin B or oral flucytosine or clotrimazole may be used.

Bronchiectasis

The essential pathological change in bronchiectasis is chronic dilatation of the bronchi. It may arise as a complication of the following conditions.

1 Measles and whooping cough

Bronchiectasis has become less common in the West since the incidence of these childhood fevers has diminished, and since antibiotics have been used freely for chest infections. The bronchi of young children, because of their small size, are easily blocked by the tenacious sputum characteristic of the bronchitis of measles and whooping cough. This produces areas of segmental collapse, with dilatation of the affected bronchi owing to increased tractive forces on their walls. At this stage the process is reversible but if allowed to persist inflammatory damage to the walls may lead to permanent bronchiectasis. The lower lobes are most commonly affected, together with the lingula on the left and the middle lobe on the right.

2 Cystic fibrosis (mucoviscidosis)

See page 115.

3 Pneumonia

Bronchiectasis may follow a bacterial pneumonia in which the bronchial walls have been involved and which has healed by fibrosis. Tuberculous lung infection frequently has coexistent endobronchitis, and fibroid tuberculosis is the commonest cause of upper lobe bronchiectasis.

4 Chronic bronchial obstruction

This may be due to tumour, foreign body or stenosis and predisposes to bronchiectasis distal to the obstruction. Pressure from enlarged and calcified glands of primary tuberculosis may cause bronchostenosis and distal bronchiectasis, and this most commonly affects the middle lobe, causing the *middle lobe* (Brock's) *syndrome* (see page 109).

5 Allergic bronchopulmonary aspergillosis

Plugging of the bronchi which occurs in this condition damages their walls and leads to a characteristic proximal bronchiectasis (see page 115).

6 Congenital bronchiectasis

This is associated with maldevelopment of acini so that there is retention of secretions and subsequent infection in poorly ventilated blind airways.

7 Kartagener's syndrome

Impaired transport of mucus owing to defective ciliary action leads to basal bronchiectasis (see page 115).

Clinical features

The clinical features of bronchiectasis are variable and depend on the extent of the disease and the degree of infection in the affected bronchi. Some patients with bronchiectasis have no symptoms at all, particularly those with bronchiectasis of the upper lobes where drainage is continuous. Such bronchiectasis is frequently the result of old tuberculous infection. In others recurrent haemoptysis, sometimes profuse, is the only symptom. Sometimes infection occurs only in the winter following upper respiratory infection and for the rest of the year the patient is well. In such patients there may no physical signs, or simply persistent crackles over the bronchiectatic lobes.

In more classical bronchiectasis there is a history of recurrent episodes of pneumonia in childhood—the first often occurring after an attack of whooping cough or measles. The patient has a cough productive of a considerable volume of purulent sputum which may sometimes contain blood. It is worse in the morning as sputum collects in the dilated bronchi during the night when the cough reflex is depressed. The sputum and breath may be foul smelling if anaerobic infection is present (see page 107). In the winter there are exacerbations of the condition with increased cough and sputum and at times fever, and recurrent attacks of pneumonia may occur.

The fingers are often clubbed. The cardinal sign is that of persistent early inspiratory coarse crackles. There will be additional signs of lung fibrosis if this is present to a significant degree, and dyspnoea and cyanosis may be present if there is respiratory insufficiency. Such is the picture of gross bronchiectasis which nowadays is rare, and the majority of patients with this disease present in less dramatic form.

Complications

Chronic bronchitis is a common accompaniment in patients with persistent severe infection. *Respiratory failure* may develop in patients with severe and progressive disease.

Patients are subject to attacks of *pneumonia*, either in the affected lobe or in another part of the lung owing to 'spillover' of infected sputum. Spread of bronchiectasis and lung fibrosis may follow.

Lung abscess or *empyema* may occur.

Cerebral abscess may result from haematogenous spread from an infected thrombus in a pulmonary venous radicle.

Amyloid disease may develop if infection has been extensive and prolonged, but is now rarely seen.

Investigations

The chest X-ray may show no abnormality; more commonly there is some increased striation in the bronchiectatic lobe owing to bronchial wall thickening and crowding of the blood vessels, and cysts with fluid levels may be seen. Abnormal shadowing will be present if there is much associated fibrosis, with compensatory emphysema in the surrounding lung. The abnormalities are often well demonstrated by CT. The diagnosis of bronchiectasis can be confirmed and its extent determined by *bronchography* (see page 95), but it is rarely required.

Treatment

Management depends on the careful assessment of the patient's history and the extent of the bronchiectasis.

Surgical treatment is rarely indicated. Young patients with a history of severe chronic infection which is not controlled by medical means can be considered for surgical treatment. The disease should be confined to one lobe, and complete bronchograms are required to exclude bronchiectasis in other parts of the lung. Surgery is contraindicated if the disease is too widespread, if there is coincident asthma or chronic bronchitis, or if there is impaired ventilatory capacity.

Treatment by postural drainage is usually remarkably effective, though clearly it cannot be curative. The severity of the symptoms is not always directly related to the anatomical extent of the bronchiectasis. They can nearly always be satisfactorily controlled and the complications largely prevented by regular and competent postural drainage. The patient is taught the position in which secretions will drain from the bronchiectatic area towards the main bronchi and the trachea. This enables sputum to be coughed up and is assisted by percussion of the chest wall. The lower lobes are affected in the majority of patients. Postural drainage for this lobe is achieved by leaning face downwards over the side of the bed with the hands on the floor. Alternatively the foot of the bed is raised on 18-inch blocks, the patient lying on his face or side, according to the segments affected. Postural drainage of the right middle lobe is achieved by placing the patient on his back with a pillow under the right side of the chest and the foot of the bed is slightly raised. With upper lobe bronchiectasis, drainage will take place if the patient is sitting up, leaning towards the unaffected side. The appropriate position must be adopted for at least ten minutes twice a day, and forcible coughing should be continued until no more sputum will come up. Drainage of the secretions can often be improved by percussion of the chest over the affected lobe. The physiotherapist or the nurse may carry out this procedure, but later the patient's relatives will have to be instructed. Alternatively, the patient can improve drainage by making a number of forced expirations ('huffing'). Postural drainage should be carried out first thing in the morning as sputum collects in the dilated bronchi during the night. It should also be performed before retiring to bed and it may be necessary to repeat it before the midday and evening meals. A hot drink given before each treatment may increase expectoration. It is not necessary for a patient to carry out postural drainage slavishly if he does not have any sputum.

Antibiotics. A course of ampicillin or tetracycline (500 mg 6-hourly) or co-trimoxazole (two tablets twice a day for one or two weeks) may be given if the purulent sputum becomes more profuse, particularly if the patient also have fever and malaise. Sometimes continuous suppressive antibiotic treatment over the winter months may be considered, or a prolonged course of high-dose ampicillin or amoxycillin (3 g daily) where sputum is persistently purulent. In patients with foul sputum there is often infection with anaerobic organisms, and penicillin and metronidazole are the antibiotics of choice. No treatment is necessary in patients whose bronchiectasis is symptomless and without evidence of infection.

Kartagener's syndrome (immotile cilia syndrome)

In Kartagener's syndrome there is tranposition of the viscera (situs inversus), poorly developed paranasal sinuses and most of the patients have rhinitis, sinusitis and chronic bronchitis; about half have bilateral basal bronchiectasis. It is inherited as an autosomal recessive. The cilia are immotile and electron microscopy of ciliary structure has demonstrated an absence of dynein arms to the microtubules. Absence of ciliary activity means that there is an even chance of foregut rotation in the fetus to the right or left. There is a generalized respiratory tract disorder due to failure of normal transport of secretions. Male patients with this disorder are infertile, as the tails of spermatozoa have the same structure as cilia and are also immotile.

Cystic fibrosis (mucoviscidosis)

In this inherited autosomal recessive disorder, bronchial secretions are abnormally viscid and lead to a spreading suppurative bronchiectasis with progressive respiratory insufficiency. A sweat test shows a diagnostic high concentration of sodium in the sweat, but this is less reliable in adults. Nowadays many patients survive until adult life and death is usually due to cor pulmonale. Bowel symptoms and malabsorption are more prominent in younger patients.

Postural drainage (see above) is the cornerstone of treatment and must be carried out regularly 2–4 times a day. It may be aided by salbutamol inhalations. Antibiotics can be given intermittently for acute exacerbations of infection or continuously when there is persistent copious sputum. Organisms most commonly present are *Staph. aureus*, *Haemophilus influenzae* and *Pseudomonas aeruginosa*. Flucloxacillin is the drug of choice for *Staph. aureus* infection; patients colonized with pseudomonas may be helped by regular use of a nebulizer containing an aminoglycoside and an anti-pseudomonal penicillin. Haemoptysis and spontaneous pneumothorax may occur. Pancreatic deficiency is discussed on page 176. Heart–lung transplantation is emerging as a treatment option.

Chronic bronchitis and emphysema

Chronic bronchitis

Great Britain has a higher mortality rate from chronic bronchitis than any other country in the world. It is a major cause of chronic disability and death, particularly in men over middle age. It is related to air pollution, cigarette smoking and the liability to viral respiratory tract infections, and is most common in outdoor manual workers in urban districts. It is a complication of the pneumoconioses (see page 124), and obesity is an aggravating factor.

In most patients chronic bronchitis and emphysema occur together and it may be difficult, in life, to decide which is making the major contribution to the patient's problems. This has led to the emergence of non-committal terms such as chronic airflow obstruction, chronic obstructive airways disease or chronic bronchitis and emphysema.

Chronic bronchitis is defined as productive cough occurring on most days for three months or more of the year, for at least two consecutive years. In the early stages there is hypertrophy of the mucous glands of bronchi, even when there is no inflammatory cell infiltration of the mucosa. In addition goblet cells replace the normal peripheral bronchial epithelium. Later, inflammatory changes in the mucosa occur with micro-abscesses and ulceration of the alveolar walls. When the sputum is mucoid bacteriological study is unrewarding. With persistently purulent sputum, and in acute exacerbations of bronchitis, *Haemophilus influenzae* and *Strep. pneumoniae* are the most common pathogens isolated.

Clinical features

The earliest symptom is probably the 'smoker's cough', with the early-morning production of non-infected mucoid sputum. This causes no disability and the patient is unlikely to seek medical advice. Later the patient complains of a winter cough with sputum, often with wheezing. At first these symptoms may only occur in episodes after a cold, which is slow to clear. Later they persist throughout the whole winter and eventually during the summer as well. There is usually a moderate amount of sputum, which may be mucoid or purulent; the latter nearly always occurs during an acute exacerbation of bronchitis, but sometimes the sputum is persistently purulent. A large volume of sputum should arouse suspicion of concomitant bronchiectasis.

The combination of chronic bronchitis and emphysema often leads to increasing dyspnoea. The patient becomes too breathless to work and finally becomes completely disabled. There is considerable variation in the degree of disablement as many patients go throughout life with chronic cough and sputum and little dyspnoea, whereas others develop severe airflow obstruction within a few years.

Examination shows wheezes due to airways narrowing; if the lungs are emphysematous with poor breath sounds the wheezing may be heard best by listening over the trachea. Early inspiratory crackles may also be heard, particularly at the lung bases. As emphysema develops it produces additional signs (see page 117). A chest X-ray may show little or no abnormality unless emphysema is severe.

Treatment

This is generally disappointing, but in certain cases considerable symptomatic improvement can be achieved. The progress of the disease is slowed by stopping smoking and perhaps by preventing, as far as possible, acute exacerbations of bronchitis and by treating them vigorously when they occur. This is more rewarding in the early case where destructive changes are not advanced and symptoms are minimal.

The smoky atmosphere of the city and dusty work should be avoided. This ideal is difficult to achieve as most patients, for financial and social reasons, cannot move to a healthier district or change their occupation. They should be strenuously urged to give up smoking as this will slow the rate of decline of lung function. They should be advised to sleep in a warm bedroom, with the windows closed in the winter, and they should stay at home in foggy weather and when they have a cold. A cold must be taken seriously, and the patient should be given a prophylactic antibiotic (see below) without delay.

Some degree of bronchospasm is often present and may be relieved by bronchodilators such as oral salbutamol or ipratropium bromide.

Prednisolone should be tried in patients with significant airflow obstruction. Eosinophils in the sputum and a family history of allergy may increase the likelihood of response. This steroid therapy should be continued only if there is striking improvement (confirmed by objective measurement such as spirometry) within a week; it is then given on the same lines as for chronic asthma, or alternatively a corticosteroid inhaler may be used.

Prophylactic antibiotics do not prevent colds, but are used to prevent the secondary bacterial infection and to cut short, or prevent, acute exacerbations of bronchitis. In a small group of patients with persistent sputum, considerable improvement can be achieved by prolonged treatment with antibiotics, from November to March. However, the majority of patients are best treated by giving them a supply of antibiotics so that they can start a course, on their own initiative, at the first signs of a cold. As *Haemophilus influenzae* and the *Strep. pneumoniae* are the common pathogens, tetracycline (1 g daily), amoxycillin (500 mg daily) or co-trimoxazole (two tablets twice daily) are appropriate. Influenza vaccination is advisable.

Heart failure in chronic bronchitis is quite common; it may be due to concurrent hypertension or coronary artery disease, or to true cor pulmonale (see page 119), or to a combination of factors.

Emphysema

Emphysema may be defined as a condition of the lungs in which there is pathological enlargement of the distal air spaces with destruction of their walls. Emphysematous bullae, which are cystic spaces of varying size, may develop, and at post mortem the lungs appear bulky as they fail to deflate. The numerous pathological classifications of emphysema are both complex and confusing. There are two main types.

1 Panacinar emphysema
There is a dilatation or destruction of the acinus. This is the lung tissue distal to the terminal bronchiole and includes the respiratory bronchioles, alveolar ducts, and alveoli.

2 Centrilobular emphysema
The dilatation or destruction is more proximal and involves the respiratory bronchioles. The emphysema is present in the centre of the lobules with the more distal part remaining unchanged. Bronchiolitis is probably the main causative factor.

Aetiology

Emphysema most commonly occurs in association with chronic bronchitis. At times it may be related to an occupational cause such as exposure to dust, and in coal miners' pneumoconiosis (see page 124) there is characteristically a centrilobular emphysema ('focal' emphysema). Occasionally it develops as a primary disease without any associated history of bronchitis, and familial cases of mainly basal emphysema are now recognized where there is a hereditary deficiency of the anti-protease *alpha-1-antitrypsin* in the blood.

The actual mechanism of production of emphysema is uncertain. Proteolytic enzymes released from leucocytes in the presence of inflammation may be important. They are more likely to be destructive to the tissues when there is deficient activity of the principal enzyme inhibitor, namely alpha-1-antitrypsin. Apart from the hereditary deficiency, alpha-1-antitrypsin activity may be affected by inhalation of cadmium fumes, and by tobacco smoke.

Emphysematous lung loses its elasticity and thus expiration requires a muscular effort on the part of the patient. Apart from the increased work involved, the forced expiration produces early closure of the airways and thus enhances the diffuse airflow obstruction already present. The chronic over-inflation of the lungs leads to an increase in the fixed volume of gas in the lungs, the residual volume, with the result that the mixing of inspired air in the lungs is less efficient. Reduction in the total surface area of the alveoli impairs the transfer of gases between the alveoli and the pulmonary capillaries (see page 94).

Two clinical types occur in severe chronic airflow obstruction, although many patients present a mixed picture. Compensatory hyperventilation may enable the patient to sustain a relatively normal PaO_2 (*pink puffers*); and because of the irregular nature of the pathological changes there is a mismatching between ventilation and perfusion (see page 94) for there are areas of comparatively normal lung where the hyperventilation prevents a rise in the $PaCO_2$. Cor pulmonale is more likely to occur when the PaO_2 is allowed to fall and the $PaCO_2$ to rise (*blue bloaters*). The suggested association of emphysema with pink puffers and chronic bronchitis with blue bloaters is not borne out by pathological studies; most patients have a combination of the two conditions.

Clinical features

The major symptom is dyspnoea. When emphysema is not too advanced there is likely to be only moderate shortness of breath on exertion. With progression of the disease the patient eventually becomes unable to walk more than a few steps. Quite frequently the breath is exhaled through pursed lips. The rate of progress of the disease is variable. Frequently it is slow, the patient reaching old age with only moderate disability. Sometimes it is rapid, the patient becoming a complete respiratory cripple by middle life. Occasionally the onset of severe disability is apparently sudden. This is usually precipitated by fog or a respiratory tract infection, the patient not admitting to significant symptoms beforehand. The symptoms of coincidental chronic bronchitis (see page 115) are commonly present at the same time.

With well-established emphysema, the chest appears over-inflated, with thoracic kyphosis, increase in the anteroposterior diameter of the chest, and horizontal ribs —a 'barrel' chest. Chest expansion is diminished, the chest being lifted up by the accessory muscles of respiration rather than expanded. The percussion note is hyper-resonant and the areas of cardiac and liver dullness are diminished. The breath sounds are faint, often with prolonged expiration. Wheezes and early inspiratory crackles may be present.

Investigations

Respiratory function tests show impaired ventilation with irreversible airflow obstruction (see page 93), increased residual volume (page 93), impaired gas transfer (page 94) and an abnormal shape to the flow–volume loop (page 94). In advanced cases, blood gas abnormalities occur (page 93) and the presence of cor pulmonale produces additional signs (page 119).

The chest X-ray may be normal unless emphysema is well developed. In such cases the lung fields appear unduly translucent with loss of the peripheral vessels. The main pulmonary arteries are large and the heart thin and vertical. Bullae may be visible as localized areas of increased translucency. The ribs are horizontal and the diaphragm depressed and flattened. The lateral film shows an enlarged retrosternal 'window' of air. Emphysema is well shown on the CT scan.

Treatment

There is no specific treatment for emphysema, and breathlessness, once developed, will persist. The patient should stop smoking in an attempt to prevent progression of the disease. Improvement in airways obstruction may be achieved by bronchodilators and by treatment of bronchial infection (see page 116) which is commonly present owing to chronic bronchitis.

Breathing exercises may help to teach the patient to breathe in a more relaxed manner and to use the lower chest and diaphragms more effectively.

Surgical treatment of large bullae in patients with generalized emphysema is problematical, as the end result is usually impossible to predict.

Spontaneous pneumothorax should be suspected if there is sudden deterioration in a patient with emphysema (see page 13).

Compensatory emphysema

When a section of lung contracts by fibrosis or collapse, or is removed surgically, the rest of that lung expands by over-inflation to fill the space. This is sometimes known as compensatory emphysema, although no destruction of alveolar walls occurs. It is not usually associated with any defect of function.

Unilateral emphysema

Unilateral translucency of a lung may be due to a large bulla or cyst, or may be due to compensatory emphysema as a result of a totally collapsed lobe in the lung on that side. It also occurs when there is over-inflation of a lung owing to partial obstruction of a major bronchus; this can produce a 'ball-valve' mechanism so that air enters on inspiration but is trapped in the lung on expiration. This is likely to be due to a bronchial neoplasm in an adult and to pressure from tuberculous glands in a child.

Unilateral emphysema (Macleod's syndrome) may follow an obliterative bronchiolitis occurring in early childhood; this arrests development of the lung which normally proceeds until the age of 8 years. The affected lung over-inflates rather than budding, with the result that it has impairment of both ventilation and perfusion; the chest X-ray shows a hypertranslucent lung with attenuated vessels and a small pulmonary artery, and an expiration film shows failure of the lung to deflate with shift of the mediastinum to the opposite side. The patient often presents in middle age at the time of coincidental bronchitis; other presenting symptoms include unexplained chest pain on that side, of haemoptysis, the latter probably related to an increased bronchial circulation. The signs are those of diminished breath sounds over the affected lung and late inspiratory crackles at the base resulting from the opening of poorly ventilated, partially deflated alveoli.

Respiratory failure

The function of the lungs may be so impaired by various diseases that there is a failure to maintain normal arterial gas tensions. Respiratory failure is defined on arterial gas levels and occurs when the PaO_2 is below 60 mmHg (8 kPa) breathing air. Type I respiratory failure is associated with a low or normal $PaCO_2$. It is caused by mismatch of ventilation and perfusion and occurs in airflow obstruction, fibrosing alveolitis, pneumonia, pneumothorax and various other conditions. In type II respiratory failure the low PaO_2 is associated with a raised $PaCO_2$ (above 50 mmHg, 7.7 kPa). This occurs when ventilation is reduced by depression of the respiratory centre or failure of the respiratory muscles. It also occurs in severe chronic bronchitis and emphysema (blue bloaters).

Patients with chronic lung disease are especially prone to respiratory failure with any added complications, such as infection or the taking of respiratory depressant drugs. Respiratory failure can occur independently of cor pulmonale, although it may precipitate it.

Clinical features

Clinical features of hypoxia are cyanosis and confusion. Hypercapnia produces warm peripheries and vasodilatation. Higher levels produce confusion, coma and papilloedema.

Treatment

Treatment of respiratory failure is directed at the underlying cause where this is possible. In some cases specific therapy will be helpful (e.g. reversal of opiate-induced respiratory depression by naloxone or bronchodilatation in asthma). Certain other general measures are also necessary.

1 Oxygen
In type I respiratory failure oxygen can be given freely to correct hypoxia as necessary. In type II respiratory failure caused by chronic airflow obstruction, oxygen can be a lethal drug. Longstanding carbon dioxide retention produces an adaptation to the effects of carbon dioxide on the respiratory centre so that hypoxia produces the main drive to respiration. Correction of the hypoxia by oxygen treatment leads to depression of respiration and further carbon dioxide retention. In these circumstances controlled concentrations such as 24% oxygen should be used and the blood gases checked soon after starting treatment. Large rises in arterial CO_2 should lead to a reduction in inspired oxygen concentration.

In chronic airflow obstruction with hypoxia and cor pulmonale, long-term home oxygen of more than 15 hours a day reduces pulmonary hypertension and improves life expectancy. This is most satisfactorily and economically delivered by oxygen concentrators rather than cylinders.

2 Respiratory stimulants
In type II respiratory failure respiratory stimulants may be helpful. When hypercapnia occurs on oxygen therapy, the addition of a respiratory stimulant such as doxapram

hydrochloride may allow the administration of a higher oxygen concentration than would otherwise be possible. Doxapram, given as an intravenous infusion of 1.5–4 mg per minute, gives less of a problem with general cerebral irritability than does nikethamide.

3 Assisted ventilation
When there is a short-term exacerbation temporary assisted ventilation must be considered. When the problem is longstanding such treatment should be carefully evaluated. It is possible to maintain such ventilation at home sometimes just for part of the day (e.g. nocturnal ventilation in patients with muscle weakness). However, in a condition such as progressive motor neurone disease or disabling chronic airflow obstruction, such an intervention may be inappropriate because of the quality of the patient's life and the difficulties of ever getting the patient off the ventilator.

4 Other treatment
In the presence of respiratory failure all other factors must be made optimal. Sputum retention should be vigorously treated with physiotherapy, diuretics given for heart failure and antibiotics for infection. Nutrition should be adequate, and certain aspects of nutrition such as the phosphate level are particularly important.

Cor pulmonale

This is heart disease secondary to disease of the lungs. It occurs most commonly with chronic bronchitis and emphysema, but also with bronchiectasis and cystic fibrosis and with diffuse fibrotic lung disease from its many causes such as sarcoidosis, the pneumoconioses and fibrosing alveolitis. It may follow the longstanding deficient ventilation of severe kyphoscoliosis, or hypoventilation syndromes associated with sleep apnoea. It also occurs in primary pulmonary hypertension (see Table 2.26).

It is mostly precipitated by respiratory infection, but drugs such as hypnotics, tranquillizers and beta-blockers may be important precipitants. *Hypoxia* and carbon dioxide retention (*hypercarbia*) occur, and the abnormal gases produce impairment of renal function with retention of sodium and water, increase in blood volume and at first a rise in cardiac output. The systemic arterioles are dilated with warm extremities and bounding pulse, and dilatation of the cerebral vessels may produce headache and even papilloedema. The effect of the hypoxia on the pulmonary arterioles, however, is to produce active vasoconstriction. This, combined with obliteration of these vessels by disease and with the increase in cardiac output, produces pulmonary hypertension. It is only in the later stages of the disease—if pulmonary hypertension becomes severe, if the heart muscle is seriously affected by anoxia or in primary pulmonary hypertension—that the cardiac output falls.

Clinical features

The patient is cyanosed, with signs of chronic bronchitis and often emphysema. The extremities are warm but cyanosed, and the pulse full. The venous pressure in the neck is raised, the liver enlarged and there is dependent oedema. The heart sounds are often difficult to hear owing to the overlying over-inflated lung, but it may be possible to detect a triple rhythm. With gross enlargement of the right ventricle a right ventricular heave may be palpable and the systolic murmur of functional tricuspid regurgitation be heard, with systolic pulsation of the neck veins. Proteinuria and a raised blood urea may be present. It the cardiac output falls, the extremities become cold and the pulse small and venous congestion and oedema increase.

An electrocardiogram shows the large, sharply pointed P waves of right atrial hypertrophy, and there may be changes of right ventricular hypertrophy. The heart is usually vertical.

Chest X-ray shows dilatation of the main pulmonary arteries with cardiac enlargement. The lung fields may show evidence of emphysema, but at times the lung fields appear congested.

Treatment

This is primarily directed at improving alveolar ventilation. Physiotherapy is of prime importance to encourage the patient to cough properly and to clear the peripheral and central airways. It should be carried out frequently and if necessary during the night when hypoventilation is likely to occur.

Bronchial infection should be treated with an effective antibiotic such as amoxycillin or co-trimoxazole, and if the patient's condition warrants it antibiotics should be given parenterally.

Respiratory stimulants may be given if respiratory depression occurs. These arouse the patient, increase the ventilation and induce coughing. The use of doxapram given by continuous IV infusion in a dose of 1–4 mg per minute, depending on the patient's response, may allow the administration of higher concentrations of oxygen without harmful CO_2 retention.

Airflow obstruction can be treated by bronchodilators such as salbutamol and the anticholinergic agent ipratropium bromide by nebulizer or hand-held inhaler. A course of oral corticosteroids of IV hydrocortisone may be indicated.

Long-term *oxygen therapy* at home should be considered in cor pulmonale. It must be given for more than 15 hours daily to have a significant effect on pulmonary hypertension and on survival.

Diuretics should be given for dependent oedema and they may improve alveolar ventilation by eliminating pulmonary oedema. The blood urea and electrolytes should be monitored.

Digoxin is indicated only if atrial fibrillation is present. It is otherwise disappointing in cor pulmonale and may induce dysrhythmias.

Vasodilators such as nifedipine and captopril have been used to lower pulmonary hypertension but their place in cor pulmonale is not certain since their effect is usually not sustained.

In patients who develop severe secondary *polycythaemia* with a PCV of 60 or more, great clinical improvement can occur after adequate venesection to lower the PCV to normal levels. This is best done with simultaneous infusion of dextran or normal saline into the other arm so that there is little disturbance of the circulating volume at the time of venesection.

Sedation. All hypnotics are potentially dangerous because of the liability of producing respiratory depression. Treatment should be directed at relieving anoxia which is the cause of restlessness and mental confusion.

Sleep apnoea syndromes

Repeated cessation of airflow during the night leads to hypersomnolence in the day and to right heart failure. The apnoea may be central in origin or, more often, associated with inspiratory upper airway obstruction. Most patients snore loudly, many are obese and some have anatomical upper airway abnormalities. Systemic hypertension and psychiatric changes may occur.

Lung tumours

Secondary deposits may occur in the lungs. They vary from single 'cannonball' deposits from renal tumours to widespread small nodular deposits seen with thyroid carcinomas. Lymphangitis carcinomatosa may complicate primary or secondary tumours.

Carcinoma of the bronchus

Bronchial carcinoma is the commonest type of cancer in men, and in women its incidence now exceeds that of carcinoma of the breast.

Reports from the Royal College of Physicians and others have emphasized the importance of cigarette smoking as a major cause of this disease. There is also some evidence that the incidence is higher in those who live in the polluted atmosphere of industrial areas. An increased incidence is reported in miners exposed to dust from chromium, nickel and radioactive ores, and there is a greatly increased incidence in association with asbestos exposure. It may also arise in scar tissue from pulmonary tuberculosis or diffuse lung fibrosis. About half the tumours arise within an inch or two of the bifurcation of the trachea. The remainder are peripheral. Histologically they are classified as:

Squamous carcinoma
Adenocarcinoma
Small-cell undifferentiated (oat cell) carcinoma
Large-cell undifferentiated carcinoma

Squamous carcinoma is rather more common and the other histological types occur in roughly equal proportions.

Clinical features

A dry cough is the commonest early symptom. Recurrent haemoptysis may result from ulceration and sometimes this is the presenting symptom. Mucopurulent sputum occurs as the increase in size of the growth produces progressive bronchial obstruction, then distal infection; and shortness of breath develops with collapse of the lung segment supplied by the affected bronchus. A persistent wheeze caused by the narrowed bronchus and dull deep-seated pain are not uncommon symptoms. Some patients are symptom-free when the disease is discovered on routine chest X-ray. In others the symptoms may be related to one or other of the complications that may occur.

Complications

1 Pneumonia
The segment of lung distal to the bronchial obstruction is liable to infection. Patients may present with a segmental pneumonia, which either fails to resolve satisfactorily or recurs repeatedly in the same area of lung. Such events should always raise suspicion of an underlying carcinoma.

2 Lung collapse
Complete obstruction of a bronchus by carcinoma produces collapse of the lung segment supplied by that bronchus, and there may be symptoms of tightness in the chest and dyspnoea. The collapsed lung may become infected, causing fever and toxaemia, but there may be little or no sputum because of total bronchial obstruction. Collapse may be associated with a pleural effusion on the same side, with the result that there is no mediastinal shift. A chronic empyema may develop.

3 Lung abscess
This may develop in an area of obstructive pneumonia. When the growth is in the periphery of the lung its centre may become necrotic and be coughed up. This produces a ragged abscess cavity with walls composed of carcinomatous tissue, and which characteristically are thick and irregular when seen on a chest X-ray.

4 Superior vena caval obstruction
This results from pressure or invasion by a growth at this site. The patient may be in acute discomfort and complains of fullness in the head and face, this being worse on bending or on waking in the morning. There is swelling of the face and oedema of the upper limbs with gross non-pulsatile swelling of the neck veins, and anastomotic veins develop over the upper part of the chest. Other causes of superior vena caval obstruction include:

Aneurysm of the ascending aorta
Thrombosis of the vein
Malignant mediastinal glands
Lymphoma
Malignant thymoma
Retrosternal thyroid with haemorrhage into a cyst
Fibrosing mediastinitis
Mediastinal tuberculosis

5 Dysphagia
Difficulty in swallowing is due to compression of the oesophagus by growth or malignant glands, and at times it is a presenting symptom.

6 Pleural
Pleural effusion may be due to spread of infection from obstructive pneumonitis, when empyema may occur. Carcinoma of the bronchus must be suspected when empyema develops for no obvious cause. Malignant effusion is often, but not invariably, blood-stained. It may be due to secondary deposits, but it is more commonly due to direct extension to the pleura from a peripheral adenocarcinoma. Pain and dyspnoea are the major symptoms.

7 Cardiovascular
Atrial fibrillation may occur as a result of direct infiltra-

tion of the atria and is sometimes the presenting symptom. Spread of growth to the pericardium may produce a pericardial effusion or malignant pericardial constriction. *Thrombophlebitis migrans*, with spontaneous thromboses in the veins of the legs and arms and even the superior vena cava, is a complication of adenocarcinoma; less common is *thrombotic non-bacterial endocarditis* which may present with systemic emboli.

8 Distant metastasis

Bronchial carcinoma may metastasize to the liver, the bones, the adrenals, the brain, the skin or the lymphatic glands, the deposits causing symptoms and signs referable to the organs affected. When secondary neoplasm is suspected and the primary focus is not apparent, the lungs should be a prime area of suspicion.

9 The nervous system

Tumours occurring at the apex of the lung may involve the first rib and the lower part of the brachial plexus, producing Horner's syndrome together with pain down the arm with weakness and wasting (*Pancoast tumour*). Both laryngeal and diaphragmatic palsy may occur owing to invasion of the recurrent laryngeal and phrenic nerves. Lung cancer may present with cerebral metastases, and a chest radiograph should always be taken when a cerebral tumour is suspected.

10 Non-metastatic syndromes

(a) *Endocrine*. Occasionally tumours may produce poly-peptides which have a hormone-like activity.

Ectopic ACTH syndrome occurs with oat cell carcinoma, as well as with tumours of the thymus and pancreas. Because of the rapidity of the growth, the classic features of Cushing's syndrome may not have time to develop; muscle weakness with potassium depletion, oedema and hypertension with sodium retention and marked pigmentation may occur. Blood cortisol levels are often extremely high and fail to show diurnal variation.

Inappropriate secretion of antidiuretic-like hormone (ADH) also occurs with oat cell carcinoma, producing water retention, hyponatraemia and mental confusion.

Hypercalcaemia may be due to a parathormone-like substance or an osteoclast-stimulating factor usually produced by a squamous carcinoma. More commonly hypercalcaemia is due to extensive deposits in bone.

Polypeptides producing thyrotoxicosis and gynaeco-mastia have been reported.

(b) *Neuromyopathy*. Various disorders of nervous tissue and muscle may develop in association with lung cancer, usually with oat cell carcinoma. They may appear some considerable time before the tumour is evident. They include encephalopathies, in particular cerebellar degeneration; neuropathies; myopathic–myasthenic

syndromes (see page 210); polymyositis; and dermato-myositis.

(c) *Skeletal*. Hypertrophic pulmonary osteoarthropathy usually occurs in association with gross clubbing of the fingers, and is most commonly seen with both squamous carcinoma and adenocarcinoma; there is pain and swelling of the ankles and the lower shin and around the wrists; it may be confused with rheumatoid arthritis, but the radiograph shows typical subperiosteal new bone formation. It remits if the tumour is resected.

(d) *Renal*. Nephrotic syndrome, with albuminuria and oedema, may occur as the result of immune complexes produced by lung carcinoma.

Diagnosis

There may be no abnormal signs in the chest in spite of well-marked symptoms or obvious metastases. The changes when present may be those of collapse, pneumonia, lung abscess or pleural effusion. A combination of effusion with collapse is not uncommon. Stridor with deep breathing, or a monophonic wheeze may be present. Clubbing of the fingers is frequent. Careful examination should be made for secondary deposits in the liver and the lymphatic glands, particularly cervical and supra-clavicular.

A patient presenting with any of the above features should have a chest X-ray. This will confirm the presence of collapse, consolidation, effusion or abscess cavity, or may show a mass spreading out from the hilum, or a peripheral mass. It should be emphasized that a carcinoma may be present in spite of what appears to be a normal chest X-ray. Expert examination of the sputum for cancer cells is positive in about 80 per cent of cases.

If the diagnosis remains in doubt the patient should be bronchoscoped, and a biopsy of the suspected lesion removed for microscopy. Fibreoptic bronchoscopy (see page 95) enables biopsy and brushings to be carried out on peripheral lesions. If this is unrewarding, percutaneous needle biopsy under fluoroscopic control may be undertaken (see page 95). Biopsy of scalene nodes or of clinically enlarged glands may confirm the diagnosis. Every attempt should be made by the above measures to confirm diagnosis histologically and to exclude other pathological conditions. In addition, knowledge of the histological nature of the tumour may influence management and determine prognosis. Bronchoscopy and CT scan are essential if surgery is contemplated in order to assess the extent of the growth and its operability, and mediastinoscopy or mediastinotomy may be necessary.

Treatment

1 Surgery

The main hope of cure lies in surgical removal of the affected lobe or lung. With successful removal the five-year survival rate is about 30 per cent and is best with lobectomy for squamous carcinoma. Unfortunately, the majority of patients are inoperable when first seen; the carcinoma may be too extensive or may have already metastasized, or operation may be contraindicated because of inadequate respiratory function or serious coexistent disease. Small-cell carcinoma is generally unsuitable for surgery as in most cases this tumour can be regarded as a systemic disease by the time the diagnosis is made.

2 Radiotherapy

This can be used to produce a remission in patients unsuitable for surgery. It is unlikely to destroy the growth completely, although occasional cures do occur. It is best avoided in patients generally ill with advanced disease, or with large tumours, as it is likely to make them worse. Palliative treatment is of value in patients with superior vena caval obstruction and in those with haemoptysis or severe pain from bone metastases.

3 Chemotherapy

With small-cell (oat cell) carcinoma various regimens of intermittent treatment using multiple cytotoxic drugs have been shown to produce worthwhile remission in a proportion of cases. Occasional cures occur, but in most cases survival is only prolonged for a matter of months. The benefits of treatment have to be weighed against the side-effects. In other types of lung cancer chemotherapy has been very disappointing.

Mesothelioma

The rising incidence of this pleural tumour is believed to be related to the increased risk of exposure to asbestos dust. It may present as a pleural opacity or as a blood-stained effusion which rapidly recurs after aspiration. Pleural masses may be visible when fluid has been removed. Malignant cells may be detected in the fluid or on pleural biopsy. The tumour is often associated with severe pain as it invades the chest wall and it may grow through needle tracks or sites of pleural biopsy.

Treatment is universally ineffective for the tumour shows little response to radiotherapy or to cytotoxic drugs. Cases with recurring effusion are best treated by pleurodesis.

Alveolar cell carcinoma

Alveolar cell (bronchoalveolar) carcinoma is an uncommon tumour of the lung. Pathologically it appears as an adenocarcinoma which arises from the epithelium of the alveoli or bronchioles. It may develop in lungs previously damaged by fibrosis. An area of tumour may remain static for some time and then spread widely throughout the lungs via the bronchi and alveolar walls. Profuse bronchorrhoea from excessive mucus production is dramatic but uncommon. When the disease is advanced the patient suffers severe breathlessness and finally respiratory failure. The X-ray changes may be those of nodular shadows confined to a segment or lobe or of confluent areas of consolidation; they may be unilateral or bilateral. The diagnosis can be confirmed by sputum cytology, transbronchial biopsy or needle biopsy.

Adenoma of the bronchus

The term adenoma of the bronchus is a misnomer as the great majority are carcinoid tumours. They are mostly benign but a proportion become malignant and metastasize locally. The systemic symptoms that arise from gut carcinoid with liver metastases are rare with a bronchial lesion. A small number of adenomas are due to an *adenoid cystic carcinoma (cylindrome)*, which is a low-grade malignant tumour, or are due to an adenoma of the mucous glands. Bronchial adenoma is much less common than carcinoma and occurs rather more often in women. A rounded opacity may be seen on chest X-ray or tomograms, and the majority of the tumour may be extrabronchial as a dumb-bell extension. More commonly the chest X-ray shows collapse/consolidation of a segment or a lobe. It may present as recurrent haemoptysis or as bronchial obstruction with segmental infection. Diagnosis is confirmed by bronchoscopy and biopsy; the histology may be misinterpreted as oat cell carcinoma. The adenoma should be removed surgically, by wedge resection or lobectomy.

Hamartoma

This benign tumour of the lung is composed of a mixture of tissues normally present in the lung, particularly cartilage. It usually produces no symptoms and is discovered on the chest radiography as a rounded opacity with clear-cut edges, a 'coin' lesion. There may be areas of calcification, best seen on tomography, when it may be impossible to distinguish it from a tuberculoma. Calcified glands and calcified lesions in other sites of the lung will be in favour of tuberculoma. Otherwise the likely differential diagnoses are an isolated secondary deposit or a peripheral carcinoma of the lung. If there is doubt about the diagnosis, surgical resection may be the only certain way of establishing the nature of the lesion.

Cysts of the lung

1 Congenital cysts

These are due to maldevelopment of part of the primitive lung buds. They are lined with epithelium similar to that of the respiratory passage. They may be single or multiple.

Congenital cysts are commonly symptomless. *In infancy* a single congenital cyst may develop a valve-like mechanism, so that air enters during inspiration but cannot be expired. The cyst expands until it interferes with respiration, causing distress and cyanosis. Treatment is surgical.

Congenital cysts may become infected. Single cysts then present as a lung abscess, usually containing a large amount of fluid owing to poor bronchial drainage. Multiple cysts may be mistaken for bronchiectasis. Although antibiotics may control the infection and constitutional upset, postural drainage of the cyst is usually unsatisfactory owing to the inadequate bronchial connections; surgical excision of the infected cyst is therefore advisable when practicable.

2 Acquired cysts

These are much more common than the congenital type and are due to stretching and breaking down of alveoli. They are not lined with respiratory epithelium.

Acute lung infection, particularly staphylococcal pneumonia (see page 104), is one possible cause. Another is *pulmonary tuberculosis* with endobronchitis, which may lead to cavities with a valvular connection with the affected bronchus. They become distended and take on the characteristics of cysts (tension cysts). Additionally, in *emphysema*, localized or generalized cysts of the lung may occur.

Large bullae interfere with respiratory function, for they decrease the total alveolar surface of the lung, diminish mixing of respiratory gases and compress the remaining lung tissue. Generally the alveolar over-distension and cyst formation are so widespread in both lungs that no specific treatment is possible, but bullae can occasionally be resected or plicated using a stapler.

The pneumoconioses

Silicosis

Silicosis is due to the inhalation of fine particles of free silica. It occurs in coal miners, and in the granite and sandstone industries, in metal foundries, in various grinding processes in which sandstone is used, and in the pottery industry.

The earliest change is the development throughout the lungs of fine, fibrotic nodules around the particles of silica. As the disease develops those nodules increase in size and coalesce until finally there are large areas of fibrosis. Tuberculosis may complicate the picture.

Clinical features

In the early stages there are no symptoms or signs and the diagnosis depends on the radiographic picture of diffuse mottling combined with a history of exposure.

The first symptom is dyspnoea on effort and later cough with mucoid sputum develops. Eventually the patient becomes severely disabled and death occurs from bronchopneumonia, tuberculosis or cor pulmonale.

Treatment

There is no specific treatment and those showing evidence of the disease must be removed from exposure to dust. *Prevention* consists of adequate exhaust ventilation, damping down the dust and personal protection by means of masks. All people exposed to silica dust should have regular chest radiographs.

Asbestosis

The inhalation of asbestos fibres, which are silicates, causes a progressive diffuse fibrosis of the lungs, particularly of the lower lobes. The disease progresses in spite of removal from exposure. Blue asbestos (crocidolite) is more destructive than white asbestos (chrysolite). The chief symptoms are cough and dyspnoea and the clinical picture is that of fibrosing alveolitis (see page 127); *asbestos bodies*, formed of asbestos fibres and fibrin, can be found on microscopy of the sputum.

Preventative measures are similar to those used in silicosis. Carcinoma of the bronchus is a common complication and malignant mesothelioma of the pleura also occurs. Calcified pleural plaques and acute pleural reactions also occur in workers exposed to asbestos dust.

There is no specific treatment for asbestosis, but prednisolone may produce some symptomatic relief.

Coal miners' pneumoconiosis

A special type of pneumoconiosis affects miners who inhale coal dust, rather than rock dust which produces silicosis. In the UK it is most prevalent in the South Wales coalfields.

1 Simple pneumoconiosis
Radiographically there are diffuse linear shadows at first. Later, scattered small nodules up to 5 mm in diameter develop, often with surrounding emphysema. The disease is only progressive if the worker remains exposed to dust.

2 Progressive massive fibrosis
Radiographically there are large, dense shadows mostly in the mid and upper zones, with surrounding emphysema. It probably represents a massive fibrotic response to low-grade inflammation. At times the centre undergoes necrosis and is coughed up to leave a shaggy-walled cavity. Although tuberculous infection or infection with opportunist mycobacteria may be suspected, there is no evidence that they play a part in the aetiology. It is progressive even if the subject is no longer exposed to coal dust.

3 Caplan's syndrome
This consists of discrete fibrotic nodules, some 3 cm or more in diameter, occurring in a patient with coal miners' pneumoconiosis and rheumatoid arthritis. The rheumatoid factor is present in the blood. The rheumatoid arthritis may precede the development of the lung lesions or develop some years later.

Clinical features

There are no symptoms in the early stages. In the later stages of simple pneumoconiosis and with massive fibrosis, dyspnoea on exertion is a prominent symptom. Cough and sputum, sometimes blackened by coal dust, develop and recurrent bronchitis is common. In advanced cases the patient becomes grossly disabled and death from cor pulmonale is usual.

Treatment

Of importance are adequate ventilation and reduction of dust by damping it down with water, by wet drilling and wet cutting. Masks are not very satisfactory as they interfere with the performance of heavy work. Chest X-rays at regular intervals should be carried out on all workers at risk, and those showing evidence of pneumoconiosis should be removed from further exposure to coal dust.

Byssinosis

Byssinosis is due to exposure to dust arising from the processing of cotton. It is believed to be an unusual allergic reaction of the bronchi to cotton dust. In the early stage of the disease the patient complains of dyspnoea, a constricted feeling in the chest, and cough which characteristically occurs on Mondays when the patient returns to work. Later the dyspnoea and cough become permanent and finally emphysema develops. Prevention is by adequate ventilation.

Sarcoidosis

Sarcoidosis is a granulomatous disease in which epitheloid (macrophage) cell tubercles, without caseation, are present in all the affected organs. The lesions may resolve spontaneously, but the older lesions become converted to hyalinized fibrous tissue, and if they involve vital organs such as the eye, lungs, heart or nervous system severe impairment of function may result. A similar granulomatous lesion is sometimes seen on biopsy, for example, of skin or lymph nodes, in quite unrelated conditions such as carcinoma or reticuloses. This *sarcoid reaction* must be distinguished from the disease sarcoidosis.

The aetiology of sarcoidosis is not known, but there is an immunological defect due to dysfunction of T cell lymphocytes. There is a reduced level of T cells in the blood with sequestration and activation of T4 cells in the sarcoid granulomata. There is depression of the cell-mediated delayed type of hypersensitivity response (type IV), with a negative tuberculin test.

At the humoral level, polyclonal hypergammaglobinaemia and immune complexes may occur.

Clinical features

The three commonest clinical presentations are the following:

1 *Erythema nodosum* with *bilateral hilar node enlargement*, fever and often *polyarthritis.*
2 *Routine chest X-ray.* The patient is commonly symptom-free and an apparently healthy young adult. The chest X-ray may show hilar node enlargement, or hilar nodes with pulmonary mottling, or mottling alone. If

the patient is breathless it is likely that longstanding fibrotic sarcoid will be present.

3 *Uveitis.* This may be symptomless and found on slit-lamp examination of the eye. It is commonly acute and transient. It may, however, be insidious and persistent with keratic precipitates forming in the anterior chamber, adhesion of the iris to the lens and obstruction of the angle of the anterior chamber leading to glaucoma. The choroid and retina may also be involved.

Other organs may be involved, including the spleen, lymph nodes, liver and salivary glands. Skin lesions are characteristically few, sharply defined, brownish in colour with a predilection for the face. They may persist for months or even years; they are benign, do not ulcerate and involute spontaneously, leaving either no trace or a pigmented or atrophic scar. *Lupus pernio*, a chilblain-like condition which affects the nose, ear lobes and at times the fingers, may occur.

In the nervous system, a granulomatous basal meningitis may produce pituitary lesions or cranial nerve lesions. Diabetes insipidus or hypopituitarism may develop. Cerebral deposits may occur occasionally.

Cystic bone change may occasionally occur, usually in the heads of the metacarpals and in the phalanges. Hypercalcaemia may be present, resulting from an abnormal sensitivity to vitamin D, and may be more marked in the summer months. Rarely the heart is involved, leading to arrhythmias, congestive failure or sudden death.

A few patients develop frank pulmonary tuberculosis.

Investigations

1 Chest X-ray

Pulmonary involvement is one of the main features of the disease, and it can only be assessed by following the changing radiological picture. Chest X-ray is therefore essential.

2 Tuberculin reaction

A negative tuberculin reaction supports the diagnosis. However, as one third of the patients with proved sarcoidosis give a positive reaction to 10 TU (tuberculin units) (1:1000 old tuberculin), a positive reaction does not exclude it. If a patient with sarcoidosis and a negative tuberculin reaction is treated with corticosteroids, the reaction then becomes positive; this is almost diagnostic of sarcoidosis.

3 Plasma proteins

In approximately one third of cases there is a polyclonal hypergammaglobulinaemia, with raised α_2 and/or γ globulins, indicating activity of the disease.

4 Kveim test

The intradermal injection of a saline suspension of sarcoid tissue obtained from spleen or lymph node of patients with active sarcoidosis is followed by the development of a nodule in the skin within the next six weeks. Biopsy of this nodule will show sarcoid histology. The test is positive in about 70 per cent of cases of sarcoidosis; a negative result does not exclude sarcoidosis.

5 Angiotensin converting enzyme

ACE is produced by granulomata, and raised serum levels of ACE indicate active sarcoidosis and certain other granulomatous diseases.

6 Biopsy

Biopsy of skin lesions or affected glands will confirm the diagnosis. Liver biopsy is positive in about 50 per cent of patients with sarcoidosis, even when there is no clinical evidence of involvement of the liver.

7 Fibreoptic bronchoscopy and transbronchial biopsy

These can be carried out to confirm the histology of pulmonary infiltration. *Bronchoalveolar lavage* (BAL) in patients with active pulmonary sarcoidosis will show an absolute increase in T cell lymphocytes with an increase in the T4:T8 ratio.

8 Respiratory function tests

These are only abnormal when there is marked pulmonary mottling, when the main defect is that of gas transfer (see page 94). In the later stages of pulmonary fibrosis impairment of ventilation may be marked, and cor pulmonale may develop.

9 Gallium scan

This will show increased uptake in the lungs and other sites of active disease.

Progress and treatment

There is no evidence that anti-tuberculous chemotherapy influences the course of the disease.

Steroids are indicated in uveitis because of the danger to sight, and local instillation of drops is usually sufficient. Steroids are also indicated with hypercalcaemia, because of the danger of renal failure.

Erythema nodosum and hilar node enlargement carries a good prognosis. With hilar node enlargement the great majority of patients improve spontaneously; the remainder develop pulmonary infiltration. With pulmonary infiltration 50 per cent of patients improve spontaneously; if this has not occurred within two years then it is unlikely to remit subsequently. The infiltration may then remain unchanged with little or no disability to the patient, but in a proportion it progresses to severe fibrosis with associated bronchiectasis and bullous change. These patients become respiratory cripples and eventually succumb to cor pulmonale.

No specific treatment is indicated in patients with hilar node enlargement. Steroids are usually indicated in patients with pulmonary mottling showing no sign of resolution after a year or two, and in those where respiratory function tests show impairment of gas transfer. It often produces symptomatic relief and hastens resolution, and is aimed at preventing the development of severe fibrosis. Prednisolone (30–40 mg daily) is a satisfactory starting dose. A daily maintenance dose of 5–10 mg may be required for several years, as relapse may occur if treatment is too short. Steroids have no effect on the lungs in the fibrotic stage but may help to relieve symptoms. Response to treatment is best monitored by serial chest X-rays and lung function tests, rather than serial BAL lymphocyte counts, ACE levels or gallium scans.

Once the disease has remitted it is unlikely to recur.

Pulmonary fibrosis

Generalized pulmonary fibrosis is relatively uncommon. It may result from:

1 the pneumoconioses (see page 124);
2 infiltration of the lungs by a variety of pathological processes, including sarcoidosis (page 125), and histiocytosis X;
3 extrinsic allergic alveolitis;
4 fibrosing alveolitis.

Extrinsic allergic alveolitis

This results from inhalation of organic dusts which produce a type III hypersensitivity reaction in alveolar walls with the formation of sarcoid-like granulomata; these may progress to fibrosis. A large number of allergens have now been identified as causing the disease. These include spores in mouldy hay (*Micropolyspora faeni*) causing *Farmer's lung*, and avian proteins producing *Bird fancier's lung*. Precipitins to the allergen can be detected in the patient's blood.

Clinical features

In the acute stages fever, malaise, cough and shortness of breath may occur some hours after intermittent exposure, as in Farmer's lung. It is less likely if the exposure is more continuous, as in those keeping birds as pets. After prolonged or repeated exposure, chronic symptoms develop. Breathlessness is the predominant symptom. Cough may be present but it is usually unproductive. Fine late inspiratory crackles are best heard at the bases. Clubbing may be present in chronic cases. The chest X-ray shows diffuse nodular and linear shadowing, and in longstanding cases fibrosis develops mainly in the upper zones. Respiratory function tests indicate that the main defect is that of gaseous exchange across the alveolar membrane (see gas transfer, page 94).

Treatment

Known allergens must be removed from the patient's environment. A course of corticosteroids may be very effective in tiding a patient over an acute episode; they are helpful but less effective with chronic changes.

Cryptogenic fibrosing alveolitis

In this condition (also known as idiopathic pulmonary fibrosis) there is no evidence of an allergic alveolitis and the cause is often not known. The widespread inflammation in the alveolar walls is not associated with granulomatous changes. It may occur in association with the collagen diseases such as systemic sclerosis, SLE and rheumatoid arthritis. Rheumatoid factor and antinuclear factor may be present in the blood even in the absence of such associated diseases. A similar picture of widespread pulmonary fibrosis may occur as a side-effect of some drugs, particularly cytotoxic agents.

Clinical features

Breathlessness on exertion is the striking symptom. It is associated with late inspiratory crackles without sputum, most marked at the bases, and at times associated with an inspiratory wheeze. In advanced cases the patient becomes hypoxic on exertion and even at rest. Clubbing of the fingers is common. The chest X-ray shows diffuse fibrotic changes most marked at the lung bases, with diminished lung volumes and at times honeycombing of the lungs. Respiratory function tests show a restrictive defect of ventilation with impaired gas transfer without airway obstruction (see page 94). Advanced cases become respiratory cripples with respiratory failure and cor pulmonale. The diagnosis is made from the clinical picture, chest X-ray and respiratory function tests. When there is doubt it can be confirmed by open lung biopsy.

Treatment

Corticosteroids may give symptomatic benefit and are usually required on a long-term basis. They are less effective the more advanced the condition. Cytotoxic agents may occasionally be helpful. Oxygen in the home and portable oxygen produces symptomatic relief.

Localized pulmonary fibrosis

Fibrosis of the lungs is commonly localized to one or more lobes, or even a segment of a lobe. It is usually the result of inflammation, and common causes are tuberculosis, unresolved pneumonia, chronic lung abscess and longstanding collapse. Bronchiectasis invariably develops in such fibrotic segments or lobes. Persistent infection is not common with fibrosis of the upper lobes because drainage is adequate.

Clinical features

In some patients there are no symptoms, except perhaps the history of the original illness which led to the fibrosis. This is often the case with healed, fibrotic tuberculosis of the upper lobes, and no treatment is required.

In others the clinical picture is that of the accompanying *infected bronchiectasis*, both with regard to symptoms and complications (see page 113). Diagnosis and treatment are also discussed under this section.

The physical signs of fibrosis include flattening of the chest overlying the lesion, with diminished movement, impaired percussion note, bronchial breathing, whispering pectoriloquy and bronchophony. The mediastinum is shifted towards the side of the lesion, and coarse crackles are present with associated bronchiectasis (see Fig. 3.4).

Diseases of the pleura

Dry pleurisy

This may be due to:
- (a) injury to the chest and lungs;
- (b) pneumonia;
- (c) pulmonary infarct (see page 71);
- (d) tuberculosis (this variety nearly always progresses to pleurisy with effusion);
- (e) lung abscess;
- (f) epidemic pleurodynia (Bornholm disease).

Bornholm disease is a Coxsackie virus infection which may occur in outbreaks. It affects the muscles of the chest wall and produces a primary pleurisy without lung involvement.

Clinical features

The cardinal symptom of dry pleurisy is pain, described on page 89. On examination the respirations may be short and grunting, for severe pleuritic pain limits inspiration. The diagnosis is confirmed by finding a *pleural rub*, which is a superficial grating or crunching sound related to respiratory movements. It appears to arise just under the stethoscope, which indeed it does, and characteristically comes and goes. Occasionally a pleural rub may be heard in a patient who makes no complaint of pain.

Chest X-ray may reveal underlying disease if present, but shows no specific sign of dry pleurisy.

Treatment

Bed-rest and analgesics are required. Co-codaprin or subcutaneous morphine may be used, depending on the severity of the pain. Some patients obtain relief by applying a hot-water bottle over the area. Specific treatment is that of the underlying lesion, and subsequent management will depend on this.

Pleurisy with effusion

Fluid in the pleural cavity may represent a transudate or an exudate.

1 Transudates

These occur when the osmotic pressure of the plasma is reduced (the nephrotic syndrome or cirrhosis of the liver) or when the venous pressure is high (congestive cardiac failure or constrictive pericarditis). The fluid in a transudate is usually clear and of low specific gravity. It contains less than 30 g/l of protein. Causes of pleural transudates are:
- (a) cardiac failure;
- (b) nephrotic syndrome;
- (c) cirrhosis of the liver.

2 Exudates

These occur in the presence of inflammation or neoplasm. They are of high specific gravity and their protein content is more than 30 g/l. Exudates may be clear (tuberculous, neoplastic disease). Cloudiness may be due to blood (neoplasm, pulmonary infarct) or pus cells (pneumonia or lung abscess). Causes of pleural exudates are:
- (a) tuberculosis;
- (b) pneumonia;

(c) neoplasm;

(d) subphrenic abscess;

(e) pulmonary infarction;

(f) collagen diseases, notably systemic lupus erythematosus, rheumatoid arthritis and ankylosing spondylitis;

(g) Meigs' syndrome, complicating fibroma of the ovary.

Effusion with primary tuberculosis

This is the most common type of tuberculous effusion and usually occurs between the ages of 15 and 30, and within a year of tuberculin conversion. The lesion in the lung is usually insignificant, but by involving the pleura it produces an acute inflammatory reaction with an outpouring of fluid into the pleural cavity.

Clinical features

The onset is variable. Sometimes it is acute with fever, malaise, sweating and severe pleuritic pain. Other patients have little pain but complain of vague ill-health and dyspnoea on effort. Occasionally an effusion may be found on routine examination or chest X-ray in a patient with no symptoms.

Examination shows the typical signs of effusion (see page 90). If it is large there is mediastinal shift to the opposite side, with stony dullness on percussion and absent breath sounds over the effusion.

Chest X-ray shows the effusion as an opacity at the base of the hemithorax. It obliterates the costophrenic angle and rises up into the axilla. The mediastinum may be displaced to the opposite side. It is unusual to see any intrapulmonary lesion even when the effusion has cleared.

Diagnosis

This is confirmed by aspiration of a sample of fluid. It is straw-coloured and contains cells, most of which are lymphocytes, although in the early stages polymorphs may predominate. Tubercle bacilli can be isolated from the fluid by culture in about 50 per cent of cases. Pleural biopsy using an Abrams needle stands a good chance of confirming the tuberculous histology. It is positive in about 70 per cent of cases.

The *course* is usually towards resolution. Slow absorption of a large effusion may lead to pleural fibrosis, with subsequent restriction of lung expansion and contraction of the chest wall—a 'frozen' chest. Before chemotherapy was available about 25 per cent of patients developed frank tuberculous lesions in the lungs within five years of an effusion.

Treatment

The aims are to eradicate the infection and to prevent serious residual pleural fibrosis by encouraging rapid clearing of the effusion.

Anti-tubercular drugs should be given for nine months, starting with triple chemotherapy (see page 111). Unless the effusion appears to be disappearing rapidly, aspiration should be carried out every two or three days until no further fluid can be removed. Half to one litre should be removed at each aspiration as removal of larger amounts may lead to pulmonary oedema. Fluid should be removed without delay if there is much mediastinal shift or if the patient is short of breath. Effusions which do not resolve, or which keep reforming in spite of these measures, may be treated in addition with corticosteroids. The steroid therapy need not be prolonged and must be combined with chemotherapy; prednisolone (20 mg daily, reducing to a maintenance dose of 10–15 mg daily for 6 weeks) is satisfactory.

Bed-rest is best continued until the effusion has cleared, usually within a few weeks. The patient should then make a gradual return to full activity and should remain off work for 2–3 months. Follow-up supervision with chest X-rays is essential as with other forms of tuberculosis.

Effusion with post-primary tuberculosis

Effusions may develop with post-primary pulmonary tuberculosis and usually indicate severe tuberculosis. Because of the underlying lung disease they resolve more slowly than effusions associated with primary tuberculosis, and may develop into tuberculous empyemata.

Treatment

Half to one litre of pleural fluid should be aspirated every other day until the pleural cavity is dry.

The subsequent management depends on the nature of the underlying lung disease, and will require anti-tubercular chemotherapy (see page 111).

Neoplastic pleural effusion

Malignant effusion is most commonly due to carcinoma of the bronchus. It also occurs with mesothelioma and with spread of extrathoracic growth to the pleura, such as carcinoma of the breast, stomach, kidney, ovary or testicle. Pleural effusions are not uncommon in Hodgkin's disease.

Clinical features

The degree of general ill-health is variable and depends on the extent and nature of the primary neoplasm. The effusions are often of insidious onset, but as they usually become large dyspnoea is a common symptom. The fluid usually reaccumulates rapidly after aspiration; it is often blood-stained and may contain malignant cells. Malignancy may be confirmed by pleural biopsy using an Abrams needle, or by biopsy taken at thoracoscopy.

Treatment

The patient must be kept comfortable by repeated aspiration. It is often possible to prevent reaccumulation of fluid by producing a chemical pleurodesis. It is most effectively carried out by performing thoracoscopy (when biopsies can be taken) and talc pleurodesis, followed by adequate drainage of the effusion to ensure that the pleural surfaces become adherent to each other.

Effusions associated with breast carcinoma may respond to hormone treatment.

Blood-stained effusions

Blood-stained pleural effusions are not uncommon. The chief causes are:
  (a) neoplasm—commonly bronchial carcinoma but any neoplastic effusion may be responsible (see above);
  (b) pulmonary infarct;
  (c) rarely tuberculosis.
A traumatic haemothorax that has been diluted by a pleural exudate may have the appearance of a blood-stained effusion.

Haemothorax

Haemothorax may follow trauma to the chest. It also occurs with a spontaneous pneumothorax, owing to bleeding from the tear in the lung or from tearing of pleural adhesions; it is then a haemopneumothorax. An aneurysm may leak into the pleural cavity.

Blood in the pleural cavity clots rapidly and fibrin is deposited on the pleural surfaces. Pleural reaction also

occurs, with outpouring of further fluid. If the blood is left in the pleura, organization with pleural fibrosis occurs with subsequent serious interference with lung function.

Clinical features

If the pleural bleeding is large and rapid the patient will be shocked and collapsed, with rapid pulse and respiration. There may or may not be evidence of trauma to the chest. There are signs of pleural fluid (see page 90), or in those cases complicating a pneumothorax the signs are those of both fluid and air in the chest.

Diagnosis

This is confirmed by aspiration of blood from the pleural space. It is important to distinguish between a frank haemothorax and a blood-stained effusion.

Treatment

The general treatment for internal haemorrhage should be given. Morphine may be required, the patient's blood group should be determined and a transfusion given when necessary.

The effusion should be aspirated and the pleural space kept as dry as possible by further daily aspiration. Antibiotics should be given during the period of aspirations as there is a danger of secondary infection, usually staphylococcal.

Surgical treatment is often required to remove a blood clot which cannot be evacuated by aspiration, or to control bleeding.

Empyema

Empyema may be defined as a localized collection of pus in the pleural cavity. It most commonly results from a pneumonia, usually pneumococcal lobar pneumonia, or it may be due to staphylococcal, Streptococcus milleri anaerobic infections. It may also be due to spread of infection from a lung abscess, from a subphrenic abscess, from mediastinal sepsis and from a chest wound. An underlying carcinoma may be present. Empyema may also result from tuberculous infection of the pleural cavity (see page 129). Infected serous fluid may collect in the the pleural cavity during the course of a pneumonia (*syn-pneumonic empyema*). It is not localized and it usually resolves with adequate treatment. It may, however, progress to become purulent and localized, and by this time the underlying pneumonia has resolved (*meta-pneumonic empyema*). A bronchopleural fistula may develop so that the empyema starts to be coughed up and there is both fluid and air in the pleural cavity.

Clinical features

Empyema most commonly arises one to two weeks after the start of a pneumococcal pneumonia. Instead of the temperature falling and the patient recovering, the temperature begins to rise again and takes on a remittent character. The patient looks ill, has drenching sweats and complains of malaise and anorexia.

Examination of the chest shows the signs of fluid; the mediastinum will be shifted if the collection of fluid is large. There is dullness over the fluid; classically the upper limit of the dull area rises in the axilla, but this is not constant as the fluid is often loculated. Usually there are absent or diminished breath sounds over the fluid, although—particularly in children—it is sometimes possible to hear bronchial breathing which may lead to an erroneous diagnosis of unresolved pneumonia.

Both posteroanterior and lateral chest X-rays should be taken so that the fluid may be exactly localized. The diagnosis is finally confirmed by needling the chest and withdrawing turbid fluid. In the early stages the fluid will be thin and serous, but if a true empyema develops it will become thick and purulent. The fluid should be cultured for oganisms.

Treatment

1 Infected pleural effusion

The infected effusion must be aspirated daily to keep the pleural cavity as dry as possible. Following aspiration, 600 mg of benzylpenicillin should be injected into the pleural cavity. At the same time systemic antibiotic treatment should be continued; benzylpenicillin (600 mg 6-hourly) is satisfactory unless the infecting organism is resistant to penicillin, when the appropriate antibiotic should be used. With this treatment most effusions will subside. Sometimes, however, the infection is not controlled and the aspirated fluid becomes progressively purulent.

2 True empyema

Appropriate antibiotics should be given, but treatment at this stage is primarily surgical. Surgical decortication of the lung with removal of the abscess cavity can be performed. Alternatively, resection of a portion of a rib and the insertion of a drainage tube into the most dependent part of the empyema cavity ensures the best possible drainage. The aim is complete obliteration of the empyema cavity with the minimum of pleural scarring and fixation of the lung. It is therefore essential, once a true empyema has developed, not to delay surgical drainage or the wall of the abscess cavity may become so thick and rigid that it cannot be obliterated.

The drain is left in the empyema cavity until this space has disappeared and will require shortening from time to time. If the drain falls out before the cavity has been obliterated it must be replaced gently because of the danger of causing spread of infection to the brain (resulting in cerebral abscess). Breathing exercises are given to re-expand the lung and minimize fixation. Provided the treatment is correctly carried out the results are good.

Failure of the empyema cavity to close is usually due to:

(a) too long a delay before a drainage;

(b) inadequate drainage, with pocketing of pus; it will be necessary to X-ray the cavity, outlined with radio-opaque material, to determine the correct site for drainage of the most dependent part of the cavity;

(c) failure to recognize that it is a tuberculous empyema;

(d) the presence of an underlying neoplasm.

Tuberculous empyema

Tuberculous empyema nearly always occurs in an effusion complicating post-primary pulmonary tuberculosis, and it is rare in a tuberculous effusion associated with a primary infection.

Clinical features

The degree of constitutional upset varies. Some patients appear surprisingly well considering the chest is filled with tuberculous pus. Others have evidence of toxaemia with weight loss, sweating and fever. If secondary infection occurs, particularly with *Staph. aureus*, the patient becomes severely ill. This is especially likely to occur if there is bronchopleural fistula, or may occur as a complication of repeated aspiration.

The signs are those of fluid in the chest. If a bronchopleural fistula is present then the signs of fluid and air in the chest may be detected: an area of dullness below due to the fluid, with resonance above. It may be possible by tilting the patient to demonstrate shifting dullness.

Treatment

The patient requires the usual general treatment for tuberculosis, including a full course of anti-tuberculous chemotherapy (see page 111). The chest should be aspirated every other day until it is as dry as possible and streptomycin can be instilled into the pleural cavity after aspiration. If this treatment is not successful, as it may not be, then excision of the empyema cavity and decortication of the lung, or thoracoplasty, may be required.

Spontaneous pneumothorax

Air collecting in the pleural cavity as a result of some pathological process is known as spontaneous pneumothorax. The commonest cause is the rupture of a small vesicle under the visceral pleura which allows air to pass from the lung to the pleural space. This type of pneumothorax is common in young people and more common in men than women. It is not associated with any underlying lung disease. The patient is often slim with long fingers and high arched palate. In about 10–20 per cent of patients it recurs, sometimes repeatedly.

A spontaneous pneumothorax may also complicate lung disease such as emphysema and asthma when it is due to rupture of a bulla. In addition, air may enter the pleural space from wounds of the chest wall or from a perforation of the oesophagus.

When the spontaneous pneumothorax is due to the rupture of a vesicle, the tear usually seals off rapidly and the air is absorbed from the pleural cavity over the next week or so. Occasionally a valve-like opening develops between the lung and the pleural space so that air can enter, but cannot leave the pleura; this leads to the accumulation of air in the pleural cavity and the development of a *tension pneumothorax*. This is a dangerous situation.

Clinical features

The onset is usually sudden with pain in that side of the chest, and dyspnoea. The degree of constitutional upset is variable, but some patients may be quite shocked and collapsed. Occasionally the pneumothorax is found on routine examination and no history of chest pain can be elicited.

Examination of the chest may show diminished movement of the affected side. The degree to which the mediastinum is displaced away from the side of the pneumothorax is variable and depends on the size of the pneumothorax. Tactile vocal fremitus is decreased or absent. The note to percussion is either normal or hyperresonant. On auscultation there are diminished breath sounds and absent voice sounds over the pneumothorax. An exocardial clicking sound may be heard over a small left-sided pneumothorax.

The development of a *tension pneumothorax* is suggested by increasing dyspnoea, cyanosis and distress. There will be signs of a pneumothorax with considerable mediastinal displacement.

At times a spontaneous pneumothorax may be associated with a haemothorax owing to the tearing of pleural adhesions or bleeding from the tear in the lung.

Chest X-ray shows air in the pleural cavity with a varying amount of collapse of the lung. If the lung is deeply collapsed then atelectasis may develop owing to closure of the airways by compression. There is rarely any evidence of lung disease.

Treatment

When a spontaneous pneumothorax is diagnosed within the first few hours after its onset, the patient is best admitted to hospital because of the slight but definite risk of a tension pneumothorax or haemopneumothorax developing. Rest at home for a short period is satisfactory if a pneumothorax has been present for a few days and is expanding satisfactorily.

No active treatment is required for a small or moderate sized pneumothorax unless the patient has emphysema, when distress may be out of proportion to the size of the pneumothorax. In all patients with a large or tension pneumothorax it is best to insert a catheter via a trochar through an intercostal space in the axilla into the pleural cavity, the other end being connected to an underwater seal. The patient is instructed to cough gently and thus slowly to expel the air from the pneumothorax; expansion of the lung will then take place. Moderate pneumothoraces may be reduced by inserting a cannula and aspirating the air directly via a syringe and three-way trap.

Occasionally the pneumothorax persists in spite of these measures owing to a persistent leak, in which case continuous suction can be applied to the underwater seal to encourage the visceral pleura to become adherent to the chest wall. If this fails, thoracotomy may be required. With recurrent pneumothorax pleurodesis is indicated, either by painting the pleural surfaces with a solution of silver nitrate and thus allowing the visceral and parietal pleurae to become adherent, or by thoracotomy and pleurectomy or scarification of the parietal pleura.

Mediastinal cysts and tumours

1 Swellings in the mid-mediastinum

Carcinoma of the bronchus is the commonest cause of a mediastinal mass. It may be due to direct extension of the growth or may result from infiltration and enlargement of lymph nodes.

Enlarged lymph nodes may be due to carcinomatous infiltration (commonly from the bronchus), lymphoma, sarcoidosis or tuberculosis.

Foregut cysts. Bronchogenic and enterogenous cysts may arise in the superior or lower mediastinum.

2 Swellings in the anterior mediastinum

Retrosternal goitre is usually, but not always, associated with a goitre in the neck. It lies anteriorly behind the manubrium and may compress the trachea or other structures in the superior mediastinum.

Thymic tumours may extend down in front of the heart. They are sometimes associated with myasthenia gravis. Some are malignant and may metastasize.

Dermoid cysts and teratomas usually lie anteriorly to the upper part of the heart. Dermoids may become infected and form fistulae with surround structures. Both may undergo malignant change.

Pericardial cysts are found in the lower anterior mediastinum, usually filling up the right cardiophrenic angle, and contain clear fluid (spring water cysts).

3 Swellings in posterior mediastinum

Neurofibroma and ganglioneuroma tumours usually lie on the paravertebral gutter. They seldom cause symptoms and are found on routine radiography, appearing as rounded opacities with clear-cut edges and the ribs may be splayed and thinner. Occasionally they have a dumb-bell extension through the exit foramen into the spinal canal, causing compression of the spinal cord. A neurofibroma of the first thoracic nerve often causes Horner's syndrome (see page 202).

Aortic aneurysm or aneurysmal dilatation of a pulmonary artery may appear as a mediastinal tumour.

Clinical features

Mediastinal tumours and cysts may produce no symptoms and may be found only on routine radiography. They may compress surrounding structures, causing a variety of symptoms and signs.

Investigation should include posteroanterior and lateral chest X-rays. Tomography, bronchoscopy and thyroid or CT scan may be required. Even with these investigations it is not always possible to make a definite diagnosis. Mediastinoscopy and thoracotomy may be required both for diagnosis and for treatment.

Further reading

West, J.B. (1985) *Respiratory Physiology: the Essentials*, 3rd edn. Williams & Wilkins, Baltimore.

Crofton, J. and Douglas, A. (1981) *Respiratory Disorders*. Blackwell Scientific Publications, Oxford.

4
Disorders of the Alimentary System

Introduction

Alimentary disorders are important causes of illness and death. In global terms, acute diarrhoeal illness and hepatitis B-related liver cancer are major killers. Nearer home, peptic ulcer, gallstones and the irritable bowel syndrome cause much misery, and cancers of the gut and pancreas are leading causes of death from malignant disease.

Recent technological advances include the widespread diagnostic and therapeutic use of flexible endoscopy, ultrasound and, more recently, CT scanning. There have also been important advances in medical treatment, surgical techniques and preventive medicine. H_2 blockers have revolutionized the treatment of peptic ulcer and the pharmacological treatment of gallstones is advancing slowly. Automatic stapling devices have facilitated cancer surgery, and there are now surgical alternatives to the incontinent ileostomy. The prevention of hepatitis B by vaccination has been achieved but has not yet been spread widely. The use of oral rehydration solution has reduced much of the morbidity and mortality from acute diarrhoeal disease in the underdeveloped world.

There are still numerous gaps in our knowledge. We do not know the cause of many common illnesses such as peptic ulcer, inflammatory bowel diseases and the major cancers of the alimentary tract. Environmental factors are probably all important and are waiting to be identified. The relationship between food and gut disease provides much controversy and a basis for much unorthodox medicine. There would certainly be less alimentary disease if people smoked less, drank less alcohol and ate a high-fibre diet.

Symptoms of gut and liver disease

Changes of appetite

Appetite is commonly lost in gut disease but this is rarely the presenting or sole feature. It is important to distinguish true anorexia from a reluctance to eat because food provokes distressing symptoms. Anorexia, especially for breakfast, is very common in heavy drinkers of alcohol and is often accompanied by nausea and retching. Alterations of appetite, aversion to some foods and cravings for others are well recognized in pregnancy. Anorexia is almost inevitable in the prodrome of viral hepatitis.

Alterations of appetite are characteristic of anorexia nervosa and may include bulimia (episodic overeating) in addition to self-induced vomiting and abuse of laxatives and diuretics. Anxious and depressed patients commonly suffer marked fluctuations in appetite.

Changes of weight

Slow loss of weight is common in many organic gut disorders (Table 4.1) and is usually due to reduced food

Table 4.1 Causes of weight loss

Reduced food intake and/or increased physical activity

Increased metabolic requirements (e.g. hypercatabolic response to sepsis, injury, thyrotoxicosis, diabetes mellitus)

Loss of nutrient in faeces in malabsorption

The wasting of chronic infections, inflammatory diseases and malignancy (caused by a combination of the above factors)

intake, although it may be caused by loss of nutrient in the faeces by malabsorption or by increased demand for energy.

Gain in weight is uncommon in gut disease, but patients with peptic ulcer may drink large amounts of milk or eat frequent snacks to relieve pain and thus put on weight. Excess alcohol consumption is a common cause of obesity, especially in otherwise fit young men who develop the characteristic 'beer belly'.

Oral symptoms

Patients often imagine that symptoms in the mouth indicate deep-seated and sinister abdominal disease, but this is rarely true. Many patients are over-anxious about coating of the tongue, especially the 'black hairy tongue', for which there is usually no apparent cause. Poor dental hygeine, smoking cigarettes or a pipe and chewing tobacco often cause bad breath (*halitosis*) and gingivitis. Rarely halitosis is caused by stagnation of food in a pharyngeal pouch, in achalasia and in the stomach above pyloric obstruction.

Recurrent small, painful ulcers (*aphthae*) are very common and rarely indicate internal disease. Associations between aphthae and both coeliac disease and inflammatory bowel diseases are recognized, but investigation is only warranted if there is some supporting evidence such as anaemia, weight loss or bowel disturbance.

Malnourished patients may have painful cracks at the angles of the mouth (*cheilosis*) and a sore, reddened, smooth tongue often ascribed to specific nutritional deficiencies (see Table 4.10). Similar symptoms may accompany the characteristic white buccal plaques of oral candidiasis.

The Sicca syndrome (dry mouth and dry eyes) is an autoimmune disorder, affecting salivary and lacrimal glands, which may be accompanied by a polyarthritis Sjögren's syndrome). It is found in a minority of patients with primary biliary cirrhosis (see page 184). Oral Crohn's disease occasionally causes deep painful ulcers or a curious, chronic swelling of the lips.

Behçet's syndrome includes chronic, deep oral and genital ulcers and can involve many systems including the gut. Small and large gut ulcers have been described. However, other organs are much more commonly affected such as the eye, the brain and the joints.

Gastro-oesophageal reflux

The combination of burning epigastric and retrosternal pain (heartburn, pyrosis) with reflux of bitter or sour gastric contents into the mouth clearly indicates the presence of gastro-oesophageal reflux. The symptoms usually occur after meals and are aggravated by stooping or lying flat. Nocturnal awakening is characteristic. The symptoms are eased by walking around and may be associated with cough or wheeze. Nocturnal reflux can aggravate asthma.

In uncomplicated reflux, swallowing is usually normal, but it may be uncomfortable or even painful (*odynophagia*) to drink hot fluids, alchohol or citrus fruit juices. Mucosal sensitivity can be reproduced by perfusing the oesophagus, via a fine naso-oesophageal tube, with dilute (N/10) hydrochloric acid – this so-called Bernstein test may be useful in distinguishing various forms of chest pain.

Waterbrash is the term used for the sudden filling of the mouth with tasteless fluid (saliva) and must be distinguished from reflux of bitter gastric contents into the mouth.

Dysphagia

This is true difficulty with swallowing, as distinct from pain, discomfort or a delayed sense of block in the gullet. The difficulty is apparent during the act of swallowing and may be accompanied by regurgitation of swallowed food into the mouth, usually without bitter gastric contents. The commonest causes are benign peptic stricture and carcinoma of the oesophagus (or high gastric carcinoma).

Rarer causes of dysphagia or odynophagia include specific infections by *Candida albicans* (thrush) and by the herpes simplex virus, and inflammation caused by swallowed caustics and certain drugs, especially if they are retained for long periods in the oesophagus (notable examples are KCl tablets and emepronium).

Chronic mechanical obstruction produces progressive dysphagia, initially for solids and later for liquids, and there may be sudden complete obstruction by a bolus of food or a large tablet, requiring urgent radiological and endoscopic attention.

Disorders of motor function of the pharynx and oesophagus also cause dysphagia (Table 4.2). Pharyngeal pouch (Zenker's diverticulum) is probably a complication of cricopharyngeus spasm, and dysphagia may initially be relatively inapparent as food passes into the pouch rather than down the oesophagus (see page 151). In both achalasia and pharyngeal pouch, stagnant food may accumulate and be regurgitated hours or days after consumption, threatening the lungs if this occurs at night.

Table 4.2 Types of abnormal pharyngeal/oesophageal motility

Disorders of CNS (e.g. bulbar, pseudobulbar palsy)	
Cricopharyngeus spasm ± pharyngeal pouch Diffuse oesophageal spasm	Primary muscle disorder
Achalasia Chagas' disease	Abnormal nerve plexuses
Scleroderma of oesophagus	Replacement of muscle by fibrosis

Atypical central chest pain

Severe central chest pain, bad enough to mimic the pain of ischaemic heart disease, can be produced by diffuse-oesophageal spasm, the spasm associated with so-called vigorous achalasia, bolus obstruction with food ('steak-house coronary') and possibly by spasm secondary to gastro-oesophageal reflux. Recent studies suggest that many patients admitted to medical wards with severe central chest pain and atypical ECGs have oesophageal rather than cardiac disorders. The increasing availability of oesophageal manometry (see page 150) should help to identify these patients.

Nausea and vomiting

Various causes of vomiting are classified in Table 4.3.

Uncomplicated peptic ulcer may cause intermittent vomiting with temporary relief of pain, but the vomiting of ulcer or gastric cancer is usually obstructive in nature with a characteristically large volume of foul, stale food residue unaccompanied by bile. Various forms of vomiting occur in patients after peptic ulcer surgery (see page 154).

Vomiting occurs in unrelieved intestinal obstruction (small or large gut) and the vomitus will be faecal in colour and smell if the site of obstruction is in the lower small intestine or beyond.

Table 4.3 Classification of causes of vomiting

Cerebral (e.g. migraine, raised intracranial tension)

Labyrinthine (e.g. travel sickness, labyrinthitis)

Metabolic (e.g. uraemia, hypercalcaemia)

Gastrointestinal (see text)

Psychological (see text)

Persistent nausea and vomiting without obvious explanation are usually psychological in origin and detailed psychiatric assessment will be required. Self-induced vomiting by finger may suggest a psychological cause, but patients with peptic ulcer and gastro-oesophageal reflux can relieve pain in this way.

Dyspepsia/indigestion

These are vague words which describe any sort of distress caused by meals, including pain, discomfort, nausea, distension, belching and heartburn. In general, patients with benign peptic ulcer (especially duodenal ulcer) feel more comfortable after meals, whereas those with most other common upper alimentary disorders feel worse. Common functional dyspeptic syndromes include a sense of bloating or distension in the epigastrium especially after fatty meals (fat intolerance) and the high colonic distension of one variant of the irritable bowel syndrome (see page 168).

The physiological explanations for many forms of functional dyspepsia are far from clear, but it is well established that fat delays gastric emptying and releases cholecystokinin (CCK) from the duodenal mucosa. CCK has potent motor effects on the small and large gut, and this may provide a rational explanation for the beneficial effects of a reduced fat intake in patients with these symptoms.

Gas/wind

We all swallow air with our meals and this passes rapidly through the small intestine. Bacterial metabolism of unabsorbed food residues in the colon produces the various smells of flatus and the gases generated include methane, hydrogen, carbon dioxide, indoles and hydrogen sulphide.

Belched gas (eructation) is usually odourless, except when gastric contents are stagnant as in pyloric stenosis. Excessive belching is usually caused by repeated air swallowing, but is also common in patients with gastro-oesophageal reflux.

Excessive flatus is a common complaint, but is often difficult to explain. Bacterial fermentation of large amounts of dietary fibre commonly causes excess flatus, and similar symptoms occur in alactasic subjects (see page 146) who drink milk. Some vegetables are notorious gas producers, including beans, cabbage and sprouts, but individuals vary greatly in their responses. Increased amounts of substrate for bacterial metabolism are available in patients with malabsorption, and the flatus is often particularly offensive.

Abdominal distension caused by accumulation of intestinal gas and fluid is seen in patients with intestinal obstruction. Chronic or recurrent abdominal distension and discomfort relieved by passing flatus suggests left-sided colonic pathology or the irritable bowel syndrome (see page 168). Abdominal distension is often more imagined than real and can be produced voluntarily by a combination of exaggerated lumbar lordosis and diaphragmatic contraction. This exercise can be reproduced on the examination couch and will help to reassure the patient that there is no serious intra-abdominal pathology.

Abdominal pain

Various types of abdominal pain are classified in Table 4.4.

Severe abdominal pain caused by hollow organ distension is often but not always colicky in nature (i.e. it comes in waves and makes the patient writhe or draw the knees up to the chest) and is usually accompanied by vomiting and sweating. The episodes are short-lived (i.e. they last for several hours only) and are either self-limiting or require relief by appropriate intervention.

Peritoneal inflammation is associated with marked tenderness and 'guarding' of the abdominal musculature. This is characteristic of a perforated viscus, when the onset is sudden and dramatic, and also accompanies the acute and chronic inflammatory lesions mentioned in Table 4.4.

Most types of chronic or recurrent abdominal pain are less distinctive than these, signs may be few or absent, and careful history taking is crucial. The pain of benign peptic (especially duodenal) ulcers is perhaps the most distinctive in its classic form with a periodicity over several years; that is, prolonged periods of freedom lasting weeks or months, aggravation by hunger, relief by snacks or antacids and nocturnal awakening by well-localized epigastric pain. Radiation to the back suggests a posterior duodenal ulcer beginning to penetrate the pancreas. Unfortunately, in many patients the symptoms are less typical. The pain of gastric ulcer and carcinoma tends to be aggravated by food and is often accompanied by nausea, anorexia and loss of weight.

Colonic pain can be very distinctive, although its location may be anywhere in the abdomen. It is usually either colicky or a more continuous distension and is most commonly sited in the left iliac fossa or above the pubis. The most characteristic feature is the temporary relief by passing flatus or faeces, although occasionally defaecation may aggravate the pain. This type of pain is characteristic of the irritable bowel syndrome and of uncomplicated symptomatic diverticular disease (see page 166), and the bowel habit is always abnormal, although detailed enquiry may be required to reveal this.

Spasmodic severe rectal pain (proctalgia fugax) is felt deep in the pelvis, occurs usually at night, may be helped by firm pressure on the perineum and is usually not associated with any organic rectal or sigmoid disease.

Chronic, continuous, inexorable and seemingly inexplicable, abdominal pain is much less common. Organic causes include chronic pancreatitis and carcinoma of the pancreas, right-sided colon cancer, chronic intestinal ischaemia ('intestinal angina') and retroperitoneal lesions such as lymphoma and the rare fibrosis and sarcoma. In most of these patients there will be an obviously downhill course and signs will eventually develop after several months of unremitting pain. A few patients have continuous, unexplained pain without any evidence of organic disease, they may be psychiatrically disturbed and are often very difficult to help.

Spinal pain may radiate to the abdomen if dermatomes T8–12 are affected. The pain is aggravated by certain postures, lifting and coughing and is usually associated with abnormalities on detailed spinal examination. It is not affected by eating or by defaecation. *Pancreatic* pain is characteristically felt in the epigastrium and spreads through the back. Unlike lumbar pain, it is aggravated by lying flat and may be eased by sitting up and leaning forward.

Finally, mention should be made of abnormalities of the abdominal wall itself. Operation wounds can produce chronic pain, which may be relieved by removing a retained suture or by injecting entrapped nerves with local anaesthetic or locally active corticosteroids, but this is uncommon. Chronic abdominal pain is often ascribed to adhesions from previous surgery, but this is very difficult to prove unless frank obstruction results from adhesive bands. Wide incisional hernias are usually painless, but

Table 4.4 Classification of types of abdominal pain

Hollow organ distension (e.g. gut, biliary, ureteric, uterine)

Peritoneal inflammation (e.g. perforated viscus, acute and chronic inflammatory diseases of gut and pelvic organs—appendicitis, diverticulitis, Crohn's disease, salpingitis)

Retroperitoneal lesions (e.g. pancreatic disease)

Referred pain from spine affecting dermatomes T8–12

Anterior abdominal wall problems (e.g. muscular pain, fatty hernias)

epigastric herniation of fat through defects in the linea alba can cause chronic abdominal pain which is responsive to local injection or to surgical correction. Pain of this type is aggravated by coughing or by contracting the abdominal musculature and is unaffected by food or by bowel function.

Disturbed bowel function

Most healthy people have between three bowel actions per day and three per week. More important than frequency is the consistency of faeces, the ease and completeness of evacuation and the ability to delay emptying until it is socially convenient. The quantity and consistency of faeces is determined mainly by the amount of fibre in the diet; that component of food that resists normal small intestinal digestion and passes into the colon where it is broken down to a variable extent by bacterial metabolism. Defaecation is also aided by physical activity, by adequate hydration and by a prompt response to the 'call to stool'. Frequent delays in responding to rectal distension results in a lessened awareness of rectal filling and gradual accumulation of faeces in the rectum.

1 Diarrhoea

This is best defined as an increased weight of faeces (more than 200 g per day) which are soft or watery in consistency. This may be difficult to establish from the history alone and inspection of the faeces is very helpful. True diarrhoea must be distinguished from faecal frequency and faecal impaction with overflow (Table 4.5.). Pale, bulky, offensive stools suggest steatorrhoea. Excess gas or fat makes faeces float and difficult to flush away. Acute episodes of watery diarrhoea are usually caused by anxiety, infections, alcohol or drugs and are self-limiting and rarely require symptomatic therapy. Diarrhoea that persists for more than 2–3 weeks should be investigated, although symptomatic treatment with codeine phosphate, loperamide or lomotil can be used in the meantime. These drugs should, however, be avoided if

there is continuous abdominal pain or blood and mucus in the faeces.

2 Constipation

This is the infrequent passage of hard faecal masses with straining, difficulty and often anal pain. In the bedbound elderly and in some young children, large, hard faecal masses may accumulate in the rectum with overflow and incontinence of loose faecal matter ('spurious diarrhoea'). This is due to loss of internal anal sphincter tone as a result of chronic rectal distension.

The various types of constipations are classified in Table 4.6. It is helpful to distinguish rectal constipation (the rectum is full of hard faeces on digital examination) from infrequent difficult defaecation caused by slow colonic transit and infrequent rectal filling.

Most patients with 'simple' primary constipation respond well to an increased intake of dietary fibre, with adequate fluid, provided they obey the call to stool and allow adequate time for evacuation. The hydrophilic bulking agents (Table 4.7) are very helpful if dietary measures alone do not suffice. It is important to deal appropriately with painful anorectal disorders, although a high-fibre diet and a stool softener may alleviate local symptoms considerably. Evacuant enemas may be required to initiate therapy if there is considerable faecal accumulation in the rectum. Bulking agents are not appropriate if the colon is already full of faeces even if the rectum is empty. In these patients colonic transit may be stimulated by the anthraquinone (e.g. Senokot) or

Table 4.5 Types of diarrhoea

True (increased quantity of faecal matter)
Steatorrhoea
Watery diarrhoea
Watery diarrhoea plus blood and/or mucus

False (normal or reduced amounts of faecal matter)
Faecal impaction with overflow
Frequency with small, bitty stools
Frequent passage of blood/mucus with little or no faeces
Passage of large volumes of mucus

Table 4.6 Types of constipation

Absence of primary cause, 'simple' constipation: inadequate intake of dietary fibre; dehydration; lack of exercise; failure to respond to 'call to stool'

Secondary to disease or functional disorder of colon/anus (e.g. diverticular disease, cancer, Hirschsprung's disease, painful haemorrhoids, anal fissures)

Neurological diseases affecting bowel and bladder

Metabolic diseases, especially hypothyroidism, hypercalcaemia

Drug-related (e.g. aluminium-based antacids, anti-cholinergics)

Table 4.7 Classification of laxatives

Lubricants/stool softeners (e.g. dioctyl sodium sulphosuccinate)

Bulking agents (e.g. methylcellulose, mucilagenous polysaccharides, from seeds/gums—Isogel, Fybogel)

Osmotic agents (e.g. magnesium sulphate, lactulose)

Stimulant cathartics (e.g. anthraquinones such as Senokot, bisacodyl, castor oil)

polyphenolic (e.g. bisacodyl) laxatives, but crampy, colonic pain is common. Continued use of the osmotic laxatives may be the only alternative in these difficult cases. Excessive or inappropriate use of laxatives will provoke large faecal losses of water and electrolytes and can lead to dehydration and hypokalaemia.

Gastrointestinal bleeding

1 Acute severe upper gastrointestinal bleeding

This is a common and self-evident emergency which demands immediate medical attention. Overall figures for the UK show the following percentage attribution of causes:

Duodenal ulcer	40
Gastric ulcer	20
Erosions	15
Varices	5
Mallory-Weiss	< 5
Carcinoma	< 5
Oesophagitis	< 5
Others/no cause	> 5

The amount and colour of vomited blood gives little clue to the source of the bleeding. Altered blood, often described as 'coffee grounds', indicates slower bleeding with retention of blood in the stomach for several hours before vomiting. Forceful repeated vomiting of food and fluid may be followed by fresh blood from a vertical mucosal tear at the lower end of the oesophagus (*Mallory–Weiss syndrome*), but many patients with this lesion do not give a typical history.

Haematemesis usually indicates a source of bleeding proximal to the ligament of Treitz; but bleeding from all common upper GI lesions can present with melaena (black, loose, smelly faeces) in the absence of haematemesis, and this is particularly likely to occur from duodenal ulcers. Bleeding from oesophageal varices, on the other hand, is usually profuse, alarming and mainly upwards. Bleeding from severe oesophagitis and gastric cancer is usually slow, chronic and occult.

2 Severe lower GI bleeding

Blood loss that is sufficient to produce shock is very much less common but can sometimes complicate ulcerative colitis, diverticular disease or tumours. With the aid of mesenteric arteriography, angiodysplasia in the right colon has been recognized with increasing frequency, especially in the older age group.

The colour of the blood gives a rough guide to its source, because right-sided colonic bleeding is usually dark-red and may be passed in clots. However, severe upper GI bleeding may be difficult to distinguish from proximal colonic bleeding at the bedside, the colour depending on the rate of loss and on the transit time through the remaining gut.

The passage of more modest amounts of altered blood, associated with sudden abdominal pain in an older patient, suggests a diagnosis of vascular occlusion. Superior mesenteric arterial or venous occulsion produces severe abdominal pain and haemodynamic collapse ensues rapidly. Inferior mesenteric occlusion produces a less devastating clinical picture with reversible ischaemia or infarction of the left half of the colon (ischaemic colitis).

3 Chronic occult blood loss.

This is common cause of iron-deficiency anaemia and should be considered as the likeliest explanation in men and in postmenopausal women. In the older age groups it is necessary to exclude gastric and right-sided colonic cancer, and it is important not to ascribe the bleeding to minor oesophagitis, to a duodenal ulcer with no evidence of recent bleeding, or to diverticular disease – common incidental findings in this clinical setting.

4 Rectal bleeding

Blood loss that is insufficient to cause shock or anaemia is common and normally attributed to haemorrhoids. The patient strains on hard stools and the bright-red blood is on the toilet paper and on the surface of the faeces. However the differential diagnosis must include proctitis and more sinister adenomas and cancer in the rectum and sigmoid colon. It cannot be over-stressed that rectal bleeding should be investigated to exclude these lesions, especially in those patients over 40 and when the history is relatively short.

Liver disease

Jaundice is the most distinctive symptom of liver disease, but it is also produced by haemolysis and commonly by extrahepatic biliary obstruction (Table 4.8). In most

Table 4.8 Classification of jaundice

Prehepatic
Haemolysis

Hepatic
Bilirubin transport defects (e.g. Gilbert's disease, Dubin Johnson syndrome)
Acute hepatocyte damage by viruses or drugs

Posthepatic (cholestatic)
Impaired hepatocyte excretion (e.g. drugs, posthepatitis cholestasis)
Intrahepatic biliary disease (e.g. primary biliary cirrhosis, sclerosing cholangitis)
Extrahepatic biliary obstruction by gallstones or malignancy

chronic liver diseases, except primary biliary cirrhosis, jaundice tends to be a late symptom occurring either near terminally or during acute exacerbations. Other symptoms of liver disease include upper abdominal pain due to enlargement of the liver and stretch of its capsule, generalized itching without obvious skin pathology (pruritus) in cholestatic liver disease, and recurrent bruising or nose bleeds caused by impaired blood coagulation.

The major complications of chronic liver disease, which may be its first manifestation, include ascites, variceal bleeding and encephalopathy (see page 188).

Haemolytic jaundice is relatively mild. Anaemia may be apparent; the urine does not contain bilirubin (because unconjugated bilirubin is bound to albumin in the plasma); and the stools are normal or dark because excess bilirubin enters the gut. By contrast, *cholestatic* jaundice is often severe. Conjugated bilirubin appears in large amounts in the urine and makes it dark; the faeces are pale because less bilirubin enters the gut; and pruritus is common and is ascribed to retention of conjugated bile salts in the systemic circulation and skin.

In *hepatitis-like* conditions (caused by viruses, drugs or alcohol) the picture is more complicated and variable. Haemolysis may accompany viral hepatitis which can later enter a prolonged cholestatic phase. Jaundice is usually mild or moderate and, initially at least, the urine contains excess urobilinogen rather than bilirubin and faecal colour is normal.

In extrahepatic obstruction, expecially by gallstones, infection in the biliary tree is common (*ascending cholangitis*) and leads typically to high fevers and rigors. The combination of jaundice, fever and itching strongly suggests obstruction of the extrahepatic bile duct by calculus.

In practice, these clinical distinctions can be quite difficult and many other details in the history are helpful. Occupational, drug and contact histories must be considered. Examples include leptospirosis (Weil's disease) in farmers and sewage workers; non-A, non-B viral hepatitis following transfusion of blood or blood products; hepatitis B in promiscuous homosexuals and intravenous drug abusers; and hepatitis A following ordinary social contact with other cases. A careful history of the use of drugs and alcohol is very important. In the older age group slowly progressive cholestatic jaundice with weight loss strongly suggests malignant obstruction of the biliary tree.

Conventional 'liver function tests' performed on plasma are helpful in following the course of the illness, but can be misleading at the initial stage of diagnosis. The typical changes are summarized in Table 4.9.

Congenital defects of bilirubin uptake and conjugation are relatively rare and will not discussed here. The exception is *Gilbert's syndrome*, which is characterized by a variably increased level of unconjugated bilirubin in the blood. It has no serious clinical significance, but it is important to exclude chronic haemolysis and to reassure the patient that there is no serious liver disease. All other liver function tests are normal. The prevalence of this condition is uncertain, but 1–2 per cent of otherwise normal adults have bilirubin concentrations greater than 25 μmol/l (the normal range is below 20).

Physical signs of gut and liver disease

With the exception of liver disease, signs are relatively few and nonspecific. However, much can be learnt by careful examination of the patient and a few specific diagnoses can be made on the basis of signs alone.

State of nutrition

Observed loss of weight is an important sign in many gut disorders. In children and adolescents chronic gut disease is commonly associated with failure to gain weight and height and with the delayed development of secondary sex characteristics. In older girls and young women, secondary amenorrhoea usually accompanies marked loss of weight, most notably in anorexia nervosa.

Loss of subcutaneous fat is a sign of calorie (energy) deficiency, and later the muscles become thin and eventually weak. Alcoholics, who derive much of their energy from alcohol and eat little protein, have thin muscles but well-preserved subcutaneous fat. Heavy drinkers, who continue to eat well, are overweight and the 'beer belly' in young men often indicates the cause of gastrointestinal complaints.

Specific nutritional deficiencies may be apparent but, with the exception of anaemia and oedema, they are relatively rare even in severe chronic gut disease (Table

Table 4.9 Patterns of 'liver function test' results in jaundice

	Haemolysis	Hepatitis	Cholestasis
Bilirubin			
conjugated	+	++	+++
unconjugated	+++	++	+
Transaminases	N	++++	+
Alkaline phosphatase	N	+	++++

Table 4.10 Clinical signs of specific nutritional deficiencies

Anaemia	Deficiency of Fe, folate, B_{12}
Oedema	Protein deficiency
Angular cheilosis, sore tongue	Various deficiencies, including B vitamins
Scaly red skin	Possibly zinc or essential fatty acid deficiency
Bleeding gums, skin haemorrhages	Vitamin C deficiency
Bruising, bleeding	Vitamin K deficiency
Bony tenderness, proximal myopathy	Vitamin D deficiency
Peripheral neuropathy, ocular palsies, confusion	Vitamin B_1 (thiamine) deficiency

4.10). Impaired nutrition is caused by neglect and poverty far more often than by chronic gut or liver disease, especially in the older age groups.

The state of the teeth should be examined because rotten teeth and badly fitting dentures make it impossible to chew food properly and food intake diminishes.

State of hydration

In patients with diarrhoea, vomiting and fistulous losses from the gut, dehydration and serious electrolyte deficiencies are common and readily corrected. Dehydration is indicated by thirst, loss of skin turgor, dry mouth and soft eyes. In severe cases there is hypovolaemia envinced by a rapid and weak pulse, postural hypotension and reduced venous pressure in the neck. Severe K^+ deficiency causes muscle weakness and loss of tendon reflexes. Reduced plasma levels of Ca^{++} and Mg^{++} are seen infrequently in chronic gut disease but may cause muscular hyperexcitability, tetany and even convulsions, although low levels of plasma Mg^{++} can be remarkably well tolerated.

Shock

Peripheral circulatory collapse commonly results from major gastrointestinal bleeding and is seen in very severe diarrhoea – it is common in cholera, for example. Sudden collapse in patients with jaundice or hepatic ascites suggests Gram-negative septicaemia arising from the biliary tree or from the ascitic fluid.

The hands, face, neck and chest

Finger clubbing is seen in the inflammatory bowel disease, especially Crohn's disease, and some other types of chronic diarrhoea. It may also occur in chronic liver disease.

The stigmata of chronic liver disease are well recognized and are summarized in Table 4.11. The explanation for many of these features is unknown, but they may be related to an altered balance of male/female sex hormones. Feminization with gynaecomastica, female distribution of body hair and small testes is common in males, especially if the liver disease is due to alcohol. Spider naevi are common in normal pregnancy.

Lymphadenopathy is an important sign of metastatic malignancy, especially from primary cancer of the stomach and pancreas. A particularly favoured site is behind the left sternoclavicular joint (*Virchow's node*).

Rare causes of GI blood loss include hereditary haemorrhagic telangiectasia (with characteristic vascular abnormalities on the lips and fingers) and the *Peutz-Jeghers* syndrome comprising small bowel polyps and a distinctive spotty pigmentation of the lips.

Examination of the mouth has already been stressed in relation to dentition and hydration and some specific oral diseases are mentioned on page 135. Evidence of anaemia and jaundice should always be sought.

The abdomen

Inspection may reveal obvious masses caused by tumours, inflammation (e.g. appendix mass, Crohn's disease) or huge cysts, especially arising from the ovary. A diffusely enlarged abdomen may be caused by fat, fluid, flatus, faeces or fetus and in most cases the cause is obvious. Visible peristalsis is seen if there is obstruction at the pylorus or in the lower small intestine. Large hernias will be obvious on coughing. Abdominal wall movements with respiration are absent in peritonitis and coughing aggravates the pain. Prominent abdominal wall veins may flow up towards the thorax (Budd–Chiari syndrome or IVC obstruction), or away from the umbilicus (portal hypertension).

Palpation must be gentle and systematic using light touch and then deep palpation in all four quadrants. In the acute abdomen, assessment of localized tenderness and guarding of the musculature is important. Masses must be

Table 4.11 'Stigmata' of chronic liver disease

Hands	Pink palms, Dupuytren's contracture, white nails
Skin eyes	Jaundice, spider naevi (arms, face, upper trunk)
Abdomen	Prominent veins, ascites, hepatosplenomegaly
Legs/back	Oedema
CNS	Mental impairment, constructional apraxia, flapping, tremor, increased tendon reflexes
Endocrine	Feminization in the male

characterized in terms of size, site, consistency, fixity or movement with respiration, and enlargement of liver, spleen and kidneys must be sought in all patients. In chronic liver disease, the liver is firm and often irregular in shape, but the size can vary enormously from very small to very large. Enlargement of the spleen is common and usually indicates portal hypertension. In patients with obstructive jaundice, tense palpable enlargement of the gall bladder is usually, but not always, caused by malignant obstruction of the lower end of the common bile duct (*Courvoisier's sign*).

The hernial orifices must be examined carefully in patients with acute abdominal pain, especially if intestinal obstruction is suspected. Small hernias in the epigastrium or paraumbilical region should be sought in patients with superficial pain aggravated by coughing. Tenderness (and pain) will be increased if the recti abdominis are contracted by raising the head or the legs off the bed.

In males the external genitalia should be palpated because the genitalia may be small in chronic alcoholic liver disease, and primary testicular tumours metastasize to abdominal lymph nodes and can cause deep abdominal or back pain.

Percussion of the abdomen is very useful in clarifying the contours of the liver and spleen, in determining the nature of suspected masses (solid or air filled), in detecting bladder enlargement, and in distinguishing ascites from other causes of abdominal distension.

Auscultation is particularly useful in the acute abdomen. Absence of bowel sounds suggests ileus, usually secondary to peritonitis following perforation or pancreatitis. The exaggerated, tinkling bowel sounds of intestinal obstruction are very characteristic. The gastric splash of pyloric stenosis is best heard by applying the ear to the epigastrium and gently shaking the patient. Vascular bruits can be heard over the abdominal aorta and femoral arteries in patients with severe atheroma and an epigastric bruit accentuated by sitting up is caused by the arcuate ligament of the diaphragm compressing the coeliac artery. The clinical significance of this so-called 'coeliac axis compression syndrome' is uncertain. Some tumours, especially primary hepatocellular carcinomas, are so vascular that bruits may be heard over an hepatic mass.

The anus and rectum

This is an essential part of the examination of all patients with bowel symptoms and lower abdominal pain. The patient is examined in the left lateral position with the legs well drawn up. The anal margin is inspected first for obvious skin disorders and for perianal tags so characteristic of Crohn's disease. The patients should then strain down and this may reveal the lower part of an anal fissure, prolapsing haemorrhoids or the so-called '*descending perineum syndrome*', which indicates weakness of the pelvic floor and is associated with problems of continence.

The anal canal is then examined digitally prior to deep rectal examination. An irregular painful canal usually suggests a fissure or Crohn's disease if there is much induration. The consistency of any faeces present is noted and its appearance observed later when the finger is withdrawn. The finger is swept around the pelvis and will feel the sacrum posteriorly and, anteriorly, the prostate in the male and the cervix uteri in the female – an anterior bulge above the cervix may be due to a retroverted uterus. Abnormal masses within the rectum and compressing if from without are noted along with any regions of particular tenderness. Pressure by the left hand above the pubis will often help to clarify the nature of a pelvic mass (bimanual examination). In the female a vaginal examination should be carried out if there appears to be a pelvic abnormality and if there are no contraindications.

Investigation of GI disorders

This will be discussed in relation to the main groups of symptoms and signs. In general, prolonged symptoms (that is, lasting more than about four weeks), symptoms unresponsive to simple therapy or recurrent symptoms responsive to empirical treatment should all be investigated. This is especially true if there are accompanying features such as anaemia and loss of weight or if persistent symptoms develop for the first time in the older age groups (above 50 years).

Dyspepsia/abdominal pain

The most effective investigations are upper GI endoscopy and ultrasound examination of the gall bladder and pancreas, the order depending on the nature of the presentation. Barium studies of the oesophagus, stomach and duodenum and oral cholecystography still have a role and, in many hospitals, are more generally available to GPs and non-specialists.

Upper GI endoscopy

This is generally well tolerated, but most patients are given intravenous sedation and oropharyngeal anaesthesia and need to recover in hospital for several hours. It is more accurate than barium meal in detecting oesophagitis, small gastric erosions, ulcers in a chronically deformed duodenal cap recurrent ulcers after gastric surgery, and it has the great advantage that biopsies and brushings for cytology can be taken from suspicious lesions. It is the investigation of choice in acute upper GI bleeding as soon as the patient has been resuscitated. It is a very safe procedure, provided that the initial intubation is gentle. Difficulty may indicate cricopharyngeus spasm, a pharyngeal pouch or other high oesophageal obstruction. If these are suspected clinically, it is wise to refer the patient for a barium study first.

Barium examination

Radiology has the advantage that no sedation is required, it is well tolerated and the patient can leave the hospital immediately. The barium examination is better at demonstrating the initiation of swallowing, oesophageal motility and the different types of hiatal herniation (especially the rare rolling or paraoesophageal hernia). The modern double-contrast technique is excellent at showing peptic ulcer, gastric cancer and even scattered small gastric ulcers. Once a duodenal cap is deformed by chronic ulceration, it is very difficult for the radiologist to demonstrate whether there is current active ulceration. It is important not to over-interpret the common finding of a small sliding hiatus hernia, especially if reflux of barium into the oesophagus cannot be demonstrated using appropriate manipulation.

Ultrasound

Examination of the upper abdomen by ultrasound has developed very rapidly in recent years and shows gallstones more reliably than oral cholecystography. It demands the presence of an expert radiologist and expensive equipment. There is no radiation exposure and the procedure is considered to be very safe. In relation to the pancreas, ultrasound examination may be vitiated by too much gas and by obesity, but it is usually an excellent way of showing cysts and pseudocysts. These can be drained using percutaneous techniques under ultrasound control for diagnostic or therapeutic purposes. Solid pancreatic masses may also be needled percutaneously under ultrasound control and material obtained for cytological or histological examination. Dilation and distortion of the duct system, features of chronic pancreatitis, are difficult to detect by ultrasound unless the changes are gross.

Oral cholecystography

OCG is a simple examination and is cheaper than ultrasound. Undertaken by radiographers, and usually requiring two visits to hospital, it indicates whether the cystic duct is patent and whether any stones are radiolucent or opaque, two points that are relevant to the medical management of gallstones (see page 171).

It may be vitiated by poor absorption of contrast material by the gut or impaired uptake and secretion by the liver. It is useless if the patient is jaundiced.

CT scanning

Computed tomography is particularly useful in the examination of the pancreas and other retroperitoneal structures. It is still very expensive, both in terms of staff and equipment, and is not yet widely available. It is probably superior to ultrasound in detecting solid pancreatic masses and chronic pancreatitis. The examination is easier if the patient is relatively obese since abdominal fat produces sharp tissue planes. Suspicious pancreatic masses can be needled under CT scan control for diagnostic purposes.

ERCP

In endoscopic retrograde cholangio-pancreatography, a side-viewing duodenoscope is used to pass a cannula through the ampulla of Vater. Contrast is then injected into both pancreatic and bile ducts. It is technically a difficult procedure but is becoming more generally available. It provides excellent views of the pancreatic duct system and this is invaluable if surgical treatment of chronic pancreatitis is contemplated. Duodenoscopy itself will identify most cases of ampullary carcinoma of the pancreas and biospies are easily obtained. Large carcinomas of the body and tail will usually distort the ductal anatomy, but histological material cannot be obtained.

In general, ultrasound and CT scanning are better and safer than ERCP in the diagnosis of pancreatic cancer, but as always the final choice depends on local facilities.

Bowel symtoms

Rigid sigmoidoscopy and proctoscopy

These are part of the initial examination of the patient and are undertaken without (usually) sedation or bowel cleansing. The sigmoidoscope is misnamed in the sense that it provides good views of the rectum only, the examination of the sigmoid colon can be difficult and painful in perhaps 50 per cent of patients. It is helpful to see the faeces and any mucus or blood in the unprepared bowel.

If bowel preparation proves necessary, it is probably better to proceed directly to flexible sigmoidoscopy if available (see below). The normal rectal mucosa is pale pink and thin so that the submucosal vessels are easily seen. In proctitis (colitis) the mucosa becomes redder, thicker, granular and bleeds easily when gently scraped with the instrument (friability) – the blood vessels are no longer visible. Discrete ulcers are relatively uncommon but are seen in Crohn's disease (although the rectum is often 'spared') and amoebic and other specific colitides. Tumours and polyps are easily seen and mucosal biopsies taken with relative safety.

The proctoscope is a shorter, fatter instrument which is designed for examination of the anal canal itself. It is ideal for examining haemorrhoids and fissures and, being short, can be used to obtain swabs of pus for bacteriological culture.

Flexible sigmoidoscopy

Sigmoidoscopy using fibreoptic instruments is an extension of rigid sigmoidoscopy. Current instruments are 30–60 cm long and the longer ones can reach the splenic flexure in most patients. Many patients will tolerate the procedure without sedation and can then leave immediately.

It is very useful in patients with rectal bleeding, for the initial assessment of colonic pain and altered bowel habit, for assessing the extent of ulcerative colitis and for clarifying radiological abnormalities of the sigmoid colon seen with a barium enema. Approximately 70 per cent of colonic tumors occur distal to the splenic flexture and are accessible with this instrument.

Full colonic examination

This requires a barium enema and/or colonoscopy, is unpleasant for the patient and needs meticulous bowel preparation if good views of the right half of the colon are to be obtained. It is essential in the investigation of overt lower GI bleeding and chronic occult blood loss if an adequate explanation has not been obtained by preliminary gastroscopy and flexible sigmoidoscopy. It is often required to establish the diagnosis of Crohn's disease (which often spares the left half of the colon) and to assess the proximal extent of ulcerative colitis (although flexible sigmoidoscopy may be adequate). It is often unrewarding in the investigation of nondescript chronic abdominal pain and watery diarrhoea, but carcinoma of the right side of the colon and proximal Crohn's colitis may have to be excluded is such patients. Diverticula are often better seen by barium examination than by endoscopy. However, they may not be the cause of the patient's symptoms and should not divert attention from other more sinister possibilities.

The preparation for barium enema and colonoscopy is similar and demands several days on a low-residue diet and 24 hours on clear fluids only. An oral cathartic agent (e.g. Picolax or Ex-Prep) is given on the evening before and on the morning of the examination. Colonoscopy almost always requires intravenous analgesics and sedation and an overnight admission is preferred in many units. It is a difficult technique, which needs constant practice and much experience if full examination is to be achieved. For these reasons barium enema is usually the initial examination, but, if an abnormality is found, endoscopy is almost always required in order to obtain histological material or to undertake appropriate treatment, especially removal of polyps by electrocautery.

The barium enema may be regarded as a screening test to decide whether colonoscopy is required. A good-quality negative examination combined with a satisfactory rigid sigmoidoscopy and normal rectal biopsy (in patients with diarrhoea) will exclude relevant or serious colonic disease in the vast majority of patients. Rectal biopsy from normal-looking mucosa occasionally provides evidence of more proximal Crohn's disease or reveals the changes of unusual forms of colitis (see page 164).

Gastrointestinal blood loss

Overt bleeding demands endoscopic assessment, after appropriate resuscitation, if an accurate diagnosis is to be achieved. It is usual to start with upper GI endoscopy, even in the absence of haematemesis, and then to consider the colon if no abnormality is found.

Colonoscopy may be possible if the bleeding is modest, but should be avoided if there is pain or evidence of active colitis on an initial rigid sigmoidoscopy. In severe, continued lower GI bleeding, selective visceral angiography is required to show the site of bleeding and it may reveal a vascular tumour or malformation, such as angiodysplasia.

Visceral angiography is often most helpful if bleeding is active and severe at the time. In patients with recurrent, unexplained bleeding, it can be difficult to judge the optimum timing of the procedure. An isotopic scan, using labelled red cells, is a useful guide to the presence and approximate site of active bleeding and, if positive, can be followed immediately by angiography.

Chronic occult blood loss is a much commoner problem and is confirmed by persistently positive tests for blood in normal-looking faeces. It usually demands upper GI endoscopy, barium enema or colonoscopy and small bowel radiology, in that order. A useful test, in younger patients, is an isotope scan using Pertechnetate which is taken up by gastric mucosa in a Meckel's diverticulum. This is a rare source of recurrent blood loss but is easily treated surgically.

Malabsorption

Clinical suspicion may be strengthened by abnormal laboratory test results – for example, anaemia (especially if macrocytic or of mixed cell type), depressed levels of serum folate and vitamin B_{12}, and biochemical evidence of osteomalacia or hypoalbuminaemia (although this is more commonly due to protein loss from abnormal mucosa than to malabsorption *per se*). Measurement of the fat content of faeces is unpleasant for the nursing and laboratory staff and for the patient himself, but it is still the only direct way to document fat malabsorption and to exclude this as a cause of chronic diarrhoea. To be worth while, the patient must be on a known fat intake (usually 70–100 g daily) starting at least two days before the collection begins, and he must collect accurately all faeces passed over at least three days.

Small bowel barium examination

The first investigation is radiology of the small bowel unless there is a strong pointer to pancreatic pathology. The conventional examination is the barium meal and follow-through, but this can be slow and tedious. It may reveal dilatation of intestinal loops and flocculation of barium, classic non-specific signs of malabsorption, or specific focal pathology such as Crohn's disease or diverticula. Better-quality information, especially about focal pathology, is provided by *enteroclysis*. This involves nasoduodenal intubation and the rapid infusion of a large volume of barium and water directly into the small intestine.

Small intestine mucosal biopsy

Biopsy is required to make a diagnosis of coeliac disease and a number of rarer causes of enteropathy, such as tropical spruce, Whipple's disease, intestinal lymphoma,

amyloidosis and intestinal lymphangiectasia. It should be undertaken if the barium study shows non-specific abnormalities or if there are strong pointers to coeliac disease, eg, unexplained folate deficiency, Howell Jolly bodies in the red cells (see page 354) or, rarely, unexplained osteomalacia. The conventional technique employs a suction biopsy capsule attached to a semi-stiff catheter which is passed via the mouth into the proximal jejunum under radiological control (see Fig. 4.1).

Useful information can be obtained from biopsies taken from the second part of the duodenum under direct vision at endoscopy. If duodenal biopsies prove different to interpret, a jejunal biopsy should be obtained for clarification.

Aspiration of jejunal juice can be undertaken at the same time as suction biopsy if some form of combined tube is used. The juice should be examined microscopically if giardiasis is suspected (see page 160). Bacterial culture using aerobic and anaerobic techniques will provide definitive evidence of overgrowth in patients

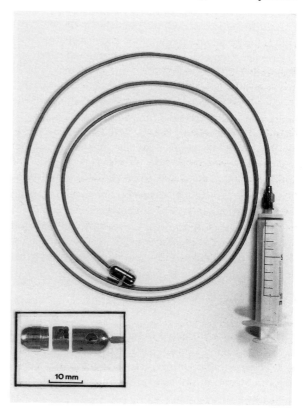

Figure 4.1 *The Watson jejunal biopsy capsule. This is mounted on a semistiff radio-opaque catheter and is advanced into the proximal jejunum under radiological control. Suction on the syringe pulls mucosa into the capsule and activates the rotating cutter.*

with abnormally slow intestinal transit or fistulous communication between large and small bowel.

Ileal function

These tests are useful in the assessment of patients with Crohn's disease and of patients after intestinal resection. The most readily available is the Schilling test, which measures vitamin B_{12} absorption in the presence of intrinsic factor. Severely impaired absorption suggests that at least 100 cm of distal ileum is diseased or has been resected (lengths of intestinal resection are notoriously difficult to assess at operation) and indicates the need for long-term vitamin B_{12} replacement therapy. Vitamin B_{12} absorption can, however, also be impaired by excessive bacterial activity in the upper small intestine.

Pancreatic exocrine function

Such tests are indicated if steatorrhoea is confirmed or obvious on clinical grounds and if the small intestine appears to be normal. Other pointers to the pancreas include heavy alcohol consumption and diabetes mellitus. The combination of steatorrhoea, diabetes and pancreatic calcification on abdominal X-ray makes formal tests of function superfluous.

The most reliable tests involve intubation of the duodenum and collection of mixed pancreatic juice and bile after a stimulus such as a mixed liquid meal (e.g. *Lundh's test*) or an intravenous injection or infusion of secretin and pancreozymin/cholecystokinin (CCK). The duodenal contents are assayed for output of enzymes (especially trypsin and lipase) and bicarbonate (following secretin infusion). In general, the tests based on hormone infusion are the more sensitive but are difficult to perform accurately. The Lundh test is much simpler but cruder, although it should identify patients with gross impairment of enzyme secretion.

Assessment of alactasia

Milk intolerance attributed to reduced levels of mucosal lactase is common in many parts of the world (especially in Mediterranean countries, Africa and India) and may occur in 5 per cent of those of North European stock. A simple trial of milk exclusion may suffice, but provocative tests using 25–50 g of lactose are often used. In alactasic subjects, lactose produces excess gas and abdominal cramps, an increased excretion of hydrogen in the breath (which can be measured with simple portable machines), and a relatively small rise (< 1.1 mmol/l) in blood glucose

concentrations. Alactasia can result from jejunal mucosal disease, especially coeliac disease, and a jejunal biopsy should be undertaken if there are any other pointers to an enteropathy.

Jaundice

The use of conventional liver function tests is summarized on page 140 and the virological diagnosis of hepatitis is referred to on page 178. This section deals with the distinction between extrahepatic obstruction of the biliary tree which requires some sort of mechanical treatment and other causes of jaundice, especially intrahepatic cholestasis. The advent of US scanning and direct cholangiography has greatly simplified the diagnostic sequence, which is summarized in Fig. 4.2.

THC (transhepatic cholangiography) is now widely practised by radiologists under local anaesthetic and sedation. A fine flexible needle is passed into the liver and contrast is injected into the dilated biliary tree under radiological control.

ERCP is an alternative diagnostic procedure and is preferred if the intrahepatic bile ducts are not obviously dilated on ultrasound and if blood coagulation is impaired.

Both techniques can be used to obtain histological or cytological material for diagnosis, to provide pre-operative drainage of a dilated biliary tree, to dilate biliary strictures and to insert stents across malignant obstructions. If ultrasound shows stones in the gall bladder and in a dilated bile duct, ERC has the distinct advantage that endoscopic sphincterotomy can be undertaken at the same time. This may allow immediate stone retrieval or later spontaneous passage of the stone(s) into the duodenum.

If ultrasound and ERC show that the extrahepatic biliary tree is normal, a liver biopsy will probably be the next investigation, especially if the jaundice shows no sign of settling spontaneously.

Liver biopsy

This is a relatively simple, but potentially dangerous, procedure which is of great value in the diagnosis and management of chronic liver disease. It allows the diagnosis of focal pathology, especially of primary and secondary malignancy.

It is advisable to undertake some scanning procedure (usually ultrasound or radio-isotope) before biopsy to assess liver size (especially if this seems to be small clinically) and to seek evidence of focal pathology. Ultra-

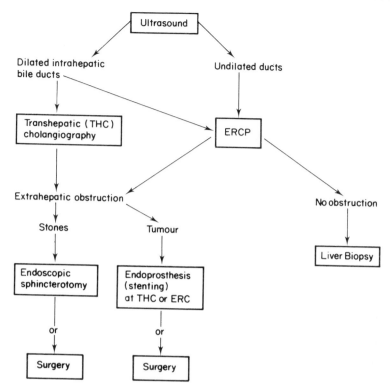

Figure 4.2 *Investigation and management of jaundice with obstructive features.*

sound-guided liver biopsy is advisable if an abnormal focus is to be sampled and is safer if the liver is unusually small or misshapen.

If the liver is thought to be diffusely abnormal, the standard percutaneous technique is used and the liver is approached through the right mid-axillary line over the middle of the area of liver dullness while the breath is held in full expiration (to bring the liver well up above the costal margin). Cutting needles (e.g. Trucut) or suction needles (e.g. Menghini) may be used.

The patient's coagulation function must be checked beforehand and any abnormalities corrected. It is advisable to have serum available for rapid cross-matching in the event of haemorrhage. The patient is kept under observation for 12–24 hours after the procedure in case there are complications.

There are no absolute contraindications to liver biopsy; but it may be impossible if coagulation problems cannot be overcome and it should not be undertaken in the presence of severe jaundice until extrahepatic biliary obstruction has been excluded – this is to obviate the risk of biliary peritonitis. Liver biopsy should be postponed until ascites has cleared.

Disorders of the oesophagus

Gastro-oesophageal reflux

Aetiology

Reflux occurs in us all and from time to time produces mild symptoms. Frequent and prolonged reflux is the result of relative incompetence of the lower oesophageal sphincter. This is more likely to occur if the sphincter lies above the diaphragm as a consequence of sliding hiatal herniation of the upper stomach. Aggravating factors include delayed gastric emptying and oesophageal motility problems which impair the clearance of refluxed gastric contents back into the stomach.

Symptomatic reflux is a very common problem and, in many patients, there is no obvious cause. Factors known to reduce lower oesophageal sphincter pressure include smoking, dietary fat, anticholinergic drugs and pregnancy (probably as a result of hormonal influences). Obesity and straining at stool are probable aggravating factors and may encourage hiatal herniation without directly affecting the competence of the lower oesophageal sphincter.

Pathology

In uncomplicated reflux there may be no macroscopic or microscopic abnormality of the oesophageal mucosa. However, oesophagitis is common in patients with more severe symptoms and is usually apparent endoscopically and, if necessary, confirmed histologically. Ulceration and stricture formation are seen in the most severe cases. There is still uncertainty about the interpretation of gastric metaplasia in the lower oesophagus. Extensive upward spread of the gastric lining is easy to recognize endoscopically (Barrett's oesophagus) and is usually associated with chronic severe reflux. It may be associated with focal peptic ulceration and probably· predisposes to the development of adenocarcinoma.

Clinical features

The usual symptoms are heartburn, reflux, odynophagia (pain on swallowing) and later obstructive dysphagia (see pages 135–136). Less common symptoms include small haematemeses, chronic occult blood loss and cough or wheeze caused by aspiration, especially at night. Physical signs are usually absent, but the patient may become anaemic from blood loss or wasted if there is dysphagia. Rarely there are tell-tale signs of systemic sclerosis (see page 251).

Diagnosis

This can be based on history alone and investigations are only required if there is doubt or if simple therapy is ineffective. Haematemesis, anaemia and dysphagia demand investigation. The relative merits of barium studies and endoscopy are discussed on page 143. The most sensitive diagnostic method is 24 h recording of oesophageal acidity using pH sensitive electrodes passed transnasally. Many systems now include portable monitors for storage of data and its subsequent retrieval and analysis by computer (ambulatory pH recording).

In general, barium studies will show the propensity to reflux (hiatal hernia and reflux of barium during screening) and complications, especially stricture. Endoscopy is required to assess the benign nature of a stricture and to clarify the source of bleeding.

The differential diagnosis is mainly from other causes of chest and epigastric pain. Differentiation from cardiac pain can be difficult and the Bernstein test is useful (see page 135). The site of pain can cause confusion with peptic ulcer and the two problems are common enough to coexist.

Complications

The most serious are peptic stricture, pulmonary aspiration and possibly cancer, especially in relation to Barrett's oesophagus.

Treatment

Some simple measures designed to reduce reflux are shown in Table 4.12.

Antacids are best taken in generous doses and in liquid form (10–20 ml) half to one hour after meals and before retiring. Alginate-containing preparations (Gaviscon and Gastrocote) are said to prevent reflux and provide a protective layer over the lower oesophageal mucosa.

H_2 receptor blockers (cimetidine, ranitidine) decrease acid production. They are certainly effective in relieving symptoms and reducing the severity of oesophagitis and should be used if simple antacid therapy fails. The need for their prolonged use should be regarded as a relative indication for anti-reflux surgery. Antacid and H_2 blocker therapy is discussed in more detail on page 153.

Metoclopramide and domperidone are dopamine antagonists, which accelerate gastric emptying and increase tone in the lower oesophageal sphincter. They relieve symptoms if taken before meals and before retiring, but may cause troublesome side-effects. This is especially true of the more centrally acting metoclopramide, which can cause distressing dystonias especially at

Table 4.12 Summary of medical management of gastro-oesophageal reflux

Reduce reflux	Weight reduction if obese
	Avoidance of straining at stool, bending at waist
	Elevation of head of bed (10–15 cm)
	Avoidance of smoking, fatty meals
	Avoidance of anti-cholinergic drugs
	Use of cholinergic drugs and dopamine antagonists
Reduce acid burden	Antacids
	Histamine (H_2) receptor blockers
Protect oesophageal mucosa	Alginate containing preparations (e.g. Gaviscon)

the extreme of age – the very young and very old. They tend to be especially effective if nausea is a troublesome symptom.

Treatment of peptic stricture

Strictures can be dilated mechanically in a number of ways, using endoscopic or radiological techniques. At endoscopy a guide wire is passed through the stricture and the scope is removed. Metal 'olives', hard rubber bougies or catheter-mounted balloons can be passed along the guide wire and through the stricture, preferably under radiological control. Dilation is usually carried out under sedation and local anaesthetic, but general anaesthetic is preferred by many surgeons and patients.

In elderly or frail patients, infrequent dilation may be a satisfactory long-term treatment, but in younger fitter patients, anti-reflux surgery should be advised in the expectation that this will prevent continued inflammation and recurrent stricture formation.

Surgical correction of reflux

The indications for surgery include chronic severe symptoms that are uncontrollable medically, the continued need for intensive medical treatment including H_2 blockers, and the development of a stricture.

The principle of surgery is to reduce hiatal herniation, to strengthen the diaphragmatic hiatus and to reduce the risk of recurrent herniation by some form of wrap of gastric fundus around the lower oesophagus. The many eponymous procedures attest to the lack of any clear superiority of one surgical method.

The major early complication of surgery is dysphagia and the inability to belch if the gastric wrap is too tight. This can usually be managed by dilatation and improves with time. Delayed recurrence of herniation and symptoms can occur, as with any form of hernia repair, and further attempts at surgery become more difficult and less likely to succeed.

Prognosis

This is good in the sense that most people respond well to medical treatment and this need not be continued indefinitely if the general measures referred to are adopted. Surgery in good hands is very effective treatment for the minority who need it. Modern dilatation techniques have improved the outlook considerably for those with strictures who are unfit for surgery. The risk of cancer seems to be very low, except perhaps in those with extensive gastric metaplasia (Barrett's oesophagus).

Carcinoma of the oesophagus

Aetiology

There are enormous geographical variations in the incidence of oesophageal cancer and it seems certain that environmental factors are largely responsible for this. In England and Wales there are approximately 4000 new cases per year or 8 per 100 000 of the population. In most cases there is no obvious explanation or recognized predisposing cause, such as chronic reflux oesophagitis, Barrett's oesophagus, achalasia or chronic iron deficiency with oesophageal web formation (*Plummer–Vinson syndrome*).

Pathology

The great majority of tumours arising in the mid and upper thirds of the oesophagus are squamous cell carcinomas. In the lower third, adenocarcinoma can arise from areas of gastric metaplasia but more commonly arises from the gastric fundus and spreads upwards. The tumours spread circumferentially and longitudinally and eventually invade locally.

Clinical features

The usual symptom is remorselessly progressive obstructive dysphagia. Pain can be produced by acute bolus obstruction or by local mediastinal spread of disease. Patients rapidly lose weight and often become anaemic from blood loss (usually occult). Metastases may be palpable in the cervical glands or in the liver.

Diagnosis

This is usually strongly suspected on barium swallow and confirmed by examination of endoscopic biospies and cytological brushings. The differential diagnosis is from benign strictures, usually caused by chronic gastro-oesophageal reflux and rarely by swallowed caustics.

Complications

Inanition and pulmonary aspiration are common. Tracheal involvement, invasion of the aorta and spread into the pericardium are relatively rare. Diagnostic or therapeutic intubation procedures may be complicated by perforation and bleeding.

Treatment

The only hope of cure of adenocarcinoma is radical surgery. Squamous cell carcinoma is radiosensitive, and radiotherapy is usually the preferred treatment for cancers arising in the upper third of the oesophagus. However, extensive oesophageal resection is feasible and a high anastomosis between the pharynx and the gastric fundus can be created in the neck.

In order to avoid fruitless surgery, it is helpful to assess operability with CT scanning and bronchoscopy.

Unfortunately, by the time of presentation most patients have inoperable tumours and only about 25 per cent of patients are suitable for surgical treatment. Palliation can be achieved by radiotherapy, but the morbidity is quite high. Most tumours are now treated palliatively by the insertion at endoscopy of short feeding tubes (endoprostheses) after initial dilatation. Again there is appreciable morbidity because the tubes can get blocked by food boluses or become dislodged and migrate into the stomach. There is considerable current interest in the use of laser photocoagulation of tumours at endoscopy. Lasers are particularly effective if there are large soft tumour masses within the lumen, and it is claimed that the quality of palliation is superior to that obtained by the placement of endoprostheses. The equipment for laser therapy is very expensive and is currently only available in a very few centres in the UK. There is no effective chemotherapy for oesophageal cancer.

Prognosis

This is very poor. Patients treated palliatively rarely survive more than a few months. Morbidity after surgery is high and mortality rates of around 30 per cent are recorded. Individual surgeons have achieved considerably lower mortality rates and there is much to be said for treating these patients in special units. Overall long-term survival after 'curative' surgery is approximately 45 per cent at one year, 20 per cent at two years and 10 per cent at five years.

Achalasia of the cardia

Aetiology

The cause of the primary neurological disturbance is unknown. A similar condition can complicate Chagas' disease, prevalent in South America, when the trypanosomal parasite damages the oesophageal nerve plexus extensively. The incidence of achalasia in the UK is approximately one case per 100 000 of the population per year.

Pathology

Ganglion cells are lost from the submucosal and myenteric plexuses at the lower end of the oesophagus. Eventually there is widespread nerve damage throughout the body of the oesophagus, which becomes progressively dilated over a period of many years. Chronic oesophagitis accompanies prolonged stagnation of food in a dilated oesophagus and may account for the small long-term risk of cancer.

Clinical features

There is usually a long history of variable dysphagia, eventually complicated by inanition in neglected cases. Regurgitation of stagnant food may produce pulmonary complications. Episodic severe chest pain is ascribed to uncoordinated muscular activity and tends to occur in the early phase of the disease ('*vigorous achalasia*').

Diagnosis

Barium swallow shows a relatively normal oesophageal contour initially and the characteristic dilatation and tortuosity only occur much later. Endoscopic appearances are normal in the early stages and the scope can usually be passed into the stomach quite easily, even though barium is held up at the tapered lower end of the oesophagus.

The abnormal motility of the oesophagus can be demonstrated by careful cineradiology while the patient swallows a bolus of food impregnated with barium. However, more accurate information is obtained by manometry, which is becoming increasingly available in specialized units. A multi-lumen tube assembly is passed via the nose into the stomach (this may prove to be difficult in achalasia) and then slowly withdrawn. Each lumen has an orifice through which pressures are measured and the orifices are placed 5 cm apart. In achalasia, there is a loss of co-ordinated peristalisis and the lower oesophageal sphincter fails to relax normally on swallowing.

The differential diagnosis is mainly from mechanical forms of dysphagia. Carcinoma can occasionally produce similar radiological appearance and manometry may fail if the assembly cannot be passed into the stomach. This has been called '*pseudo-achalasia*'. Vigorous achalasia has to be distinguished from diffuse oesophageal spasm.

Treatment

This is best achieved by the mechanical disruption of muscle fibres at the lower end of the oesophagus. This allows swallowing to occur by gravity but does not influence the disordered motor function of the oesophageal body. Heller's operation is a surgical myotomy in which the muscle is cut down to the submucosa. Various methods of forceful dilatation have been devised using air-, water- or mercury-filled balloons. There is a revival of interest in dilatation techniques, which are usually employed initially and, if successful, repeated as necessary. Myotomy can be performed if dilatation fails or is unacceptable to the patient.

Long-acting nitrates and nifedipine inhibit smooth muscle activity in the oesophagus and may provide some symptomatic relief, but mechanical methods of treatment are usually required.

The major complication of successful therapy is gastro-oesophageal reflux because the sphincter is disrupted. This can be severe because oesophageal clearance of refluxed material is grossly impaired. It may be necessary to undertake anti-reflux surgery later.

Diffuse oesophageal spasm

Aetiology

The cause of the disordered motility is unknown and the prevalence of this condition is uncertain.

Clinical features

There is episodic severe chest pain occasionally associated with dysphagia. Conventional barium swallow and endoscopy are normal, but cineradiology of swallowing may show disordered peristalsis, especially if the patient has symptoms at the time. Oesophageal manometry is abnormal and typically there is high-pressure uncoordinated activity. It may be possible to provoke this with an anti-cholinesterase drug such as edrophonium and reproduce the patient's symptoms at the same time. Normal relaxation of the lower oesophageal sphincter excludes achalasia.

The main differential diagnosis is from cardiac pain, especially if there is no obvious disturbance of swallowing.

Treatment

As with achalasia, long- or short-acting nitrates or nifedipine may be used to reduce muscular activity in much the same way as they are used in treating angina. For the occasional severe attack, some relief may be obtained by the sublingual application of glyceryl trinitrate in spray or tablet form or nifedipine as a crushed capsule. Response to treatment is difficult to evaluate or to predict, but most patients come to no harm especially if they are reassured that the symptom does not arise in the heart.

Cricopharyngeus spasm and pharyngeal pouch

Aetiology

The cause of the spasm is unknown, but the pouch arises as a pulsion diverticulum through the posterior gap between the oblique fibres of the inferior constrictor muscle and the horizontal fibres of cricopharyngeus.

Clinical features

There may be variable difficulty with swallowing, but most food goes down the right way, while some accumulates and stagnates in the pouch, which slowly enlarges to the left of the midline. Pouch contents will regurgitate from time to time and this may produce cough and pulmonary aspiration. Pouches may be palpable or visible in the neck and occasionally they can reach a large size and extend down into the mediastinum.

Diagnosis

This is by barium radiology with particular emphasis on the pharyngeal phase of swallowing. Endoscopy is potentially dangerous and the diagnosis may be suggested by difficulty in passing the 'scope into the oesophagus. The common *globus hystericus*, or sense of lump in the throat, is not clearly related to and may even be relieved by swallowing. This is usually a psychological problem. It may be caused by increased tone in the cricopharyngeus muscle, but muscular coordination during swallowing is normal.

Treatment

It is necessary to perform a myotomy of the cricopharyngeus muscle and to excise the pouch. Occasionally myotomy alone is successful if dysphagia is the dominant symptom and if the pouch is small (or absent).

Scleroderma (see page 251)

This rare multisystem disorder (systemic sclerosis) can slowly destroy the oesophageal musculature, which is replaced by fibrous tissue. Peristalsis becomes weak and eventually disappears completely. There is dysphagia and often troublesome reflux oesophagitis, because refluxed acid is not adequately cleared. Oesophageal strictures may occur. There is no specific treatment and nasogastric tube feeding may eventually be required.

Para-oesophageal hiatal hernia (rolling)

This uncommon form of hiatal herniation may be a chance finding on chest X-ray or at endoscopy or barium meal. Occasionally it may present acutely with severe chest pain and dysphagia if the herniated portion of stomach becomes twisted or strangulated. It is usually seen in older patients and probably does not cause chronic mild symptoms. If a patient has a large hernia and any difficulty with swallowing or reflux symptoms, then surgical treatment should be undertaken.

Gastroduodenal disorders

Peptic ulcer

Aetiology

A mucosal break in the stomach or proximal duodenum represents a temporary victory by offensive factors in gastric juice (especially acid and pepsin) over the defensive properties of the mucosa (production of mucus and antral and duodenal secretion of small amounts of bicarbonate). Reflux of duodenal contents into the stomach provides additional noxious agents (especially bile salts), which may be implicated in the development of gastritis and gastric ulcer. The overriding importance of acid is shown by the healing properties of strong anti-secretory agents and the absence of peptic ulcer in patients who fail to secrete acid (e.g. pernicious anaemia). However, most patients with peptic ulcer produce amounts of acid which are within the normal range, and anti-secretory agents do not heal all ulcers. Acid is necessary for ulceration, but impairment of mucosal resistance is clearly important, especially in patients with gastric ulcer who tend to have lower acid outputs than those with duodenal ulcer.

Genetic and environmental factors are responsible for the development of peptic ulcers but are largely unidentified. No certain noxious agents in food have been identified and it is possible that some foods have a protective role. There are striking geographical variations in the prevalence of peptic ulcers and in the distribution between gastric and duodenal types.

In the developed world, duodenal ulcer is commoner than gastric ulcer and occurs at a younger age. Gastric ulcer becomes relatively commoner in the elderly and the use of non-steroid anti-inflammatory drugs may account for an increasing admission rate for perforated peptic ulcer in elderly women, against a background of a sharp fall in admissions to hospital for peptic ulcer over the last 20 years. Part of this fall is due to improved medical management rather than to decreasing prevalence.

The prevalence of peptic ulcer is difficult to determine, because minor digestive disturbances are not investigated and ulcers may be asymptomatic. Moreover, ulcers come and go over prolonged periods. Prevalence rates of 6 per cent for men and 2 per cent for women in the London area were obtained 20 years ago and duodenal ulcer was 2–3 times commoner than gastric ulcer. The prevalence of peptic ulcer is higher in Scotland and the North of England than in the South. Although its prevalence and severity may be declining, peptic ulcer remains a common disease in the UK.

Smoking cigarettes is probably an aggravating and not a causative factor, and alcohol consumption has not been implicated in the pathogenesis of chronic peptic ulcer (as opposed to acute transient gastric damage).

The relationship between stressful life events and ulcer disease is unclear, but the stress of serious illness and injury is sometimes associated with acute gastric and duodenal ulceration ('stress ulcers').

Pathology

The lesions may be superficial or deep, large or small, single or multiple, acute or chronic. Common sites of chronic single ulcers are on the lesser curve, in the antrum, pyloric channel and first part of duodenum. Multiple ulcers tend to be acute, superficial and widely scattered over the gastric mucosa. The duodenal mucosa may be diffusely inflamed with many tiny superficial ulcers (duodenitis), and this pattern may coexist with a single chronic ulcer crater. Acute, multiple ulcers are related to acute gastric injury by drugs, alcohol and perhaps stress and are clinically quite distinct from the more common chronic ulcers. Most patients have either duodenal or gastric ulcers; but the two can coexist, in which case the gastric ulcer is usually situated in or close to the pyloric channel.

The histophathological features are not in any way

specific or distinctive. Chronic inflammatory changes are seen in the mucosa near gastric ulcers and various forms of intestinal metaplasia have been described.

Clinical features

The commonest symptom is pain and the main features have already been described (see page 137). Vomiting and weight loss are common with uncomplicated gastric ulcers. The major complications include the vomiting of pyloric stenosis, haematemesis and melaena and sudden perforation with peritonitis. Physical signs in the uncomplicated case are usually limited to epigastric tenderness.

Diagnosis

This depends on barium meal and/or gastroscopy, as discussed on page 143. Gastric ulcers should be biopsied to exclude malignancy, but this is not relevant to the management of duodenal ulcer. The differential diagnosis is wide and has been discussed in the section on investigating dyspepsia and abdominal pain (page 142). Zollinger–Ellison syndrome is described on page 156.

Medical management

1 General measures

These are summarized in Table 4.13. Smoking should be prohibited because ulcers heal more slowly in smokers than in non-smokers. Sensible eating habits should be encouraged, with regular meals and the avoidance of long periods without food. Symptoms may be relieved by milk and snacks, but there is no evidence that the once fashionable gastric diets (mainly steamed fish and milk) are of any real value in healing ulcers. Large volumes of milk combined with generous quantities of sodium bicarbonate or calcium carbonate were in the past responsible for hypercalcaemia and renal failure ('*milk–alkali*

Table 4.13 Summary of medical management of peptic ulcer

General measures	Avoidance of smoking, aspirin, non-steroid anti-inflammatory drugs, corticosteroids; 'sensible' eating habits
Antacids/anti-secretory agents	Histamine H_2 receptor blockers; selective anti-cholinergics (e.g. pirenzipine)
Mucosal protective agents	Sucralfate, De Nol (bismuth complex)

syndrome'), but this is rarely seen now with modern medical management. Prolonged bed-rest certainly accelerates healing but is rarely necessary.

2 Antacid therapy

This should be used first for symptomatic relief. To be effective in healing, large volumes of a soluble preparation have to be given one hour after meals and on retiring (e.g. 100–200 ml daily), but smaller doses will usually provide symptomatic relief and may be taken in tablet form. There are numerous preparations and many contain several compounds in order to improve palatability and reduce the risk of complications. In general, magnesium-containing antacids produce diarrhoea and could lead to magnesium intoxication in patients with renal failure. Aluminium-containing compounds tend to produce constipation and sequester phosphate in the gut, and they could lead to phosphate depletion (they are used for this purpose in patients with chronic renal failure). Calcium carbonate and sodium bicarbonate are seldom used now. Some antacid mixtures contain large amounts of sodium and should be used with caution in patients with heart failure and other causes of fluid retention. In view of all these problems and the availability of more effective and acceptable drugs, antacids are seldom now the main therapy for chronic peptic ulcer, unless symptoms are mild and intermittent.

3 Histamine-2 receptor blockers

The advent of cimetidine in 1976 revolutionized the treatment of peptic ulcer. This drug and its successors provide remarkably safe, simple and effective treatment of gastric and duodenal ulcers, but they remain relatively expensive and should be used with some circumspection. It is unnecessary to demand endoscopic assessment before prescribing these drugs, but their continued use over long periods (months) or their frequent use in shorter courses should be delayed until a diagnosis has been made. One worry in the older age groups is that these drugs may mask the symptoms of gastric cancer and lead to a delay in diagnosis.

It is usual to treat symptoms for a month or so with the full dose of cimetidine 400 mg b.d. or ranitidine 150 mg b.d. (there is evidence that a single night-time dose is as effective). The dose can then be halved to a 'maintenance' dose and this should be continued for a variable period by trial and error. Symptoms are often controlled within days, and 60–80 per cent of ulcers can be expected to heal completely within six weeks. Up to 80–90 per cent will heal if treatment is continued for 12 weeks, but healing rates are slower for gastric than for duodenal ulcers. Relapse rates are unfortunately high (probably more than 50 per cent over one year) after the treatment is withdrawn, but not all relapses are symptomatic or necessarily harmful to the patient, and symptomatic relapses can usually be controlled easily with another course of the drug.

The long-term treatment of duodenal ulcers with H_2 blockers is empirical and it is doubtful whether endoscopic follow-up is of much help in management. The management of a gastric ulcer is different, because endoscopic follow-up is required to ensure that the ulcer has healed and is not malignant (repeat endoscopy, biopsy and cytology at 6–8 weeks and again at 12–16 weeks if healing is slow), and because treatment is relatively less effective and alternative drugs are more likely to be required.

The choice of H_2 blocker is determined partly by cost and partly by consideration of the potential side-effects of cimetidine (Table 4.14). Ranitidine is the drug of choice for long-term use in males and for short-term use in patients taking drugs whose metabolism is impaired by cimetidine.

4 Mucosal protective agents

A number of drugs heal ulcers as effectively as H_2 blockers, without inhibiting acid secretion, and in various ways protect the mucosa. They can promote healing of ulcers, which fail to respond adequately to H_2 blockers, and this probably applies particularly to gastric ulcers. Their precise mode of action is uncertain. Two commonly used drugs are sucralfate (a complex of aluminium hydroxide and sulphated sucrose) and DeNol (a potassium citrate bismuth chelate), and current trials are in progress of orally administered prostaglandin derivatives. Sucralfate is given twice daily over 1–2 months and the only side-effect is mild constipation. DeNol is now given in tablet form, again twice daily and colours the stools black. It should not be used in long courses for fear of bismuth accumulation and is best avoided in renal failure. There is some evidence that relapse rates after withdrawal of these drugs are less than those observed after withdrawal of H_2 blockers.

Carbenoxolone is now rarely used because of its aldosterone like side-effects.

Table 4.14 Side-effects of cimetidine and ranitidine

	Cimetidine	Ranitidine
Impairs cytochrome p450 oxidase	Yes	No
Anti-androgenic	Yes	Probably no
Mental confusion	Yes	No
Arrhythmias	Yes	Rare, if at all

Surgical management of uncomplicated ulcer

The relative indications are continued distressing symptoms in spite of full medical measures and the continued need to take H_2 blockers if surgery can safely be offered as an alternative. Operation rates for peptic ulcer fell dramatically in the years following the introduction of cimetidine; but there is evidence of a renewed rise, perhaps reflecting an understandable reluctance to take medication indefinitely. Surgery tends to be offered when gastric ulcers fail to heal in a few weeks, but this reflects concern over the possibility of malignancy as well as the poorer prognosis of unhealed gastric lesions in terms of complications.

Surgery is designed to reduce gastric acid secretion. The older operations of partial gastrectomy, vagotomy and antrectomy were undoubtedly very successful, but at the expense of sometimes distressing side-effects. Vagotomy is better tolerated but has a higher rate of ulcer recurrence. A balance has to be struck between the risk of serious side-effects and the risk of recurrent ulcer, but the latter is probably preferable as recurrent ulcers may respond well to medical treatment. Highly selective vagotomy is theoretically the most attractive operation for duodenal ulcers, but recurrence rates as high as 20 per cent have been reported. Gastric ulcers can also be treated by this operation; but there has always been reluctance to leave a gastric lesion *in situ* (for fear of malignancy), and most surgeons still perform a limited gastrectomy with removal of the antrum and the more physiological Bilroth I anastomosis if the proximal duodenum is healthy.

Patients can reasonably expect a 90–95 per cent success rate in terms of complete or considerable relief of symptoms, but side-effects may be distressing (at least temporarily) in up to 5 per cent of patients. Table 4.15 shows the most usual symptoms following surgery. Vomiting may be part of the '*small stomach syndrome*' with post-prandial pain and fullness and early satiety.

Table 4.15 Symptoms after peptic ulcer surgery

'Small stomach syndrome'	Early satiety, food-induced pain and vomiting
Rapid transit of food into intestine	Early dumping syndrome; reactive hypoglycaemia; postvagotomy diarrhoea
Reflux of bile into stomach	Bile-vomiting syndrome
Impaired luminal digestion	Steatorrhoea
Long-term problems	Loss of weight; anaemia (Fe, B_{12} deficiency); osteomalacia

This usually responds simply to reducing the size and increasing the frequency of meals. A rarer but more distressing problem is bile vomiting which occurs particularly in patients who have a gastrojejunostomy. Copious vomiting of bile rather than food occurs after meals and is ascribed to the passage of large amounts of proximal duodenal contents through the gastric remnant. It can be very difficult to control and may occasionally justify a second bile-diverting procedure (especially the Roux-en-Y conversion). In well-selected patients, this can be very successful.

A change in bowel habit is common after all types of gastric surgery, but it is usually a mild increase in faecal frequency and bulk which may not be unwelcome to the patient. A modest degree of steatorrhoea is common, especially after gastric resection, and is not surprising in view of the gross disturbance of gastric emptying and the impaired mixing of food with pancreatico-biliary secretions. This can be helped, if necessary, by some restriction of dietary fat and occasionally by the use of pancreatic enzyme replacements (see page 174).

Severe watery diarrhoea, often intermittent, is an occasional complication of truncal vagotomy and pyloroplasty and is much less of a problem after highly selective vagotomy. The mechanism is unclear, but it seems to be related in some patients to the rapid transit of intestinal contents into the colon after meals. Under these circumstances, bile salts can be swept into the colon where they exert a direct cathartic effect. In approximately 50 per cent of these patients, the diarrhoea will respond well to the bile acid binding agent cholestryamine.

The term *'dumping syndrome'* is applied to two different physiological disturbances, which result from the rapid entry of gastric contents into the small intestine and the rapid absorption of carbohydrate. Early dumping occurs within 30 minutes of eating and is characterized by faintness, palpitations, abdominal distension and sometimes later fluid diarrhoea. Postural hypotension and temporary haemoconcentration may occur and suggest a shift of fluid from plasma into the gut lumen. Release of vasoactive materials from the gut may also produce vasodilatation. Treatment can be difficult and the usual advice is to reduce the intake of fluid with meals and to avoid sweet drinks and carbohydrate-rich foods, which would promote the osmotic attraction of fluid into the gut lumen. Hypoglycaemic symptoms may develop after a delay of 1–2 hours and result from excessive insulin release in response to rapid absorption of glucose from the gut. Again a relatively low carbohydrate diet and the avoidance of sweet drinks may prevent this symptom. Agents which delay gastric emptying and retard the absorption of carbohydrate (e.g. guar gum) may help to prevent both types of dumping problem.

Loss of weight is common after gastric resection but is less marked after vagotomy. It is usually caused by reduced food intake rather than by malabsorption and preoperative weight may never be regained. Iron deficiency anaemia is the commonest long-term nutritional deficiency seen after gastric surgery and responds well to inorganic ferrous salts. Vitamin B_{12} may eventually be malabsorbed as a result of chronic inflammation of the remnant of gastric mucosa with consequent loss of the capacity to secrete intrinsic factor (IF). Osteomalacia, due to vitamin D deficiency, is an occasional consequence of previous resection.

Complications

Acute superficial ulcers can bleed, occasionally profusely. Deep ulcers can bleed, often profusely, can perforate through the gut wall and can obstruct the pylorus or an operative stoma.

Acute upper gastrointestinal haemorrhage is a common emergency. The immediate priorities are to assess the severity of blood loss, to institute appropriate resuscitative measures, and then to find the source of the bleeding. Blood transfusion is required urgently to treat shock and is ideally monitored by measurement of central venous pressure. Blood should also be transfused if the Hb falls below 10 g/dl or if bleeding continues. Gastroscopy should be undertaken within 12–24 hours of admission, but after the patient has been resuscitated. No food or fluid should be given by mouth until the timing of endoscopy has been agreed; otherwise the patient can eat normally if the haemodynamic condition is stable.

Bleeding from multiple superficial ulcers usually settles spontaneously and rarely requires surgery. Intravenous cimetidine and continuous alkalinization of the stomach with two-hourly antacids may be helpful. Recurrent bleeding from a chronic ulcer crater is likely if endoscopy shows tell-tale features such as an adherent clot or the so-called 'visible vessel' – a pink or bluish bulge in the base of the crater. Such patients should be considered for emergency surgery or some form of electrocoagulation or photocoagulation therapy by laser if the facilities are available. Surgical or other intervention is probably advisable in the over-60s unless there is a really serious contraindication, because mortality is much higher in the older age groups. However, there is still considerable debate about the wisdom and timing of surgery in this common problem, and it is impossible to lay down firm rules. Relatively clear guidelines for surgery are the need to replace more than four units of blood and undoubted continued or recurrent bleeding, as judged by external blood loss or difficulty in maintaining the CVP (nasogastric tube aspiration is not very helpful and is best avoided). Intravenous cimetidine is probably of little use in stemming serious bleeding from a chronic crater but is widely prescribed.

Perforation of a deep ulcer crater usually presents with sudden severe pain and board-like abdominal rigidity. An erect chest X-ray will show free gas under the diaphragms. Treatment requires nasogastric aspiration, intravenous fluids and analgesics followed by surgery after appropriate resuscitative measures have been carried out. Perforations can close spontaneously, and nonoperative treatment is sometimes appropriate if there is delay in recognizing that a perforation has occurred.

Pyloric stenosis causes a characteristic form of vomiting with distinctive physical signs, which have been described. The patient may be wasted if the condition has been neglected and is often dehydrated and alkalotic. The typical biochemical disturbance is a low plasma chloride, a high bicarbonate and a raised pH and somewhat raised PCO_2. Fluid depletion leads to sodium retention in the kidneys at the expense of potassium and hydrogen ions. This may produce hypokalaemia and a paradoxically acid urine. Nasogastric aspiration, initially using a wide-bore tube and repeated lavage, will relieve gastric distress, and intravenous saline supplemented by KCl will usually correct the biochemical abnormalities quite easily. Endoscopic assessment can be undertaken after lavage has cleared the stomach of gross contamination by food. Treatment is usually surgical, although rarely relatively acute ulcers with much surrounding oedema will subside rapidly with medical treatment.

Prognosis

The prognosis of benign peptic ulcer disease is good in the sense that deaths are infrequent and diminishing and modern medical treatment is effective and improving. There is every chance that even more effective treatment will be available, with the advent of a new generation of drugs which can block acid secretion almost completely by proton pump inhibition (e.g. omeprazole).

Zollinger–Ellison syndrome (gastrinoma)

This rare condition is caused by a gastrin-producing tumour arising from islet cells of the pancreas. In over 50 per cent of cases the tumour is malignant and can metastasize, but the natural history is a long one. Gastric

secretion of acid is greatly increased and produces severe ulcer disease in the stomach, the duodenum and even in the jejunum. Chronic diarrhoea is common and may even be the presenting symptom. Ulcer complications are frequent and recurrent ulcer is invariable after all forms of surgery other than total gastrectomy. Very large dose of H_2 blockers (e.g. 2–5 g of cimetidine daily) may be required to control symptoms and reduce acid secretion.

The diagnosis should be considered in patients with ulcers involving the more distal duodenum, in patients with ulcers and diarrhoea, and in patients with recurrent ulceration after conventional gastric surgery, especially if further surgery is planned. Another clue might be the finding of hypercalcaemia because there is an association with hyperparathyroidism in type I multiple endocrine adenomatosis. The most important diagnostic step is to measure the fasting serum gastrin, which is usually grossly raised. Tests of gastric acid secretion should also be undertaken – a very high basal acid output (above 15 mmol H^+/h) is the most characteristic abnormality. It is advisable then to search for tumour with appropriate scanning techniques in case resection can be undertaken. Otherwise treatment consists of large doses of H_2 blockers or the removal of the end-organ (i.e. total gastrectomy).

Gastric cancer

Aetiology

Adenocarcinoma of the stomach accounts for almost 10 per cent of all cancers in the UK, although its incidence is declining. There are approximately 28 male and 19 female deaths from this cancer per 100 000 of the UK population annually. Mortality rates are lower in the USA and much higher in Japan and other parts of the Far East. It is almost certain that dietary carcinogens play a crucial role in pathogensis. Epidemiological evidence from Japan has implicated highly salted food as a causative factor. Genetic factors are also important as shown by studies of family history.

Certain chronic gastric lesions predispose to cancer and include the atrophy of pernicious anaemia and some types of intestinal metaplasia associated with chronic gastritis and benign gastric ulcers.

Pathology

Adenocarcinomas arise in all parts of the stomach. They are usually single, spreading lesions, which grow into the lumen, infiltrate the wall and penetrate beyond its confines. The term early gastric cancer is applied to lesions confined to the mucosa and submucosa and which, if resected, can carry a remarkably good prognosis. It is clearly important to try to recognize this lesion, but the clinical, radiological and even endoscopic features may be minor. Unfortunately gastric cancer is often recognized at an advanced stage when there has already been metastatic spread to local and distant lymph nodes and to the liver.

Clinical features

The usual symptoms are epigastric pain, nausea and anorexia in a patient over the age of 55, and the history is short. A high fundic lesion can cause obstructive dysphagia and a distal antral lesion may obstruct the pylorus and produce vomiting. Loss of weight and anaemia are common. Physical signs include wasting, palpable metastases in the neck or liver and occasionally a palpable gastric mass.

Diagnosis

This depends on barium meal and gastroscopy with biopsy and cytology. The major differential diagnosis is between a benign gastric ulcer and a flat ulcerating malignancy and histological examination is crucial. A rarity is a gastric lymphoma, which may carry a better prognosis if treated with appropriate chemotherapy.

Complications

These are bleeding and obstruction. Chronic loss of protein-rich fluid from the mucosal surface can produce marked hypoalbuminaema and present as oedema.

Treatment

The best (but small) hope of cure is radical surgical excision. This may necessitate total gastrectomy if the lesion is in the mid or upper third of the stomach. Preliminary CT scanning helps to determine operability and may reduce the need for fruitless laparotomy. If the lesion is judged to be inoperable, palliative surgery may still be worth while, especially to by-pass an obstructing antral lesion. Resection of a tumour may occasionally be justified, even if metastases are present, in order to relieve distressing gastric symptoms, anaemia or protein loss.

Non-surgical palliation is very limited in its scope. Conventional radiotherapy is ineffective, but some success has been achieved with fast neutron irradiation.

There is no established chemotherapy programme, although multicentre trials continue in many parts of the world.

Prognosis

This remains poor and patients rarely survive more than a few months unless radical resection is possible. Fewer than a third of patients are suitable for 'curative' resection and, of those, five-year survival figures are 30 per cent or less. By contrast, resection of early gastric cancer produces an 80 per cent chance of surviving five years or more.

Other gastric lesions

Chronic gastritis

This is an endoscopic and histological diagnosis and its symptomatic significance is uncertain. It can be induced by duodenogastric reflux (e.g. postoperatively) and the excessive and continued use of alcohol, aspirin, spicy foods, etc., is often implicated but without good evidence. Current interest relates to the possible role of infection with a campylobacter-like organism now called *Campylobacter pyloris*. The main significance of chronic gastritis is its probable relation to the development of gastric ulcer and cancer.

Autoimmune destruction of the specialized gastric mucosa of the body and fundus is the basis of pernicious anaemia (see page 360).

Benign tumours of the stomach

These are rare and include adenoma and leiomyoma. They are usually chance findings but may bleed and cause anaemia if the surface is ulcerated. They require removal at endoscopy or by surgery, unless they are very small, because both types can become malignant.

Menetrier's disease

This is a rare condition of unknown cause in which there is massive hypertrophy of the non-specialized part of the gastric epithelium. The mucosa becomes grossly folded or polypoid in appearance and histological differentiation from multiple adenomatous polyps requires deep biopsies at endoscopy. The presentation is with pain and hypoalbuminaemic oedema – it is a well-recognized cause of protein loss from the mucosa (protein-losing gastropathy). Treatment is by surgical excision, although self-limiting cases have been described. There is probably an increased risk of later adenocarcinoma.

Disorders of the small intestine

Coeliac disease
(Gluten-sensitive enteropathy, coeliac sprue)

Aetiology

This a diffuse enteropathy, which affects the proximal small intestine more than the distal and is caused by a sensitivity to dietary gluten. Gluten is the water-insoluble protein found in wheat, barley, rye and oats but not in rice. The condition probably starts when wheat-based foods are introduced after the baby is weaned from milk. Transient sensitivity to gluten has been described in infants; but in true coeliac disease the sensitivity is life-long although clinical presentation can be remarkably variable and delayed. Acquired sensitivity in later life has never been described. The mechanism of gluten sensitivity remains uncertain but is thought to involve local cell-mediated immune responses in the intestinal mucosa.

The disease is far commoner in the developed world than elsewhere, the highest recorded prevalence being in the UK (1 in 2000) and in the west of Ireland (1 in 500 or even less).

Genetic factors are undoubtedly important as shown by family studies and a well-established association with the genetic marker HLA-B8.

Pathology

The jejunal mucosa becomes relatively or completely flat with loss of villi, deep crypts and a marked cellular infiltrate into the lamina propria. The enterocytes (mucosal absorptive cells) are flattened, lymphocytes infiltrate the mucosal surface and there is evidence of increased mitotic activity in the crypts.

Clinical features

It is rare to see patients with severe steatorrhoea and malnutrition. However, diarrhoea and steatorrhoea may be prominent, anaemia is common and the patients are often underweight. Infants and young children are characteristically miserable and pot-bellied. Older children fail to grow normally and their development is delayed. There is a tendency for symptoms to improve in later

adolescence but problems can develop again at any age.

Adults usually present with anaemia or bowel symptoms in their twenties or thirties. They tend to be thinner and shorter than the rest of their family, but may be perfectly well developed. Osteomalacia, owing to vitamin D deficiency, is an unusual presentation.

Diagnosis

This depends on jejunal biopsy (see page 145). Important indications for jejunal biopsy include evidence of mixed deficiency anaemia and folate depletion (page 360). Indeed, the folate status (serum and red cell levels) is probably the best screening test for coeliac disease, even in the absence of overt anaemia. Hyposplenism, as shown by Howell–Jolly bodies in the red blood cells, is a well-recognized but unexplained feature of coeliac disease.

The differential diagnosis is from other causes of anaemia and malabsorption as discussed on page 145. Histological differentiation from other forms of enteropathy may be difficult, and the biopsy may have to be repeated after periods of gluten challenge or gluten withdrawal.

Complications

These tend to occur in older adults (after many years of continuous gluten exposure) and include benign ulceration, strictures and small intestinal lymphoma. There is an increased risk of adenocarcinoma of the small intestine (an otherwise rare tumour) and curiously also of carcinoma of the oesophagus. It is uncertain whether prolonged avoidance of dietary gluten will prevent these complications.

Treatment

This involves strict dietary exclusion of gluten and should ideally be encouraged for life. Many gluten-free products are available on prescription and patients can bake their own bread using gluten-free flours. The Coeliac Society provides patients with useful dietary and other advice. Anaemia should be corrected with iron and/or folate as appropriate. Vitamin B_{12} deficiency is rare in coeliac disease because the lower ileum is usually not involved. Vitamin D therapy will be required for symptomatic osteomalacia.

The patients often feel better quickly (within weeks or even days), but improvement may be slow and perseverance is needed. It is important to repeat the jejunal biopsy after approximately six months to ensure that the histological abnormalities are improving. In most patients the mucosa will return completely to normal and this proves that the diagnosis is correct. Persistent diarrhoea may be helped in the early stages by milk exclusion, because lactase levels are often very low in the grossly abnormal mucosa (secondary hypolactasia, see page 146).

It is unusual to meet patients who fail to respond symptomatically and histologically to a gluten-free diet. In such patients it is necessary to ensure strict dietary compliance and to exclude the complications listed above by small gut radiology and, if appropriate, laparotomy. Corticosteriod therapy will produce rapid symptomatic benefit and histological improvement in coeliac disease even if the patient continues to eat gluten. It is justified if the patient is making poor progress on a gluten-free diet alone.

Prognosis

This is usually excellent if the patient adheres to the diet, but unfortunately the long-term risk of lymphoma and carcinoma remains. The magnitude of this risk is uncertain but is probably less than 10 per cent.

Dermatitis herpetiformis

This chronic, distinctive itchy rash is closely associated with coeliac disease. Approximately 70 per cent of patients have a jejunal mucosa which is indistinguishable from that of coeliac disease. Gluten restriction will allow the mucosa to heal and the skin lesions may also improve or disappear. It is curious that overt malabsorption and anaemia are rare in patients and many prefer to continue normal diet, because the skin lesions can usually be controlled more readily by dapsone therapy. The risk of malignancy is similar to that of coeliac disease.

Tropical sprue

Aetiology

This is an enteropathy, which involves the jejunum and ileum and is probably caused by abnormal bacterial activity in the intestinal lumen. It is endemic in parts of India, the Far East and the Caribbean and can be acquired by those travelling through these areas. The term 'temperate sprue' has been applied to a similar but milder illness acquired during travel through less tropical places such as the Middle East and Northern India. Malnutrition and parasitic infestation of the small intestine can produce mucosal abnormalities leading to diarrhoea and malab-

sorption. This makes an exact definition of tropical sprue difficult, if not impossible, and it is unlikely that a single cause will be identified.

Pathology

There is blunting and thickening of the villi, which are usually short and irregular, but which rarely disappear completely. The lamina propria is heavily infiltrated with chronic inflammatory cells.

Clinical Features

The disease may present acutely and occur in epidemics. More commonly the illness is chronic with diarrhoea, steatorrhoea, anorexia, weakness and loss of appetite. Loss of weight and anaemia are common and folate depletion occurs in a few weeks. Diagnosis depends on jejunal biopsy, and the different diagnosis is from other forms of chronic enteropathy (see page 145).

Treatment

Folic acid replacement and broad-spectrum antibiotics (e.g. tetracycline) are usually given in combination with success. Vitamin B_{12} malabsorption occurs, but deficiency is rare because of the large stores in the liver.

Prognosis

This is usually good and, in most patients returning from the tropics permanently, full recovery can be expected.

Whipple's disease

This very rare disease is caused by a bacillus which invades the small intestine and other parts of the body (for example the heart and brain). The intestinal mucosa is diffusely abnormal and the lamina propria is packed with large macrophages full of material which is stained by the periodic acid Schiff reagent (PAS-positive). Electron microscopy shows that this material consists of bacterial bodies, but the organism has not yet been cultured and identified.

The disease typically affects older men who present with the symptoms of chronic malabsorption and who often, in addition, have lymphadenopathy and polyarthropathy. The condition, which used to be invariably fatal, does respond to protracted antibiotic therapy.

Giardiasis

A number of chronic infections can damage the small intestine and lead to diarrhoea and malabsorption, but the only one that is at all commonly seen in the West is that caused by *Giardia lamblia*. Less common organisms are becoming increasingly recognized as causes of chronic diarrhoea and malabsorption, especially in patients with impaired immunity (e.g. *Campylobacter*, *Strongyloides* and *Cryptosporidium*).

Aetiology

Giardia lamblia is a flagellate protozoan which infests the upper intestine and can cause variable inflammatory changes in the mucosa, occasionally as severe as that seen in coeliac disease. The encysted form is passed in the faeces. Infection is acquired from contaminated food and water and is endemic in many parts of the tropical and sub-tropical world and in parts of Eastern Europe and the USSR.

Clinical features

The usual symptoms of any chronic mild malabsorption are present — steatorrhoea, weight loss and usually anorexia and malaise. Diagnosis may be revealed by the presence of cysts in a faecal sample, but this is not always reliable. Aspiration of duodenal or jejunal juice is more reliable because the flagellate forms can be recognized easily by direct microscopy of suitably stained fluid. It is advisable to take a jejunal biopsy at the same time, because the organism can be identified in conventionally prepared histological sections and may also be seen by examining smears of the mucosal surface.

Treatment

Metronidazole is the drug of choice and is usually given in a dose of 1200 mg daily for 7 days or 2 g daily for 3 days; side-effects are common with the higher doses. Resistance is unusual and other drugs are available including tinidazole and mepacrine.

Prognosis

Response to therapy is usually excellent but recurrent infections can occur in travellers. Patients with immunological abnormalities (for example, congenital and acquired immunoglobulin deficiencies) are prone to recurrent episodes of infection even in the absence of foreign travel and will need repeated courses of antibiotic therapy.

Tumours of the small intestine

These are all rather rare and will not be discussed in detail. They can obstruct the lumen by intussusception and can bleed and usually require surgical resection. Benign polyps are usually hamartomatous (e.g. Peutz–Jeghers syndrome) or adenomatous and may accompany colonic polyposis (see page 168). Adenocarcinoma is rare and may complicate coeliac disease (page 158) and Crohn's disease (page 161). Ileal carcinoid tumours are less rare and, although potentially malignant, have a long natural history. Their main importance is the propensity for large metastatic masses in the liver to produce the carcinoid syndrome (page 192).

The small intestine may be involved in abdominal Hodgkin's disease and non-Hodgkin's lymphoma, but the lymph nodes and spleen are the major sites of abdominal disease. Focal or diffuse intestinal lymphoma is usually a complication of coeliac disease (see page 158), but it does occur as a primary phenomenon, especially in parts of the Middle East and North Africa where it is the commonest recognized cause of chronic malabsorption.

Mediterranean lymphoma and alpha-chain disease

Aetiology

This diffuse lymphomatous process is thought to be a sequel to recurrent or chronic gut infections or infestations. It occurs in parts of the world where gut infection and malnutrition are common, but seems to be associated more with subtropical than tropical areas. Accurate figures of prevalence are not available.

Pathology

There is diffuse mucosal and submucosal infiltration with lymphocytes, plasma cells and histocytes and variable distortion and destruction of the villous architecture.

Clinical features

There are the usual clinical features of chronic malabsorption, often with finger clubbing, loss of weight and a downhill course over several months. Laboratory tests are non-specifically abnormal, but may reveal high concentrations of isolated heavy chains of IgA in the serum if sought by immunological methods. This variant is usually referred to as alpha-chain disease. Small bowel radiology is focally or diffusely abnormal without specific features, and the diagnosis is based on jejunal biopsy or on histological material obtained at laparotomy.

Treatment

In the early stages broad-spectrum antibiotics may be helpful or even curative, suggesting that gut bacteria are in some way responsible for initiating the illness. Once the disease becomes established, chemotherapy is required as for other lymphomatous conditions. Surgical excision is not feasible because the disease involves much of the small intestine, but radiotherapy has been used with some success in advanced disease.

The prognosis is generally regarded as poor even with aggressive chemotherapy, but accurate follow-up data are not available.

Disorders of intestinal motility

Apart from the common types of 'functional' diarrhoea and abdominal pain (see irritable bowel syndrome, page 168), disorders of structure impairing motility are uncommon; they include jejunal diverticulosis, scleroderma, diffuse infiltrative disorders such as amyloidosis, and strictures caused by focal ischaemia as in the various forms of vasculitis. Intestinal transit can be sluggish in untreated coeliac disease (see page 158) and is often abnormal in Crohn's disease (page 161).

The major consequences of impaired intestinal transit are chronic pain, abdominal distension and, often, malabsorption resulting from overgrowth of colonic type bacteria in dilated upper intestine. The diagnosis is based on small bowel radiology and treatment is often unsatisfactory. Strictures or short lengths of diseased intestine are best treated by surgical resection. If the intestine is diffusely abnormal, surgery is not feasible; treatment with broad-spectrum antibiotics is often effective but may be required on an indefinite and empirical basis. Intestinal bacteria have numerous metabolic effects on food residues and can damage the intestinal mucosa. Most notably they interfere with the absorption of vitamin B_{12} and deconjugate bile acids and thus impair the absorption of fats and fat-soluble vitamins.

Chronic non-specific inflammatory bowel diseases

The above term conventionally refers to Crohn's disease and ulcerative colitis. It is convenient to consider them together because there are points of similarity although many notable differences. They are both diseases of unknown origin, affect mainly young adults, produce considerable chronic morbidity but relatively little mortality and are treated empirically with a variety of medical and surgical methods. The management of these two disorders forms a considerable part of gastroenterological practice (medical and surgical) throughout Northern Europe and North America. In many other parts of the world, they are considered to be uncommon or even rare.

Crohn's disease

Aetiology

There have been numerous speculations about infective agents and immunological responses to food or bacterial antigens in the gut lumen. The distinctive histology has led to much interest in the possible role of atypical mycobacteria, and a specific myocobacterial infection in cattle is known to cause a similar chronic granulomatous disorder of the small intestine.

Although environmental factors must be of great importance, genetic factors are also important as shown by family studies and the prevalence of the histocompatibility antigen HLA B27. There is a genetic association with both ulcerative colitis and with ankylosing spondylitis.

Prevalence rates vary in different parts of the developed world. In the UK there are 25–35 cases per 100 000 of the population with an annual incidence of new cases of 2–5 per 100 000.

Pathology

The disease can affect all parts of the GI tract including the mouth and, very commonly, the anus. The typical lesion is focal mucosal oedema often with a cobblestone appearance accompanied by linear ulcers or fissures. Superficial aphthous ulcers may represent the first phase of the disease. There is a great tendency for abnormal intestine to adhere to other intestinal loops and to the abdominal wall. Large inflammatory masses are often produced and may become infected with gut organisms to produce abscesses. Fistulae commonly form between segments of small and large bowel, in the perianal region and with bladder, vagina and skin.

The commonest sites of involvement are the lower ileum and the right side of the colon. Extensive colitis is, however, well recognized although the rectum may be relatively spared.

Histologically there is deep submucosal, patchy chronic inflammation with relative preservation of the surface layer of mucosal cells. Granulomatous collections of lymphocytes and histocytes, sometimes with giant cells, are the most distinctive feature but are by no means always present.

Clinical features

These are variable and depend on the site of involvement and the age of the patient. Abdominal pain is the most common symptom and bowel disturbance, with predominant diarrhoea, is usual but not invariable. Loss of weight and in childhood failure to grow are common features, and there are often a variety of other nutritional disturbances including anaemia and hypoalbuminaemia. Physical examination may reveal abdominal masses and tell-tale signs at the anus, especially thick skin tags, induration of the anal canal, chronic anal fissure and evidence of present or past perianal sepsis.

In fewer than 10 per cent of cases there may be present or past evidence of various extraintestinal manifestations, including acute monarthritis or oligoarthritis affecting major joints, acute iritis, erythema nodosum and a distinctive necrotizing lesion on the legs and feet called pyoderma gangrenosum. Sacroiliitis is occasionally evident clinically as pain and tenderness over these joints, and the patient may have ankylosing spondylitis. These features are all shared with ulcerative colitis and are usually associated with extensive colonic rather than small intestinal involvement.

Small intestinal disease can present acutely with intestinal obstruction. Diffuse small intestinal disease is relatively uncommon but can produce all the features of chronic malabsorption. Small-gut strictures can cause chronic partial obstruction and bacterial overgrowth in the upper small intestine.

Diagnosis

This is based on small and large gut radiology, which defines the extent of the disease and shows the distinctive focal, ulcerating lesions, strictures and fistulae. Histological diagnosis is obtained by endoscopy of the large bowel or by surgical resection, especially of focal small intestinal lesions.

Differential diagnosis

Acute ileal Crohn's disease may be confused with an acute self-limiting ileitis caused by *Yersinia enterocolitica*. This illness resembles acute appendicitis and may be strongly suspected at laparotomy if the ileum is red and thick and the regional lymph nodes are inflamed (acute mesenteric adenitis). The ileum should not be resected, although a normal appendix can be safely removed, because the disease should remit spontaneously or with appropriate antibacterial therapy (e.g. gentamicin or tetracycline). The diagnosis is usually confirmed by finding a rising titre of antibodies in the serum, although a positive faecal culture is sometimes obtained.

Extensive Crohn's colitis may be difficult to distinguish from ulcerative colitis, especially if the rectum is involved. Right-sided colitis and ileitis can be caused by mycobacterium tuberculosis, and so this must be borne in mind in patients from the underdeveloped world and especially the Indian subcontinent. There may be evidence of pulmonary involvement on chest X-ray, and characteristic histology can be obtained by endoscopic biopsy although bacteriological culture often fails. Stool examination for mycobacteria is fruitless. Diagnosis of tuberculosis commonly depends on histological examination of resected gut.

Rectal and anal disease may require differentiation from the various specific infections in this area (e.g. chlamydial proctitis, lymphogranuloma venereum and rectal schistosomiasis). However, most patients with anal fissures and perianal sepsis have no underlying chronic inflammatory bowel disease.

Complications

These are numerous and include obstruction (common), abscess formation (common) and severe bleeding (rare). Free perforation into the peritoneal cavity is distinctly unusual. Toxic dilatation of extensively diseased colon, with risk of perforation, has been described but is much less common than in ulcerative colitis.

Treatment

The management of Crohn's disease is summarized in Table 4.16. Corticosteroids are the most effective medical weapon and should be used if the patient is 'toxic' (for example, obviously unwell, with fever, with tachycardia,

Table 4.16 Summary of the management of Crohn's disease

Nutritional support if underweight or anorexic

Correction of specific nutritional deficiencies, especially anaemia

Relief of symptoms (e.g. with analgesics, anti-diarrhoeal agents)

Anti-inflammatory drugs (e.g. corticosteroids),
   sulphasalazine (in colonic disease),
   metronidazole (especially for perianal sepsis),
   azathioprine (especially for its 'steroid-sparing' effect),

Surgery (drainage of abscesses, relief of obstruction, resection
   of all or most of the disease)

or losing weight) and has features of active inflammatory disease (inflammatory mass, anaemia, high white blood cell count and ESR, active joint, skin or eye disease). In such patients it is imperative to ensure that the illness is not caused by a septic complication rather than by the primary disease itself. The diagnosis of intra-abdominal or pelvic abscess can be very difficult in Crohn's disease and may be facilitated by the use of ultrasound and various isotopic techniques (e.g. the use of labelled leucocytes).

Symptoms often recur after an initially good response to a standard course of corticosteroids as the dose is reduced or after the drug is withdrawn. In these patients, continuous low-dose treatment may be required (e.g. 5–10 mg of prednisolone daily or 10–20 mg on alternate days) and the effective dose may be less if simultaneous treatment with azathioprine (2 mg/kg) is given.

Sulphasalazine (as used in ulcerative colitis) is a moderately effective anti-inflammatory drug for the less ill patient with predominantly colonic disease. Metronidazole is probably as effective as salazopyrine but is less well tolerated as long-term treatment. It has particular value in the treatment of serious perianal disease, especially if complicated by sepsis.

Surgical treatment is reserved for the treatment of complications, because it is never curative. Common procedures are drainage of abscesses and resection of short segments of small intestine causing obstruction or fistulation. Defunctioning ileostomy or colostomy allows distal disease to settle and is occasionally indicated in the management of large inflammatory masses and of severe perianal disease. Gut continuity can be restored later, although disease activity is likely to increase afterwards.

Patients with complicated disease are often ill and malnourished and frequently require nutritional support in the form of sip supplements, nasogastric or intravenous feeding according to tolerance and the severity and extent of small intestinal involvement. The use of low-residue liquid diets or, in sicker patients, intravenous feeding, will allow distal disease to settle with relief of symptoms and sometimes closure of fistulae.

Major colonic resection for extensive colitis, with or without ileorectal anastomosis, is justified in patients with poorly controlled symptoms and little or no small gut involvement. Ileostomy losses of fluid, electrolytes and nutrient are greater than after comparable operations for ulcerative colitis and can pose major problems of management.

Extensive small gut resection is complicated by diarrhoea, steatorrhoea and other features of malabsorption. After ileal resection, vitamin B_{12} absorption is impaired and long-term replacement therapy is often required. Bile salt malabsorption produces watery diarrhoea which will usually respond to cholestyramine (4–16 g daily) if the colon is relatively healthy.

Prognosis

There is much morbidity and most patients require some form of surgery, which may have to be repeated over the years. Nevertheless, long periods of relatively good health are possible and deaths directly attributable to Crohn's disease are infrequent. Actuarial analysis does, however, show that the mortality rate in patients with Crohn's disease is approximately twice than in suitably matched control subjects.

Ulcerative colitis (UC)

Aetiology

This is unknown but genetic factors are involved as discussed on page 161. Many infective agents produce an acute illness morphologically indistinguishable from acute ulcerative colitis, and it may be that some cases of so-called UC are in fact self-limiting specific colonic infections. However, typical UC is a chronic disease, although it is tempting to speculate that it can be initiated by specific infections.

Prevalence rates are higher than those of Crohn's disease and are relatively stable at 80–100 cases per 100 000 of the population in the UK. Annual incidence rates are 5–15 per 100 000. As with Crohn's disease, UC is seldom recognized in parts of the world where specific gut infections are very common.

Pathology

UC typically affects the rectum and spreads proximally to involve part or all of the colon. It is a diffuse, superficial inflammation which damages the mucosal cells on the surface and lining the crypts. The disease often remains localized to the distal third of the colon or to the rectum (*proctitis*). In severe extensive disease, the inflammation may spread more deeply and damage or destroy parts of the muscle wall. This leads to dilatation of the colon and the threat of perforation.

All these changes are non-specific and the diagnosis of UC is only established by exclusion of specific infections and by the passage of time.

In active superficial disease, ulceration is often inapparent macroscopically. In severe, chronic disease with deeper inflammation, there may be extensive areas of ulceration with islands of surviving mucosa, often heaped up into pseudopolyps.

Premalignant changes in the mucosal cells may be found in longstanding chronic, extensive disease and there is a serious risk of local and later invasive adenocarcinoma (see page 167).

Clinical features

The typical symtpoms are bloody diarrhoea and crampy abdominal discomfort relieved by defaecation. Pain is seldom severe. In severe, acute illness the patient may rapidly become dehydrated, anaemic and weak. Marked faecal frequency, fever and tachycardia with abdominal tenderness and, sometimes, distension indicate the need for urgent admission.

Most attacks are less severe and tend to come and go without obvious explanation. There may be a precipitating factor such as stress, an infection or perhaps the use of antibiotics or analgesics. Attacks are usually brought under control or settle spontaneously within a few weeks and there may be long periods of good health.

Patients with distal UC, and especially proctitis, often have marked faecal frequency and bleeding but little faecal material is passed and hard faecal masses can accumulate in the healthy colon above (proximal constipation). The patient is seldom ill, but may become anaemic.

Diagnosis

This is usually apparent at the initial examination with the rigid sigmoidoscope. The mucosa is bright red and may be oozing blood, especially if it is scraped gently with the instrument. In proctitis, healthy mucosa will be seen proximally. The lumen usually contains blood, mucopus and a variable amount and consistency of faecal material depending on the extent and severity of the disease. Luminal contents should be sampled for urgent bacteriological examination in an acute severe attack.

The extent of the disease is assessed by flexible endoscopy and barium enema as discussed on pages 143–144. It is, however, dangerous and unnecessary to undertake these examinations in the acute, severe attack and the required information can be obtained from an abdominal X-ray. This often shows the extent of disease quite clearly, indicates the presence of solid faeces and whether the colon is dilated.

Differential diagnosis

This is usually from acute specific colitis, although in more chronic disease the differential diagnosis from extensive Crohn's colitis can be difficult. Proctoscopy will differentiate haemorrhoids from distal proctitis.

Faecal material and, if present, pus must be examined bacteriologically for salmonellae, shigellae and campylobacters and microscopically for *Entamoeba histolytica*. In patients recently treated with antibiotics, the faeces should also be examined for *Clostridium difficile* and its toxin and occasionally the macroscopic appearances of *pseudomembranous colitis* will be seen, with patchy inflammation and adherent white plaques. Antibiotics commonly incriminated include lincomycin, clindamycin, ampicillin and other broad-spectrum agents.

Rectal biopsy should be undertaken particularly in cases where the macroscopic abnormality is atypical or mild. Indeed, obvious microscopic abnormality has been described in some patients with diarrhoea and normal endoscopy ('microscopic colitis'). It is not clear whether this is a variant of UC, but the symptoms may respond to anti-inflammatory drugs.

Complications

The major complication of the acute, severe attack is colonic dilation followed by perforation. Profuse colonic bleeding, sufficient to produce shock, is very rare. Colonic cancer is a long-term risk (see page 167). The extraintestinal manifestations of the disease, affecting especially the joints, skin and eyes, are mentioned in relation to Crohn's disease on page 161.

Various forms of hepatobiliary disease may complicate UC and are less frequently associated with Crohn's disease. These include pericholangitis, sclerosing cholangitis and cholangiocarcinoma (see page 172).

Treatment

Topical and systemic corticosteroids provide most effective treatment for the acute attack. Sulphasalazine (Salazopyrin) is a weaker anti-inflammatory drug and is particularly indicated for the long-term prevention of acute relapses of the disease. Azathioprine is best reserved for its steroid-sparing effect and is much less commonly required in UC than in Crohn's disease.

Supportive treatment includes the use of faecal bulking or softening agents (see page 138) in patients with distal colitis and proximal constipation and the correction of iron deficiency anaemia. Anti-diarrhoeal agents should be avoided in the severe, acute attack for fear of masking symptoms and, possibly, precipitating colonic dilation. Non-steroidal anti-inflammatory drugs and antibiotics can aggravate or precipitate colitis and should be used sparingly or avoided. There is no evidence that dietary factors are important, but a low-residue diet is usually considered prudent in patients with severe diarrhoea, whereas a high-residue diet may prevent proximal constipation. Milk exclusion may help a very small minority of sufferers, but whether this relates to previously unrecognized lactase deficiency or is a true 'allergic colitis' remains unclear.

Most attacks of colitis can be handled on an outpatient basis, with a course of topical steroids for disease confined to the left half of the colon or of oral prednisolone for more extensive disease. Liquid enemas of various prednisolone preparations (e.g. Predsol, Predenema) are self administered at night for a few weeks until bleeding and diarrhoea stop. A foam preparation of hydrocortisone (Colifoam) is a convenient alternative, which many patients prefer. A typical course of oral prednisolone would start at around 30 mg (approximately 0.5 mg/kg) reducing by 5 mg every two weeks over the next 6–10 weeks, or faster if the symptoms are controlled rapidly. Topical and systemic steroids should be withdrawn completely if the attack is brought into complete remission as judged both by symptoms and endoscopic appearances. The minority of patients with chronic, grumbling disease may require low-dose alternate-day steroid therapy (enemas or tablets) for prolonged periods, but this is uncommon and colectomy would probably be a preferred alternative.

Sulphasalazine is usually started during the acute attack and then continued for a prolonged period in the hope of maintaining a remission. Unfortunately side-effects are common, especially with the usually recommended doses of 2–3 g daily, and it is advisable to start with a lower dose. Common problems are dyspepsia (which may be averted by using an enteric-coated preparation), headache and skin rash. More serious side-effects are haemolytic anaemia (with Heinz bodies in the red cells), impairment of folate metabolism, agranulocytosis and, rarely, widespread erythema multiforme. Reversible infertility in the male is a recently recognized side-effect. These are attributed to the sulphapyridine moiety of the drug, and new preparations of 5-aminosalicylic acid (e.g. mesalazine) can now be prescribed to patients who are intolerant of sulphasalazine. It is uncertain for how long sulphasalazine should be taken after the last attack; periods of one or two years are recommended and the drug should be withdrawn empirically after that. Recurrent attacks would then indicate the need for indefinite treatment.

The acute, severe attack of UC should be managed in hospital with intravenous corticosteroids in a dose of at least 60 mg daily of prednisolone or equivalent. A light diet may be taken if there are no serious abdominal signs and no evidence of colonic dilation on X-ray. However, in most cases it is preferable to give all the fluid and electrolyte requirements intravenously. Transfusions of blood and albumin are often needed to correct anaemia and hypoalbuminaemia respectively. Unless the attack settles very rapidly (within 48 hours) the next step would be to start intravenous feeding using a centrally placed feeding line. Most patients will improve markedly during 5–7 days of intensive treatment of this sort, but close observation is essential and must include daily abdominal X-ray to detect colonic dilation. Failure to improve, the development of serious abdominal signs and dilation of the colon (transverse colon diameter more than 5.5 cm) are the usual indications for urgent colectomy (see below). However, if the response is favourable and rapid, the patient should be able to resume normal eating and drinking after 5–7 days; prednisolone can be then given orally in a dose of 40 mg daily, reducing later to 30 mg and less according to progress.

Surgery

This is required for the acute, severe attack which fails to respond to the above measures, and for chronic unremitting symptoms especially if most or all of the colon is involved. A less common indication is the finding of premalignant changes in the mucosa during long-term surveillance for cancer (see page 167).

Total colectomy is always required, as lesser resections are invariably followed by recurrent disease in the remaining colon. In the acutely ill patient, the rectum is left behind in order to minimize risks. In the otherwise fit patient, the colon and rectum can be removed as a one-stage panproctocolectomy with permanent ileostomy. In recent years, there has been much interest in alternatives to the conventional, incontinent ileostomy which requires a permanent bag. Those include the so-called continent ileostomy and, more recently, various forms of ileo-anal anastomosis with the creation of a neorectum from several adjacent loops of ileum.

Ileostomy after colectomy is usually very well tolerated once the patient learns how to use the bag and care for the skin. Specially qualified stomatherapy nurses provide invaluable care and advice. The major risk is of salt and water depletion because relatively large volumes of fluid are lost (500–1000 ml/day). Patients should be advised to take extra water and salt in very hot weather and during temporary bouts of diarrhoea. There is a long-term risk of uric acid stones in the renal tract, because of the passage of relatively small volumes of concentrated urine.

Prognosis

This is good, provided that acute attacks are treated effectively and that colon cancer is prevented. Patients at risk of cancer are those with chronic disease affecting all or most of the colon for eight or more years, especially if symptoms have been frequent and troublesome during this period.

These patients should have annual colonoscopy with multiple biopsies. The finding of early cancer or severe dysplasia (if confirmed) should lead to total pan-proctocolectomy, with every hope of cure or prevention.

Long-term survival in ulcerative colitis is only slightly less than that of suitably matched controls.

Other disorders of the large intestine

Diverticular disease

Aetiology

Diverticula are very common throughout the developed world in the older age groups. They are thought to result from a low-fibre diet associated with slow colon transit and high intraluminal colonic pressures. There is evidence that the disease is becoming commoner in parts of the less developed world where people have adopted the Western low-fibre diet. Current changes in the Western diet towards more fibre and less refined sugar may reduce the prevalence of the disease in the future.

Prevalence figures based on barium enema and necropsy vary considerably, but in the Western World fewer than 5 per cent of people aged below 40 have diverticula, whereas more than 30 per cent of those aged 60 and above are affected.

Pathology

The disease affects the sigmoid and descending colon particularly, but all parts can be involved. The affected segments show marked hypertrophy of the circular layer of colon muscle. The pouches are formed by pulsion through tiny defects in the circular muscle and gaps where major blood vessels penetrate and emerge between the longitudinal taeniae on the anti-mesenteric surface of the colon.

In uncomplicated disease no other pathological process is evident, but acute inflammation may ensue and lead to abscess formation, fistulation or free perforation. Chronic narrowing of the lumen, especially of the sigmoid colon, is common.

Clinical features

The condition is commonly silent and is often found by chance. The most common symptoms are those of colonic pain and altered bowel habit as described on page 137. The patient tends to constipation with small, misshapen, bitty stools. There are often short episodes of diarrhoea, but prolonged painless diarrhoea should never be attributed to diverticula. Bleeding is uncommon, but rarely can be severe and demands exclusion of other pathology.

In acute diverticulitis there is continuous pain, tenderness, fever and a mass can often be felt in the lower abdomen or pelvis. Abscess formation is accompanied by severe illness with a swinging pyrexia, and perforation by the rapid development of peritonitis. Fistulation can present with pneumaturia, recurrent urinary infections or the passage of faeces per vagina.

Diagnosis

This is by barium enema examination. Flexible endoscopy tends to underestimate the extent of the problem and can be difficult if the sigmoid lumen is very narrow and tortuous. In patients with acute symptoms, both procedures should be avoided for fear of aggravating the inflammation and producing a perforation. If there is marked local tenderness or a mass, an ultrasound exam-ination will help to decide whether an abscess has formed and, in difficult cases, an isotope-labelled white cell scan may be helpful.

Differential diagnosis

The symptoms in uncomplicated disease are very similar to those of the irritable bowel syndrome (see page 168), but the latter is common in the under-40s and should not be diagnosed in the older age group without full investigation. Localized disease, especially in the sigmoid colon, can coexist with adenocarcinoma or Crohn's disease. If the barium enema is at all equivocal, flexible endoscopy and biopsy should be carried out.

The common mistake is to ascribe symptoms to diverticula, when the fault lies elsewhere, simply because they are so common.

Treatment

Symptomatic, uncomplicated disease usually responds to a high-fibre diet supplemented if necessary by faecal bulking agents and anti-spasmodics, as discussed on page 169 in relation to the irritable bowel syndrome.

Acute diverticulitis is treated with broad-spectrum antibiotics, such as ampicillin, and will require intravenous fluids and bed-rest in hospital if the patient is ill with serious abdominal signs.

Perforation is an acute emergency, which requires resuscitation, surgical drainage of the peritoneal cavity and the creation of a defunctioning colostomy. Fistula formation can only be treated by resecting the affected segment of colon, and the anastomoses may require protection by a temporary defunctioning colostomy.

In general, resection of a segment of colon for diverticular disease should only be undertaken if there are or have been serious, well-documented complications. Chronic colonic pain and bowel disturbances are not usually cured by local resection.

Prognosis

This is excellent in most cases. However, chronic symptoms can be difficult to treat, and acute complications threaten life and may require multiple operations with all their attendant risks.

Adenoma and adenocarcinoma

Aetiology

Bowel cancer is one of the commonest cancers in the developed world. The annual incidence in the UK is about 30 per 100 000 of the population.

It is thought that many cancers arise in adenomas, which can be present in the colon for years beforehand. Other precancerous lesions include chronic ulcerative colitis (see page 163), familial polyposis coli (page 168), colonic schistosomiasis and possibly Crohn's colitis.

Genetic and environmental factors are important, but poorly defined. Dietary factors, especially fat, have been implicated by epidemiological studies. Bile salts are cocarcinogens in experimental colon cancer and have been much studied in the human disease.

Pathology

Adenomas can arise anywhere in the colon and are frequently multiple. Probably 70 per cent arise distal to the splenic flexure. There are commonly polypoid and may have long stalks. Malignant change and invasion can be impossible to determine unless the whole adenoma is removed from its stalk. Malignant transformation is rare until adenomas are more than 2 cm in diameter.

Adenocarcinoma arises more often in the left than the right half of the colon, and about 50 per cent of all bowel cancers are to be found in the rectum. They are ulcerating or fungating growths which later penetrate the bowel wall, invade local structures and spread more widely. The famous Dukes' classification of tumour spread is widely used in relation to prognosis (Table 4.17). Because adenomas are often multiple, it is not uncommon for several primary adenocarcinomas to arise in one colon, both simultaneously and after an interval of many years.

Clinical features

Adenomas are commonly symptomless but may ulcerate and bleed or, if large and pedunculated, can intussuscept or even appear at the anus.

Adenocarcinoma in the left side of the colon presents with blood loss (overt or occult), with altered bowel habit and with colonic or rectal pain. Right-sided cancer tends to be more silent and presents typically with iron-deficiency anaemia and, less commonly, with chronic pain. There may be a palpable abdominal or rectal mass and the liver is commonly involved by metastatic disease.

Table 4.17 Dukes' classification of large bowel cancer

Stage A	No spread beyond muscularis mucosa
Stage B	Spread beyond muscularis but no lymph nodes involved
Stage C	Spread to regional lymph nodes or beyond

Diagnosis

A barium enema will usually show typical or suspicious features of cancer, but the sigmoid colon can be very difficult to examine and the caecum and ascending colon are often contaminated by faeces. Endoscopic examination and biopsy are required to confirm the diagnosis, to determine the distribution of any adenomas and to exclude additional primary cancers.

Adenocarcinoma has to be distinguished from diverticular disease, in the sigmoid colon especially, and on the right side may be mistaken for inflammatory lesions such as Crohn's disease and tuberculosis. A further differential diagnosis is from the various forms of colonic polyps, which are summarized in Table 4.18. Histological clarification is essential.

Complications

These are obstruction, especially of the colon by left-sided cancers, and less commonly perforation and severe, acute bleeding. Untreated rectal cancer can penetrate widely within the pelvis, invading the bladder and vagina and causing intractable pain.

Treatment

Adenomas can usually be removed by electrocautery at colonoscopy if they are pedunculated and small. Larger, sessile lesions can be removed piecemeal at several sessions but much skill and care is required. It is essential to destroy the stalks and bases of larger adenomas to ensure that no malignant or premalignant tissue remains.

Adenocarcinoma is treated by wide surgical excision of bowel along with the mesenteric lymph nodes. Continuity of the bowel can often be restored at a one-stage operation, unless there has been a complication such as obstruction or perforation. Cancers in the lower half of the rectum used to be treated by total proctectomy and permanent colostomy and this may still be necessary if the lesion is very low. The newer stapling devices have enabled surgeons to perform much lower rectal anastomoses in recent years, with relative ease and safety and without impairing the prognosis.

The adjuvant roles of chemotherapy and radiotherapy are still being assessed in multicentre clinical trials. Inoperable carcinoma has a very poor outlook, but useful palliation can sometimes be achieved by laser therapy at endoscopy if the facilities and skills are available. Resection should, however, always be undertaken if feasible, even in the presence of obvious metastases in lymph nodes or liver, because of the appalling consequences of leaving untreated tumour behind.

Prognosis

The prognosis of adenomas is good provided that they are excised when still small and that the whole colon is subjected to regular and complete endoscopic surveillance (every 2–5 years).

The prognosis of adenocarcinoma depends on its spread at the time of excision and on the histological grade of malignancy. Current UK figures relating five-year survival to the Dukes' classification are as follows:

Stage A	80–100 per cent
Stage B	60–70 per cent
Stage C	25–35 per cent

Polyposis coli

This is a confusing suject which is summarized in Table 4.18. Most serious are the adenomatous polyps because of the high risk of cancer. The others are important to recognize, because they can be confused with adenomas and give rise to unnecessary alarm. They can all bleed and, if multiple, can cause disturbance of bowel function.

Familial polyposis coli has autosomal dominant inheritance. Polyps develop at 20–40 years of age and families must be screened for asymptomatic cases. Established cases should be treated by total colectomy at an early stage if cancer is to be avoided. If the rectum is not removed, endoscopic surveillance and cautery of recurrent polyps are required. *Gardner's syndrome* is a rare variant where polyposis is associated with osteomas, sebaceous cysts, abnormalities of the teeth and soft tissue tumours.

Irritable bowel syndrome (IBS)

Although the symptoms are mainly colonic, this should be regarded as a disorder affecting all parts of the gut. It

Table 4.18 Classification of intestinal polyps

Type	Solitary form	Multiple form
Neoplastic	Adenoma	Familial adenomatous polyposis coli
Hamartomatous	Juvenile polyps	Peutz–Jeghers syndrome (mainly small gut)
Inflammatory	Benign lymphoid polyps	Pseudopolyposis in colitis

can be defined as the association of abdominal pain with bowel disturbance in the absence of any structural disease and can thus be distinguished from other disorders of function such as non-ulcer dyspepsia, 'simple' constipation and painless chronic diarrhoea. Clearly such a definition is quite arbitrary but it is useful in practice.

Aetiology and prevalence

Symptoms of this sort are remarkably common and studies of the 'normal' population reveal that up to 30 per cent of subjects have symptoms of this type quite frequently but most do not complain (fortunately!). In gastroenterological clinics at least 50 per cent of all new patients have no evidence of organic disease and many will be diagnosed with more or less confidence as IBS.

The cause is unknown and often assumed to be entirely psychological. Episodes can be provoked by all the usual stresses of life and a minority of patients are or will become overtly depressed. It is not uncommon for there to be many other symptoms such as migraine, vague and variable problems with breathing and swallowing, palpitations and other features of anxiety.

The possibility that symptoms are caused by intolerance of certain foods has received much recent attention. Such intolerance is unlikely to be caused by true allergy and IBS patients are not notably atopic.

Typical IBS symptoms can follow acute gut infections, such as amoebic dysentry, and can coexist with those of chronic disease, which may act as trigger factors (e.g. ulcerative colitis).

Clinical features and diagnosis

The pain can occur anywhere in the abdomen or in the flanks (Fig. 4.3). Careful history taking and inspection of the stools may be required to clarify the true nature of the

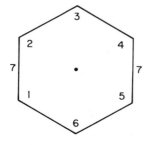

Figure 4.3 *Sites of pain in the irritable bowel syndrome. Mimicry: (1) appendix, ovarian problems; (2) gallstones; (3) peptic ulcer; (4) gas in stomach; (5, commonest site) diverticular disease; (6) uterine problems; (7, flanks) lumbar, renal problems.*

bowel disturbance. Most patients present in early or middle adult life and often have a history going back to adolescence or childhood.

Examination is often negative, but common findings include a thickened, tender colon in the left iliac fossa, small bitty stools on digital examination, marked spasm of the lower colon on endoscopy, and excessive haustration of the left colon on barium enema. Inflation of the colon with air at endoscopy may reproduce the patient's symptoms accurately.

How far the patient is investigated depends on how typical the symptoms are, the patient's age and the duration of the problem. A patient presenting over the age of 40 for the first time must have at least a rigid sigmoidoscopy and barium enema. In younger patients, loss of weight or anaemia should raise the suspicion of Crohn's disease and lead to fuller investigations.

The differential diagnosis is from diverticular disease and colon cancer in the older age groups and from Crohn's disease in the younger. The less typical variants shown in Fig. 4.3 have a wide differential diagnosis.

Complications

These may arise as a result of overzealous and inappropriate investigations or treatment, including the risks of unnecessary surgery. In a small minority, serious depressive illness may be overlooked, with a remote risk of suicide.

Treatment

The first phase is reassurance, explanation and encouragement. It is important to come to a decision, offer a diagnosis and treat. Confidence is lost if investigations continue to be requested or if other opinions are sought.

The second phase is to try to improve bowel habit and this usually means giving advice about a high-fibre diet if the patient is constipated or has the typical 'spastic' bowel habit. If this is unsuccessful, faecal bulking agents (see page 138) are often helpful. Anti-diarrhoeal agents should be avoided unless the patient has continuous watery diarrhoea without pain. If these measures improve bowel function but do not relieve pain, colon anti-spasmodics should be prescribed such as mebeverine and anticholinergic drugs (e.g. propantheline, dicyclomine). The latter, however, are likely to produce side-effects, especially dryness of the mouth.

Most patients will respond more or less completely to these simple measures. An interview with an interested psychiatrist may be very helpful in the small minority of subjects who are extremely difficult to treat.

Exclusion diets should not be recommended unless the patients can be closely followed by a doctor or dietitian with special interest and expertise. Their use remains controversial at present.

Prognosis

Symptoms are likely to recur over many years and probably fewer than 50 per cent of sufferers ever go into complete remission. However, the majority learn to live and cope with their symptoms and few suffer from any permanent disability.

Disorders of the biliary tract

Gallstones

Aetiology

Most gallstones are composed of cholesterol and relatively small amounts of inorganic salts and organic debris (mucus, desquamated cells etc.). A minority (about 10 per cent) contain enough calcium salts to be opaque on an abdominal X-ray. In patients with chronic haemolytic anaemia, the main ingredient of the stones is calcium bilirubinate and they are almost black in colour.

Cholesterol stones develop when the concentration of cholesterol in gallbladder bile is high relative to the concentrations of bile acids and phospholipids, which normally keep cholesterol in solution. Bile acids are the end products of cholesterol metabolism in the liver, and subtle alterations of this metabolic pathway have been demonstrated in the livers of patients with gallstones. Stasis and infection of gallbladder bile are usually secondary to gallstones but may encourage their further growth.

Gallstones are extremely prevalent, and associated factors include the female sex, increasing age, obesity and parity. Ultrasound studies in asymptomatic subjects suggest that they occur in more than 10 per cent of women over the age of 40 and they are common incidental findings at post mortem. Other risk factors include drugs, such as clofibrate and oestrogen-containing contraceptives, some hyperlipidaemic states and ileal resection.

Pathology

Gallstones are found primarily in the gallbladder and commonly migrate into the biliary tree where they can cause many complications. They rarely arise *de novo* in the bile duct unless that is chronically obstructed. The stones are often multiple and can reach a very large size.

Acute and chronic inflammatory changes in the gallbladder and biliary tree are secondary to obstruction by gallstones. The gallbladder wall is commonly thickened by both fibrosis and muscular hypertrophy and the mucosa can be extensively damaged or destroyed.

Clinical features

The typical symptom of uncomplicated stones is the pain of biliary colic (see page 137). It is unwise to ascribe the common flatulent dyspepsia and fat intolerance to stones in the absence of other evidence. Biliary colic, although commonly felt over the gallbladder, may spread across the abdomen or chest and may last intensely for long periods (hours) in spite of the name. The essential clues are great severity and intermittent discrete attacks.

Other symptoms are those of complications and include obstructive jaundice with or without cholangitis (see page 146) and acute pancreatitis (page 172). Acute cholecystitis is associated with marked local tenderness, guarding and fever. It can be complicated by secondary infection with pus formation (empyema of the gallbladder) and septicaemia. The patient is very ill with high fever and marked tenderness over the gallbladder.

Diagnosis

This is made by ultrasound or oral cholecystography in the uncomplicated case (see page 143). In acute cholecystitis, the cystic duct is usually obstructed and this can be revealed by a gamma camera following the injection of a radiopharmaceutical (e.g. HIDA), which is taken up by the liver and secreted into bile.

The differential diagnosis is from the many causes of severe abdominal pain, dyspepsia and jaundice already discussed.

Complications

These are summarized in Table 4.19. Fistulation can lead to calculous obstruction of the ileum (gallstone ileus). Adenocarcinoma of the gallbladder is uncommon but almost always arises in a chronically diseased gallblader.

Treatment

The conventional treatment is cholecystectomy with, if appropriate, exploration of the bile duct.

Current medical treatment is suitable for patients who

Table 4.19 Complications of gallstones

Acute cholecystitis Empyema of gallbladder }	Superadded infection
Obstructive jaundice Cholangitis Acute pancreatitis }	Stone passing through CBD
Fistulation into small gut Adenocarcinoma of gallbladder }	Rare

have relatively small, non-opaque stones in a well-functioning gallbladder, as defined by oral cholecystography. Treatment consists of the long-term (1–2 years) use of oral bile acids (chenodeoxycholic acid or ursodeoxycholic acid), which expand the bile acid pool and enhance the solubility of cholesterol in bile. This treatment is suitable for a minority of patients with gallbladder problems, especially those who have uncomplicated disease and who are frail or unfit for surgery. There is a continuing search for new agents that can dissolve stones safely and more rapidly. One such agent monoctanoin, can be infused through a surgically created T-tube over stones retained in the common bile duct. Moderate-sized gallstones (10–15 mm diameter) can dissolve in 7–10 days.

Stones in the bile ducts are, however, more commonly treated now by endoscopic sphincterotomy, as mentioned on page 146. In skilled hands, this is a safe and effective procedure and is particularly indicated in patients who have already had a cholecystectomy. Ascending cholangitis is an urgent indication for this procedure.

Acute cholecystitis may be treated conservatively with intravenous fluids, nasogastric suction, pain relief and antibiotics followed later by elective cholecystectomy when the inflammation has settled. However, many surgeons consider that early cholecystectomy is safe and preferable . Empyema of the gallbladder demands urgent drainage, often by cholecystotomy alone in a frail elderly patient.

Prognosis

The complications of gallstones are a major threat to health and life, especially in the elderly. However, more than 50 per cent of subjects with asymptomatic stones will probably suffer no serious consequences and prophylactic cholecystectomy is not recommended. Adenocarcinoma of the gallbladder has a low prevalence and is usually disregarded in considering the wisdom of cholecystectomy for stones. When it does occur it tends to be diagnosed late and carry a poor prognosis. However, early cancer may be found incidentally at cholecystectomy for stones and the outlook is then much better.

Sclerosing cholangitis

Aetiology

This uncommon disorder is being increasingly recognized since the advent of ERCP. It is usually associated with ulcerative colitis (much less often with Crohn's disease) and may also occur as part of a more widespread chronic, inflammatory, fibrosing process affecting especially the retroperitoneal tissues and mediastinum. The cause is unknown.

Pathology

There is diffuse or patchy chronic inflammation with fibrosis affecting all or most of the extrahepatic biliary tree and spreading along its intrahepatic branches.

Clinical features

The features are those of chronic obstructive jaundice which may be complicated by cholangitis. In early cases there may be episodes of cholangitis with long periods of apparently good health, but liver function tests will be persistently abnormal.

Diagnosis

This is now made by ERCP (see page 143) or other forms of direct cholangiography, which show irregular narrowing and dilatation of the biliary tree. The differential diagnosis is from all other types of obstructive jaundice and, if the lesion is focal, from cholangiocarcinoma which may coexist.

Treatment

Corticosteroids are often tried but are usually ineffective. Cholangitis is treated by suitable antibiotics. Symptomatic treatment includes the use of cholestyramine for itching and a low-fat diet for steatorrhoea and the appropriate use of fat soluble vitamins as in primary biliary cirrhosis (see page 184). Surgical treatment is often disappointing and, in severe cases, liver transplantation may be the only hope of prolonged survival.

Prognosis

This is generally regarded as poor, because treatment may be impractical or ineffective and because there is a long-term risk of cholangiocarcinoma (see below). However, the condition is being increasingly recognized at an early stage owing to the more widespread use of ERCP in patients with inflammatory bowel disease and persistently abnormal liver function tests. It seems that the natural history is one of very slow progression over many years.

Cholangiocarcinoma

Aetiology

This is a relatively rare tumour arising from the epithelium of the biliary tract. The best recognized association is with sclerosing cholangitis and inflammatory bowel disease, but it is also described in patients suffering from chronic infestation of the biliary tree with the liver fluke *Clinorchis sinensis* prevalent in the Far East.

Clinical features

The patient presents with obstructive jaundice, which may be complicated by cholangitis. Diagnosis is by direct cholangiography and by obtaining material for cytology and histology. This may be possible by the transhepatic route or during ERCP, but is often only feasible at surgery.

Treatment

Surgical excision is worth attempting if the lesion is the common bile duct. A low lesion near the ampulla will require a Whipple's resection of the head of pancreas and duodenum (see page 175). A high lesion arising in the hepatic ducts near the porta is very difficult to treat surgically, but may be managed by some form of dilation and 'stenting' (i.e. placement of an internal drainage tube) using the transhepatic or endoscopic approach.

Prognosis

Progression of the tumour is relatively slow and spread is usually local. Some patients will survive for up to two years even after palliative treatment alone. However, median survival times are only about six months and attempts at curative surgery are well worth while, especially if the lesion is at the lower end of the common bile duct.

Functional disorders

Intermittent abdominal pain, suggesting biliary colic with negative investigations, is sometimes ascribed to disturbances of the sphincter of Oddi (biliary dyskinesia) or to probably innocent anatomical abnormalities of the gallbladder (e.g. adenomyomatosis, cholesterolosis). Biliary pressures can now be measured at ERCP and there is evidence that intermittent papillary obstruction does occur. It is tempting to remove an anatomically abnormal gallbladder (without stones) or to undertake endoscopic sphincterotomy in these patients, but such treatment is often ineffective and carries its own risks. Many of these patients have the 'hepatic flexure syndrome' variant of the irritable bowel syndrome and should be treated accordingly (see page 168).

However, since functional disorders of the gut are so common, it seems probable that subtle disturbances of biliary function can produce a variety of digestive complaints.

Disorders of the pancreas

Acute pancreatitis

Aetiology

See Table 4.20. The best recognized cause is reflux of bile into the pancreatic duct secondary to the migration of stones through the bile duct. An alcoholic binge rarely

Table 4.20 Causes of pancreatitis

Gallstones, especially acute and recurrent acute

Alcohol, especially chronic and chronic relapsing

Other
    virus infections (e.g. mumps)
    hyperlipidaemia
    hypercalcaemia
    drugs (e.g. azathioprine, some diuretics)
    secondary to pancreatic cancer
    haemochromatosis (chronic pancreatitis)
Trauma

induces an attack but can produce an acute relapse of chronic pancreatitis. The other associations listed in the table are poorly understood and in many patients no clear explanation is found. Specific infections, especially with the mumps virus, are well-recognized but rare causes of severe disease. Trauma is an occasional cause and severance of the main duct can produce major complications.

Pathology

The pancreas is acutely inflamed and sometimes severely haemorrhagic. Full recovery of structure is possible after a moderately severe, uncomplicated attack. Typically there is widespread 'fat necrosis' of the omentum and mesentery — white plaques that are thought to be formed by the deposition of calcium salts of fatty acids, liberated by the local action of lipase.

In severe attacks, there can be extensive necrosis and sloughing of pancreatic tissue with secondary infection and abscess formation. Enzymes leaking into the peritoneal lesser sac and beyond may produce a chemical peritonitis with accumulation of fluid rich in pancreatic enzymes ('pancreatic ascites'). More localized leaks of pancreatic juice in and near the pancreas lead to the formation of *pseudocysts* which, unlike true cysts, are not lined with an epithelium but simply by adjacent tissues and later by a firm fibrous wall.

Clinical features

This is usually an acute abdominal crisis of considerable severity. Typical pancreatic pain (see page 137) develops often quite suddenly after a rich meal or a drinking bout and is accompanied by sweating, vomiting and later by vascular collapse and shock in a severe case.

Examination reveals marked abdominal tenderness with guarding, especially in the epigastrium, and later distention and ileus. A severe attack may be marked by bruising in the left flank. Hypoxia and dyspnoea may occur as part of respiratory distress syndrome caused by increased permeability of pulmonary capillaries.

Diagnosis

The cardinal investigation is the measurement of amylase or other pancreatic enzymes in the serum. Amylase levels rise rapidly in the first few hours of the attack and fall slowly over the next few days. Serum amylase is occasionally raised in diabetic ketosis and in perforated peptic

ulcer, but rarely to the levels seen in acute pancreatitis. The levels may be misleadingly low in patients with acute replases of severe chronic pancreatitis.

Having made a diagnosis, the cause should be sought and this will include investigation of the biliary tree. In most cases this is undertaken by ultrasound when the attack has settled and, in recurrent disease, by direct cholangiography. ERCP should be avoided in or soon after acute pancreatitis because it may produce a recurrence or introduce infection into a pseudocyst. It is useful in recurrent disease to define the anatomy of the pancreatic duct (in case surgery is required) and, particularly, to exclude stones in the common bile duct.

The differential diagnosis is from all the other causes of the acute abdomen, but especially from perforation and infarction of bowel in view of the severity of the clinical presentation.

Complications

See Table 4.21. Pseudocysts, ascites and left pleural effusions are quite common. Pancreatic necrosis and sloughing are rarer. Severe bleeding can occur into the duodenum if major arteries are affected by local inflammation and necrosis.

Treatment

This is supportive and as yet no specific therapy has been shown to be effective. The usual measures are nasogastric suction, intravenous fluids and parenteral analgesics. Hypoxia should be looked for and treated by continuous oxygen therapy. Oral fluid and food are not allowed until pain and abdominal signs subside and gastric aspirates decline. Hypotension requires the infusion of plasma expanders and CVP monitoring. Blood transfusion may be required for anaemia secondary to extensive haemorrhage. Transient hypocalcaemia and hyperglycaemia often require correction. Antibiotics are not given routinely but will be required if features of abscess or septicaemia

Table 4.21 Complications of acute pancreatitis

Hypotension $\longrightarrow$ Renal failure
Pulmonary alveolar damage $\longrightarrow$ shock lung
Pleural effusions
Pseudocysts
Pancreatic ascites
Pancreatic necrosis/abscess
Metabolic
   hyperglycaemia
   hypocalcaemia

develop. Renal failure may require temporary haemo-dialysis. Pseudocysts, ascites and abscesses should be drained, and it is now usually possible to do this per-cutaneously under ultrasound control. Surgery is usually reserved for very ill patients who have extensive pancreatic necrosis or inadequately drained abscesses. It is necessary to remove all necrotic tissue and leave wide drainage tubes in the pancreatic bed.

Prognosis

The disease carries an appreciable mortality and figures vary from 5 to 20 per cent. The course can be slow with much morbidity, but ultimately full recovery of pancreatic structure and function can occur.

Attacks may recur, especially if treatable causes such as gallstones or hypercalcaemia are ignored, but also when no obvious cause is apparent. In such cases abnormalities of the pancreatic duct may be amenable to surgical correction and should be sought by ERCP.

Chronic pancreatitis

Aetiology

Most cases are caused by chronic, excessive alcohol consumption. Uncommon causes include haemochroma-totis (see page 185), and in the tropics malnutrition is thought to lead to chronic pancreatic damage. Cystic fibrosis is a cause of chronic pancreatic exocrine failure and is discussed on page 176.

Pathology

The pancreas is irreversibly damaged with loss of exocrine and endocrine cells, disruption of the normal ductular anatomy and much fibrosis. The main ducts are irregularly dilated and contain proteinaceous plugs derived from the protein-rich exocrine secretion. Calc-ification of the plugs produces radio-opaque stones, and patchy calcification of the parenchyma is common, especially in alcoholics.

Clinical features

The disease may be silent for long periods and present with complications such as diabetes mellitus and pancreatic steatorrhoea. However, pain is the characteris-tic feature and it can be acute and relapsing or chronic and unremitting. The distribution of pancreatic pain is

discussed on page 137. Patients with chronic pain may become addicted to strong analgesics.

Intermittent or even continuous obstructive jaundice can be produced by swelling or fibrosis of the pancreatic head.

The many features of chronic alcohol abuse may be apparent, and further complications are of endocrine and exocrine failure and of addiction to analgesic and narcotic drugs.

Diagnosis

Abdominal X-ray may reveal distinctive pancreatic calc-ification. Pancreatic function is assessed by a glucose tolerance test and by a tube test of pancreatic exocrine secretion (see page 146). Pancreatic structure is best assessed by ERCP, but ultrasound or CT scanning can give useful information and avoid the risks of pan-creatography.

Pancreatic steatorrhoea is often gross and the faecal fat excretion can be more than ten times greater than the upper limit of normal, a level rarely seen in other forms of malabsorption.

The differential diagnosis is from the many other causes of chronic abdominal pain (see page 137) and malabsorption (page 145). In patients with obstructive jaundice, differentiation from pancreatic cancer can be very difficult even at surgery (page 175).

Treatment

The most important measure, if relevant, is to advise complete and permanent abstinence from alcohol, but compliance is often poor. Analgesics should be used sparingly and, in severe cases, percutaneous coeliac plexus block may be effective in relieving pain, although it is not without risk. If pain proves intractable, ERP may show a ductular abnormality that can be treated surgically; for example, a distended duct may be drained into a jejunal loop. Occasionally total pancreatectomy is undertaken in desperate cases, especially if function has been lost.

Diabetes mellitus will require insulin treatment (see page 323) and symptomatic steatorrhoea will respond to restriction of dietary fat and replacement of pancreatic enzymes. Enzyme therapy is difficult, however, because the various preparations available are unpalatable and have to be taken in large doses with every meal (e.g. 3–6 capsules of Pancrex V forte with meals). The enzymes are also irreversibly damaged by a gastric pH lower than 4, and so it is usual to add cimetidine or ranitidine to try to avoid this. Newer preparations are more acceptable (e.g. Creon).

Patients often eat well and maintain their weight even if steatorrhoea is marked, unless there is much pain or overt diabetes mellitus. Reduction of fat intake alone to 40–60 g daily may be remarkably effective in relieving diarrhoea. If the appetite is poor or if there is marked loss of weight, calorie supplements will be required. Medium-chain triglyerides (MCT) are absorbed in the absence of pancreatic lipase and provide a valuable source of calories. MCT is available as an oil for cooking and in various powdered forms.

Prognosis

This is good in terms of survival, but severe chronic pain may require surgical intervention with its attendant risks.

Carcinoma

Aetiology

This is a common cancer and the incidence is increasing. In Europe and North America there are 9–10 cases per 100 000 of the population annually.

There are no certain causes, although food factors such as soya protein and coffee have been implicated. The disease is commoner in smokers and in diabetics. There are no known genetic associations and chronic pancreatitis is not thought to be a predisposing cause.

Pathology

This is an adenocarcinoma arising from the ductular epithelium or the exocrine acini. It can occur in any part of the gland but those arising in the ampulla and head are commoner than those in the body and tail. Ampullary carcinoma arises from the mucosa which lines the short length of duct common to the biliary and pancreatic systems and which spreads over an area of the duodenum around the common orifice.

The tumour spreads widely, invading local structures and metastasizing to the liver and regional lymph nodes.

Clinical features

The commonest presentation is obstructive jaundice when the lesion is at the ampulla or in the head. This tends to be steadily progressive and, although it may be painless, pancreatic pain develops in most cases.

Cancer in the body or tail causes chronic pancreatic pain, which can defy diagnosis for months until the tumour reaches a large size.

Occasionally the tumour presents with a complication such as duodenal obstruction. Extensive pancreatic damage can lead to diabetes mellitus or steatorrhoea. Transient migratory thrombophlebitis is a rare and unexplained clinical association.

Physical examination may reveal a mass caused by a large tumour in the body or tail or an enlarged, tense gallbladder in association with obstructive jaundice (*Courvoisier's sign*).

Diagnosis

This is usually revealed during the investigation of jaundice or by ultrasound or CT scanning for abdominal pain. Histological confirmation is obtained percutaneously (see page 143) or at surgery. Pancreatic histology can be difficult to interpret, even if obtained at surgery, because some tumours produce a lot of surrounding inflammation and fibrosis.

The differential diagnosis is from the many causes of abdominal pain and obstructive jaundice. The differentiation from chronic pancreatitis can prove very difficult.

Complications

The main ones are obstructive jaundice, duodenal obstruction, pancreatic failure and, rarely, compression of the superior mesenteric artery with small intestinal ischaemia or infarction.

Treatment

The only possibility of cure is surgical resection, but this is rarely feasible except when the tumour is confined to the head or ampulla and produces jaundice relatively early. The preferred procedure is Whipple's excision which involves resection of the head of the pancreas and the C loop of duodenum with gastrojejunostomy. Separate anastomoses between the bile and pancreatic ducts and a loop of jejunum are created.

Surgical palliation of jaundice is commonly necessary, and cholecystojejunostomy is usually performed along with a gastrojejunostomy in case of later duodenal obstruction. The placement of stents using the endoscopic or transhepatic routes is becoming an increasingly popular alternative to the surgical palliation of jaundice.

For severe pancreatic pain in untreatable cancer, coeliac plexus block is often very effective and it can be undertaken at surgery or percutaneously.

Radiotherapy is not used and chemotherapy has not yet found an established place in treatment, although life can be prolonged by a few weeks or months.

Prognosis

This is still very poor and few patients survive more than six months. Whipple's resection for ampullary carcinoma can produce a 30–40% chance of surviving for five years; but cancer at other sites is associated with a much poorer survival rate even when resection is feasible.

Functional tumours

These rare tumours arise from the pancreatic islets, are usually single or multiple adenomas, and come to attention because symptoms result from the increased amounts of hormone(s) being produced. The commonest example is insulinoma (see page 326), and gastrinoma (Zollinger–Ellison syndrome) is described on page 156. Rarer tumours include those producing glucagon and VIP (vasoactive intestinal polypeptide). The glucagonoma syndrome includes a characteristic rash and mild diabetes mellitus. VIPomas produce severe chronic diarrhoea.

Cystic fibrosis (mucoviscidosis) (see page 115)

Aetiology

This congenital lesion is inherited in an autosomal recessive fashion and is the commonest serious disorder of this type in the UK with a prevalence of approximately 1:2000 births. The genetics of this disorder are discussed on page 487.

Pathology

The characteristic abnormality is the increased viscosity of pancreatic juice, and this also applies to the bronchial and intestinal secretions and to bile. The pancreas and lungs are damaged by the stasis of their viscous contents, by rupture of small ducts under pressure and, in the case of the lung, by recurrent infections of the bronchial tree. Retention cysts full of viscous bile may be found in the liver and this may eventually lead to secondary biliary cirrhosis and portal hypertension.

Clinical features

These are variable and depend very much on the age of

presentation. Soon after birth the intestine may be obstructed by thick plugs of inspissated meconium. In infancy and early childhood, the major problem is of recurrent, severe chest infections that may lead to bronchiectasis. Pancreatic exocrine failure with steatorrhoea becomes a problem later in childhood and can interfere with growth and development.

It used to be rare for these patients to survive into adolescence or adulthood, but survival is now possible with improved antibiotics and postural drainage for chest infections.

Diagnosis

This is usually suggested by the characteristic history and confirmed by the high concentrations of sodium and chloride in sweat. This can lead to salt depletion in hot weather.

Pancreatic exocrine function can be assessed in the usual way (see page 146). Glucose intolerance is relatively infrequent in younger patients but does occur later as a result of progressive pancreatic damage.

The differential diagnosis is from other forms of malabsorption in childhood, especially coeliac disease and the rarer pancreatic disorders of childhood. However, the serious nature of the chest infections usually draws attention to the correct diagnosis.

Treatment and prognosis

Pancreatic enzyme replacement therapy is given as described on page 175. Chest infections are treated with antibiotics and postural drainage. Dietary advice is required to ensure an adequate intake of calories and nitrogen. The prognosis appears to be improving steadily and increasing survival into adulthood can be predicted.

Diseases of the liver

Acute liver disease usually presents with jaundice or a transient disturbance of biochemical tests of liver function. As a working definition, all evidence of liver disease should resolve within six months. Chronic liver disease may follow an overt episode of acute disease, but usually presents in a number of other ways including non-specific symptoms, abnormal signs or biochemical test results or with complications (bleeding, ascites, encephalopathy).

Viral hepatitis

Aetiology

See Table 4.22. Non-A, non-B hepatitis is a diagnosis by exclusion. The yellow fever virus produces an acute hepatitis and is transmitted from man to man by the mosquito.

HAV is spread mainly by the oral, faecal route. HBV and CMV are spread by transfusion or injection of contaminated blood or by contact with infected blood, saliva or semen. EBV is spread mainly by direct oral contact, whereas HSV lies dormant for years but can be activated by a number of stresses or spontaneously. There are probably several non-A, non-B hepatitis viruses with different routes of infection.

A more recently discovered incomplete virus is called the delta agent (or delta virus). It is known to infect patients who are already carrying the virus of hepatitis B, and may produce a sudden deterioration of liver function in patients with acute or chronic hepatitis B.

Epidemiology

Hepatitis A is endemic in many parts of the world and outbreaks occur in closed institutions when contaminated food (e.g. uncooked shellfish) is consumed. Hepatitis B occurs all over the world, but the prevalence of viral markers in 'healthy' subjects is remarkably variable, as the following list shows:

Northern Europe and USA	0.1–0.5 per cent
Southern Europe and Japan	2–5 per cent
South Africa and Far East	10–15 per cent

In many parts of the underdeveloped world and in the Far East, hepatitis B infection is probably acquired during childbirth or infancy and there is strong evidence linking this to the subsequent development of hepatocellular cancer (see page 191).

Pathology

The viruses all produce a similar abnormality, with en-largement of the liver, diffuse lobular necrosis and acute inflammation predominantly near the central veins. In severe cases there is massive destruction of the lobules with shrinking of the liver ('acute yellow atrophy') but, if the patient survives, the liver can recover completely. However, there may be irreversible damage to the liver architecture even during an apparently mild attack. This will heal by nodular regeneration, fibrosis and cirrhosis (post-necrotic scarring or post-hepatitis cirrhosis). Sometimes a more chronic, active inflammatory and necrotic process ensues and leads to the clinical and histopathological entity of chronic active hepatitis (see page 183).

These longer-term complications of hepatitis are most likely to follow hepatitis B infection, which may be mild clinically or asymptomatic. It seems to be exceptionally rare for HAV, EBV or CMV to produce chronic liver disease. The chronicity of non-A, non-B hepatitis will remain uncertain until a marker of this diasease becomes available.

Clinical features

The various types of viral hepatitis have distinctively different incubation periods. Hepatitis A has an incubation period of 20–40 days and hepatitis B 40–140 days. There appear to be both short and long incubation periods for the different clinical types of non-A, non-B hepatitis. Symptomatic cases present with a non-specific, febrile illness and rather characteristic aversion to food and cigarettes. There may be pain over an enlarging liver. Jaundice develops after a week or so and usually subsides slowly over the next few weeks. There is often consider-able malaise and nausea which can outlast the jaundice by weeks or rarely months. The patient may enter a choles-tatic phase with deepening jaundice and itching, which can be prolonged.

Physical signs are usually restricted to jaundice and modest, tender enlargement of the liver. Liver function tests will show marked elevation of the transaminases with rather more modest increase in the alkaline phospha-tase. Serum albumin is usually well maintained, but blood coagulation tests are abnormal in all but the mildest cases. In EBV infection there are usually other signs of infectious mononucleosis (glandular fever, page 421). In herpes simplex infection there may be obvious signs of the virus around the mouth or evidence of infection elsewhere (e.g. encephalitis, page 418).

Diagnosis

This is confirmed by appropriate serological tests on the

Table 4.22 Viruses causing hepatitis

Hepatitis A virus (HAV)
Hepatitis B virus (HBV)
Non-A non-B hepatitis (NANB)
Cytomegalovirus (CMV)
Epstein–Barr virus (EBV)
Herpes simplex virus (HSV)
Yellow fever virus

plasma. The characteristic time sequence of the main abnormalities in acute hepatitis A and B is shown in Fig. 4.4. As with all infections, only IgM antibodies indicate that the infection is current or recent.

In patients with evidence of acute hepatitis B (i.e. positive B surface antigen), it is advisable to determine whether another marker of this virus—the e antigen—is present in the serum. Its presence indicates continuing viral replication in the liver cells, high infectivity of the blood and a continuing risk of progressive liver disease. The development of antibodies to this antigen heralds an improved prognosis.

Differential diagnosis

Viral hepatitis must be distinguished from drug-induced

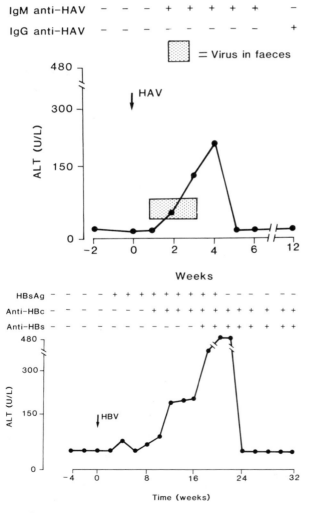

jaundice (see page 179), other causes of infective jaundice such as leptospirosis (page 427) and non-specific ascending cholangitis (page 171) and, especially if cholestasis is marked, all the many causes of obstructive jaundice (page 140).

Complications

The major acute complications are bleeding as a result of impaired coagulation and the rapid development (over days) of encephalopathy, hypoglycaemia and oliguric renal failure (fulminant hepatic failure). The remote complications of hepatitis B (and probably non-A, non-B hepatitis) include chronic active hepatitis, cirrhosis and hepatocellular carcinoma (see page 191).

Treatment

This is supportive in the expectation that resolution will occur over several weeks. There is much current interest in the use of antiviral drugs and interferon in the management of hepatitis B, but this is still at the stage of clinical research. Acyclovir is usually given to patients with severe local and systemic herpes simplex infections. There is no evidence that corticosteroids are helpful and they are best avoided—their use in hastening the resolution of severe cholestasis is controversial.

In most cases, supportive therapy merely means a light, palatable diet and bed-rest if the patient feels weak. Enforced bed-rest is of no benefit. Alcohol should be avoided completely at least until liver function tests have returned to normal. All unnecessary drugs should be with-held, especially those that are known to be potentially hepatotoxic. In more severe cases, intravenous hydration may be required and blood glucose levels must be maintained with adequate intravenous administration. Sedatives should be avoided for fear of masking encephalopathy. The best early guide to prognosis is the prothrombin time. Infusions of fresh frozen plasma will correct a prolonged prothrombin time and should only be given if there is active bleeding.

In severe acute liver failure, full intensive care will be required. Early referral to a specialist liver centre carries the best hope of recovery. Various techniques may be helpful, including charcoal haemoperfusion and intracranial pressure monitoring. Emergency liver transplantation is being evaluated.

Prognosis

This is usually excellent in hepatitis A and in infections

Figure 4.4   *Time course and serological responses to hepatitis A and B virus infections. (ALT = alanine aminotransferase).*

with EBV and CMV, although there may be a prolonged period of morbidity. Generalized HSV infection has a high mortality rate and the risk of developing the remote complications of hepatitis B is uncertain.

Fulminant hepatic failure is very rare and carries a poor prognosis which depends on the criteria used to define the condition. If the patient is drowsy and confused, the chances of survival are less than 30 per cent. However, those who recover from fulminant hepatitis are not at increased risk of chronic liver disease.

Preventive aspects

Care must be taken with venepuncture and the handling of blood and other body fluids in the laboratory. Faeces must be treated with antiseptic fluid and disposed of carefully. Strict barrier nursing is not essential if these precautions are taken. Attendants must sterilise their own hands before handling food. Ideally patients should be treated out of hospital or in separate sidewards or cubicles if admission is necessary.

If contamination occurs, passive immunization with immunoglobulin (for hepatitis A) or hyperimmune immunoglobulin (for hepatitis B) should be undertaken as soon as possible. This is particularly important for contacts of hepatitis cases if the patient has e antigen in the serum.

Active immunization against hepatitis B is now available, using a vaccine derived from viral capsular material. It is given to dental, medical and nursing personnel on a selective basis and is effective in preventing the spread of infection among high-risk homosexuals.

Chemicals, drugs and the liver

Aetiology

Many drugs and chemicals can damage the liver (ethyl alcohol will be considered in the next section). The precise mechanism of action is often uncertain. Some reactions are dose-related and predictable, suggesting a direct toxic effect on the liver (e.g. carbon tetrachloride, chloroform, paracetamol). Most drug reactions are idiosyncratic, unpredictable and can be produced by very low doses. A classification of the major drugs responsible for liver disease is shown in Table 4.23.

In the case of acute paracetamol (acetaminophen) poisoning the mechanism of action and protection has been established. Glutathione within the hepatocyte plays a protective role and is consumed by the products of paracetamol metabolism. These toxic products denature intracellular proteins and destroy the liver cells. This understanding has led to rational treatment (see page 508).

Pathology

Some drugs produce hepatocellular necrosis and the lesions resemble those of viral hepatitis (hepatitis-like reactions). Others produce predominant bile stasis with damage to the excretory membrane of the hepatocyte and accumulation of bile plugs in distended canaliculi (cholestatic reactions). There may be various combinations of both reactions. There are sometimes features of an acute allergic response with eosinophil leucocyte infiltration into the portal tracts in addition to other acute inflammatory features.

Exceptionally, chronic liver disease may ensue and a lesion resembling chronic active hepatitis has been described following the use of oxyphenisatin (a laxative now withdrawn), methyldopa and other drugs. Some drugs can produce chronic portal tract fibrosis without

Table 4.23 Liver damage caused by drugs

Predictable (dose-dependent)

Liver cell necrosis:
    paracetamol (acetaminophen)
    carbon tetrachloride, trichlorethylene
    tetracycline, ferrous salts in excess

Cholestasis*
    oestrogens
    anabolic steroids
    17α-alkyl-substituted androgens

Unpredictable (rare, not dependent on dose)

Liver cell necrosis:
    antituberculous drugs
    (especially isoniazid, rifampicin, pyrazinamide)
    monoamine oxidase inhibitors (e.g. iproniazid)
    halothane
    and many others

Cholestasis:
    phenothiazines (especially chlorpromazine)
    erythromycin estolate
    tricyclic antidepressants

Hepatic vein thrombosis
(Budd–Chiari syndrome):
    oral contraceptives
Benign hepatic adenomas:
    oral contraceptives
Microvesicular fatty change:
    sodium valproate

*Clinically apparent only in a minority.

any initial inflammatory reaction (e.g. methotrexate used in treating psoriasis). These chronic drug-related lesions will often improve slowly following withdrawal of the drug.

Clinical features

There is usually either an acute hepatitis-like illness or a cholestatic syndrome with any or all of the clinical features that have already been described. Occasionally there is evidence of generalized allergy with skin rashes and bronchospasm.

Jaundice after an operation may result from infection, from drugs or from the anaesthetic agent *halothane*. This has been a remarkably controversial matter and a suitable, reasonably cheap alternative to halothane has not yet found wide acceptance. The risk is greatest in patients who have several general anaesthetics within short intervals (less than six months). The clinical picture is of an acute hepatitis-like illness with fever, which can rarely progress to fulminant hepatic failure and death.

Paracetamol (acetaminophen) poisoning has a well-defined clinical pattern with a slow evolution of clinical and laboratory abnormalities over 48 hours after ingestion. Elevation of the transaminases and prolongation of the prothrombin time precede the onset of encephalopathy and bleeding by several days. Early use of methionine or acetylcysteine (see page 588) is crucial if severe liver disease is to be prevented. Once liver damage is established, these drugs are useless and progression to liver failure may be unavoidable.

Diagnosis

This is based almost entirely on the drug history and the exclusion of other causes of jaundice. There may be other features to suggest an allergic illness (e.g. rashes, bronchospasm). Liver biopsy may show features very suggestive of drug damage but is often not necessary if the drugs can be withdrawn and if the patient recovers quite rapidly. Rechallenge with the drug following recovery is sometimes justifiable, but potentially dangerous, and is the only way to establish the relationship with cetainty.

The differential diagnosis is from all other causes of jaundice. It is especially important to exclude virus infection and extrahepatic obstruction if there are cholestatic features (see page 140).

Complications

Acute hepatitis-like lesions can progress to acute liver

failure and death. Prolonged cholestasis may lead to steatorrhoea and deficiency of fat-soluble vitamins.

Treatment

All potentially culpable drugs must be withdrawn. In some cases (for example, rifampicin in the treatment of tuberculosis), it may be justifiable to ignore mild disturbances of liver function because they can resolve even if treatment is continued. In the cholestatic syndrome associated with the contraceptive pill, the condition will resolve if very-low-oestrogen or progesterogen-only preparations are substituted. Otherwise the patient is treated in the same supportive way as for viral hepatitis and intensive care may be required. Prolonged cholestatic jaundice usually requires the parenteral use of fat-soluble vitamins and oral cholestyramine for itching.

Prognosis

This is usually excellent provided the drug is withdrawn completely. Full recovery of liver structure and function can be predicted in the vast majority of cases. Prognosis regarding the outcome of acute damage by paracetamol can be predicted with some accuracy by blood levels of the drug over the first 12 hours after its ingestion and, subsequently, by repeated measurements of prothombin time.

(Ethyl) alcohol and the liver
Aetiology

Alcohol is the most familiar liver toxin and its first metabolite, acetaldehyde, is probably the compound which damages the liver cell directly. Acute alcohol poisoning produces a predictable and rapidly reversible acute liver injury, which is usually inapparent clinically if the liver was initially healthy. The continued ingestion of large amounts of alcohol over many years (60 g daily in males, 30 g in females) is associated with a number of different clinical syndromes. There is considerable variation in individual susceptibility and this is probably determined genetically.

It is helpful to remember that a standard drink (a half pint of beer, a single unit of spirits or a small glass of wine or sherry) contains about 10 g of alcohol. It cannot be assumed that a lower consumption is totally safe, and some organs, especially the brain, may suffer subtle damage in the absence of any evidence of disease of the liver or other organs.

Pathology

There are several types of liver injury depending on the amount of alcohol consumed and the chronicity of the habit. In fatty liver (steatosis) the hepatocytes are swollen by collections of intracellular fat which form large globules displacing the nucleus. This is usually a subacute process with little or no inflammation and is completely reversible if the patient stops drinking. Acute alcoholic hepatitis is a severe inflammatory and necrotic process affecting the lobules diffusely with relatively little fatty change. This is again fully reversible, but if the patient has repeated bouts of hepatitis, the liver architecture is damaged permanently and cirrhosis will result.

Alcoholic cirrhosis usually develops insidiously without overt episodes of acute hepatitis. There is variable inflammation, necrosis and fat accumulation and a frequent feature is Mallory's hyaline—an eosinophilic material, which accumulates in damaged hepatocytes.

Clinical features

Simple steatosis is often asymptomatic and may present with hepatomegaly or abnormal liver function tests as chance findings.

Acute alcoholic hepatitis is a severe illness with fever, nausea and vomiting, jaundice and tender hepatomegaly. The condition can progress to liver failure with bleeding and encephalopathy. The liver function tests show elevation of transaminases, although rarely to levels as high as those seen in viral hepatitis. There are often other features of alcohol abuse such as poor nutrition and withdrawal symptoms, especially convulsions and delirium tremens.

Chronic alcoholic cirrhosis presents insidiously with non-specific symptoms and the gradual development of the characteristic signs of chronic liver disease (see Table 4.11). Feminization with gynaecomastia and impotence are common in the male. The course is eventually that of slow deterioration, if drinking continues, with the later development of complications. These patients are prone to acute and chronic infections in the lungs, ascitic fluid and elsewhere. Malnutrition is common with loss of muscle bulk, weakness and the development of specific deficiencies, especially of folic acid and thiamine (vitamin B_1).

Diagnosis

This depends on the finding of clinical or laboratory evidence of acute or chronic liver disease in a known or suspected heavy drinker. The taking of an alcohol history requires experience since most patients underestimate and some deny consumption. Liver biopsy is required to determine the type and severity of the liver disease and to indicate its likely reversibility if the patient stops drinking.

The combination of macrocytosis and a raised gamma-glutamyl transferase (γ-GT) liver suggests heavy alcohol consumption, and the measurement of blood alcohol will confirm the suspicion if the sample is taken at an appropriate time. In a cooperative patient a period of abstinence will often clarify the nature of biochemical abnormalities of liver function.

Differential diagnosis

A fatty liver can be produced by obesity, diabetes mellitus and by severe malnutrition. Acute alcoholic hepatitis must be distinguished from viral and drug-induced hepatitis. There is typically a heavy neutrophil infiltrate into the lobules in alcoholic disease, but liver biopsy may not be feasible if the patient is ill with disturbed coagulation tests.

Alcoholic cirrhosis must be distinguished from the other identifiable forms of chronic liver disease, especially those related to hepatitis B and autoimmune phenomena. There may be confusion with haemochromatosis because alcoholics tend to accumulate iron in the liver (see page 185).

Complications

Acute alcoholic hepatitis or an acute exacerbation of chronic alcoholic liver disease can lead to acute liver failure and a fatal outcome. Superadded infections, including tuberculosis, are common and may be lethal if not treated vigorously.

The major complications of chronic liver disease are discussed on page 187.

Treatment

Alcohol withdrawal is the essence of treatment, irrespective of the stage of the disease or the severity of its complications. In the acutely ill patient, it is important to recognize and treat hypoglycaemia, thiamine deficiency and infections, especially of the chest and of any ascitic fluid. Full supportive therapy for acute liver failure may be required as discussed on page 178. The treatment of ascites, encephalopathy and variceal bleeding are described on pages 187–189.

A severely agitated patient will require careful sedation with chlormethiazole or chlordiazepoxide which should then be tailed off over 6–7 days.

How much alcohol should a patient be 'allowed' to drink after he has recovered from an acute episode of hepatic dysfunction? The ideal answer is none at all, especially if there is evidence of chronic liver damage. Patients whose livers have recovered could presumably tolerate moderate amounts of alcohol with impunity (for example, below 40 g daily in men and 20 g in women). However, the major risk is that this level of consumption will not be maintained with the passage of time and the resumption of full social and business activities.

Prognosis

This depends entirely on the ability of the patient to abstain. Fatty liver and acute hepatitis carry very good prognoses if the patient survives the acute illness and abstains. The course of chronic disease can be modified by abstinence, although cirrhosis itself is by definition irreversible. However, the progress of the disease can be halted and it is always worth trying very hard to achieve abstinence. In patients presenting with major complications, prognosis is poor and the chance of survival to five years is no more than 10 per cent, or less if drinking continues.

Cholestasis of pregnancy

Aetiology

The condition occurs in the last three months of pregnancy and remits after delivery. It is an idiosyncratic reaction to a rise in circulating oestrogens and can be reproduced in sensitive women by oestrogen-containing contraceptives. The prevalence of the sensitivity shows marked geographic variation and is notably common in Scandinavia.

Clinical features

These is itching and mild jaundice with elevation of the serum alkaline phosphatase. There are no histophalogical features of note. The condition is usually quite mild, although the itching can be intense. The condition will probably recur in future pregnancies.

The prognosis is good and chronic liver disease does not ensue. Future contraception should be achieved with progestogen-only pills or by other methods.

Fatty liver of pregnancy

Aetiology

This poorly understood and rare entity develops during the last three months of pregnancy. It usually occurs spontaneously although it can be provoked by drugs —most notably by tetracyclines. It is probably aggravated rather than caused by the impaired nutrition that can accompany prolonged vomiting during pregnancy. The histopathological features are distinctive: a microvesicular distribution of tiny fat globules within the hepatocyte, a feature shared with Reye's syndrome and sodium valproate hepatotoxicity. Since aspirin sensitivity has been proposed as a cause of Reye's syndrome, it is possible that fatty liver of pregnancy is also a hypersensitivity phenomenon.

Clinical features

The onset is insidious with malaise, anorexia and vomiting followed by progressive deterioration of liver function. Jaundice is often delayed and mild. Coagulopathy and encephalopathy may ensue rapidly after a week or more of prolonged severe vomiting. Death from acute liver failure will follow, although it may be averted by prompt recognition of the syndrome and induction of labour. Following delivery recovery of liver function is rapid and complete.

Treatment

Full supportive therapy as described on page 178 and prompt delivery of the fetus are required. The prognosis is usually regarded as very bad, but it seems likely that mild cases may be missed and recovery is now undoubtedly commoner than it was. The long-term prognosis is excellent after successful delivery.

Budd–Chiari syndrome

Aetiology

This is produced by occlusion of the hepatic veins by thrombosis, by tumour or occasionally by webs in the upper inferior vena cava. Venous thrombosis may be caused by the contraceptive pill and by hypercoagulable states such as polycythaemia vera. Tumours may compress from without or obstruct from within by intraluminal spread.

Pathology

The liver enlarges and there is haemorrhagic necrosis of the central parts of the liver lobules. Venous collaterals develop, but in spite of this portal pressure rises and, in survivors, cirrhosis may ensue as complete resolution of the lesion is unlikely.

Clinical features

In classical cases, there is hepatic enlargement with pain and rapidly developing ascites over a period of days or weeks. The time course is, however, variable, and in some patients only part of the hepatic venous system is occluded giving a more chronic and less dramatic clinical picture. The liver is enlarged or tender with variable ascites and later splenomegaly will be apparent. The ascitic fluid has no distinctive features and a variable protein content.

The isotope liver scan may show a relatively normal or large caudate lobe with grossly impaired uptake elsewhere. Ultrasound will reveal characteristic venous collaterals. The liver histology is very distinctive and clear proof can be provided by hepatic venography

Treatment

The underlying disease should be corrected where possible. Anticoagulants or thrombolytic therapy have not met with much success. Surgery or angioplasty may be helpful in patients with caval webs. Most patients are treated with the various supportive measures outlined elsewhere for complicated liver disease.

Prognosis

This is usually poor with about 50 per cent of the patients dying within a year from liver failure or bleeding varices. However, long-term survival is possible and depends, in part, on the nature of the underlying cause if any. Liver transplantation has been used successfully in several patients.

Chronic active hepatitis
Aetiology

This is most commonly produced by viruses (especially hepatitis B and perhaps non-A, non-B hepatitis) and by autoimmune phenomena which often affect other organs or systems. A similar clinical syndrome can be produced by Wilson's disease (see page 186). Some drugs have been implicated, including methyldopa and the now withdrawn laxative oxyphenisatin.

Pathology

There is diffuse lobular inflammation and necrosis of hepatocytes. A distinctive feature is the breakdown of the boundary zone between the lobules and the portal tracts (limiting plate) as inflammatory cells infiltrate the lobules and surround small islands of hepatocytes. The activity of the necrosis and inflammation can be greatly modified by treatment; but if it is unchecked, permanent damage to the liver architecture will result with the usual risks of nodular regeneration and bands of fibrosis (i.e. cirrhosis, page 181).

Clinical features

During an active episode there is malaise, jaundice, hepatomegaly and biochemical evidence of acute hepatocellular necrosis (i.e. marked elevation of the transaminases). Acute liver failure may, rarely, ensue with coagulopathy and encephalopathy. In most cases, the symptoms are milder and persist for months or years with variable jaundice and disturbances of biochemical tests.

The autoimmune type of disease affects mainly middle-aged women and there is often evidence of inflammatory disease of other organs (for example, the thyroid and joints).

Diagnosis

This is based on clinical and biochemical evidence of chronic remitting and relapsing liver disease in a person who has evidence of past viral infection or autoimmune phenomena. Past viral B infection is indicated by the carriage of hepatitis B surface antigen (HBsAg) or by antibodies to the surface or core antigens. The commonest autoimmune markers are anti-nuclear, smooth muscle, liver and kidney microsomal antibodies. Liver biopsy is required to establish a firm diagnosis and to indicate the severity of the disease and its potential reversibility. There is a rather poor correlation between symptoms, the elevation of transaminases and the histological abnormality.

Differential diagnosis

In a young person (under 30) Wilson's disease (see page 186) must be excluded. *Chronic persistent hepatitis* is the name given to a similar but very much milder illness. It is often asymptomatic, the biochemical disturbances are mild and histologically the inflammation is confined to the portal tract. This may progress to more florid active hepatitis and it is probably part of the same illness, although formerly regarded as always having an excellent prognosis.

Complications

The main risks are the development of an acute episode of severe liver failure and, after a very variable and often prolonged period of time (5–10 years), all the complications of end-stage disease (see page 187).

Treatment

There is no established treatment for the disease induced by hepatitis B virus, and corticosteroids are best avoided. If there is evidence of active viral replication, antiviral agents such as interferon and adenosine arabinoside may be helpful in halting progression of the disease, but such treatment is still at the experimental stage. Once viral replication has ceased, however, the disease may become self-perpetuating perhaps as a result of immunological disturbance. This type of chronic hepatitis can run a relatively silent clinical course until complications develop.

The autoimmune disease produces more clinical and biochemical disturbances, which usually respond very well and quickly to corticosteroids. There can be remarkable histological resolution, but steroid withdrawal is often followed by relapses which may be more difficult to treat. It is exceptional for permanent resolution to follow short courses of steroids and long-term treatment is usually advised. In view of the risks incurred by this, azathioprine is often added for its 'steroid-sparing' effect in order to keep the dose of prednisolone below 10 mg daily. The course of the disease is monitored by biochemical tests and ideally by liver biopsy.

Prognosis

This used to be considered grave with progression to death over a 5–7 year period. However, this applied to untreated florid autoimmune disease and use of anti-inflammatory drugs has improved the outlook considerably. Milder cases are now being treated and long survival can be predicted.

The prognosis of prolonged liver disease after hepatitis B is less certain and may improve with the use of antiviral drugs in the future.

Primary biliary cirrhosis

Aetiology

This relatively rare disease has an autoimmune basis but the initiating trigger factor is not known. Environmental factors (including drugs) have been implicated, and the disease's great predilection for women suggests a role for female sex hormones.

Pathology

The histopathological features in typical cases include chronic inflammation around the small bile ducts in the portal tracts, small granulomas and a marked accumulation of copper within the hepatocytes. The duct epithelium is ultimately destroyed, but lobular architecture is preserved for long periods with relatively little damage to the hepatocytes. In the later stages of the disease, the hepatocytes are damaged and the lobular architecture is eventually destroyed, leading to cirrhosis (the name of the disease is misleading because cirrhosis is a late feature).

Clinical features

The most distinctive features are chronic itching and jaundice in a middle-aged woman. The disease is often diagnosed in asymptomatic patients in whom the laboratory abnormalities are discovered by chance.

In severe longstanding disease, there are deep jaundice, marked pigmentation and all the stigmata of chronic liver disease (see Table 4.11). Hypercholesterolaemia is common and may be shown clinically by xanthelasmas or xanthomas. Well-recognized clinical associations include the Sicca syndrome, dry eyes and dry mouth, caused by immunological damage to the lacrimal and salivary glands, and renal tubular abnormalities.

Steatorrhoea is common but seldom severe, but fat-soluble vitamin deficiency may arise and lead to bleeding, osteomalacia and, rarely, night blindness. Bone pains and vertebral collapse are caused by vitamin D deficiency and accelerated osteoporosis, the reason for the latter being uncertain.

Diagnosis

This is suggested by the finding of greatly raised alkaline phosphatase, hypercholesterolaemia and a positive anti-mitochrondrial antibody in the serum. The latter is positive in 95 per cent of cases. Liver biopsy is needed to confirm the diagnosis.

If the history is short and jaundice prominent, other causes of obstructive jaundice must be excluded (see page 140). After more prolonged illness the differential diagnosis is narrower and includes sclerosing cholangitis and cholangiocarcinoma (page 172). In atypical cases, especially if the anti-mitochrondrial antibody is negative, ERCP should be undertaken to exclude biliary tract pathology.

Complications

These include fat-soluble vitamin deficiencies, portal hypertension and ultimately liver failure. As with all chronic liver disease, malignant transformation may occur. Gallstones are common in chronic liver disease and, by migration, may cause sudden deterioration.

Treatment

There is no known effective therapy. Corticosteroids are ineffective and contraindicated in view of the frequency of oesteoporosis. Azathioprine produces a marginal improvement in survival. Pencillamine will reduce the amount of copper in the liver but it does not seem to produce prolonged clinical benefit. Moreover, side-effects are common and often lead to withdrawal of therapy. Cyclosporin is currently under trial.

Treatment is therefore supportive and includes the use of cholestyramine for itching, a low-fat diet for steatorrhoea and fat-soluble vitamin replacement. The vitamins are most conveniently given in large intramuscular doses every two months, but the new preparation alfacalcidol is effective orally.

End-stage disease with incipient liver failure is now being treated by liver transplantation in carefully selected patients, and this possibility should be considered in otherwise fit and relatively young patients whose condition is obviously deteriorating.

Prognosis

The natural history is of very slow progression over many years and it is being increasingly recognized in its milder or subclinical forms. Once symptoms develop the median survival time is approximately 5–6 years. Malignant transformation is uncommon and death is usually caused by variceal bleeding or liver failure.

Haemochromatosis

Aetiology

This terms applies to a rare familial disorder in which the intestine absorbs iron excessively because the normal regulatory mechanism is ineffective. It is inherited as an autosomal recessive trait and there is an association with histocompatibility antigens HLA A3 and B14.

Pathology

There is a slow accumulation of iron in the liver, pancreas, heart and testes. Pigmentation of the skin is caused by the accumulation of melanin rather than iron itself.

In the liver, iron accumulates in hepatocytes and in reticuloendothelial cells within the portal tracts. Eventually the hepatocytes are damaged and undergo necrosis, with little active inflammation. Finally lobular architecture is destroyed with resultant cirrhosis, but this can take many years even after clinical features have become apparent. Similar damage to and fibrosis of the pancreas is evident in most cases.

Clinical features

The disease presents in males in middle age (30–50 years) and in females considerably later because of the menstrual losses of iron during the reproductive years. There are usually mild non-specific symptoms with slow liver enlargement. The skin becomes progressively pigmented and insulin-dependent diabetes develops eventually ('bronze diabetes'). Joint symptoms may be troublesome and the knees are commonly affected. Loss of libido and feminization occur frequently. In severe untreated disease there may be clinically overt heart disease with arrhythmias and congestive cardiac failure. The liver function tests are variably abnormal without any distinctive features.

Diagnosis

There is characteristically a raised serum iron with a normal iron binding capacity, so that iron saturation is high. Serum ferritin levels are very high. Liver biopsy with special iron stains is required to make a firm diagnosis, to assess the extent of iron accumulation and liver cell damage, and to give some idea about reversibility and prognosis.

Differential diagnosis

The main differential diagnosis is from other causes of iron overload. Excess hepatic iron is commonly seen in alcoholic liver disease, owing to increased iron intake (for example, from certain wines) and inappropriately high absorption rates. However, the total accumulation of iron in the body is far less than that seen in haemochromatosis.

Iron accumulates to excess in chronic haemolytic anaemia, after years of inappropriate iron therapy and in patients who require repeated blood transfusions.

Complications

To the usual complications of chronic liver disease are added diabetes mellitus and cardiac failure. Joint disease and testicular failure are common. There seems to be a particularly high risk of hepatocellular carcinoma.

Treatment

The only effective treatment is to remove iron by venesection and to keep body iron stores near normal by repeated venesection over the years. Iron chelating agents are much less effective in quantitative terms and require systemic administration. Subcutaneous infusions of desferrioxamine are given to patients with chronic haematological disorders to prevent iron accumulation.

One unit of blood contains approximately 250 mg of elemental iron. Haemochromatosis may cause a total accumulation of 20–40 g of iron compared with the normal store of about 4 g. Therefore venesections at the rate of one unit every two weeks will be required for one or two years to rid the body of its excess iron. Treatment is monitored by measurement of haemoglobin (to avoid anaemia) and serum ferritin and life-long observation is required.

Prognosis

This is good with a chance of long survival if the condition is detected early and treated conscientiously. The risk of hepatocellular carcinoma (see page 191) may not, however, be averted by venesection.

It is important to persuade other family members, especially males, to have tests of liver function, serum iron and ferritin. If these are abnormal, a liver biopsy should be performed and venesection started in the hope of preventing disease later.

Wilson's disease (hepatolenticular degeneration)

Aetiology

In this rare disease, copper accumulates to excess in the liver and in certain parts of the brain and other organs. The primary abnormality is unknown, but there is usually a deficiency of the plasma protein caeruloplasmin, which is responsible for the transport of copper in the blood. There is also impaired excretion of copper in bile. The condition is inherited as an autosomal recessive trait.

Clinical features

The main features are hepatic and cerebral. The hepatic manifestations are variable and include progression to cirrhosis with all the usual long-term complications, a more symptomatic disease resembling chronic active hepatitis clinically and histologically and an acute fulminating illness presenting as acute hepatic failure. The onset of overt liver disease is usually before the age of 15 years.

The neurological features include extrapyramidal tract signs and slowly developing dementia and tend to occur later in adolescence. The main diagnostic features are the distinctive deposition of copper around the periphery of the cornea (*Kayser–Fleischer rings*) best seen by slit-lamp examination, depressed level of serum caeruloplasmin, variable serum copper and increased urinary copper excretion. Orcein staining of liver biopsy material shows considerable accumulation of copper binding protein in the hepatocytes.

Treatment and prognosis

Penicillamine is the drug of choice. It chelates copper and increases its urinary excretion. Treatment is life-long, but it may be complicated by side-effects, which are usually dose-related and reversible. These include skin rashes and heavy proteinuria.

The prognosis has improved considerably since the introduction of penicillamine and survival for many years is now possible. Liver transplantation has been employed, with reversal of the biochemical abnormality.

Genetic counselling and tracing of relatives. Young relatives should be examined clinically and biochemically for evidence of liver and neurological disease at a presymptomatic stage so that early treatment can be started. Patients reaching the reproductive years will require advice about procreation. Successful pregnancy has been reported in women taking penicillamine continuously.

Complications of chronic liver disease

Ascites

Aetiology

The combination of hypoalbuminaemia and portal hypertension allows the retention of sodium and water in the extravascular space, and especially in the peritoneal cavity where the portal capillary pressure is raised. The reduction in circulating volume encourages renin release by the kidney and this stimulates aldosterone production and intense renal conservation of sodium (secondary aldosteronism). The retained sodium does not, however, restore the circulating plasma volume and oliguric renal failure may ensue.

Clinical features

Ascites is often very gross indeed, when 10–20 litres may have accumulated, with relatively little dependent oedema in the legs or over the sacrum. In severe cases, especially if there has been vigorous diuretic therapy, the patient may be hypovolaemic with a low blood pressure, depressed venous pressure in the neck and oliguria. The umbilicus may be everted and there are often venous collaterals over the distended abdomen, indicating portal hypertension.

Differential diagnosis

The many causes of ascites (Table 4.24) are usually excluded on clinical grounds and by suitable examination of the ascitic fluid obtained at an initial small-volume paracentesis (50 ml). In hepatic cases the ultimate diagnosis usually requires liver biopsy, which is generally not advisable until the ascites has cleared. However,

Table 4.24 Causes of ascites

Primary liver disease, including Budd–Chiari syndrome
Abdominal malignancy
Infection, especially tuberculosis
Pancreatic ascites
Chylo ascites due to lymphatic block
'Cardiac cirrhosis'
Hypothyroidism

laparoscopically or ultrasonically guided biopsies may be obtained with greater safety (see page 146).

Malignancy and peritoneal infection can complicate longstanding liver disease, so initial cytological and bacteriological examination of ascitic fluid is required even when a firm diagnosis of chronic liver disease is already well established. Pancreatic ascites occasionally develops in heavy drinkers and is indicated by a high amylase concentration in the fluid.

Ascites is rare in acute or subacute liver disease. Its rapid development suggests the possibility of hepatic venous thrombosis (Budd–Chiari syndrome, page 182). In chronic liver disease the sudden onset of ascites might suggest portal vein occlusion, especially if infection and malignancy are excluded.

Treatment

The mainstays of treatment are the restriction of sodium and water intake and the careful use of diuretics. Forty eight hours of bed-rest and observation will establish a baseline weight, allow time to exclude problems requiring specific treatment, especially infection, and permit measurement of urinary flow and sodium losses. Salt should not be added to the ward diet and fluid intake should be restricted to less than 1500 ml daily if the serum sodium concentration is below 130 mmol/l (this usually indicates impaired excretion of 'free water'). The need for greater restriction of salt and water intake will be determined by the measured urinary losses and by a falling level of serum sodium.

Spironolactone is the diuretic of choice and should be introduced on the second day at a dose of 50 mg daily, doubling every two days to 200 mg daily and by 100 mg increments thereafter according to response as measured by careful daily weighing and urinary outputs (including sodium concentration). The ideal rate of weight loss is 0.5 kg a day, and a greater rate should be avoided for fear of producing hypovolaemia and impaired renal function. Urinary sodium concentrations below 20 mmol/l indicate intense salt conservation and the need to increase the dose of spironolactone. If the urinary concentration is higher, additional salt and water losses will only be achieved by a more proximally acting diuretic such as frusemide or a thiazide. Serum potassium concentrations must be closely monitored and levels in the range 4–5 mmol/l should be maintained by oral supplementation. Tissue potassium depletion is common in these patients and will be aggravated by the use of proximally acting diuretics (especially if spironolactone is not being used simultaneously).

Most patients will respond to this treatment, but additional measures may be required. It may be necessary to enforce a strict 22 mmol sodium intake. If the ascites is very tense, a slow paracentesis of 4–5 litres will relieve distress without harm. Repeated paracenteses should be avoided unless some of the protein lost is replaced by infusions of salt-poor albumin (e.g. 40 g daily IV). Albumin infusion is also appropriate if the patient becomes hypotensive and oliguric because this will re-expand the circulating volume and should improve renal function. The infused albumin has a relatively short half-life (7–8 days) so the benefits will be short-lived and, moreover, it is very expensive.

In very resistant cases it is possible to insert a shunt between the peritoneal cavity and the great veins of the neck (e.g. a *LaVeen shunt*). This can be dramatically effective in promoting diuresis; but it carries many hazards, including cardiac failure and intravascular co-agulation. Truly resistant ascites is fortunately rare if the patient complies with the regimen and if complicating factors have been excluded. Non-steroidal anti-inflammatory drugs may make ascites resistant to treatment and should be withdrawn if possible. A high albumin concentration in the ascitic fluid (above 20 g/l) would indicate the need to search again for malignancy, infection and pancreatic disease.

Prognosis

This is usually good if the patient complies with treatment and if the progression of the underlying liver disease can be halted, for example by abstaining from alcohol or by the use of corticosteroids in patients with chronic active hepatitis. Poor response to the above measures and the development of other complications will, however, indicate a poor overall prognosis with little chance of surviving for more than a few months.

Hepatic (portal–systemic) encephalopathy

Aetiology

This reversible cerebral syndrome is caused by the accumulation of a number of nitrogenous compounds, which would normally be detoxified and excreted by the healthy liver. It is especially likely to occur if there is major shunting of portal venous blood directly into the systemic circulation. Surgical shunts are now created much less commonly than in the past, but numerous small shunts can develop spontaneously during the development of cirrhosis.

Ammonia has been the most widely studied putative neurotoxin and plasma levels of ammonia are high in these patients. However, there is a poor correlation between the level of ammonia and the severity of the encephalopathy. Other candidates include more complex amines with false neurotransmitter properties (e.g. octopamine), which can interfere with the action of true neurotransmitters such as noradrenaline and dopamine.

Clinical features

Minor changes include somnolence, impaired memory for recent events and a characteristic difficulty with spatial orientation as shown by an impaired ability to draw shapes such as five-pointed stars, clock faces etc.

In more severe cases somnolence can progress to stupor or even coma. The physical signs include a distinctive oral fetor, flapping tremor of the outstretched hands and symmetrical hyperreflexia with variable plantar responses.

There may be clinical or laboratory evidence of a precipitating cause, such as constipation, inappropriate use of sedatives, a recent gastrointestinal haemorrhage, hypokalaemia or an infection in the lungs, urinary tract or in ascitic fluid.

Differential diagnosis

There is nothing absolutely pathognomonic, and similar encephalopathic features can be observed in other metabolic disorders (for example, renal and respiratory failure). Signs of chronic liver disease and high blood ammonia concentration would strongly suggest the diagnosis. Its severity can fluctuate markedly depending on the nature of the precipitating cause, if any, and on the treatment given.

There are characteristic EEG abnormalities, especially increased slow frequency activity, but this cannot be regarded as diagnostic.

In the neglected alcoholic patient, there are many possible sources of confusion, including withdrawal symptoms, hypoglycaemia, cerebral abscess, subdural haematoma and vitamin B_1 deficiency, and careful assessment and exclusion of focal pathology are required.

Treatment

The first essential is to try to identify any precipitating cause which can be corrected. Sedatives and opiates must be withdrawn and severe constipation corrected with a phosphate enema and oral lactulose. Gastrointestinal bleeding must be identified, hypovolaemia corrected and residual blood in the gut expelled by purgation. Hypokalaemia and other metabolic disturbances must be sought and corrected. Infections must be treated with appropriate antibiotics.

Otherwise the mainstays of treatment are a low-protein (40–60 g), high-energy diet accompanied by gentle daily purgation with lactulose (40–60 ml daily as required). It may be necessary to feed the patient via a nasogastric tube or even intravenously initially and an intake of approximately 2000 non-protein calories should be encouraged. Antibiotics, especially neomycin, have been much used in an attempt to suppress bacterial production of toxic nitrogenous compounds in the gut. Neomycin 2–4 g daily can be very effective but, if used for long periods, can damage the kidneys and the inner ear. It may be used in conjunction with lactulose in more resistant cases.

Prognosis

As with ascites, this depends on the nature of the underlying liver disease and whether it can be arrested, on the patient's compliance with dietary and drug regimens, and on whether a correctable precipitating cause can be identified. Many patients survived for long periods (years) after portocaval shunt operations but had chronic encephalopathy which greatly reduced the quality of their lives and led to the recent disenchantment with this type of surgery.

Bleeding from oesophageal varices

Aetiology

The pathological processes of hepatic fibrosis and cirrhosis produce profound effects on the hepatic circulation, leading to portal hypertension and the opening up of collateral vessels between the portal and systemic venous systems. Collaterals develop most notably along the submucosa of the oesophagus and stomach (varices) and, less frequently, deep to the anorectal mucosal junction as haemorrhoids.

Other causes of varices include hepatic venous obstruction (Budd–Chiari syndrome) and portal vein obstruction. The Budd–Chiari syndrome is a relatively acute illness (see page 182) with predominant ascites, and varices only develop later if survival is prolonged. Portal vein thrombosis may complicate cirrhosis or can occur as an isolated entity especially in the neonatal period as a result of sepsis spreading along the umbilical vein to the

porta hepatis. This is the commonest cause of childhood varices.

Fibrosis of the portal tracts without true cirrhosis is characteristic of hepatic schistosomiasis and is the commonest cause of varices in parts of the world where this disease is prevalent, such as in Egypt, parts of South America and in the Far East.

Clinical features

The bleeding is usually sudden and severe, without any obvious precipitating cause. Gastro-oesophageal reflux and oesophagitis are often invoked as aggravating factors and, if present, should be treated appropriately. There is almost always marked enlargement of the spleen and usually other features of chronic liver disease depending on the cause of the portal hypertension.

Differential diagnosis

This is from other causes of severe upper GI bleeding and depends on gastroscopy, which should be undertaken as soon as possible after initial resuscitation. Varices often coexist with ulcers and diffuse gastric erosions, and it is always necessary to undertake gastroscopy even when varices are known to be present in order to exclude other sources of blood loss.

Treatment

See Table 4.25. The first priority is to restore and maintain the circulating blood volume, with CVP monitoring. Lactulose orally and enemas should be given if bleeding produces encephalopathy.

If the bleeding continues after admission, vasopressin should be given either as a bolus (20 units in 200 ml of 5% glucose infused over 20 minutes) or as a continuous infusion (0.4 units/minute) into a peripheral vein over about two hours. This constricts the splanchnic arterioles and reduces portal pressure but produces significant side-effects, including gut colic and hypertension. Nitroglycerin can be added to the infusion to reduce these side-effects. It can be dangerous in patients with ischaemic heart disease and slow continuous infusion is probably the safer method of administration. The use of vasopressin allows time to prepare the *Sengstaken–Blakemore* tube (Fig. 4.5), which should be passed with minimal sedation into the stomach through the mouth. Meticulous attention to detail is required and there are many hazards in its use. Successful balloon tamponade will usually control bleeding and after about 24 hours the balloons

Table 4.25 Summary of management of variceal haemorrhage

Resuscitation
↓
Vasopressin (bolus or infusion)
↓
Sengstaken tube for 24–48 hours (if bleeding persists)
↓
Sclerotherapy (preferably after bleeding has stopped)
↓
Surgical stapling of varices (if bleeding persists)

Long-term
Repeated endoscopic sclerotherapy
or
Portocaval shunt surgery (now rare and
in very well-selected cases only)

should be deflated and the tube later withdrawn. Gastroscopy is repeated at the time of withdrawal so that the varices can be injected with sclerosant (2–3 ml of ethanolamine oleate into each varix under direct vision). This usually prevents further bleeding and the procedure is repeated every one or two weeks until the varices are thrombosed. Endoscopy is repeated at regular intervals thereafter (every 3–6 months) and any recurrences are reinjected in the hope of preventing further bleeding.

Sclerotherapy may be impractical during active bleeding. If the Sengstaken tube is ineffective, a surgical approach is usually required. The currently favoured procedure is to ligate the submucosal veins at the gastro-oesophageal junction with an automatic stapling device inserted from below through a gastrotomy incision. This should control bleeding for a few months but varices tend to recur and will require sclerotherapy at subsequent gastroscopy.

Prognosis

The outlook is good if bleeding can be controlled and if the underlying functional reserve of the liver is adequate. All too often, bleeding precipitates encephalopathy and an acute deterioration of liver function as shown by impaired coagulation, jaundice and ascites. In such patients, even if the bleeding can be controlled, the prognosis is very poor.

Bleeding can be prevented by various portal decompression operations (portacaval shunts), but these are much less frequently performed now in the UK, although still popular in the USA. Drugs (e.g. propranolol) can lower portal pressure and are being evaluated in the prevention of variceal bleeding.

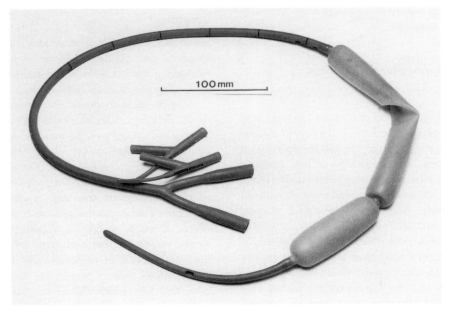

100 mm

Figure 4.5 *A Sengstaken–Blakemore tube. The distal balloon is inflated with contrast material in the stomach, the proximal with air in the oesophagus. The proximal port is continuously aspirated to prevent inhalation of saliva. The distal port is used for gastric aspiration and for the administration of drugs.*

Malignant disease of the liver

Primary hepatocellular carcinoma

Aetiology

This tumour is common in the global sense, and in parts of the underdeveloped world it is the commonest form of cancer (Table 4.26). It almost always develops in an abnormal liver, usually with evidence of pre-existing cirrhosis, although this may not have been apparent clinically. In much of the world there is a close relationship between the prevalence of hepatitis B in the community and the incidence of hepatocellular carcinoma (HCC). Viral DNA is integrated into the nuclear material of the host's liver cells and is found in the cancer cells.

However, other chronic liver diseases predispose to primary carcinoma without any evidence of previous hepatitis B infection. This applies especially to patients with alcoholic cirrhosis and haemochromatosis, but no chronic liver disease is exempt. Men with chronic liver disease are affected far more commonly than women. Aflatoxin may be an important aetiological factor in parts of the world where food is subject to fungal contamination.

Clinical features

Enlargement of the liver, accompanied by continuous pain caused by stretch of the liver capsule, suggests the presence of a liver tumour, if the patient is known to have chronic liver disease or to be a carrier of hepatitis B markers. In patients with decompensated chronic liver disease, there is usually a rapid deterioration of liver failure.

There is commonly a low-grade fever and tenderness and a vascular bruit may be heard over a palpable mass. The most helpful laboratory test is the serum alpha-feto-protein (α-FP). This is not specific for HCC but, using sensitive radio-immunoassay, 70–90 per cent of patients with HCC and cirrhosis will have detectable alpha-feto-protein, and in most patients the levels will be very high. In HCC without cirrhosis, α-FP is elevated in only 50 per cent of cases.

Imaging techniques, especially ultrasound and CT scanning, will define the extent and number of tumours and will allow guided biopsy for histological diagnosis. Images can be difficult to interpret if the tumour is multifocal and arises in a very non-homogeneous liver. Ascitic fluid, if present, is often blood-stained and must be examined cytologically for neoplastic cells. However, diagnosis generally depends on adequate liver biopsy.

Treatment

Primary HCC is often slowly growing and can remain confined to one lobe of the liver for long periods (months) so that surgical excision must be considered if the patient is relatively young and otherwise fit. It is unlikely that the rest of the liver will be absolutely normal histologically and, provided that there is good overall liver function, cirrhosis is not an absolute contraindication to surgery. Careful preoperative assessement will include CT scanning and hepatic arteriography to determine the limits of the tumour. In well-selected cases, 20–50 per cent five-year survivals can be expected in those who survive the immediate postoperative period. This outlook can be improved if sufferers are detected at an early and even asymptomatic stage. Screening programmes based on α-FP have been introduced in parts of the world where HCC is common and medical services are sophisticated (e.g. Hong Kong).

Medical treatment for HCC is not well established, but tumours will respond to a number of regimens, which usually include adriamycin and 5-fluorouracil. Clinical trials continue and so firm guidelines cannot yet be given.

Prognosis

This is very poor if the tumour is not resectable and survival beyond a few months cannot be expected. Resection does, however, offer a real hope of cure, and liver transplantation may eventually become more widely available for patients in whom resection is not possible.

Metastatic tumours

In general, metastatic tumours are treated by chemotherapy or hormonal therapy if appropriate, and prolonged survival can be achieved for example in breast cancer and in lymphoma. For many patients with the

Table 4.26 Incidence rates of primary liver cancer

Area	Rate per 100 000 males per year
Mozambique	98
China	17
S. Africa	14
UK USA Central America	2–3

common carcinomas arising from the gut, pancreas or lungs, no treatment other than simple palliation is available. Surgical excision of a solitary metastasis or metastases confined to one lobe of the liver is undertaken occasionally (for example, for colonic adenocarcinoma or renal carcinoma).

Carcinoid tumours and the carcinoid syndrome

Aetiology

These tumours arise from enterochromaffin cells situated in the gut, bronchial mucosa and elsewhere. The commonest site is the appendix, where they are found incidentally during appendicectomy and usually have no sinister long-term significance.

Clinical features

Localized tumours in the ileum (the second commonest site) can obstruct the lumen or bleed if the mucosa is ulcerated. Spread to the liver is frequent (30–60 per cent) and the metastases are large and multiple. The carcinoid syndrome is almost always associated with large hepatic metastases. The natural history is of slow progression over many years.

Functional tumours produce 5-hydroxytryptamine, bradykinin and other vasoactive compounds. The symptoms are facial flushing, abdominal cramps and diarrhoea and, less commonly, asthma and right-sided heart failure secondary to valvular changes. The symptoms are often intermittent but can persist with permanent changes in facial colour.

The diagnosis is based on the finding of a big liver with ultrasonic evidence of multiple tumour deposits. The urinary excretion of 5-hydroxyindole acetic acid (5HIAA) —a metabolite of 5-hydroxytryptamine—is greatly increased. Ultrasonically-guided liver biopsy will enable a firm histological diagnosis to be made. Not all carcinoid tumours are functional (for example, those arising from stomach and rectum are usually not) and, in such cases, histology is required to differentiate the lesions from the much commoner metastatic carcinoma.

Treatment

Pharmacological treatment using antagonists of 5-hydroxytryptamine (e.g. cyproheptadine) or inhibitors of its synthesis (e.g. parachlorophenyl-alanine) can be helpful, but in severe cases treatment designed to reduce tumour bulk is usually more satisfactory if feasible. Ultrasound, CT scan and hepatic angiography indicate whether limited hepatic resection is feasible, and this is probably the treatment of choice.

An alternative approach is embolotherapy with boluses of gel foam or wire coils, injected at arteriography, in the hope of reducing by necrosis the size of some of the larger deposits. There is a risk of producing a massive release of vasoactive compounds and pharmacological blockade must be achieved before the procedure is undertaken.

Radiotherapy and cytotoxic drugs are relatively ineffective and seldom used.

Prognosis

This is relatively good, compared with carcinoma, but the carcinoid syndrome can be distressing and very difficult to treat. Survival is very variable, but in one large series the median survival was eight years (range 1–20 years).

Further reading

Bouchier, I.A.D., Allan, R.N., Hodgson, H.J.F. and Keighley, M.R.B. (1984) *Textbook of Gastroenterology*. Ballière Tindall, London.

Sherlock, S. (1981) *Diseases of the Liver and Biliary System*, 6th edn. Blackwell Scientific Publications, Oxford.

Sherman, D.J.C. and Finlayson, N.D.C. (1982) *Diseases of the Gastrointestinal Tract and Liver*. Churchill Livingstone, Edinburgh.

Wright, R., Alberti, K.G.M.M., Karran, S. and Millward-Sadler (1979) *Liver and Biliary Disease*. W.B. Saunders, London.

5
Disorders of the Nervous System

Introduction

The evaluation and management of neurological problems follows the traditional medical approach of a history, examination and investigation leading to a diagnosis and followed by treatment.

The most important part of the initial assessment is the history, the diagnosis being evident in the majority of patients from the history alone. After the initial assessment, the answer to the question 'where is the lesion' should be clear. The history sometimes gives a precise answer and nearly always indicates the general area, and the examination provides more precise localization. The answer to the question falls into one of three categories:

1 The history and physical signs can all be explained by a lesion at one location, that is a single focal lesion.
2 It is necessary to postulate more than one focal lesion.
3 It is a system disease.

For example, a patient with a unilateral third cranial nerve palsy and a contralateral hemiplegia need only have a single lesion in the midbrain at the level of the third cranial nerve nucleus. If this patients also had unilateral amblyopia with optic atrophy, it would be necessary to postulate at least two lesions, one in the optic nerve and the other in the brain stem. Lesions at two different sites are not necessarily due to the same pathology, as is likely in this example. Many neurological conditions are neither focal nor multifocal, but affect the whole system, as in motor neurone disease, and these can be conveniently described as system diseases.

Having determined the location of the lesion, the next step is to determine its nature. The history and examination may give the answer and should give a differential diagnosis. Further investigation may be required and the choice of tests depends on the shortlist of diagnostic possibilities. Usually the simpler tests are carried out first and the more complicated tests subsequently until a diagnosis is made or a plan of management determined.

Investigations

The investigation of neurological problems uses the full range of diagnostic tools available to medicine, but some of the more specialized investigative procedures will be considered here.

Plain X-rays

1 Skull
Plain skull X-rays have been largely replaced by CT scanning; but where this is not readily available skull X-rays are useful for skull fractures, sinus disease, and bony erosions including enlargement of pituitary fossa and the internal auditory meati.

2 Spine
Cervical spine X-rays give valuable information in patients with cervical spondylosis, and it may be necessary to include lateral views in flexion and extension as well as oblique views to show the foramina. Similar information is available from lumbar and thoracic spinal X-rays. Plain X-rays may also show rib erosions, cervical ribs, congenital fusion of the vertebrae and narrow spinal canals.

Computerized X-ray tomography

The development of computerized tomography of the brain has been described as the greatest advance in the use of X-rays since their discovery by Röntgen in 1895. A narrow pulsed beam of X-rays is passed through the brain and a detector records the amount that is transmitted. The X-ray source and its corresponding detector is rotated around the head. From the data obtained the absorption coefficient or X-ray density of small volumes of brain can be computed. The resulting composite picture clearly shows any structure whose X-ray density varies from that of calcium at one extreme to that of fat at the other.

It is therefore possible to delineate tumours, abscesses, haematomas, infarcts and cerebral oedema. The ventricles are clearly seen so it is possible to say whether or not they are dilated or displaced and whether or not there is evidence of cortical atrophy. Tumours that are isodense with brain may not be seen, but their presence may be inferred from distortion of normal structures. Many tumours are enhanced following the intravenous injection of an iodine-containing contrast material, since this makes the blood vessels appear denser than normal and if it extravasates it may increase the apparent density of tumours.

The CT scan is a rapid, accurate, reliable and atraumatic method of visualizing the intracranial contents and it is associated with a low radiation dose. Early CT scanners were less reliable in showing abnormalities in the posterior fossa and in demonstrating small lesions lying close to the base of the skull. However, the latest generation of high-definition machines provide very much better images. The use of these machines has considerably reduced the need for other diagnostic procedures, particularly pneumoencephalography.

Magnetic resonance imaging

This new imaging technique (also called nuclear magnetic resonance) provides very detailed images. The images are constructed by CT techniques from the radio-frequency signal that is emitted as electron orbits return to normal, having been displaced by an electromagnetic force applied to the patient by powerful magnets. In the brain, the difference between grey and white matter is particularly well shown and small lesions of white matter are easily seen. The widespread small lesions in multiple sclerosis are particularly well demonstrated. It is possible to reconstruct the image in any plane, and, unlike X-ray CT scans, the image is not distorted by the partial volume effect close to bone and can therefore provide excellent pictures close to the floor of the skull and in the posterior fossa. It has the additional advantage of being non-invasive and does not expose the patient to X-irradiation. Since clear films of the spinal column and spinal cord can be obtained, it is possible that this technique will eventually replace conventional myelography, although

at present the definition of nerve roots in the cervical region is less satisfactory. Good visualization of lumbar roots is obtainable.

CSF analysis

Lumbar puncture for CSF analysis may be diagnostic in all forms of meningitis and meningoencephalitis. Carcinomatous meningitis may be diagnosed from the morphology of cells obtained by lumbar puncture, and the analysis of CSF proteins, including protein immunoelectrophoresis, may be helpful in the diagnosis of multiple sclerosis.

Cerebral angiography

The carotid and vertebral arterial system can be visualized by injection of a radio-opaque dye and rapid-sequence X-rays to show the arterial, capillary and venous stages. This is usually done by femoral catheterization and then by selective catheterization of the artery of interest, although it can be carried out by direct arterial puncture. Angiography is indicated if the diagnosis on the CT scan is in doubt, if it appears to be a vascular lesion, particularly a cerebral angioma, or if detailed anatomy of the vascular tree is required by a surgeon planning operative intervention.

A recent advance in this field is the development of digital computerization of the image from which can be subtracted the digitalized data from a plain skull film, thus giving a subtraction image. This subtraction technique allows visualization of very weak concentrations of contrast medium so that arteries and veins can be seen following intravenous injection. Intravenous injection opacifies all the arteries and veins which may make interpretation difficult, but very-high-definition films can be obtained following the intra-arterial injection of very small volumes of contrast material. It seems likely that most angiography will be carried out using these techniques in the future.

Doppler ultrasonic angiology

This can be used to measure the velocity of red blood cells. It shows the direction of flow and turbulence and is used to assess the carotid arteries. B-mode scanning shows an image of the artery.

Pneumoencephalography

In this investigation air is used as a contrast medium displacing CSF in the ventricular system and cerebral subarachnoid spaces following lumbar injection. This investigation has been completely replaced by CT scans and magnetic resonance imaging.

Electroencephalography

The EEG provides valuable information in patients with all forms of epilepsy and in many forms of encephalopathy, including toxic, metabolic, inflammatory and degenerative diseases. It is of no value in the assessment of space-occupying lesions.

Isotope scans

Isotope brain scans using technetium have been largely replaced by CT scans and magnetic resonance imaging. Where these investigations are not available the isotope brain scan may provide useful information in subdural haematoma and multiple metastases. Isotope cisternography may be a useful test in patients with communicating hydrocephalus (see page 196).

Intellectual function and dementia

Tests of intellectual function

A formal psychometric analysis of intelligence provides quantitative information and can be used to follow progress. Simple bedside testing provides useful clinical information, but appropriate allowance must be made for educational background.

1 Orientation
The patient is asked the day of the week, the date, the month, the year, where he is at the moment and his home address.

2 Memory
Tests of memory are conveniently divided into three groups:
(a) *Immediate recall.* The patient is asked to repeat a sequence of random numbers, first forwards (normal more than six) and then backwards (normal four or more).
(b) *The five-minutes memory test.* This is usually carried out with a name, an address and a flower. The number of errors and the total number of words should be recorded.
(c) *Long-term memory.* Questions may include items from the patient's past or items of national importance and should be adjusted to the patient's educational level and social background.

3 Learning
The patient should be asked to learn the Babcock sentence by repeating it after the examiner as often as necessary to get it word perfect; this should be achieved in less than five attempts.
4 Calculation
The patient is asked to subtract seven from a hundred and continue to subtract seven from the result; the time taken and number of errors should be recorded. This is usually called 'serial sevens'.

Dementia (see also page 468)

Dementia is a deterioration in the intellectual function of the brain as a result of organic disease. It is a sign and sometimes a symptom, but it is not a diagnosis.

About 50 per cent of elderly patients with dementia have Alzheimer's disease, about 20 per cent have cerebrovascular disease alone and about 20 per cent have a combination of these two degenerative diseases. The remaining 10 per cent are divided among a wide range of conditions, including syphilis, Jakob–Creutzfeldt disease, low-pressure hydrocephalus, Huntington's chorea, tumours, progressive multifocal leucoencephalopathy, toxic and deficiency diseases, including alcohol, vitamins B_1, B_6 and B_{12} and myxoedema.

It is usually easy to identify patients with the typical features of the two principal causes of dementia—Alzheimer's disease and vascular disease—but they are not mutually exclusive and in the elderly they often occur together.

Alzheimer's disease

The cause of this progressive cerebral degeneration is unknown, but cholinergic pathways are the most severely affected. It may occur at any age and is more common in women and in the elderly.

It presents with a very slow insidious onset of mental deterioration, often starting with memory impairment. The presenting features may suggest lateralization to one hemisphere, but focal deficits do not occur and epilepsy is unusual. Alzheimer's disease has a characteristic pathological appearance with neurofibrillary tangles and argyrophilic plaques.

Vascular disease

Cerebrovascular disease rarely causes dementia under the age of 60 without clear evidence of generalized vascular disease, particularly systemic hypertension. Dementia may result from strokes and the subsequent deterioration may be stepwise as further infarcts occur. Vascular disease may also cause a more insidious dementia without clinically evident infarcts. Men are much more frequently affected than women and insight is often preserved.

Binswanger's disease is a vascular leucoencephalopathy nearly always associated with hypertension. There is a characteristic appearance on the CT scan with low-density areas in the frontal periventricular white matter.

Communicating hydrocephalus (formally called low-pressure hydrocephalus) is caused by an obstruction to CSF pathways outside the ventricular system, usually at the tentorial hiatus or at the longitudinal sinus. The history of dementia is often short and may be associated with a clearly identifiable cause such as head injury, subarachnoid haemorrhage, meningitis or following surgical intervention in the posterior fossa. The classical triad is dementia with akinesia, incontinence and a gait apraxia. The CT scan shows markedly dilated ventricles including the third and fourth ventricles, and lack of CSF over the surface as the brain is pushed out against the skull. If a suitable isotope is injected into the lumbar theca, it enters the ventricular system and stays there for 48–72 hours, whereas in the normal subject the isotope would be distributed according to the CSF flow over the surface of the brain to be cleared through the longitudinal sinus. Patients who show these characteristic clinical features and investigations, particularly if they have a clear cause for the condition, usually respond very well to ventriculo-atrial or ventriculo-peritoneal shunts.

Investigation of dementia

Although the chances of finding a treatable cause are small, it is important to attempt a precise aetiological or pathological diagnosis and to exclude the treatable conditions, particularly in younger patients.

This should include a search for space-occupying lesions, toxic, metabolic and deficiency states, and tests for syphilis. Special tests should include electroencephalography and a CT scan. Exceptionally a brain biopsy is required to establish a diagnosis. CSF analysis may be appropriate in certain cases.

The cerebral hemispheres

The dominant hemisphere and language

This is the left hemisphere in all right-handed patients and in about 50 per cent of left-handed patients. The dominant hemisphere is concerned with all forms of language.

All *language inputs* are processed in Wernicke's area, which is at the posterior end of the superior temporal gyrus. It receives input from the primary visual cortex for reading, semaphore and other visual forms of language and from the primary auditory cortex for speech, morse code and auditory forms of language. It may also receive information from the somatosensory cortex for the interpretation of Braille.

A lesion of the primary visual cortex causes blindness, but a lesion of the pathway between the visual cortex and Wernicke's area causes dyslexia; in patients with this condition, comprehension of the spoken word is preserved. Information going initially to the right hemisphere has to cross the corpus callosum to reach Wernicke's area, so that a lesion affecting the left visual cortex and the posterior part of the corpus callosum causes a right homonymous hemianopia and dyslexia because of interruption of information from the right visual cortex to Wernicke's area.

Lesions of Wernicke's area cause loss of ability to understand any form of language input (Wernicke's aphasia; fluent, receptive or sensory aphasia). The patient can still speak clearly and fluently, but since there is no auditory feedback cannot understand what he is saying and is unaware of any errors he may make. This usually produces fluent nonsense.

All *language output* arises in Broca's area and is then relayed to the motor cortex for speech and writing. If a lesion is confined to Broca's area and Wernicke's area is intact, comprehension is preserved but the patient is unable to express himself (Broca's aphasia; non-fluent, expressive or motor aphasia). If he attempts a word and gets it wrong, he is immediately aware of the error and attempts to correct it. This produces a halting, non-fluent dysphasia, which in mild cases may consist of some hesitation only, while in the more severe cases there may be no speech at all.

Both Wernicke's area and Broca's area, together with their connecting pathways, are supplied by the middle cerebral artery and an infarct in this territory is the commonest cause of dysphasia; tumours are the next commonest cause. Anterior lesions are more likely to cause non-fluent dysphasia and posterior lesions cause fluent dysphasia.

Gerstmann's syndrome is caused by a lesion of the dominant angular gyrus and consists of finger agnosia, right/left disorientation, dysgraphia, dyscalculia and dyslexia.

The non-dominant hemisphere and spatial orientation

The non-dominant hemisphere is concerned with spatial awareness, both personal and extrapersonal, at a higher level than the primary sensory cortex concerned with vision, hearing and somatosensory information. This is the reason why patients with a right hemisphere lesion may show a striking neglect of the left side of the body and ignore objects in the left visual field out of proportion to the sensory and visual loss. Lesions of the left hemisphere may cause some sensory extinction, but neglect or denial of the right side of the body is unusual. This loss of spatial orientation causes difficulty in dressing (dressing dyspraxia) and difficulty in finding the way in a familiar environment (topographical amnesia).

The cranial nerves

The olfactory nerve (I)

This is the only cranial nerve in the anterior fossa. Numerous small fibres arising in the mucosa in the roof of the nasal cavity pass through the cribriform plate to reach the olfactory bulb, which is continuous posteriorly with the olfactory tract lying in the olfactory groove. Just above the anterior clinoid processes there is a partial decussation. Lesions behind this decussation cannot cause a unilateral or complete loss of the sense of smell. The sensory cortex for smell is in the uncus on the medial aspect of the temporal lobe.

This pathway serves all smell and this includes all flavour; only the cruder sensations of salt, sweet, bitter and acid are relayed through the chorda tympani and glossopharyngeal nerves.

Apparent loss of the sense of smell may be due to nasal obstruction. It is important, therefore, to determine that the airway is clear before testing smell on both sides separately with a mild non-irritant odour. There may be temporary loss of smell as a result of acute or chronic rhinitis, but the commonest cause is head injury, particularly occipital head injuries. If the penetrating fibres through the cribriform plate are sheared, the loss of smell is permanent. If continuity exists they may recover. Unilateral or bilateral anosmia may be an early sign in tumours in the floor of the anterior fossa, in particular, olfactory groove meningiomas.

The optic nerve (II)

Changes in visual acuity imply some abnormality of macula vision. There may, of course, be a distortion of information reaching the macula owing to refractive errors or lens opacities. It is important, therefore, to test visual acuity with the refractive errors corrected. Impairment of visual acuity may also be due to a lesion affecting the macula fibres in the optic nerve. Lesions behind the chiasm always affect the vision in both eyes.

Lesions of the visual pathways causing visual field defects can be accurately localized owing to the anatomical arrangement of the visual fibres as they traverse the length of the brain to the visual cortex.

1 Retinal lesions
The raised intraocular pressure associated with glaucoma first affects the superficial retinal fibres which come from the periphery, with resultant loss of peripheral vision (tunnel vision). Infarction of small bundles of retinal fibres causes arcuate scotomata.

2 Loss of one visual field
This must be due to disease of the optic nerve. Small lesions cause unilateral scotomata or defects and are best delineated with a small red object. The commonest cause is retrobulbar neuritis (disseminated sclerosis).

3 Lesions affecting the chiasm
Central compression damages the decussating fibres and causes a bitemporal field defect; in the early stages this may be bilateral temporal scotomata, which are often asymmetrical. Later the more typical bitemporal hemianopia develops. The commonest cause is a chromaphobe adenoma of the pituitary. There are usually some features of hypopituitarism of hypothalamic dysfunction, either clinically or on laboratory investigation. Eosinophilic tumours may also cause chiasmal compression, but the clinical features of acromegaly are usually obvious. Basophil adenomas produce florid Cushing's disease before they become sufficiently large to compress the chiasm. Craniopharyngiomas produce a similar visual field defect; calcification can often be seen in the tumour on plain X-ray.

4 Lesions of the visual pathways
Behind the chiasm these cause homonymous hemianopia. The nearer the visual cortex, the more congruous the defect. The fibres of the optic radiation are widely separated shortly after leaving the lateral geniculate ganglion, so that lesions of the temporal lobe may cause an upper quadrantic defect and lesions above the Sylvian fissure a lower quadrantic defect. Macula sparing may occur in vascular lesions of the cortex because the cortical area concerned with macula vision receives its supply from more than one main cerebral artery.

With ophthalmoscopy the retina with its blood supply and the optic disc can be visualized directly. In addition the cornea, lens, anterior and posterior chambers can be examined.

Papillitis and papilloedema

The optic disc may be oedematous and appear swollen. If this is due to an inflammatory process of the nerve head (the same pathology as retrobulbar neuritis) it is called papillitis and vision is affected early and severely. There are no other retinal changes and no haemorrhages. If the swelling is caused by raised intracranial pressure or systemic hypertension, it is called papilloedema and the vision is not affected apart from enlargement of the blind spot. In severe cases of papilloedema the pressure may occlude the arterial supply and cause attacks of amblyopia, which occasionally results in permanent blindness. The presence of hypertensive retinal changes and a markedly elevated systemic blood pressure or the presence of retinal haemorrhages with preservation of vision clearly distinguishes papilloedema from papillitis, but in many patients the appearance of the fundus is indistinguishable. Raised intracranial pressure may be accompanied by headache and vomiting and, if acute, by altered consciousness.

Pseudopapilloedema

Occasionally patients are found to have the appearance of papilloedema but with no evidence of raised intracranial pressure. This swelling of the nerve head is a congenital abnormality. The differentiation from papilloedema may be extremely difficult and many require a CT brain scan and fluorescein angiography.

Optic atrophy

Optic atrophy refers to an appearance of the optic disc, which loses its normal pink/yellow colour and assumes a grey/white appearance. There is usually reduced visual acuity or a field defect. The terms primary optic atrophy, secondary optic atrophy and consecutive optic atrophy are purely descriptive and have no pathological connotation. Primary optic atrophy implies a clearly demarcated pale disc with normal retina and blood vessels. It is caused by any lesion of the optic nerve, the commonest of which is retrobulbar neuritis; but it may follow compression by tumours or be the result of toxic (quinine, tobacco, methyl alcohol) or deficiency states (vitamin B_{12}). Secondary optic atrophy implies a pale disc with a hazy outline, which follows swelling of the nerve head (papilloedema or papillitis). Consecutive optic atrophy implies a pale disc where the cause of the atrophy can be seen in the fundus (retinitis pigmentosa, syphilis).

The oculomotor, trochlear and abducent nerves (III, IV and VI)

Disorders of the oculomotor system can be divided into upper motor neurone lesions (disorders of gaze), lower motor neurone lesions (disorders of the third, fourth and sixth cranial nerves) and internuclear lesions (a mixture of upper and lower motor neurone disorders with vestibular or cerebellar components).

(a) Gaze palsies

Gaze palsies result from upper motor neurone lesions of the oculomotor system and, in common with all upper motor neurone lesions, it is the movement which is affected, not the action of individual muscles—in this case conjugate eye movement. There are centres concerned with gaze both in cortex and in the brain stem.

The cortex

There are two cortical gaze centres in each hemisphere. The *frontal eye field* in the premotor cortex is responsible for scanning and roving eye movements and is the site of conscious voluntary control of eye movement. As with the control of other movements, one hemisphere is responsible for the opposite side of the body and the contralateral extrapersonal space; the left frontal eye field therefore directs eye movement to the right, and vice versa. The effect of destruction and excitation can therefore be predicted:
(a) *Destruction* (e.g. infarction)—transient paralysis of gaze to the opposite side. Occasionally deviation of the eyes to the side of the lesion may be seen.
(b) *Excitation* (e.g. epilepsy)—deviation of the eyes and usually the head to the opposite side (frontal adversive seizure).
Following and reflex eye movements are not affected by lesions of the frontal eye field, and optokinetic nystagmus is normal.

The *occipital eye field* in the visual association cortex is responsible for following, pursuit and reflex eye movements. It is intimately associated with the visual pathways and lesions in this area are usually associated with a field defect. In destructive lesions (infarction or tumour) there is a full range of voluntary movements but inability to follow or locate objects. Examination is usually complicated by the associated field defect. Optokinetic nystagmus is impaired.

The brain stem

There are two areas in the brain stem concerned with conjugate eye movements.

1 Upper midbrain and vertical eye movements

There is no precise centre for vertical eye movement but the pathways concerned must lie at and above the level of the third nerve nucleus in the region of the posterior commissure. Lesions in the pretectal region (pinealomas) pressing on the superior corpora quadragemini cause defects of upward gaze (*Parinaud's syndrome*).

2 Pons and horizontal eye movements

There are two pontine gaze centres situated close to the sixth nerve nuclei on either side and responsible for gaze to the same side; this function is mediated through the pontine paramedian reticular formation (BPRF).

Examination for gaze palsies should include both voluntary and following movements as well as tests for optokinetic nystagmus.

(b) The cranial nerves and eye movements

Third cranial nerve

The third cranial nerve nucleus lies ventrally in the periductal grey matter in the midbrain at the level of the superior corpora quadragemini and the red nucleus. It is a large nucleus with clear grouping of nerve cells responsible for the different muscles innervated. Nearby is the Edinger–Westphal nucleus whose parasympathetic fibres run with the third nerve. The nerve runs forwards through the red nucleus and the medial part of the basis pedunculi emerging close to the midline in the interpeduncular fossa. The two nerves pass on either side of the basilar artery between the posterior cerebral artery above and the superior cerebellar artery below. The nerve lies just below the posterior communicating artery throughout its length and passes laterally over the internal carotid artery to enter the cavernous sinus where it lies on the lateral wall. It passes through the superior orbital fissure and divides into two main branches—the superior branch to the superior rectus and levator palpebrae superioris and the inferior branch to the medial rectus, inferior rectus and the inferior oblique. The parasympathetic nerves travel with the inferior branch. A complete third-nerve palsy comprises a fixed dilated pupil due to the unopposed action of the sympathetic, ptosis due to involvement of levator palpebrae superioris, and

a fully abducted eye due to the unopposed action of sixth nerve.

Fourth cranial nerve

The fourth cranial nerve lies ventrally in the periductal grey matter nearly at the junction of the midbrain and pons and at the level of the inferior corpora quadragemini. The nerve runs round the aqueduct and decussates in the superior medullary velum. The nerve then passes round the cerebral peduncle below the tentorium, the posterior cerebral artery lying just above the tentorium. Like the third nerve, it passes between the posterior cerebral artery and the superior cerebellar artery, crosses the apex of the petrous temporal bone just above and medial to Meckel's cave, and enters the cavernous sinus lying on the lateral wall below the third nerve. It then passes through the superior orbital fissure to supply the superior oblique muscle. A fourth-nerve palsy causes vertical diplopia, maximal on downward gaze with the affected eye adducted.

Sixth cranial nerve

The sixth cranial nerve nucleus lies in the lower pons close to the midline and near the floor of the fourth ventricle. The fibres of the seventh nerve are wrapped around the sixth nerve nucleus and this forms a small hump in the floor of the fourth ventricle, the facial colliculus. The nerve runs forward to emerge at the pontomedullary junction near the midline. It runs up the clivus in front of the pons parallel to the basilar artery and then at the tentorial hiatus it turns forwards to enter the cavernous sinus where it lies below the internal carotid artery. From the cavernous sinus it passes through the superior orbital fissure to supply the lateral rectus muscle.

A sixth-nerve palsy causes horizontal diplopia, maximal on gaze to the affected side.

(c) Lesions and their effects

All three nerves may be damaged by brain-stem tumours and vascular disease. The extramedullary part of the nerve trunks between the brain stem and the cavernous sinus are vulnerable to granulomatous meningitis (tuberculosis and sarcoid), meningovascular syphilis and nasopharyngeal carcinoma. The intracavernous course of these nerves may be damaged in cavernous sinus thrombosis, carotid aneurysm and pituitary tumours. The superior orbital fissure may be encroached by sphenoidal ridge meningiomas and the nerves may be damaged in the intraorbital part of their course by orbital tumours. In addition the nerves may be damaged by involvement of their vasa-nervorum in diabetes, hypertension and collagen vascular disease (polyarteritis nodosa and giant cell arteritis).

Lesions of the third nerve

Intramedullary lesions

Nerve nucleus. Lesions of the nuclei are usually bilateral because they lie close together. The commonest cause is pressure from above by tumours of the pineal gland or gliomas (*Parinaud's syndrome*).

The nerve trunk and red nucleus (Benedikt's syndrome). The combination of a third-nerve palsy and a contralateral flapping tremor with ataxia of the arm and hand is usually due to vascular disease, disseminated sclerosis or a tumour.

Nerve trunk and cerebral peduncle (Weber's syndrome). A combination of a third-nerve palsy and a contralateral hemiplegia is usually of vascular origin.

2 Extramedullary lesions

Bilateral third-nerve palsies and tetraparesis may result from any large space-occupying lesion in the interpeduncular fossa. The third-nerve may be damaged by aneurysm at either end of the posterior communicating artery, although the internal carotid/posterior communicating aneurysms are very much more common.

Lesions of the fourth nerve

Isolated lesions of the fourth cranial nerve are rare and are usually due to trauma, diabetes, granulomatous meningitis, syphilis or collagen vascular disease.

Lesions of the sixth nerve

Lesions affecting the nucleus almost always involve the seventh cranial nerve, and since these nerves then follow quite separate pathways, a combination of a sixth and seventh lower motor neurone lesion is likely to be at this level.

Sixth cranial nerve and contralateral hemiplegia (*Raymond–Cestan* syndrome) is directly analogous to Weber's syndrome.

The nerve trunk is very vulnerable when it crosses the free edge of the tentorium, and it may be damaged here if the brain stem is distorted by a space-occupying lesion in the opposite hemisphere (a false localising sign) or if there is displacement of the brain stem through the tentorial hiatus (coning).

Internuclear ophthalmoplegias

A combination of upper motor neurone lesions usually associated with evidence of cerebellar or vestibular involvement (nystagmus) is common because of the wide spatial separation of the third, fourth and sixth nerve nuclei from the upper midbrain to the lower pons, the separation of mechanisms controlling vertical and horizontal conjugate movement and the intimate relationship of vestibular and cerebellar function to eye movement. There are many possible combinations; patients may develop a series of different combinations of signs during the course of an illness, particularly in progressive lesions such as pontine glioma. However, there are two principal combinations of signs.

1 Anterior internuclear ophthalmoplegia

(Superior or upper, Harris's sign). There is normal convergence but a failure to adduct on lateral gaze with nystagmus in the abducting eye. The lesion lies between the fourth nerve nucleus and sixth nerve nucleus and involves the medial longitudinal bundle. It is almost always due to disseminated sclerosis.

2 Posterior internuclear ophthalmoplegia

(inferior or lower). This is the opposite of an anterior internuclear ophthalmoplegia and there is failure to abduct on lateral gaze with nystagmus in the adducting eye. The lesion lies at or just below the sixth nerve-nucleus.

Diplopia

The analysis of diplopia depends on a knowledge of the precise actions of the extraocular muscles. The medial walls of the two orbits are nearly parallel and the lateral walls are roughly at right angles to each other. Since the muscles are inserted into a fibrous ring at the apex of the orbit, the muscle cone is at an angle of about 23° to the optical axis. It is evident therefore, that the lateral and medial recti only move the eye in the horizontal plane, but the superior and inferior recti only become pure elevators or depressors when the optical axis is the same as the muscle-cone axis, that is when the eye is 23° abducted, so that the line of pull of the muscle lies over the optical axis of the globe. Similarly the superior and inferior oblique muscles are only pure elevators or depressors when the eye is adducted since the origin or effective origin of the oblique muscles is antero-medial to the eye. When the eye is abducted the oblique muscles produce rotation only around the optical axis but no vertical movement, and similarly the superior and inferior recti rotate the eye without elevation or depression when the eye is adducted.

The reason why patients see double when one muscle is not functioning is that the normal eye moves to keep the image on the macula, but the image falls progressively further round the retina away from the macula in the palsied eye. The brain projects this false image further away from its true position and the degree of separation of the images is directly proportional to the distance from the macula. It follows, therefore, that the direction of maximal separation of the images is in the direction of action of the affected muscle, and it also follows that the distal image is always the false one. In this context, distal means furthest away from a point straight in front of the eyes.

When a patient complains of double vision he should be asked the direction in which the separation of the images is maximal and whether the separation is in the horizontal or vertical plane. Since the distal image is always the false one, covering one eye will show which eye is giving rise to the false image. In horizontal diplopia, this will reveal whether the double vision is due to one medial rectus or the other lateral rectus. The situation is complicated in vertical diplopia because two muscles are used to elevate and two to depress the eye. First determine whether the diplopia is maximal on upward or downward gaze, then determine which eye is responsible for the false image. This reduces the possibility to two muscles, then determine whether the diplopia is maximal with the affected eye abducted (a rectus palsy) or adducted (an oblique palsy). To summarize:

1 *The direction of maximal separation of the images is the direction of action of the affected muscle.*
2 *The peripheral image is always the false one.*
3 *In vertical diplopia, separation of the images is maximal when the affected eye is adducted in oblique palsies and when abducted with rectus palsies.*

The cause of diplopia is often obvious, such as a complete sixth or third nerve lesion. But it may be difficult in partial lesions and in detecting multiple lesions without proper examination. The full range of movement should be tested with both eyes open and each eye separately with the cover test to determine which eye is fixing. When diplopia has been present for some time the false image may be suppressed and the patient loses the double vision. When there is already a marked disparity in the visual acuity of the two eyes, the patient may still prefer to fix with the eye with the better visual acuity, even if its movement is impaired.

Nystagmus

Accurate and stable eye fixation normally occurs despite constant movement of both the observer and the object. Fixation on a moving object while the observer remains still is achieved by the parieto-occipital eye field and ocular fixation. Compensation for movement of the observer is through a sensitive feedback mechanism from the vestibular system and to a lesser extent from the proprioceptive system via the cerebellum. A lesion affecting any one of these mechanisms, visual fixation, vestibular and cerebellar pathways, can give rise to nystagmus.

Nystagmus is the jerky eye movement due to a failure to maintain fixation; the eye drifts away from the object so that a rapid voluntary movement is required to regain fixation.

1 Ocular nystagmus
This is due to a defect of fixation and is, therefore, seen with small central scotomata, general depression of visual acuity (usually congenital), miner's nystagmus and other defects of the macula. It usually takes the form of a fine oscillatory movement without clear fast and slow components, it is present in all directions of gaze, including gaze ahead, and may be only visible on ophthalmoscopic examination as a fine tremor (jelly nystagmus).

2 Vestibular nystagmus
Disturbance of the vestibular mechanism is the commonest and most important cause of nystagmus and may be due to a lesion of the vestibular end organ or its central connections. Nystagmus due to vestibular end organ disease is always associated with vertigo and habituates after a few weeks. Nystagmus not associated with any other features which persists for more than a few weeks must be due to a central lesion.

3 Cerebellar nystagmus
The cerebellum is concerned with the maintenance of ocular fixation and this is in part related to information from the proprioceptive system in the neck. Unilateral lesions of the cerebellum may produce nystagmus, particularly if it affects the deep nuclei. Midline and degenerative lesions usually do not cause nystagmus, probably because the balance between the two sides is not disturbed.

4 Brain-stem or central nystagmus
Lesions of the vestibular and cerebellar pathways in the brain stem may cause nystagmus. This is often lateralised but may be bilateral and vertical nystagmus only occurs in brain stem lesions.

Examination. The patient should be asked to follow an object, both vertically and to either side. The object must be held at or beyond the near point, so that the patient does not have to converge and the extremes of movement should be within binocular vision.

Nystagmoid movements of no significance may be seen if these precautions are not followed. The direction of nystagmus is recorded as the direction of the quick component, even though the quick component is the voluntary overriding attempt at fixation and a slow drift to the resting position is the abnormal movement. If nystagmus is not present on gaze ahead but has to be elicited, it is always in the direction of gaze. The degree of nystagmus should be recorded: first-degree nystagmus to the left is nystagmus only on gaze to the left, second-degree nystagmus to the left is nystagmus to the left on gaze ahead, and third-degree nystagmus to the left is nystagmus to the left on gaze to the right. In unconscious patients vestibular lesions or stimulation by caloric testing causes tonic conjugate deviation, because there is no conscious effort to override this.

The pupil

The pupillary muscles are arranged both *concentrically* (the sphincter pupilli, which receives its parasympathetic nerve supply from the ciliary ganglion via the short ciliary nerves) and *radially* (the dilator pupilli, which is innervated by sympathetic fibres via the nasociliary nerve).

The pupil of one eye constricts when that eye is exposed to light (the direct reaction) and at the same time the pupil of the other eye also constricts (the consensual reaction). Dilatation occurs in the dark. The *afferent* pathway is via the optic nerve to the lateral geniculate ganglion and then through the brain stem to the third-nerve nuclei on both sides. The *efferent* pathway runs from the Edinger–Westphal nucleus via the third nerve to the ciliary ganglion.

Fixation on an object within the near point requires convergence of the optical axes, and this is associated with pupillary constriction. The *afferent* pathway is with the visual fibres to the occipital cortex, and the *efferent* pathway is from the Edinger–Westphal nucleus.

1 Vascular and hyaline degeneration

This is common in old age and may give rise to pupils which are small, unequal, irregular and relatively immobile.

2 The myotonic pupil

This is dilated and shows a very slow reaction to light and convergence. It may be necessary to keep the patient in the dark for some time before testing the light reflex and to ask the patient to fix on a near object for several minutes to show the contraction with convergence. This condition occurs much more commonly in women and is often of sudden onset. It is thought to be due to a post-ganglionic lesion in the efferent parasympathetic

pathway. The defect is permanent but does not carry any other pathological connotation. The myotonic pupil may be found in conjunction with absence of tendon reflexes (the *Holmes–Adie syndrome*).

3 Horner's syndrome

This consists of pupillary constriction, slight ptosis, and failure to sweat on the same side of the face. The syndrome results from a lesion anywhere in the sympathetic pathway from the hypothalamus down through the lateral part of the pons and medulla, and Clarke's column in the lateral column of the cervical cord. The fibres then emerge at the level of the first thoracic segment to relay in the cervical sympathetic genglion and then pass up in a plexus on the carotid artery to be distributed throughout the territory of the external and internal carotid arteries. It is, therefore, a poor localizing sign, but a good lateralizing sign because the pathway does remain ipsilateral throughout its course.

4 Argyll Robertson pupils

The pupils are small, unequal, eccentric and irregular. They do not react to light but do constrict on convergence. The lesion is thought to affect the afferent pathway in the midbrain. It is almost always due to syphilis.

5 The afferent pupillary defect

This is a useful sign in patients with an optic nerve lesion, such as retrobulbar neuritis. The ipsilateral direct reaction and the contralateral consensual reaction are impaired because of the lesion in the afferent pathway, but the consensual reaction following exposure of the other eye to light is brisk, since the efferent pathway functions normally. If a light is shone alternately into both eyes the affected eye will show only the consensual reaction and, therefore, follows the constriction and dilatation of the normal eye, so that when the light is removed from the normal to the affected eye the pupil is seen to dilate.

The trigeminal nerve (V)

The trigeminal nerve has three major peripheral branches. The *ophthalmic* branch supplies the eye via the nasociliary nerve, the forehead and the scalp as far back as the vertex. A small strip extends down the bridge of the nose. The fibres pass back through the roof of the orbit, through the superior orbital foramen, along the lateral wall of the cavernous sinus to reach the gasserian ganglion situated in Meckel's cave at the apex of the petrous temporal bone.

The *maxillary* branch supplies the lower eyelid, the side of the nose, the cheek and the upper lip. It extends laterally only to a line approximately between the outer canthus of the eye and the side of the mouth. The fibres pass through the maxilla and enter the anteromedial aspect of the middle cranial fossa via the foramen rotundum to reach the gasserian ganglion.

The *mandibular* branch supplied the lower lip and chin, a thin strip lateral to the maxillary division but sparing an area of three fingers from the angle of the jaw; it supplies the upper part of the tragus and adjoining parts of the pinna and a variable area of adjacent scalp on the side of the head. The fibres pass back through the pterygoid fossa and reach the gasserian ganglion via the foramen ovale, which lies just below the ganglion.

The *motor division* travels with the mandibular branch and supplies muscles of mastication, particularly the lateral pterygoid.

Distal lesions usually affect one branch only because of the wide separation of the three main branches distal to the ganglion. Lesions of the nerve proximal to the ganglion, as it crosses the anterior end of the cerebello-pontine angle to enter the mid pons, affect all three divisions to some extent. The earliest sign of a lesion of the pathway between the main sensory nucleus and the gasserian ganglion is loss of the corneal reflex. Lesions below mid pons affect only the descending tract or its decussating fibres, which relay the sensations of pain and temperature. The arrangement of fibres in the descending tract results in 'onion skin' loss of sensation of the face from compressive lesions, with the snout area nearest the main sensory nucleus and the most peripheral of the 'onion skins' extending down into the upper cervical region. Lesions of the descending tract may cause diminution but not loss of the corneal reflex.

Intramedullary lesions affecting the trigeminal nerve include syringobulbia, demyelinating disease, tumours and infarcts. Extra medullary intracranial causes include lesions in the cerebellar pontine angle, such as acoustic neuromas, meningiomas and trigeminal neuromas, granulomatous meningitis (tuberculosis, sarcoid and syphilis) and nasopharyngeal carcinoma eroding the base of the skull.

(a) Pain in the face

There are many causes of facial pain and these need to be differentiated carefully as the treatments are often quite different.

Idiopathic trigeminal neuralgia (tic douloureux)

The cause of this condition is unknown. It may occur at any age but becomes more common with increasing age.

In young patients it may be a sign of multiple sclerosis.

The pain is always *confined to the distribution of the trigeminal nerve*, usually affecting either the third or second divisions or both; involvement of the first division alone is rare. Involvement of both sides is quite exceptional.

The pain is *paroxysmal* and usually described as a brief, stabbing, lancinating or shooting pain. It is usually extremely severe, lasting for a few seconds only but may be repeated frequently. It is always *precipitated* and patients may describe a trigger point which is particularly sensitive. Trigger stimuli include touch, washing or shaving, facial movement, eating and drinking hot or cold liquids. During particularly severe bouts, patients may not be able to speak, eat or drink.

Patients usually have frequent stabs of pain over a short period of time and may then have minutes or hours of freedom before the next bout. These paroxysms occur over several weeks before complete remission. The pain always returns but the interval may vary from months to years. The periods of remission tend to become shorter and bouts of pain more severe and longer. A few patients never show remission. The pain always remains paroxysmal and never becomes constant. There are *never any abnormal signs*.

The only effective medication is carbamazepine and this will control the pain in almost all patients, at least initially. Treatment should be started with 300 mg a day in divided doses and increased as required up to a total dose of 1200 mg a day. The development of a rash is an idiosyncratic side-effect and the medication should be stopped. Dose-dependent side-effects include unsteadiness, vertigo and nausea and these can be relieved by reducing the dose. In some patients this treatment is ineffective or becomes so with repeated exacerbations. For these reasons, or because the patient is unable to tolerate the medication, it may be necessary to destroy the trigeminal nerve. To be effective the lesion must be at or proximal to the gasserian ganglion as lesions distal to the ganglion cause only temporary relief of symptoms and are usually unsatisfactory. The ganglion may be reached through the cheek and foramen ovale and injected with phenol or alcohol, or destroyed with a radio-frequency probe or cryoprobe. The sensory root may be divided between the ganglion and the pons following craniotomy, in which case an attempt may be made to preserve the corneal reflex by a partial root section. If this is done properly, the analgesia and the relief of pain are permanent. After partial lesions a few patients complain of unpleasant sensations in the face (anaesthesia dolorosa). Most patients quickly become accustomed to a numb face, but they must always exercise great care to prevent corneal ulceration and should wear glasses with a side-piece to protect the eye. They should also be warned against nasal ulceration.

Symptomatic trigeminal neuralgia

This condition may be clinically indistinguishable from idiopathic trigeminal neuralgia with precisely the same features and no detectable neurological deficit. If any abnormal signs are found (usually an impaired corneal reflex) it cannot be idiopathic trigeminal neuralgia and there is an underlying abnormality such as disseminated sclerosis, a congenital vascular anomaly, a neoplasm in the cerebellar pontine angle, or nasopharyngeal carcinoma.

A number of patients have been found to have an aberrant artery which impinges on the trigeminal nerve root. This can be surgically separated and the root decompressed, with relief of symptoms without damage to the trigeminal nerve. Such patients usually have atypical features such as persisting pain, a pain which is not obviously triggered and some persisting neurological deficit. The absence of these features does not exclude the possibility of an aberrant artery.

Atypical facial pain

This condition commonly occurs in middle-aged women. No organic cause is ever found and it is thought to be largely if not completely psychosomatic. The patient complains of constant aching pain, usually in the jaw, which does not vary much throughout the day and persists for weeks or months. It is often helped by the use of tricyclic antidepressent drugs.

Temporomandicular joint dysfunction

This can cause an aching pain in the mandible which is usually worse with chewing.

Facial migraine

This is a rare manifestation of migraine in which the patient experiences episodic facial pain usually without other migrainous manifestations.

Periodic migrainous neuralgia

See page 227.

(b) Trigeminal neuropathy

Patients with this condition develop numbness, which may be confined to one of the divisions of the trigeminal nerve. The motor division is usually spared. The sensory deficit evolves over days or weeks and usually persists. In some patients the onset is associated with pain but this does not resemble trigeminal neuralgia. It is a benign condition but it is important to exclude other causes of trigeminal sensory loss.

The facial nerve (VII)

The facial nerve nucleus lies in the floor of the fourth ventricle in the lower pons; the fibres pass round the sixth nerve nucleus forming a small hump in the floor of the fourth ventricle, the facial colliculus, and then run laterally to emerge from the pons near its lower border. They cross the cerebello-pontine angle with the nervus intermedius (secretomotor to the lacrymal gland and taste fibres from the anterior two-thirds of the tongue) and the eighth nerve. All three nerves pass through the internal auditory meatus into the internal auditory canal to the geniculate ganglion. The eighth nerve leaves at this point, and shortly afterwards the chorda tympani and the nerve to stapedius also leave the facial nerve, which finally emerges from the skull through the stylomastoid foramen. It divides in the parotid gland to supply all the muscles of facial expression.

Unilateral upper motor neurone lesions of the facial nerve cause quite marked weakness of the lower half of the face with the relative sparing of the upper half. This is because the supranuclear pathways for the muscles of the forehead and around the eyes are bilateral. Upper motor neurone lesions also cause greater impairment of voluntary movement than of involuntary and emotional movement. Strokes and hemisphere tumours are common causes.

Lower motor neurone lesions cause weakness of all facial muscles. The site of the lesion can often be accurately located because of involvement of associated structures:

1 Lesions of the nuclei are nearly always associated with an ipsilateral sixth-nerve palsy.
2 Lesions in the cerebellar pontine angle are usually associated with eighth-nerve and chorda tympani involvement. In addition the corneal reflex may be absent owing to fifth-nerve involvement and there may be cerebellar signs.
3 Lesions in the internal auditory canal as far as the geniculate ganglion may also be associated with lesions of the eighth nerve and chorda tympani, and

there may also be hyperacusis owing to paralysis of the stapedius muscle.

In the brain stem, tumours and vascular lesions are the commonest causes of seventh-nerve damage. The facial nerve is the most frequently affected cranial nerve in the Guillain–Barré syndrome. It may also be damaged in operations on the parotid salivery gland, and involvement with sarcoidosis may cause bilateral lesions. The commonest cause of a lower motor neurone lesion of the seventh nerve is, however, Bell's palsy.

Bell's palsy

Bell's palsy is an acute lower motor neurone palsy of the facial nerve of unknown aetiology. The occurrence in some patients of hypercusis or loss of taste on the anterior two-thirds of the tongue implies that the nerve may be involved at different levels within the petrous temporal bone. The onset may be sudden or develop over several hours, rarely more than a day or so. The onset may be associated with some pain in or behind the ear. About 50 per cent of patients make a complete recovery, although this may take weeks or months. Some patients start to improve within a few days but it is possible to make a complete recovery even if the improvement does not start for six to eight weeks. Some estimate of the prognosis can be made from electromyography after one month.

Treatment with steroids should be started within 24 hours of the onset of symptoms. Prednisolone (60–80 mg a day) for two or three days, followed by a rapidly diminishing dose over two or three weeks, is a suitable regimen.

Ramsay–Hunt syndrome

This is due to infection of the seventh nerve by herpes zoster. The syndrome consists of herpetic vesicles on the soft palate and in the external auditory meatus and may include deafness, facial palsy and trigeminal nerve involvement.

The acoustic vestibular nerve (VIII)

The acoustic and vestibular parts of the eighth nerve serve quite separate functions. The acoustic nerve arises in the cochlea and the vestibular nerve in the semicircular canals and otolith. Both pass down the internal auditory canal with the seventh nerve and chorda tympani, they cross the cerebello-pontine angle and enter the brain stem at the ponto-medullary junction. The nuclei are situated in the region of the inferior cerebellar peduncle.

From the cochlear nuclei some fibes decussate in the trapezoid body and ascend in the lateral lemniscus, and some fibres ascend in the ipsilateral lateral lemniscus, so that there is bilateral representation of hearing at supranuclear level.

Hearing acuity should be tested and, if deafness is found, it is then necessary to determine whether this is due to middle-ear disease affecting the ear ossicles (conductive deafness) or whether it is due to a lesion of the nerve (perceptive deafness). Normally air conduction is better than bone conduction and this difference is preserved in perceptive deafness; but in conductive deafness bone conduction appears louder than air conduction because it bypasses the ear ossicles. Perceptive deafness due to intramedullary lesions is unusual and may be associated with other brain-stem or long-tract signs; lesions of the cerebello-pontine angle (acoustic neuroma, trigeminal neuroma, meningioma and cholesteatoma) may be associated with fifth- and seventh-nerve palsies and cerebellar signs; lesions in the petrous temporal bone (Paget's disease) may be associated with a facial palsy and impaired taste.

Vestibular nuclei are connected to the cerebellar hemisphere on the same side, to the third, fourth and sixth nerves via the medial longitudinal bundle, via the vestibular spinal tract to centres in the cord, and via the ipsilateral lateral lemniscus to the cortex.

Vestibular function is assessed by the caloric test, in which the ear is syringed with water above and below body temperature. This stimulates movement of endolymph in the semicircular canals and causes nystagmus. A standard technique is used and should always be followed. The duration of the nystagmus is timed.

Acute vestibular lesions cause vertigo and disequilibrium. Vertigo which is solely related to changes in position indicates disease of the otolith, although it may occasionally occur in some posterior fossa lesions.

Vestibular neuronitis

This is an acute vestibular disturbance with nausea, vomiting and unsteady gait, which develops over a few hours and may be completely prostrating for a day or two before passing off over a few more days. Most patients have a liability to vertigo on rapid head movement for several weeks or even months.

Menière's disease

Patients with this condition suffer recurrent attacks of vertigo with vomiting and prostration, associated with tinnitus, which is usually more persistent, and progressive deafness. During the acute attack patients usually have nystagmus, but this disappears during remission. The treatment is symptomatic with intramuscular or oral phenothiazines. The aetiology is unknown.

The glossopharyngeal nerve (IX)

This is a mixed motor and sensory nerve, which arises in the medulla and leaves the skull through the jugular foramen with the vagus and the spinal accessory nerves and supplies the stylopharyngeus muscle. Sensory fibres carry all forms of sensation, including taste, from the posterior third of the tongue, the tonsillar fossa and the pharynx. Parasympathetic fibres from the inferior salivery nucleus also travel with the glossopharyngeal nerve but leave it within the skull to supply the parotid gland via the otic ganglion.

Isolated lesions of the glossopharyngeal nerve are rare; lesions at the jugular foramen also involve the vagus and accessory nerves.

Glossopharyngeal neuralgia

This is a condition similar to trigeminal neuralgia (see page 203) but the pain is felt in the distribution of the glossopharyngeal nerve and is precipitated by eating and swallowing. Pain may also be felt deep in the ear. The treatment is also with carbamazepine. If this fails to control the pain, the nerve should be surgically divided.

The vagus (X)

The nuclei of this motor and sensory nerve are situated in the medulla. The nerve leaves the skull through the jugular foramen and it lies in the carotid sheath in the neck. It is the motor supply to the pharyngeal and laryngeal muscles and it carries the parasympathetic supply to the thoracic and abdominal viscera. Sensory fibres carry sensation from the larynx. Lesions of the vagus nerve result in paralysis of the soft palate, the pharynx and the larynx, with a curtain movement of the uvula away from the side of the lesion on phonation.

The spinal accessory nerve (XI)

The nuclei of this motor nerve lie in the lower medulla and upper part of the spinal cord. The nerve emerges from the medulla and spinal cord in a continuous line of rootlets. The spinal rootlets unite to form a trunk which ascends through the foramen magnum to join the cranial rootlets. The nerve leaves the skull through the jugular foramen with the vagus. The cranial fibres are distributed to the pharynx and larynx. The spinal fibres descend to supply the sternomastoids and the upper fibres of trapezius.

The hypoglossal nerve (XII)

The nucleus lies in the dorsal part of the lower medulla and the nerve leaves the skull through the hypoglossal foramen (the anterior condylar canal) and supplies the muscles of the tongue.

Lesions of the twelfth nerve cause wasting, fasciculation and weakness of the ipsilateral side of the tongue, and the tongue deviates to the affected side on protrusion.

Dysarthria

Dysarthria may occur in any lesion of the motor pathway to the bulbar muscles. Because the pathways are bilateral above the bulbar nuclei, a unilateral upper motor neurone lesion only causes temporary dysarthria. Dysarthria occurs in pseudobulbar palsy (upper motor neurone lesions) and in bulbar palsies (lower motor neurone lesions). Dysarthria may also occur in extra pyramidal and cerebellar lesions, myasthenia gravis and in some diseases of muscle.

It is necessary only to determine that the patient has dysarthria, since the physical signs will indicate the cause.

Bulbar and pseudobulbar palsies

The lower cranial nerves (IX–XII) arise from a chain of motor nuclei in the medulla and emerge as an almost continuous line of rootlets. The ninth, tenth and eleventh nerves all leave the skull through the jugular foramen. This anatomical arrangement means that these nerves are often affected together.

A *bulbar palsy* is a lower motor neurone lesion affecting the cranial nerves whose nuclei lie in the bulb (the medulla). The commonest causes include syringobulbia, motor neurone disease and vascular lesions. The nerves may be affected outside the medulla in diphtheria and the Guillain–Barrè syndrome. Tumours in the region of the jugular foramen may affect the ninth, tenth and eleventh nerves, and these include nasopharyngeal carcinoma, meningioma and glomus jugulari tumours.

Patients with bulbar palsy complain of dysarthria and dysphagia, and fluids may regurgitate through the nose when they attempt to swallow. Signs include loss of taste and sensation on the posterior third of the tongue and in the tonsillar fossa (IX), paralysis of the vocal cords (X), weakness of the sternomastoid and upper fibres of trapezius (XI) and, if the twelfth cranial nerve is involved, there may be wasting and fibrillation of the tongue.

Patients with *pseudobulbar palsy* have the same complaints and difficulties as patients with a bulbar palsy, but it is due to an upper motor neurone lesion of the bulbar muscles. The upper motor neurone pathways must be affected on both sides because the pathways are bilateral. Causes include motor neurone disease, vascular lesions (usually associated with hypertension) and multiple sclerosis. Signs include a brisk jaw jerk and a slow-moving spastic tongue. The plantar responses are usually extensor.

The motor system

The motor system comprises the upper motor neurone pathway, the lower motor neurone, the myoneural junction and muscle.

Cortex

The upper motor neurone pathway arises in the precentral gyrus. Lesions strictly confined to the motor cortex give rise to a characteristic pattern of motor deficit. There is weakness of all movements of the affected part, there may be some wasting but there is no tone or reflex change (cortical pattern of motor deficit). Because of the wide extent of the motor cortex with the face/hand area laterally and the foot area medially, a single lesion only produces these signs in a relatively small part of the body, perhaps the hand or the foot. Large lesions necessarily involve subcortical structures and this produces a different pattern.

The pyramidal tract

The upper motor neurone pathway descends from the precentral gyrus and is gathered into a compact bundle at the internal capsule, so that lesions at this level tend to produce a complete hemiplegia, including the face. Any lesion above the midbrain will affect the cranial nerves on the same side as the hemiplegia. Some fibres cross the midline in the midbrain, pons and upper medulla to supply the contralateral cranial nerve nuclei. A lesion, therefore, of a cranial nerve on one side, together with a contralateral hemiplegia, accurately locates the site of the lesion to the level of that cranial nerve nucleus. In the lower part of the medulla, just above the level of the foramen magnum, the pyramidal tract decussates from its anterior position in the brain stem to the lateral column of the cord on the opposite side.

Lesions of the pyramidal tract cause spasticity, which is an increase in muscle tone that is not uniform throughout the range of movement and does not affect both directions of movement equally. There may be flaccidity after an acute pyramidal tract lesion owing to 'spinal shock', and spasticity may only develop later. Conversely, marked spasticity without much weakness is a sure sign of chronicity. Lesions of the pyramidal tract cause a characteristic distribution of muscle weakness. All the muscles may be weak on the affected side, but in the upper limb the extensors are much more affected than the flexors and in the lower limb the flexors are much more affected than the extensors. It is important, therefore, to test shoulder abduction, elbow extension, wrist and finger extension and finger abduction in the upper limb, and hip flexion, knee flexion and ankle dorsiflexion in the lower limb; these movements are always weaker than their antagonists.

The reflexes are all pathologically brisk. Reflexes that are normally only just obtainable may be very brisk, such as the digital reflex, and there may be clonus, particularly at the ankle. The cutaneous reflexes (the abdominal and cremasteric reflexes) are reduced or abolished on the affected side and the plantar response is extensor.

The lower motor neurone

The lower motor neurone, arising in the anterior horn cells of the spinal cord, is the final common pathway to muscle. Lesions anywhere in this pathway cause wasting and weakness. The reflexes are absent owing to disruption of the efferent limb of the reflex arc. The nearer the lesion is to the spinal cord, the more likely is fasciculation to be found in the affected muscles. It is, therefore, very common in anterior horn cell lesions, frequently seen in root lesions and rare in peripheral nerve lesions (see under disorders of the peripheral nervous system).

Motor neurone disease

This is a progressive degeneration of the motor pathways in the central nervous system. It may affect any part of the pathway from the motor cortex to the anterior horn cells. It usually occurs between the ages of 50 and 70 and is extremely rare before the mid thirties. Men are affected more often than women. The clinical signs are strictly confined to the motor system and there are never any sensory signs or sphincter disturbance. The disease usually presents with one of three groups of symptoms —progressive bulbar palsy, amyotrophic lateral sclerosis or progressive muscular atrophy—but any combination may occur and eventually all these features are usually present.

Progressive bulbar palsy

This is progressive degeneration of the motor nuclei in the medulla, causing a lower motor neurone bulbar palsy (see page 206). A wasted fibrillating tongue is the most important sign. This is the form with the worst prognosis and patients seldom survive more than eighteen months after the diagnosis is made.

Amyotrophic lateral sclerosis

This is the most common presentation of motor neurone disease and, as the name implies, it is due to a combination of wasting and weakness, often most obvious in the hands, and pyramidal tract involvement, often most prominent in the legs. The finding of upper motor neurone signs with widespread fasciculation is a characteristic feature. The prognosis from diagnosis is usually less than five years and this is largely determined by the development of bulbar signs.

Progressive muscular atrophy

In this form of motor neurone disease there is a slowly progressive lower motor neurone involvement of the arms and legs with wasting and weakness. This is the form with the best prognosis and patients may survive from five to fifteen years; again, the length of survival depends largely on whether or not the bulbar muscles become involved.

The diagnosis is often clear on clinical grounds alone but it may be confirmed by electromyography. No treatment is known to influence the course of the condition.

Spinal muscular atrophy

There is a group of genetically determined degenerations of the lower motor neurone which produce a symmetrical wasting and weakness of muscles, often with fasciculation.

Werdnig–Hoffman disease

This is the commonest form and occurs in infancy. Survival is usually a matter of months.

Kugelberg–Welander syndrome

This presents at any age with wasting and weakness of the arms and legs and is slowly progressive. It appears to be inherited by an autosomal recessive mechanism. The condition probably accounts for most patients previously thought to have a 'limb girdle dystrophy' (see page 210). Some patients show widespread fasciculation. The diagnosis can be confirmed by EMG and muscle biopsy, but the interpretation may be complicated by the fact that secondary myopathic change commonly occurs.

The neuromuscular junction

The arrival of a nerve impulse at the neuromuscular junction causes the release of acetylcholine. The acetylcholine crosses the cleft between nerve and muscle and becomes attached to the acetylcholine receptor in the motor end-plate, causing depolarization and subsequent contraction of the muscle. The acetylcholine is rapidly destroyed by cholinesterase or taken up by nerve endings, and the motor end-plate repolarizes.

Procaine and botulinus toxins inhibit the release of acetylcholine, whereas guanidine increases the release of acetylcholine. Physostigmine, neostigmine and pyridostigmine inhibit cholinesterase and allow the acetylcholine to accumulate, perpetuating its action. Curare, tubocurarine and galamine act as competitive inhibitors by reacting with the acetylcholine receptors on the end-plate, producing a conduction block.

Myasthenia gravis

Myasthenia gravis is an immunological disease with damage of the acetylcholine receptors by antibody, which not only blocks the receptor sites but also causes degeneration of the receptors. The characteristic feature of this disease is abnormal fatiguability of striated muscle with rapid recovery after rest.

It may occur at any age but most commonly affects women in the second and third decades. Children born of myasthenic mothers may show evidence of myasthenia for some days after birth because the mother's antibodies cross the placenta. There is a much higher incidence of thyrotoxicosis in patients with myasthenia than can be accounted for by chance.

Clinical features

The condition does not affect all striated muscle equally and, although electromyography may show evidence of widespread disease, it may be quite localized clinically. It commonly affects the external ocular, bulbar, neck and limb girdle muscles. The onset is often gradual and fluctuating. Patients may complain of diplopia, dysphagia, dysarthria and difficulty in chewing, and these symptoms may all show marked variability. Patients, for example, may have difficulty in completing a meal or only develop ptosis and diplopia in the evening.

Examination shows no wasting or fasciculation. The most striking feature is undue fatiguability, which can be shown by asking the patient to raise the arm above the head 30 times and demonstrating the development of weakness as a result. Normal power returns after a few moments of rest.

Diagnosis

The diagnosis can be confirmed by intravenous edrophonium. This is a short-acting anticholinesterase drug which may give a dramatic response for up to two or three minutes. Atropine should be administered first, followed by a test dose of 1 mg of intravenous edrophonium; if no undue reaction occurs, a further 9 mg may be injected.

The response to edrophonium is often disappointing in ocular and bulbar myasthenia and a negative test does not exclude these varieties of myasthenia. Confirmation of the diagnosis may be obtained from electromyography, which shows the characteristic decrease in evoked response with faradic stimulation. Single-fibre recording shows an increase in jitter, demonstrating instability of neuromuscular junctions within one motor unit. Thyroid function tests should be carried out because of the association with thyrotoxicosis, and it is important to look for an associated thymoma with chest X-ray and CT of the mediastinum.

Skeletal muscle antibodies may be elevated, and are almost always elevated if there is an underlying thymoma. Acetylcholine receptor antibody is usually elevated, but the level does not show an obvious relationship to the severity of the disease.

Treatment

Anticholinesterase drugs have been the basis of treatment since their use was first described in 1934 and remain the initial treatment of choice for limb myasthenia. Treatment should be started with pyridostigmine (60 mg t.d.s.) and increased as necessary. Some patients require up to 600 mg a day. The half-life of pyridostigmine is about four hours. It may be helpful ocasionally to use the shorter-acting neostigmine bromide with a half-life of 1½ hours when a short-lived boost is required, such as just before a meal in patients with bulbar myasthenia, but it is usually easier to stabilize the patient on pyridostigmine alone.

Although increasing the dose results in increasing strength initially, a plateau is soon reached and further increase results in progressive weakness due to conduction block. A patient who deteriorates while on treatment may be having either a myasthenic or a cholinergic crisis. These can be distinguished by intravenous edrophonium, which can also be used to determine whether a patient is on an optimal dose of drugs. Ocular and bulbar myasthenia often respond poorly to anticholinesterase drugs and in these patients steroids are the treatment of choice. In contrast to the usual use of steroids, it is important to start with a small dose and make gradual increments until a therapeutic effect is achieved. Large doses given initially may precipitate a myasthenic crisis. It is usually possible to control symptoms satisfactorily with a modest dose of steroid, which may be given on alternate days to minimize the long-term side-effects.

If these measures fail to control the patient's symptoms, thymectomy should be considered; and it is better to carry out this procedure sooner rather than later, particularly if immunosuppressive drugs are used in the treatment of limb myasthenia. Patients with a thymoma or thymic hyperplasia have a worse prognosis than those with a normal thymus. Thymectomy appears to make patients more responsive subsequently to anticholinesterase drugs and immunosuppression, and this may be related to a reduction in the amount of circulating antibody. The amount of circulating antibody can be temporarily reduced by plasmapheresis and this may be helpful as a short-term measure while awaiting a response from immunosuppression. It may, for example, be enough to keep a patient off a ventilator during a critical time. If large doses of steroids are required to keep control or it is likely that this treatment would need to be continued for a long time, the steroid should be combined with an immunosuppressive drug such as azathioprine.

Myasthenic syndrome

This condition (the *Eaton–Lambert* syndrome) usually complicates oat-cell carcinoma of the bronchus, but it has been described with other tumours. The weakness may precede clinical evidence of the carcinoma by months or years. The patient complains of weakness after exertion, but examination shows weakness of proximal limb girdle muscles which improves after exercise. The reflexes are almost always depressed or absent, unlike true myasthenia. The edrophonium test is usually positive but anticholinesterase drugs given therapeutically have little or no effect. The diagnosis can be confirmed by electromyography. The condition responds to guanidine hydrochloride given orally.

Diseases of muscle

Diseases of muscle may be conveniently divided into the congenital genetically determined abnormalities, which carry the generic name of muscular dystrophy, and acquired diseases.

Muscular dystrophies

These are classified according to their clinical picture and mode of inheritance.

Sex-linked pseudohypertrophic muscular dystrophy (Duchenne and Becker dystrophy)

This is due to a sex-linked recessive gene or genes, although there is a high rate of new mutations. The abnormality becomes apparent at about the age of three, with difficulty in walking and climbing stairs owing to proximal leg weakness. Some pseudohypertrophy is very common and principally affects the calf muscles. Although termed pseudohypertrophy, there is, in fact, enlargement of individual muscle fibres. The condition is slowly progressive, patients become chairbound between the age of eight and ten and die at around the age of fifteen, usually from respiratory and cardiac causes. During the later years of his life the patient suffers progressive deformity, particularly of the chest. There is no treatment; but female carriers can often be identified and, if they become pregnant, the sex of the child can be determined by amniocentesis.

The Becker type of muscular dystrophy is a more benign form of the Duchenne type and constitutes about 10 per cent of cases. The condition may develop at any age up to about 25 and patients may not become chairbound for another 25 years.

Autosomal dominant facioscapulohumeral muscular dystrophy

This condition affects both sexes equally and usually presents in adolescence with facial involvement, followed shortly by weakness of the shoulder girdle muscles. It may follow a very prolonged, indolent course and the patients may never become chairbound.

Limb girdle dystrophy

This is not a clinical entity and the majority of patients with this condition have the Kugelberg–Welander syndrome.

Mitochondrial myopathy

Mitochondrial abnormalities can produce a wide range of clinical conditions, including a myopathy associated with a characteristic muscle biopsy. This condition may present as a pure ocular myopathy. The patients usually present with ptosis and subsequently develop a bilateral external ophthalmoplegia over many years. Although the condition may be confined to the ocular muscles, some patients show weakness of facial and shoulder girdle muscles and others show evidence of degeneration in other parts of the nervous system.

Myotonic syndromes

Myotonia is the persistence of muscle contraction after voluntary effort has ceased and is well demonstrated by difficulty in relaxing the grip after vigorous contraction. Percussion of a muscle belly causes a localized area of contraction, which relaxes slowly (myotonic dimpling).

1 Dystrophia myotonica

This is a widespread dystrophic condition, not only affecting muscle. There is an autosomal dominant inheritance with onset usually in adolescence and early adult life. It appears to show the phenomenon of anticipation within a family, with each succeeding generation showing more widespread abnormalities. The first member of the family to be affected with this condition may have cataracts alone and the fully developed picture may not present for two or three generations.

The fully developed syndrome consists of frontal baldness, wasting of the masseter, temporal and sternomastoid muscles, facial weakness with ptosis, posterior capsular cataracts and a distal myopathy with wasting and weakness, starting in the hands and later involving the feet, gonadal atrophy—as shown by small testes in the male and menstrual irregularity in the female—and impaired production of thyroid hormone and insulin.

2 Myotonia congenita (Thomsen's disease)

Patients show widespread myotonia from birth. There is usually hypertrophy of muscles, giving the appearance of a Little Hercules. The condition is usually dominantly inherited.

Acquired disorders of muscle

These can be conveniently divided into primary inflammatory disorders of muscle (polymyositis) and those myopathies which complicate systemic disease, though this may be an artificial distinction.

Polymyositis (see page 253)

This is a group of conditions associated with weakness of proximal muscles which is usually painless and is probably due to an autoimmune mechanism. One muscle group constantly affected in polymyositis, which may be spared in other myopathies, are the neck extensors. It may occur at any age and usually follows a very prolonged relapsing and remittent course. *Raynaud's syndrome* is a common association in younger patients, and there may be a characteristic rash (*dermatomyositis*). There is an association with occult neoplasm and this increases with age; there is usually a loss of reflexes in these patients. The diagnosis is made by the characteristic clinical picture, EMG and muscle biopsy. The ESR is usually raised, as are the muscle enzymes such as creative phosphokinase (CPK).

The majority of patients respond to steroids, which may need to be continued for several years. Patients who require continued high-dose steroid medication may benefit from an alternate-day regimen or the addition of immunosuppressive drugs, such as azathioprine.

Myopathies complicating systemic disease

Inflammatory conditions of muscle may complicate sarcoidosis, rheumatoid arthritis, polyarthritis nodosa, disseminated lupus erythematosus and scleroderma.

A proximal limb girdle myopathy may complicate steroid therapy, thyrotoxicosis and occasionally myxoedema. Diabetic amyotrophy is not a myopathy but describes the wasting that follows a neuropathy principally affecting the femoral nerve.

Polymyalgia rheumatica is described on page 259.

The sensory system

Pathways for the different modalities of sensation have separate courses in different parts of the nervous system, so that lesions at various levels produce characteristic patterns of sensory deficit.

Peripheral nerve lesions

The area of sensory loss in a peripheral nerve lesion is fairly constant. It may be associated with dysaesthesia, such as pins and needles, tingling or burning sensations. The triple response is abolished.

Root lesions

The autonomous area of skin supplied by a single root may be extremely small, so that even a complete lesion may not produce any detectable sensory loss; this is because of overlap from adjacent dermatomes. Conversely, the rash of herpes zoster may be found over a relatively large area, since vesicles occur where there is any contribution from one nerve root.

Sensory pathways in spinal cord

After entering the spinal cord through the dorsal root, there is a separation of fibres, with those responsible for pain and temperature crossing the midline to reach the contralateral spinothalamic tract in the anterior white matter of the cord, and those fibres concerned with touch and position sense travelling in the ipsilateral posterior columns to the gracile and cuneate nuclei in the lower medulla. Fibres from these nuclei decussate to form the medial lemniscus and lie in close association with the spinothalamic tract; so that the pathways for all sensation lie on the same side of the brain stem. These pathways are joined by the fibres from the fifth-nerve nucleus, the quintothalamic tract. The sensory pathways then pass up to the thalamus, where all sensory information from one half of the body is relayed to the cortex. The pain pathways above the thalamus are very extensive, so that localized lesions of the main sensory radiation cause marked loss of light touch and position sense with relative preservation of pain.

The basal ganglia and extrapyramidal system

There are two principal non-pyramidal systems concerned with control of movement, the cerebellum and the extrapyramidal system. Disorders of the basal ganglia and extrapyramidal system can cause a wide variety of movement disorders.

Parkinson's disease

Clinical features

James Parkinson first described paralysis agitans in 1817. Its three principal characteristics are an increase in muscle tone (rigidity), slowness of movement (bradykinesia) and a characteristic tremor.

1 Rigidity
This form of hypertonus must be distinguished from spasticity. In rigidity the increase in tone is present throughout the range of movement and in both directions.

2 Bradykinesia
The slowness of voluntary movement is out of proportion to the degree of rigidity and patients have difficulty in initiating and carrying out coordinated movements.

3 Tremor
This is present at rest and inhibited by movement. It may also be temporarily inhibited by conscious effort.

Parkinson's disease may develop at any age but is much commoner after the fifth decade. The patient may present either with rigidity and bradykinesia and little or no tremor, or with an obvious tremor which may be confined to one limb with little or no rigidity and brady-kinesia. All three features eventually develop. The condition is slowly progressive over many years. Early features include loss of facial expression, a monotonous speech and loss of associated movements, such as swinging the arms when walking.

The disease is caused by the degeneration of dopa-minergic pathways in the basal ganglia, principally in the globus pallidus and substantia nigra. These structures are found to be relatively deficient in dopamine in patients with Parkinson's disease.

Treatment

The aim of treatment is to increase the dopamine levels in the brain. Dopamine cannot be given orally because it does not cross the blood–brain barrier. Dopa is its immediate precursor but only the laevo form (levodopa) crosses the blood–brain barrier. More than 90 per cent of an orally administered dose of dopa is destroyed outside the brain by dopa decarboxylase. It is usual, therefore, to administer levodopa, together with a proportionate amount of a decarboxylase inhibitor, which itself does not cross the blood–brain barrier but inhibits the extra-cerebral decarboxylation of levodopa. This combination makes more levodopa available in the brain and consider-ably reduces systemic side-effects (Table 5.1).

When using lower doses of levodopa it is usually necessary to use a preparation with a 4:1 ratio in order to achieve satisfactory peripheral decarboxylase inhibition. The 10:1 ratio gives a satisfactory inhibition in the majority of patients at higher dose levels. Treatment should be started with Sinemet Plus half a tablet t.d.s. and gradually increased according to response. Most patients achieve a satisfactory response on less than one tablet of Sinemet-275 t.d.s. Since the half-life of levodopa is only about four hours, a smoother response may be obtained by multiple divided doses.

The response to levodopa is often dramatic and the patients may be able to return to a relatively normal life. It does not, however, alter the long-term prognosis and over the years it tends to become less effective, often producing unacceptable side-effects at a lower dosage. The principal dose-limiting side-effect is orofacial dyskinesia and other dystonic and choreiform movements affecting the limbs. This is dose-dependent and disappears with reduction in dosage. The reduction of the effect of levodopa with time may be partly due to the loss of the enzyme which converts dopa to dopamine. This loss of response may occur after 5–7 years of treatment with levodopa and has led to the suggestion that treatment in younger patients should be initiated with anticholinergic drugs and only changed to levodopa when these become ineffective. In this way the problems associated with long-term levodopa therapy may be postponed by several years.

Table 5.1 Combinations of levodopa and dopa-decarboxylase inhibitors*

Sinemet Plus	Levodopa 100 mg + carbidopa 25 mg
Sinemet 110	Levodopa 100 mg + carbidopa 10 mg
Sinemet 275	Levodopa 250 mg + carbidopa 25 mg
Madopar 62.5	Levodopa 50 mg + benserazide 12.5 mg
Madopar 125	Levodopa 100 mg + benserazide 25 mg
Madopar 250	Levodopa 200 mg + benserazide 50 mg

*Sinemet are scored tablets, Madopar are capsules.

It may also be possible to postpone starting levodopa therapy by the use of selegiline or amantadine. There is some controversy over delaying the onset of levodopa therapy, and some authorities think that the development of intolerance to levodopa is related to the severity of the disease and not necessarily to the duration of treatment. Until this point has been determined it seems sensible to postpone the onset of levodopa therapy by using alternative medication but not to deny the patient the benefit of levodopa unreasonably.

Normally the dopaminergic pathways are in balance with the cholinergic pathways. If a satisfactory response cannot be obtained by increasing the dopa levels in the brain, the balance between these two systems may be restored by inhibition of the cholinergic system. The use of anticholinergic drugs is well established and was the mainstay of treatment before the advent of levodopa. The most effective is benzhexol which is available in tablets containing 2 and 5 mg. It may be given in addition to levodopa in a dose of between 6 and 15 mg a day. Orphenadrine may be better tolerated. Benztropine, methixene and procyclidine have similar properties. Side-effects include dry mouth, blurred vision and, commonly in older patients, confusion and hallucinations.

The biggest problem in the management of Parkinson's disease now is dealing with patients who no longer respond to levodopa. Problems include hallucinations and confusion, unacceptable dyskinesia, wide fluctuations in performance from gross dyskinesia to akinesia (the on–off phenomenon), as well as painful dystonic movements. The first step is to try and smooth out the levodopa dosage with multiple divided doses throughout the day, keeping the total dose to a level which does not cause confusion and hallucinations. The next step is to add the monoamine oxidase B inhibitor selegiline; this results in a delay in the clearance of levodopa and, because of its long effect, can be given as a single daily dose of either 5 or 10 mg. A useful response may also be obtained from amantadine which appears to promote the release of levodopa from the synaptic vesicles. The dose is 100 mg b.d. Unfortuntely many patients find the beneficial effect of amantadine to be short-lived.

Some additional response may be obtained by using the dopamine agonist bromocriptine which acts directly on dopaminergic receptors. It has a half-life of about eight hours and may therefore be used to provide a background dopamine stimulation to which a suitable amount of levodopa can be added. The initial dose is 2.5 mg b.d., which may be increased slowly to 40–60 mg a day according to response. Occasionally marked postural hypotension occurs after the smallest dose so that a test dose of 1.75 mg should be given in the evening before starting treatment.

Physiotherapy can often result in considerable improvement in the performance of patients with Parkinson's disease; and when it is combined with help and advice from occupational therapists, patients are often able to continue to lead an independent existence where this might otherwise not be possible.

Stereotactic thalamotomy, once commonly performed, is now rarely necessary in view of the response of Parkinson's disease to levodopa. However, it remains suitable for younger patients who have a unilateral tremor and little in the way of bradykinesia and rigidity and in whom there are no general medical contraindictions to surgery, such as hypertension. Surgery does not affect the subsequent response to levodopa.

Other causes of the Parkinsonian syndrome

In the 1920s there was a pandemic of encephalitis thought to be of viral origin, although a virus was never isolated (encephalitis lethargica). This resulted in a very large number of patients with a Parkinsonian syndrome, post-encephalitic Parkinsonian. These patients had all the characteristic features of Parkinson's disease; in addition there was usually evidence of cortical damage from the encephalitis, and this seems to make these patients peculiarly susceptible to levodopa preparations, so that very small doses cause unacceptable mental confusion. They were also subject to oculogyric crises. Since no authenticated cases of this encephalitis have occurred since the 1920s, the condition is becoming extremely rare.

Vascular disease does not cause a true Parkinsonian syndrome, but extrapyramidal signs may occur in patients with vascular disease, often associated with pseudobulbar palsy.

Chorea

Choreiform movements are involuntary movements which resemble part of a coordinated intended movement, and patients may be able to disguise the fact that movement is involuntary.

1 Sydenham's chorea

This occurs in children in association with acute rheumatism. It is usually a benign condition and most patients recover within a few weeks.

2 Chorea gravidarum

A similar clinical picture may occur during pregnancy and

some patients develop chorea on the contraceptive pill.

3 Chorea following stroke

Choreiform movements may occur after cerebrovascular lesions, particularly in the elderly. There may be an obvious association with a stroke or the chorea may develop without such an obvious cause. The onset is sudden and unilateral. The chorea may persist but does not progress.

4 Huntington's chorea

This condition is inherited as an autosomal dominant and is characterized by chorea and progressing dementia. The new mutation rate is very low so that a positive family history is usually obtainable. Although evidence of the disease may appear at any age it is most common in middle age and usually after the reproductive period, so that patients often have children and grandchildren before the diagnosis is made. In children it may present with widespread rigidity mimicking an extrapyramidal disorder (rigid Huntington's).

The condition may present with either involuntary movements or with dementia, but the former is more common. The combination of involuntary movement and dementia is strongly suggestive of this condition. If the family history is known to the patient, the depression associated with the development of involuntary movements is often mistaken for dementia. The diagnosis is confirmed by obtaining a positive family history. There are no specific investigations but the CT brain scan shows a characteristic dilatation of the lateral ventricles due to atrophy of the caudate nuclei. Tetrabenazine may be effective in reducing the abnormal movements.

Torsion dystonia

This is a disorder of the basal ganglia of unknown aetiology. The onset is usually gradual, starting at any age, and the characteristic features are strong intermittent uncontrollable contractions of voluntary muscle. There is a wide spectrum of presentation, from dystonia musculorum deformans presenting in childhood and resulting in considerable deformity over the years, to fragmentary forms, including spasmodic torticollis and writer's cramp. There is no effective treatment but anticholinergic drugs may be of some benefit.

The cerebellum

The cerebellar hemispheres are concerned with coordination of movement on the same side of the body. Coordination depends on the smooth contraction of one group of muscles (agonists), the equally smooth relaxation of the opposing muscles (antagonists), and the maintained contraction of other muscles to support the part of the body concerned. The central part of the cerebellum, the vermis, is concerned with equilibrium and maintains balance when the centre of gravity changes.

Signs of cerebellar disease

1 Nystagmus

See page 201.

2 Dysarthria

The coordination of the muscles of speech are affected (see page 206).

3 Intention tremor

Attempts at fine coordinated movement produce a tremor, which is worse at the completion of the movement and may be demonstrated by the finger/nose test and the heel/knee/shin test. Occasionally there may be a flapping tremor at rest. A cerebellar tremor on the same side as pyramidal tract involvement indicates a contralateral lesion between the red nucleus and the thalamus.

4 Disequilibrium

This is caused by a lesion of the vermis or bilateral hemisphere disease. There may be a marked disturbance of gait without any evidence of ataxia or other physical signs.

Lesions of the cerebellum and its connections

The cerebellar pathways are frequently affected in disseminated sclerosis. Space-occupying lesions of the posterior fossa usually cause some cerebellar signs and there may also be involvement of the brain stem. The volume of the posterior fossa is relatively small, so that small lesions may obstruct CSF pathways and produce hydrocephalus.

The patients presenting with the slow insiduous onset of a cerebellar syndrome may have a cerebellar degeneration. Usually no cause is found, but it may be a complication of myxoedema, alcoholism, some drugs (e.g. phenytoin) and as a non-metastatic manifestation of an occult neoplasm, in which case the reflexes are usually depressed or absent.

The spinal cord

The spinal cord is a segmental structure. The location of

a lesion within the cord can be determined by finding the highest affected segment. This level may be motor, sensory or reflex. A motor level would give lower motor neurone signs at the affected segment owing to involvement of the anterior horn cells and the emerging motor root, and upper motor neurone signs below this on the same side. A sensory level would give loss of all forms of sensation at the affected level owing to involvement of the dorsal root and its entry zone, impairment of pain and temperature sense below this level on the opposite side owing to involvement of the crossed spinothalamic tract, and impairment of light touch and joint position sense on the same side owing to involvement of the uncrossed posterior columns. A reflex level is the absence of a reflex at the level of a lesion owing to interruption of the reflex arc and brisk reflexes below this on the same side with an extensor plantar response owing to involvement of the pyramidal tract.

Hemisection of the cord world, therefore, produce lower motor neurone weakness, absent reflex and impairment of all forms of sensation at the level of the lesion on the same side. Below this level there would be ipsilateral pyramidal tract signs with brisk reflexes and impairment of touch and proprioception, while on the contralateral side there would be impairment of pain and temperature appreciation. This is the *Brown–Séquard syndrome* and is seldom seen in its complete form. Partial forms due to compression are quite common and usually associated with bilateral pyramidal involvement, often asymmetrical.

The causes of focal disease of the spinal cord may be conveniently divided into extradural and intradural. Intradural lesions are either extramedullary or intramedullary. The commonest extradural cause is prolapse of an intervertebral disc in the cervical region. Cord compression occurs earlier in patients with congenital narrowing of the cervical canal, and hypertrophy of the ligamentum flavum posteriorly may also narrow the canal. Other causes include vertebral collapse due to osteoporosis or metastases, myeloma, tuberculosis (Pott's disease) and subluxation.

Intradural extramedullary lesions include meningitis and arachnoiditis, meningioma and neurofibroma.

Intramedullary lesions include glioma, ependymoma, transverse myelitis, which may be caused by multiple sclerosis, radiation myelitis, vascular lesions (thrombosis of the anterior spinal artery) and herpes zoster.

Management

Any patient developing a focal lesion of the spinal cord must be assumed to have cord compression until proved otherwise. The patient should be investigated as a matter of urgency. Plain X-rays should be followed by myelography, and this is preferably carried out in a neurosurgical unit so that decompression can follow the investigation immediately if a compressive lesion is found. In many patients a good recovery will occur if surgery is performed without delay.

Syringobulbia, syringomyelia and hydromyelia

The majority of patients with syringomyelia have a developmental abnormality in the region of the foramen magnum with prolapse of the cerebellar tonsils through the foramen magnum (tonsillar ectopia), which obstructs the normal outflow of CSF from the fourth ventricle. This may be associated with adhesions which further impede the flow of CSF. The upper end of the central canal of the cord is kept patent by the normal pulse pressure waves in the ventricular system, and dilates. Eventually, the ependymal lining of the central canal ruptures and there is an extravasation of CSF into the surrounding central grey matter. These outpouchings dissect up and down to produce the typical syrinx seen on cross-section which may not obviously show a connection with the central canal. The first symptoms and signs are nearly always in the cervical cord and the condition may remain localized, but the whole cord may become affected. Rarely a syrinx will develop as a result of trauma to the cord and dissection occurs up or down from the level of the lesion.

Clinical features

The early involvement of the central grey matter interrupting the decussating pain and temperature fibres and the reflex arc determines the cardinal signs of syringomyelia, which are:

1 dissociated cutaneous loss: loss of pain and temperature sensation with preservation of touch;
2 loss of reflexes.

As the lesion becomes more extensive, so there may be involvement of the anterior horn cells with wasting of the small hand muscles, involvement of the pyramidal tracts with development of upper motor neurone signs in the legs, involvement of Clarke's column with a Horner's syndrome and finally, in the late stages, involvement of the posterior columns. Syringomyelia is probably the commonest cause of Charcot joints in the upper limbs;

this is a painless arthropathy due to loss of pain appreciation and results in gross disorganization of joints. Despite
this, pain is not an uncommon symptom in syringomyelia.

Upward dissection of a syrinx may extend into the
medulla (syringobulbia) causing a bulbar palsy (see page
206).

Treatment

Although syringomyelia is usually progressive, it need
not be so and it may follow a very indolent course. If
there is no evidence of progression then intervention is
not indicated. If tonsillar ectopia can be demonstrated by
myelography, CT scanning or NMR and there is no
evidence of adhesions, the treatment of choice is decompression by enlargement of the foramen magnum and a
laminectomy of C1 and C2. The presence of adhesions is
a contraindication to this procedure. Occasionally a
syrinx may be drained by a shunt into the peritoneum.

Spinal root and peripheral nerve lesions

Lesions at different levels in the lower motor neurone
produce characteristic patterns of neurological deficit.

The *motor distribution* of peripheral nerves is very
constant, so that a lesion of one nerve causes weakness
in a particular and specific combination of muscles. The
level of the lesion can be predicted from the muscles
affected and a knowledge of the levels of which the main
branches arise; these may, of course, be affected without
involvement of the main trunk. The motor distribution of
roots is much less specific and most muscles receive some
contribution from several roots; it is, however, important
to know the principal contribution.

The *cutaneous distribution* of peripheral nerves is also
fairly specific, although there is some variability and
overlap. The cutaneous distribution of roots is extremely
variable and there is considerable overlap (Table 5.2). The
autonomous area for a single root may be so small that
a complete lesion may not cause any detectable sensory
loss; whereas the rash of herpes zoster, which occurs
wherever there is any contribution from the affected root,
involves a relatively large area.

Root lesions

Intravertebral disc prolapse and osteophytes

A nerve root may be affected in the spinal canal by a

Table 5.2 Principal 'root values' of selected muscles in the arms and legs

Root	Muscle	Reflex
C5	Deltoid	+
C5/6	Biceps	+
C6	Brachioradialis	+
	Extensor carpi radialis	
C7	Triceps	+
	Extensor digitorum	+
C8	The finger flexors	+
T1	The small hand muscles	
L1/2	Iliopsoas	
L2/3	Adductors	+
L3/4	Quadriceps	+
L4	Tibialis anterior	
L4/5	Tibialis posterior	
L5	Extensor hallucis longus	
L5/S1	Peronei	
S1	Gastrocnemius and soleus	+

lateral disc protrusion or as it enters the exit foramina by
osteophytes, and these are usually associated with
chronic disc degeneration and a narrow disc space. These
lesions occur at sites of greatest spinal mobility and are,
therefore, frequently found in midcervical and lower
lumbar regions. Thoracic disc prolapse is a rare cause of
spinal cord compression and does not occur without plain
X-ray changes. In the cervical spine the root emerges
above the vertebral body of the same number and is
affected by disc prolapse at the same level. For example,
the C7 root is affected by the C6/7 disc. Since there are
eight cervical roots and only seven cervical vertebrae,
this relationship changes below C7, and in the thoracic
and lumbar spins the root emerges below the corresponding vertebral body. In the lumbar spine a root is affected
by the disc at one level above its exit. For example, the
L5 root is affected by disc protrusion between L4 and L5,
although it emerges between L5 and S1.

Disc herniation causing root compression may occur at
any age and usually presents acutely with pain, which
may be severe. The pain of a root lesion is felt in the
myotome and not in the dermatome, so that the pain of
a C7 root lesion is felt in triceps and in the forearm
extensors and sometimes in pectoralis major. Numbness
and dysaesthesia is felt in the dermatome. Depression or
loss of a reflex at the appropriate level is an early sign in
root lesions.

Radiography of the spine may show narrow disc
spaces, osteophytes, subluxation or vertebral collapse,
though the plain X-ray changes often do not accord with
clinical evaluation or with the level of maximal compression as determined by myelography. In younger

patients with acute disc prolapse, X-rays are usually normal. Myelography is only indicated if the diagnosis is in doubt or if surgery is contemplated. Surgery is indicated for pain or increasing neurological deficit. Painless stable deficit seldom improves after surgery.

Herpes zoster (shingles)

See page 418.

Tumours

Tumours affecting the cervical roots are rare. Neurofibromata (see page 233) may occur and produce a characteristic enlargement of the foramina on plain X-rays.

Trauma

Cervical roots may be avulsed from the spinal cord by traction and the commonest cause of this is motor-cycle accidents. If the roots are completely avulsed there is a characteristic myelographic appearance and recovery does not occur. If continuity of the roots is preserved, some recovery is possible.

Plexus lesions

Brachial plexus

1 Ruck sack palsy
This is due to traction on the upper trunk from heavy and badly adjusted back-packs. The nerves remain in continuity and recovery is usually complete.

2 Trauma
Any part of the plexus may be damaged by trauma. Lesions of the upper part of the brachial plexus (C5, C6 and the upper trunk) are nearly always traumatic, but lesions of the lower part of the plexus (C8, T1 and the lower trunk) are less often due to trauma and are usually due to malignant infiltration or to the thoracic outlet syndrome.

3 Malignant infiltration
This may be due to apical lung carcinoma (*Pancoast's tumour*) or to local metastatic spread from mammary carcinoma. A slowly progressive weakness develops in the small hand muscles (T1) and spreads to involve the finger flexors (C8). There is usually pain and sensory loss in the medial aspect of the forearm (T1). Horner's syndrome commonly occurs by involvement of the cervical sympathetic ganglia.

4 Thoracic outlet syndrome
The lower trunk of the brachial plexus may be angulated over a cervical rib, together with the subclavian artery. Patients may present with a neurological deficit or with vascular symptoms or a combination. Neurological signs and symptoms predominate with the small rudimentary ribs which continue into a fibrous band, and vascular features predominate in the large well-formed bony cervical ribs.

Cervical ribs are quite common and only rarely cause symptoms. Neurological features commonly present in young women with the insidious onset of wasting and weakness of the small hand muscles, often accompanied by pain; a bruit may be heard over the subclavian artery. Other causes of a thoracic outlet syndrome include compression of the neurovascular bundle between scalenus anterior and the first rib.

5 Neuralgic amyotrophy (brachial neuralgia).
This is an inflammatory neuropathy principally affecting branches of the brachial plexus. A characteristic feature is the dense involvement of some muscles and sparing of others within the same myotome. It commonly occurs in young adults and pain is usually a prominent feature at onset. A few days later weakness develops and later there may be quite marked wasting. The pain usually subsides in a week or so, but the weakness may persist for months, often with incomplete recovery, so that some wasting may be permanent.

Lumbosacral plexus

Malignant infiltration is by far the commonest cause, often due to spread from carcinoma of the cervix or uterus. It may also occur in the lymphomas. A radiculogram may be necessary to distinguish these conditions from intraspinal lesions. Lesions of the lumbosacral plexus are best demonstrated by a CT scan.

Peripheral nerve lesions

A *mononeuropathy* is a lesion of a single peripheral nerve. *Mononeuritis multiplex* is involvement of more than one peripheral nerve and this is associated with polyarteritis nodosa, amyloid, systemic lupus erythematosus and rheumatoid arthritis. *Polyneuropathy* (see page 219) is symmetrical involvement of all peripheral nerves.

Peripheral nerves may be damaged by external compression or by internal entrapment. Other causes include trauma, fractures, operations, penetrating injuries and injections.

Compression usually occurs where a nerve lies

between skin and bone, unprotected by soft tissue; for example, the ulnar nerve at the elbow and the common peroneal nerve at the head of the fibula. This anatomical arrangement means that some nerves are particularly prone to damage at certain sites, particularly if pressure is maintained for long periods without change in posture.

Entrapment usually occurs where a nerve passes through a fascial plane or down a fibro-osseous tunnel; for example, the median nerve in the carpal tunnel.

The lateral cutaneous nerve of the thigh may be trapped under the lateral end of the inguinal ligament. Patients complain of an area of pain and paraesthesia with numbness on the lateral aspect of the thigh just above the knee (*meralgia paraesthetica*). The area never extends across the midline anteriorly or below the knee. It is more likely to occur in obese, middle-aged patients and weight reduction may be the only treatment necessary. Local steroid injections are sometimes effective; decompression is occasionally required.

A localized lesion of the femoral nerve may occur in diabetes (diabetic amyotrophy). Apparently spontaneous haematomas may also affect the femoral nerve, and this occurs in patients with bleeding diathesis or in patients who are on anticoagulant treatment.

Electromyography and nerve condition studies may be helpful to localize the precise site of the lesion and quantify the severity of the lesion.

The median nerve

The *carpal tunnel syndrome* is the commonest mononeuropathy and is due to compression of the median nerve as it passes through the carpal tunnel in the flexor retinaculum. There is usually no associated systemic disease, but the carpal tunnel syndrome may occur in rheumatoid arthritis, myxoedema, acromegaly, oedema, pregnancy and obesity. It is much more common in women and usually affects the dominant hand first. Patients complain of pain and paraesthesia which may wake them at night and they may shake the hand out of bed to obtain relief. Symptoms are brought on or aggravated by use, particularly activities which require gripping. In the early stages there may be no detectable deficit but, as the condition progresses, weakness of abductor pollicis brevis may develop with difficulty in fine manipulation. The earliest sensory deficit is usually widening of two-point discrimination. Abnormal signs are strictly confined to median nerve territory, but symptoms may occur in all digits and there may also be pain in the forearm.

Splinting, diuretics and local steroid injections may relieve the symptoms and may be the only treatment necessary for self-limiting conditions, such as pregnancy. In more severe cases, particularly if there is sensory loss or progressive weakness, surgical decompression is necessary. Pain and intermittent symptoms are relieved immediately, and the continuous symptoms may resolve with time but wasting of abductor pollicis brevis may never recover.

In *anterior interosseus palsy* a lesion of the anterior interosseus nerve produces weakness of the flexor pollicis longus, flexor digitorum profundus 1 and 2 and pronator quadratus. There is no sensory loss. Spontaneous recovery usually occurs, but the nerve should be explored if recovery is delayed beyond three months.

The ulnar nerve

Lesions of the unlar nerve occur at four sites: behind the medial epicondyle, in the cubital tunnel, at the wrist, and in the hand.

The elbow is a classic site for a compressive lesion. Damage occurs if the groove is shallow and particularly if there has been damage to the elbow joint by a previous fracture. Sometimes the nerve may override the medial epicondyle in full flexion. These patients present with a slowly progressive deficit which may be predominantly motor or sensory. The nerve is usually thickened. Involvement of the ulnar innervated long flexors (flexors digitorum profundus 3 and 4) is rather variable; if it is affected, the lesion must be at the elbow.

In mild cases it may be sufficient to advise against full elbow flexion and leaning on the elbow. In more severe cases, or where the lesion is clearly progressing, it may be necessary to transpose the nerve anteriorly.

The *cubital tunnel syndrome* is an entrapment neuropathy of the ulnar nerve in the foreaem flexor group. Clinically it is similar to the lesion at the elbow, but flexor digitorum profundus is not affected. Simple decompression is all that is necessary.

At the wrist the nerve may be compressed by a ganglion in Guyon's canal.

In the hand the deep motor branch may be compressed against the pisiform and the hamate if the hand is used as a mallet. The sensory branches are always spared and the motor supply to the hypothenar eminence may also be spared or less affected than the other ulnar innervated small hand muscles.

The radial nerve

The commonest sites for radial nerve lesions are in the

arm and in the extensor muscles affecting the posterior interosseus branch.

Crutch palsy is due to compression of the radial nerve above the spiral groove by long crutches when the weight is taken in the axilla. *Saturday-night palsy* is due to compression of the radial nerve in the upper part of the arm and is caused by resting the arm against a sharp edge for a prolonged period; triceps is usually spared. Both these lesions produce weakness of brachioradials, wrist and finger drop and weakness of the long thumb extensors and abductor. There may be dysaesthesis in the distribution of the superficial radial nerve.

Posterior interosseus palsy is caused by entrapment of the posterior interosseus nerve in the forearm extensor group. It presents with weakness of finger and thumb extension but the radial wrist extensor and brachioradials is spared and there is no sensory loss. These lesions usually do not recover spontaneously and should be explored without delay.

Sciatic nerve lesions

The sciatic nerve may be damaged by apparently spontaneous haematomas and misplaced injections.

The common peroneal nerve is relatively unprotected as it traverses the lateral aspect of the head of the fibula and may be compressed at this site. Patients present with a painless foot drop and may complain of numbness or paraesthesia on the lateral aspect of the foot (*common peroneal palsy*). Examination shows weakness of dorsiflexion and eversion of the foot and weakness of extensor hallucis longus. Inversion and plantar flexion are normal and the ankle jerk is preserved. In the majority of patients, where the lesion is due to simple compression, recovery occurs within a few weeks. If the weakness progresses or fails to resolve in a month or two or if there is any obvious local lesion, surgical exploration may be required.

Polyneuropathy

Polyneuritis or polyneuropathy is the term used to describe symmetrical involvement of all the peripheral nerves. The longest nerves are affected first so that signs and symptoms start in the feet and progress proximally, later involving the hands. The majority of patients have both motor and sensory signs and symptoms but some neuropathies are predominantly motor and others predominantly sensory.

The earliest symptoms are usually persistent tingling and numbness of the hands and feet, accompanied by peripheral weakness. The signs accord with the symptoms with uniform distal weakness, absent reflexes and a characteristic 'glove-and-stocking' sensory impairment. In some patients the weakness is more proximal. Pathologically there are two main groups, the *demyelinating neuropathies* and the *axonal neuropathies*.

The striking feature of demyelinating neuropathies is the slowing of conduction velocity. Causes include diabetes, the Guillain–Barré syndrome, carcinomatous neuropathy, hypertrophic neuropathy, metachromatic leucodystrophy and diphtheria.

Nerve conduction velocity may be relatively preserved in the early stages of an axonal neuropathy owing to normal conduction in unaffected fibres. Causes include alcoholism, porphyria, isoniazid, vincristine and thalidomide.

This differentiation is only valid in the early stages and eventually both myelin and axons are affected. This mixed pattern is commonly seen is diabetes and lead poisoning.

Acute infective polyneuropathy (Guillain–Barré syndrome)

This predominantly motor demyelinating neuropathy usually follows an upper repiratory tract infection by a week or so. The infection may be due to a wide range of organisms, including glandular fever, cytomegalovirus infection and mycoplasma infection. It may occur in either sex and at any age. It develops rapidly from onset, reaching its maximum within a few days. The paralysis may affect all four limbs and endanger respiration. Patients with progressive symptoms should be transferred immediately to a centre where artificial ventilation is available. Facial weakness occurs in most patients but any of the cranial nerves may be involved.

Autonomic involvement is common with labile blood pressure and cardiac involvement, and this is the cause of death in a number of patients with this condition.

It is unlikely that this is a single disease entity, but the diagnosis can be made on clinical grounds and supported by the demonstration of marked slowing of peripheral nerve conduction. CSF analysis shows characteristic changes with a markedly elevated CSF protein owing to involvement of the spinal roots with a normal cell count. Even in severe cases, it is not usually necessary to ventilate the patient for more than two or three weeks. With modern methods of artificial ventilation there is no reason why patients should not survive this critical period. Recovery can be quite prolonged, extending from six months to two years, but this is not incompatible with a complete restoration of function. Nerve conduction abnormalities usually persist, but a residual deficit detectable clinically only occurs in around 30 per cent of cases and this is usually not of great significance. Temporary relapses may punctuate return to activity.

Patients still progressing in the early stages must be transferred immediately to a unit where ventilation and cardiac monitoring is available. Plasmaphoresis may be of some benefit in the acute stages and may produce sufficient short-term benefit to keep a patient off a ventilator. Steroids are now known to be of no benefit and there is some evidence that they may actually retard progress, although they are of value in the chronic relapsing form of this disease.

Infections

Infections of the nervous system may be divided into acute and chronic infections of the meninges (meningitis) and of the brain parenchyma (encephalitis) and further divided into the bacterial or pyogenic infections, including fungal infections, and the viral infections.

Acute pyogenic meningitis is discussed on page 425.

Chronic meningitis

Many organisms can cause a subacute or chronic meningitis and this may also be the consequence of inadequate treatment of organisms usually associated with acute meningitis. Tuberculosis, syphilis and the cryptococcus are important causes.

Tuberculous meningitis

In most patients this is the consequence of rupture of a small tuberculous brain abscess, which in turn is the result of blood-borne infection. A chronic granulomatous basal meningitis develops. Most patients have evidence of tuberculosis elsewhere, usually in the lung. Dissemination may occur spontaneously or the organism may be released by the use of systemic steroids. The onset is insidious, often with several weeks of vague ill health, sometimes with confusional episodes. Because of this the diagnosis is often delayed. Eventually the patient develops headache often with vomiting, convulsions may occur and the patient becomes drowsy or even delirious. There is usually a low-grade fever. Papilloedema is a late development but choroidal tubercles may be seen quite

early in the course of the illness. Cranial nerve palsies are quite common.

Lumbar puncture shows CSF under increased pressure; it is usually clear initially but on standing develops a fine 'cobweb clot'. Analysis shows a lymphocytosis with increased protein and a reduced sugar level. In the more acute forms there may be an initial polymorphonuclear leucocytosis, but this changes to a predominant lymphocytosis. A low CSF chloride, once thought to be characteristic of this condition, is a measure of the amount of vomiting. The tubercle bacilli may be found by direct staining and this, of course, confirms the diagnosis; but in the majority of cases the organism is not seen and culture may not be positive for several weeks, which often results in further delay in diagnosis and treatment.

It is usually necessary, therefore, to start *treatment* on the basis of a high index of clinical suspicion, rather than on a confirmed diagnosis. The difficulty of antibiotic treatment is the poor penetration of the most suitable agents into the CSF. Isoniazid in doses of 10 mg/kg/day, combined with pyridoxine 10 mg daily to avoid polyneuritis, is the most useful drug. This may be combined with rifampicin (12 mg/kg/day) and pyrazinamide (30 mg/kg) orally. The latter (maximum dose 3 g) penetrates well into the CSF. In addition, oral ethambutol or intramuscular streptomycin may be given initially. Betamethasone (2.0 g q.i.d.) is often given for the first few weeks of treatment to minimise reactive fibrosis in the meninges but its usefulness is unproven.

Cryptococcal meningitis

Cryptococcus neoformans is a fungus which may cause a chronic meningitis. This may escape detection unless special stains are requested. Amphotericin B and 5-fluocytosine are effective treatments.

Sarcoidosis, syphilis and carcinoma may all cause a chronic basal meningitis.

Acute viral meningitis (lymphocytic meningitis)

Viral infections are seldom confined to the meninges and usually cause a meningoencephalitis. This may be produced by a wide variety of organisms including mumps, glandular fever, some Coxsackie and echo viruses, poliomyelitis and the virus of acute lymphocytic choriomeningitis. The clinical picture is similar with acute or subacute onset of meningitis. In the early stages CSF analysis shows both polymorphs and lymphocytes but, after a few days, it becomes purely lymphocytic and this is associated with a normal glucose level. There may be diagnostic difficulty in distinguishing this from tuberculous meningitis, when acid-fast bacilli have not been found in the CSF. The CSF sugar is not a reliable distinguishing feature. There may be other signs which help with the diagnosis, such as pharyngitis and lymphadenopathy in glandular fever and swelling of the salivary glands with mumps. There is no specific treatment, but the prognosis is good with the majority of patients making a complete recovery.

Pyogenic encephalitis (brain abscess)

Intracranial abscess may be extradural and secondary to osteitis of the skull or intracerebral, usually as a result of blood-borne infection. Subdural and subarachnoid abscesses are rare. Cerebral abscess due to spread of infection from middle ear disease was once common, but with effective early control of this condition, cerebral abscess is now a rare complication.

A cerebral abscess starts as a localized area of cerebritis, which later breaks down with pus formation. An encapsulated abscess then develops and may go on to act as a progressive space-occupying lesion.

Causes include spread from middle-ear disease, septicaemia, particularly in patients on steroids and immunosuppressive drugs, acute infective endocarditis and fractures of the skull. If the intracranial abscess is secondary to infection elsewhere, this is usually in the lungs. The onset may be acute or chronic, there is often evidence of infection elsewhere, there may be focal signs, there is usually headache and fever and there may be papilloedema. Most patients have a leucocytosis and the organism may be cultured from the blood. Patients may rapidly deteriorate and investigation and treatment is, therefore, a matter of some urgency. Lumbar puncture should be avoided because of the risk of herniation. The EEG is always abnormal and usually shows high-amplitude slow activity over the abscess. Computerized tomography is the definitive investigation. The treatment is neurosurgical.

Acute viral encephalitis

A wide range of both DNA and RNA viruses may cause encephalitis. The onset may be acute or subacute with confusion, drowsiness, hallucinations and abnormal movements suggesting basal ganglia involvement. The EEG is always abnormal. The CSF may be either normal or show a lymphocytosis. The causative agent is identified by a rising antibody titre.

Encephalitis lethargica was almost certainly viral in origin and produced a pandemic between 1915 and 1925 in the form of an acute encephalitic illness. It was followed in a large number of patients by post-encephalitic Parkinsoniam; no definite cases have occurred since then.

Herpes simplex encephalitis (see also page 418)

Herpes simplex may cause an acute necrotizing encephalitis which usually starts in one temporal lobe and a few days later affects the other temporal lobe. It is the commonest cause of severe encephalitis in the UK. Epilepsy may be a presenting feature. The patient is usually seriously ill within a few days. The EEG is abnormal in the early stages and between the second and the twelfth day may show periodic complexes with relative attenuation of activity between; in severe cases this precedes marked flattening of the record on that side. Changes in the other temporal lobe follow the first affected side by a few days. CT scan shows low-density areas in the temporal lobe, indicative of oedema. The diagnosis can be confirmed by biopsy and the virus identified by immunofluorescence, electron microscopy and culture and also by the demonstration of a rising antibody titre, although this takes longer.

Treatment should be started as soon as possible with systemic acyclovir, and it may also be necessary to give betamethasone to reduce cerebral oedema. It was once thought that herpes simplex encephalitis was uniformly fatal, but it is now clear that milder causes do occur and the course of the illness may be modified by treatment. Patients are often left with a dense memory defect and dysphasia.

Poliomyelitis

The development of polio vaccinces has dramatically altered the incidence of this disease, but outbreaks still occur from time to time. The portal of entry is thought to be the nasopharynx and there is an incubation period of about two weeks. In epidemics there is evidence that many patients are infected and have only a mild 'flu-like' illness; only a small proportion of patients develop paralysis, which usually progresses rapidly over a few days. The extent and the degree of the paralysis are extremely variable. The commonest cause of death is from respiratory paralysis, either as a consequence of bulbar nuclei involvement or from paralysis of the muscles of respiration. The mortality decreased considerably with the introduction of better methods of artificial respiration. Some recovery usually occurs but this is often incomplete.

Rabies (see also page 447)

Infection by the rabies virus may follow the bite of an infected animal because the virus is found in large quantities in the saliva and a bite is an effective innoculation. The disease is endemic in many parts of the world, including most of the continent of Europe. Although widespread among wildlife, most cases of human infection are due to dog bites. The virus travels to the brain along nerve trunks, so that the incubation period depends on the distance from the bite to the brain (usually between one and two months). An early symptom is pharyngeal spasm brought on by drinking and this seems to lead to marked hydrophobia. The disease is almost invariably fatal. No cases of infection between human contacts have been reported.

The use of modern diploid vaccines is very effective in treating patients who have been infected. The vaccination should be given as soon as possible after exposure to the virus.

Chronic viral encephalopathies

Subacute sclerosing panencephalitis

This disease is now known to be due to the measles virus and may develop months or even years after an attack of measles. It is slowly progressive over months or years and is nearly always fatal. Initially, there are signs of intellectual deterioration, accompanied by myoclonic jerks and occasionally by fits. The patient gradually becomes more demented. The EEG may show a repetitive burst suppression pattern. The diagnosis can be confirmed by finding an elevated measles antibody titre in the CSF.

Progressive multifocal leucoencephalopathy

This is an opportunistic viral encephalopathy which occurs in patients whose immunological competence is impaired. Associated conditions include the reticuloses and sarcoidosis. The infection causes foci of demyelination in the white matter of the brain. The clinical course is one of progression over months and the disease is usually fatal. Occasionally, patients survive for some years. The CT scan shows a characteristic appearance and the diagnosis can be confirmed by cerebral biopsy. Antiviral agents may be of value if given early.

Jakob–Creutzfeld disease (subacute spongiform encephalopathy)

This is due to a slow virus whose transmissability has been demonstrated in humans. The incubation period is several years. Patients present with a rapidly developing dementia, associated with extrapyramidal features and myoclonus. The EEG is abnormal and may show a burst-suppression pattern. The condition is invariably fatal, usually within six months.

Neurosyphilis

The nervous system is involved in *secondary syphilis*. Invasion of the meninges by the spirochaete produces the symptoms of meningitis. Examination may show papilloedema and neck stiffness. These symptoms resolve, together with the other features of secondary syphilis, and there may be no further clinical manifestation. Fewer than 10 per cent of patients later develop tertiary neurosyphilis and this may follow the original infection by many years.

Tertiary neurosyphilis classically presents as one of three clinical syndromes: meningovascular syphilis, tabes dorsalis or general paralysis of the insane (GPI). In addition there may be gumma formation and optic atrophy. These typical and well-known presentations are relatively rare now and this may be because of the widespread use of penicillin. It is now more common to find positive serological tests for syphilis in patients with a wide variety of neurological signs and symptoms which are not immediately suggestive of this disease. It is important to carry out these tests in all patients with otherwise unexplained central nervous system disease, particularly as it is treatable.

Meningovascular syphilis

This is due to an endarteritis affecting meningeal vessels and cerebral vessels. It may present as a basal granulomatous meningitis with cranial nerve palsies and obstruction to CSF pathways. Local syphilitic granulomas (gumma) may present as space-occupying lesions either in the subarachnoid space or in the brain itself.

Meningovascular syphilis affecting the spinal cord can cause a transverse myelitis. The CSF is abnormal with a raised protein and an increased immunoglobulin fraction, lymphocytosis and positive serological tests for syphilis.

Tabes dorsalis

In this form of neurosyphilis there is progressive demyelination and atrophy of the posterior roots, the root entry zone and the posterior columns. The decussating pain and temperature fibres are also involved but the spinothalamic tracts do not show demyelination because they comprise second-order neurones.

The presenting symptoms include pain, paraesthesia, sensory ataxia and bladder disturbance. In more advanced cases there may be rectal incontinence, impotence, neurogenic ulcers and neuropathic joints (*Charcot joints*).

Lightning pains are common and characteristic. They occur without obvious provocation and are described as momentary sharp stabs of pain affecting one spot, as if stabbed by a knife. The affected spot is usually in the thigh, calf or ankle.

The pupils are usually small, irregular in outline and unreactive to light, but contract normally on convergence (Argyll Robertson pupils). Cutaneous hypoalgesia is often found in the legs and over the trunk anteriorly and down the medial aspects of both arms, as well as across the nose. The deep tendon reflexes are absent, there is loss of light touch, vibration and position sense, particularly in the legs, loss of deep pain appreciation and impairment of pain sensation, often accompanied by a prolonged delay in appreciating stimuli.

There may be trophic ulcers on the feet and neuropathic joints may develop owing to loss of sensation; the shoulders, spine, hip, knees and ankles are commonly involved. There is gross disorganization of the joint, which is nearly always painless. The CSF is usually abnormal.

General paralysis of the insane (GPI)

This is a chronic spirochaetal meningoencephalitis, and the spirochaete may be isolated from the brain. The presenting features are those of dementia and personality change, and epilepsy may be an early symptom. Examination shows the features of dementia, often associated with a dysarthria, tremors of the hands, lips and tongue, a spastic paraparesis with extensor plantar responses, optic atrophy and Argyll Robertson pupils. The CSF is abnormal.

Syphilitic optic atrophy

This may occur as an isolated manifestation of neurosyphilis or it may accompany any of the other clinical syndromes. The funduscopic appearance may be that of a primary optic atrophy or there may be evidence of syphilitic choroidoretinitis.

Treatment. The treatment of all forms of neurosyphilis is by intramuscular procaine penicillin 1 g daily for three weeks. A *Herxheimer reaction* is rare but can be prevented by covering the first few days of treatment with oral steroids.

Sarcoidosis

Sarcoidosis may affect any part of the nervous system but the meninges and peripheral nerves are the most frequently involved. Sarcoid may cause a chronic granulomatous basal meningitis often associated with cranial nerve palsies. There may be hypothalamic, pituitary and chiasmal involvement.

Intracranial sarcoid granulomas are rare and tend to occur in the hypothalamus. The meningitis may result in obstruction of CSF pathways with raised intracranial pressure and papilloedema. There may be direct involvement of the optic nerve as well as retinal lesions and uveitis. The peripheral nervous system may also be affected with polyneuritis and there may be direct involvement of muscle (sarcoid myopathy).

Although neurological sarcoid is usually associated with evidence of sarcoidosis elsewhere, it may be confined to the nervous system. The CSF is usually abnormal, often with a markedly raised protein and a few lymphocytes.

The condition usually runs a fluctuating low-grade course and may be modified by steroids.

Acquired immunodeficiency syndrome (AIDS)

A very wide range of neurological abnormalities has been described in patients with AIDS, extending from an encephalopathy to a peripheral neuropathy. In addition AIDS patients are particularly prone to opportunistic infections which may affect the nervous system. The diagnosis should be considered in all patients presenting with atypical syndromes, particularly in those groups known to be at risk. Progressive dementia appears to be a common late phenomenon in AIDS.

Epilepsy

Epilepsy is the clinical manifestation of a paroxysmal electrochemical disturbance in the brain. The attacks are of sudden onset and brief duration. Heredity is an important factor and it may be that what is inherited is the epileptic threshold. Patients with the lowest threshold would be prone to spontaneous attacks and show the features of idiopathic (generalized, centrencephalic or major) epilepsy (see below). Those with a slightly higher threshold would only develop epilepsy if the brain was damaged by birth trauma, tumours, angiomas, head injury, infections, vascular disease, poisons and drugs, anoxia, congenital abnormalities, degenerative conditions and inborn or acquired errors of metabolism. The higher the threshold, the less likely that these conditions would cause epilepsy. Patients with the highest thresholds would be unlikely to develop epilepsy whatever the cerebral insult. This concept explains why some patients develop epilepsy and others with apparently similar conditions do not.

It is convenient to divide epilepsy in adults into two main groups, the generalized and the focal. This also applies to children, but there are many other factors to consider, partly because the maturing brain reacts differently from the adult brain and partly because children are subject to different diseases and hazards.

Epilepsy and driving

A single epileptic attack does not constitute epilepsy, which is by definition a liability to attacks. The law in the UK does not allow patients who have had more than one attack to drive until they have been attack-free for more than two years.

A single attack of epilepsy with an abnormal EEG is considered to indicate a liability to epilepsy.

If the attacks are nocturnal (i.e. while asleep) and continue to be solely nocturnal for more than three years, then a driving licence is allowed.

The regulations are much stricter for HGV and PSV licences and any attack after the age of five permanently excludes these licences.

Focal epilepsy (simple and complex partial seizures)

The term implies that the attacks arise from a focal discharge. The attack may take any form from a brief focal event to a major convulsive seizure, and this is a continuum.

1 Aura

A focal discharge may cause a brief focal disturbance usually called an aura, although it need not proceed any further. The nature of the attack depends on the location of the focus. Examples include a curious smell, usually unidentifiable and often unpleasant (uncinate attacks), a brief flash of light, a formed visual hallucination, auditory hallucination, *déjà vu* experiences, twitching of the thumb and index finger, abdominal sensations, feelings of fear and panic, and numerous others. Nothing else develops and consciousness is preserved.

2 Epilepsia partialis continua

Rarely a persisting focal discharge may cause a focal attack which continues for hours or days.

3 Aura with Jacksonian march

A focal disturbance causing symptoms, such as twitching of the thumb and index finger, may spread across the cortex, causing twitching of the hand, face and arm in sequence. Consciousness need not be lost.

4 Aura with loss of consciousness

If the disturbance becomes generalized, consciousness may be lost. This is often very brief and not associated with any convulsive features. Sudden loss of consciousness without a clinically identifiable aura does not exclude the presence of a focus, since the focal event may have been too brief to identify or have occurred in a part of the brain which is not symptomatically eloquent.

5 Aura, loss of consciousness and convulsive seizure

The sequence outlined so far may finish with a major tonic–clonic seizure, often with tongue-biting and incontinence.

Treatment is effective in controlling the later stages of this progression, the initial focal event itself being the most refractory.

Generalized epilepsy

In patients with a low epileptic threshold, the whole brain may discharge synchronously and the EEG shows a characteristic spike and wave pattern. This is not necessarily associated with loss of consciousness unless it lasts for several seconds. The clinical manifestations range from a brief absence to a major convulsive seizure (*grand mal*). Many patients diagnosed as having *petit mal* suffer from a minor form of generalized epilepsy. The term *petit mal* should either be abandoned or reserved for the classical absence attacks of adolescence associated with three per second spike and wave in the EEG. The differentiation is important because true *petit mal* requires different medication.

Diagnosis

The diagnosis of epilepsy is made on the history alone. The account of a witness is often helpful since there are usually no abnormal signs. In developing focal lesions, such as a brain tumour, persisting signs may not appear for several years. Occasionally focal signs persist after the attack (*Todd's paralysis*), but this term should only be used when the signs resolve within 24 hours. In adults this strongly implies an underlying structural lesion.

Investigation

In addition to a full clinical examination, all patients with epilepsy should have an EEG and, in the absence of any focal features, a lateral skull X-ray. When epilepsy develops later in life and in patients with focal features, either clinically or on the EEG, further investigation may be necessary and a CT scan is the most appropriate. Serological tests for syphilis, a chest X-ray and serum calcium estimation should also be done.

Treatment

The object of treatment is to control the attacks so that the patient may lead a normal life, and this can be achieved in the majority of patients.

The biggest advance in recent years has been the development of methods of measuring *anticonvulsant blood levels*, and this has profoundly affected the management of patients with epilepsy. The blood level cannot be predicted from the oral dose. Epilepsy can be controlled in over 80 per cent of patients by the use of a single drug, provided the blood level is maintained in the upper part of the therapeutic range. The therapeutic range is arbitrarily derived; levels below the lower limit usually have little effect and levels above the upper limit

are often associated with signs of toxicity; though it is, of course, the patient who requires treatment and not the blood level.

Drug treatment, however successful, is not a cure and patients may have to continue regular medication for many years. Since there may be no immediate consequence if a dose is missed, compliance is often poor. Medication given in one or two doses a day considerably improves compliance. Three doses a day necessitates taking tablets to school or work and is to be avoided. Dose frequency depends on the biological half-life of the drug, and all the major anticonvulsants have half-lives long enough to allow a twice-daily regimen.

Drug interactions are particularly important for patients on long-term treatment, and it may be necessary to advise patients accordingly. Drug combinations in a single preparation should not be used, since it is not possible to vary the doses independently.

Some basic data about the more commonly used drugs are given in Table 5.3. Patients should be started on one drug in moderate dose (for example, the initial figure in the table under 'usual daily dose range'). If the attacks are controlled, no further action is required. If attacks continue, the blood level should be measured and the dose adjusted, bearing in mind that it takes 2–3 weeks for most drug blood levels to stabilize. If attacks continue despite a blood level in the upper part of the therapeutic range, a different drug should be either substituted or added and the process repeated.

Phenytoin

Hydroxylation of phenytoin in the liver is a saturable process, so that a small dose increment can result in a considerable rise in blood level. It is unwise, therefore, to

Table 5.3 Anticonvulsive drugs

Preparations	Tablet or capsule size (mg)	Usual daily dose range (mg)	Therapeutic range (mg/l)	Approx. half-life (h)	Usual dose frequency
Phenytoin	25				b.d.
	50	200–400	0–16	12–40	or
	100				daily
Carbamazepine	100				
	200	200–1200	4–14	9–20	b.d.
	400				
Sodium valproate	200	600–3000	40–100	7–9	b.d.
	500				
Primidone	250	500–1500	< 14	5–15	b.d.
Phenobarbitone	15				
	30				
	60	30–90	9–25	75–108	daily
	100				

increase the dose of phenytoin by more than 25 or 50 mg when the daily dose exceeds 300 mg. In some patients, the addition of only 25 mg may convert a subtherapeutic blood level to a toxic level. The long half-life of phenytoin means that it need be given only once a day.

Dose-related side-effects include nystagmus, ataxia and dysequilibrium. Gingival hyperplasia may occur in children, and hirsuitism may be a problem in young women. Some patients are allergic to the drug and develop a rash.

2 Sodium valproate

This drug has a short blood half-life of about eight hours, but it is reasonable to give the drug twice a day since the anticonvulsant effect seems to last much longer. The short half-life also makes blood level measurements difficult to assess, unless taken at a fixed time after a dose (perhaps two hours).

Gastrointestinal upset is a common early side-effect but often improves with continuing medication. Hair loss occasionally occurs, and some patients develop a fine tremor.

3 Carbamazepine

This drug is probably the treatment of choice for women of child-bearing age or who are likely to enter the child-bearing age during the course of treatment, as it is the least likely to be associated with fetal abnormalities. Side-effects include unsteadiness, sedation and headache.

4 Clonazepam and clobazam

These two benzodiazepines are effective anticonvulsants, but they may show drug fatigue which limits use, and both drugs cause sedation.

5 Primidone

A variable proportion of an oral dose of primidone is converted into phenobarbitone. There is, therefore, no reason to use a combination of primidone and phenobarbitone. Patients who are stabilized on primidone alone show a ratio of phenobarbitone to primidone which exceeds 2:1. If the primidone level exceeds the phenobarbitone level, it can be concluded that compliance is poor.

The dose of primidone must be gradually increased, starting with 125 mg at night and increasing every three or four days to a therapeutic dose. If this is not done a number of patients will develop acute nausea, vomiting and unsteadiness which may also occur as a toxic side-effect.

6 Phenobarbitone

Although still very widely used, phenobarbitone is no longer a treatment of first choice in adult patients with epilepsy. It may cause behavioural disturbance in children, the sedation is unacceptable to young adults and it may contribute to depression in the middle-aged. Blood levels should not normally exceed 25 mg/l, especially in children, but many patients who have been stabilized on this drug for many years tolerate much higher levels without signs of toxicity. Withdrawal of the drug should be gradual owing to the risk of precipitating fits.

Status epilepticus

Status epilepticus is a series of major attacks without full recovery between seizures. This is a dangerous condition with a high mortality and requires urgent treatment.

The priority is to stop the attack, and this is best done with an intravenous injection of diazepam (10–20 mg) or clonazapam (1–2 mg). It should not be given intramuscularly or diluted in intravenous infusion fluids. The diazepam injection may be repreated and is often all that is necessary.

Control must be maintained; if attacks recur less than an hour or two after more than two or three injections of diazepam, the patient must be transferred to an intensive care unit where methods of artificial ventilation are available. Chlormethiazole may be used by slow intravenous infusion, and this may be combined with paralysis and ventilation. While paralysed and ventilated the patient's brain activity may be monitored by electro-encephalography.

Epilepsy in pregnancy

Phenytoin is a powerful liver enzyme inducer and when used in patients on the combined contraceptive pill it is necessary to prescribe a preparation containing at least 50 µg of oestrogen.

There is an increased risk of fetal abnormalities in children of patients with epilepsy and this risk is increased by medication, particularly combinations of drugs. There is about fivefold increase in the risk of cleft palate and cardiac abnormalities in children born to mothers with epilepsy on phenytoin; carbamazepine may be a safer drug to use in pregnancy. Phenobarbitone should be avoided, and sodium valproate has been associated with neural tube defects.

In the majority of patients with epilepsy it is important to maintain their anticonvulsant drugs during pregnancy, but it also important to ensure that the blood levels are within the therapeutic range. As pregnancy advances the blood levels of most anticonvulsants fall; this is partly dilutional and partly due to more rapid clearance. It is, however, very rarely necessary to increase the dose during pregnancy, but if this is done, the dose must be reduced after delivery.

Most anticonvulsant drugs are excreted in small quantities in breast milk; but breast feeding is not contraindicated except for patients on phenobarbitone, which tends to cause drowsiness in the infant.

The risks of a child born to a patient with epilepsy of developing the same condition is only slightly greater than chance. If there is also a history of epilepsy in the father's family, the risk rises considerably.

Migraine

Clinical features

Migraine is a paroxysmal headache which may be clearly lateralized, but not necessarily always to the same side, or it may be generalized. The headache may be preceded by an 'aura' which can take many forms, the most common of which are a variety of visual disturbances such as fortification spectra, flashing lights or hemianopic defects. There may be numbness or tingling of the face and arms, weakness of one side of the body and, occasionally, dysphasia. These symptoms usually evolve over a few minutes and last for between 15 and 25 minutes. The headache starts towards the end of the aura and usually builds up to a maximum over an hour or so. It may remain severe for several hours and the whole attack is over in 6–12 hours; occasionally, attacks last a day or two. The headache is often accompanied by nausea and vomiting, photophobia and noise intolerance. The frequency of migraine is very variable, ranging from weekly to yearly; but about once a month is common and attacks are often related to menstruation.

Pathophysiology

The aura stage of migraine is associated with cerebral vasoconstriction and it is likely that all patients go through this stage, even though it may not be clinically identifiable. The headache stage is associated with noncerebral cranial vasodilation. The cause of migraine is unknown, but there is probably a genetic factor because there is often a family history.

Treatment

1 Avoidance of aggravating or precipitating factors.

Some patients are able to identify a major aggravating or precipitating factor and it is much easier to avoid this than to take medication. Only a few patients are sensitive to food substances and these are usually the tyramine-containing foods; but chocolate and citrus fruits are also potent aggravating factors in some patients. The contraceptive pill usually aggravates migraine and, though it may be reasonable to take simple treatment for the migraine, if severe attacks persist then alternative methods of contraception should be used. The contraceptive pill is contraindicated in patients who repeatedly have the same aura. The commonest cause of an aggravation of migraine in middle age is the development of hypertension. The menopause is often associated with a change in the pattern of attacks. Other aggravating factors include stress and anxiety, alcohol, relaxation (weekend migraine) and the menstrual cycle.

2 Treatment of the acute attack

The simplest treatment for an attack of migraine is a combination of soluble aspirin or an equivalent mild analgesic, taken together with metoclopramide (10 mg). The metoclopramide promotes the absorption of aspirin and is useful for its antiemetic effect. Some patients benefit from the use of Migraleve (a mixture of analgesics and an antiemetic). If these measures fail, an ergotamine preparation may be used and these are available either sublingually, to swallow, by inhalation or by suppository. Patients who have very occasional but very severe attacks may best be treated with a single large dose of a sedative and sleep the attack off.

3 Prophylaxis

This is the most effective form of treatment for patients who have frequent attacks and may, of course, be combined with treatment for the acute attack; a number of drugs are effective:

on vascular smooth muscle, clonidine 25 μg t.d.s.
on vascular innervation, propranolol starting with 10 mg t.d.s.
by serotonin antagonism, pizotifen up to 3 mg a day
on psychological factors, tricyclic antidepressants (amitriptyline 25–50 mg at night).

Migrainous neuralgia

This is a paroxysmal vascular headache but is otherwise different from migraine. It is much more frequent in men than in women and the attacks are not preceded by an aura. Attacks occur in clusters (hence *'cluster headache'*), the patient usually having one or two attacks a day for several weeks before a remission, which may last for months. The attacks are sharply localized to one supra and reto-oribital region and it may spread to the cheek.

The pain is very intense and lasts for about an hour. The attack is associated with watering of the eye and blocking of the nose on the same side; subsequently the nose runs. In severe attacks there may be a Horner's syndrome (ptosis and a small pupil—see page 202), and this occasionally persists between attacks. The attacks often occur at the same time every day and may waken the patient from sleep.

The most effective treatment is an ergotamine suppository containing 2 mg either daily or twice a day up to 5 suppositories weekly.

Beta-blockade with propranolol and the serotonin antagonist methysergide may also be effective prophylaxis in some patients. Alcohol should be avoided as this often precipitates attacks during clusters.

Cerebrovascular disease

Intracranial haemorrhage

Extradural haemorrhage

This may occur after head injury and is due to the fracture line crossing a meningeal artery, usually the middle meningeal artery. The initial head injury is of sufficient severity to cause loss of consciousness, from which the patient often recovers. The bleeding is arterial, so that the haematoma forms over several hours, causing gradually increasing coma and in the later stages progressing to hemiplegia with fixed dilated pupils. Removal of the haematoma is life-saving.

There may be no *lucid interval* if the initial injury is particularly severe. In suspected cases burr-holes should be made as a matter of urgency. The prognosis is related to the promptness of treatment, which should not be postponed until the patient is transferred to a neurosurgical unit if this is likely to result in undue delay. The haematoma can be demonstrated by a CT scan or by carotid angiography.

Subdural haemorrhage

Subdural haematomas also follow head injuries but the injury may be quite slight and the history of trauma may be unobtainable. The haematoma is due to venous bleeding and it may take days or weeks to form. It usually occurs in the young and the elderly. The presenting feature may be headache or epilepsy. Later there are periods of fluctuating drowsiness leading to coma, and there may be clear lateralizing signs or evidence of brainstem compression. The haematoma may be demonstrated by a CT scan, though there is a stage at which the haematoma is isodense with brain. If unilateral, there will be displacement of the ventricles but, if bilateral, there may be no shift of midline structures. However, in such patients, the ventricles appear unusually small and the cerebral sulci are not very prominent. An isotope scan may be positive and the haematoma can be demonstrated by angiography.

Treatment. Small subdural collections, in the absence of any physical signs or symptoms or evolving clinical picture, may be left to resolve; otherwise the treatment is by surgical evacuation of the clot.

Subarachnoid haemorrhage

This is usually due to the rupture of a berry aneurysm or bleeding from an arteriovenous malformation, and it most commonly occurs in middle life. The onset is usually abrupt with severe headache and often with loss of consciousness. Subsequently, the patient complains of severe occipital headache and this is often accompanied by vomiting. Examination may show subhyaloid haemorrhages and there is marked neck stiffness. Focal signs, such as aphasia, a visual field defect or hemiparesis may occur either because the bleeding is partly intracerebral and partly subarachnoid or because of associated spasm of major cerebral arteries. The clinical diagnosis can be confirmed by a CT brain scan, which may also show the aneurysm. If this investigation is not available, lumbar puncture may show CSF under pressure and a diagnostic feature is xanthochromia.

1 Cerebral aneurysm

There are several different sorts of cerebral aneurysm, but the one most likely to cause subarachnoid haemorrhage is a berry aneurysm, which is due to a congenital defect of the arterial wall at major branches. Berry aneurysms are commonly found around the Circle of Willis, particularly on the internal carotid artery at the origin of the posterior communicating artery. Other common sites are on the anterior communicating artery and at the trifurcation of the middle cerebral artery. Aneurysms at either end of the posterior communicating artery may be associated with a third nerve palsy.

The fusiform aneurysms associated with degenerative vascular disease and hypertension and large saccular aneurysms seldom rupture and usually present with compression of cranial nerves.

2 Cerebral angioma

This is a congenital arteriovenous malformation which, although present from birth, may not give rise to symptoms until the second or third decade. Patients may complain of headache which is usually worse with exercise. It may present with subarachnoid haemorrhage, in which case the bleeding is usually less than occurs with the rupture of a berry aneurysm and often recurs. It may also present with epilepsy or with a very progressive hemipareis. A bruit may be heard over the mastoids or orbits and a venous hum may be heard in the neck.

Investigation

If a patient survives the rupture of a berry aneurysm, investigations to find the source of the bleeding should be undertaken as soon as the patient has made a reasonable recovery. Patients are at risk from rebleeding at any time and there is no safe period. Bilateral carotid and vertebral angiography should therefore be undertaken as soon as possible with a view to a surgical approach to the aneurysm if such be found. After about six weeks the risk of rebleeding is about the same as the risks of surgery. No cause for the subarachnoid haemorrhage is found in about 20 per cent of cases.

Intracerebral haemorrhage

This is nearly always associated with systemic hypertension and the commonest cause is the rupture of a Charcot–Bouchard aneurysm. These microaneurysms occur on the short perforating arteries arising from the Circle of Willis and the lenticulostriate arteries. For this reason cerebral haemorrhage usually occurs in the internal capsule, corpus striatum, upper brain stem and thalamus. The onset is usually abrupt and the rapidly expanding lesion may cause loss of consciousness at or shortly after onset. The destruction of brain tissue and the site of the lesion usually results in severe deficit and recovery is often poor. It is not uncommon for the haemorrhage to rupture into the lateral ventricles. Surgical evacuation of the clot is usually disappointing.

Cerebral ischaemia

Cerebral ischaemia or infarction occurs when a cerebral artery is occluded by thrombus or embolus.

The important risk factors in cerebrovascular disease are hypertension, diabetes, hyperlipidaemia, syphilis, a haemoglobin above 15 g/dl or a PCV above 45 per cent and the contraceptive pill. A cerebral thrombosis is unusual in young patients and in menstruating women. If a stroke occurs in these two groups, it is likely either to be an embolism from the heart or in association with one or more major risk factors. These risk factors need to be assessed in all patients with stroke and, if found, treated accordingly.

Cerebral thrombosis

The onset is usually less abrupt than cerebral haemorrhage and the neurological defect may take several hours to evolve. This often occurs overnight and the patient wakes with a completed stroke. Occlusion is due to the formation of clot at a site where the artery is already narrowed by an atheromatous plaque. Occasionally a thrombus forms in a segment of inflamed artery (arteritis); causes include giant-cell arteritis, syphilis, polyarteritis nodosa and systemic lupus erythematosus.

Cerebral embolism

Emboli to the brain may arise from any part of the vascular tree from the heart to the major cerebral vessels. The commonest sites are the heart and the carotid bifurcation.

1 Emboli from the heart may arise from mural thrombi which form as the result of myocardial infarction or in the atria as a result of atrial fibrillation. In both cases the embolus consists of formed blood clot. In bacterial endocarditis, pieces of heart valve may break away to form emboli.
2 The carotid bifurcation is a common site for atheromatous plaque formation. This may produce any degree of carotid stenosis to complete occlusion and at any stage in this process the surface of the plaque may ulcerate, giving rise to emboli of atheromatous debris, including cholesterol crystals. Platelets aggregate on the raw surface and many form platelet emboli. This process may also occur at the origin of the cerebral arteries from the aorta and in the carotid syphon.

Whatever the source of the embolus, the onset is abrupt, though the deficit may subsequently increase or repeated emboli may give rise to a 'stuttering hemiplegia' or 'stroke in evolution'. If an embolus impacts in a cerebral artery and subsequently fragments, the resulting transient neurological deficit is called a *'transient ischaemic attack'* (TIA) and is usually due to a platelet embolus. By international convention, TIAs resolve completely in less than 24 hours. Any attack which results in permanent neurological deficit is known as a *completed stroke*. If the deficit lasts longer than 24 hours but recovers completely, it is known as reversible ischaemic neurological deficit (RIND).

The clinical syndrome that results from cerebral embolism depends on which artery is involved, and for descriptive purposes the area of brain involved is identified by its feeding artery. Occlusion of the main trunk of the middle cerebral artery causes damage in its entire territory, with motor and sensory deficit on one side of the body associated with aphasia if the dominant hemisphere is affected, and a homonymous hemianopia due to involvement of the optic radiation. Fragmentary forms of this syndrome occur with embolization of more distant branches.

The *carotid artery syndrome* consists of attacks of ipsilateral amblyopia and attacks with contralateral long tract signs, and is due to emboli from the carotid artery to the ophthalmic artery and middle cerebral artery. The emboli may be seen traversing the retinal circulation. If the eye and the brain are affected at the same time the cause is more likely to be a perfusion failure due to a tight carotid stenosis or occlusion.

About 30 per cent of patients who have transient ischaemic attacks develop a completed stroke within three years and this may occur after only a few attacks. These patients should be investigated with a view to endarterectomy if a surgically treatable lesion is found. Vertebrobasilar transient ischaemic attacks should be managed conservatively since they have a better prognosis than those in carotid territory and since most of the vertebrobasilar system is not accessible for surgery. A bruit over the appropriate carotid bifurcation is a strong indication of stenosis of the artery at that site and considerably increases the chances of finding an operative lesion. Initial screening may be carried out with Doppler ultrasonic angiology. Useful information may also be obtained from digital subtraction angiograms which produce images of the arteries following intravenous injection of contrast. This technique is particularly useful in identifying occluded arteries and major stenoses. The definitive investigation is still by arteriography, usually performed by femoral catheterization and subsequent selective catheterization of the appropriate vessels.

If emboli are thought to arise in the heart, the patient should be anticoagulated. Emboli arising more distally in patients not suitable for surgery may be treated with antiplatelet drugs, such as aspirin 300 mg daily.

Any consideration of surgery must take account of the operative mortality and morbidity of carotid endarterectomy. It is doubtful if the operation should be performed if the combined mortality and morbidity exceeds 5 per cent.

Management of a completed stroke

About 50 per cent of patients who have a hemiplegic stroke make a good recovery, about 25 per cent die within the next month and the remainder are left severely disabled.

The immediate treatment consists of good nursing care with particular attention to the avoidance of chest infection and the management of urinary retention if it occurs. Although the blood pressure may be quite high in the hours after a stroke, it usually settles in a few days and treatment which causes a precipitous fall in pressure should be avoided. Dehydration must be prevented as it increases the tendency to thrombosis. Rehabilitation by physiotherapists and, if necessary, speech therapists should be commenced as soon as possible, as vigorous early treatment probably decreases subsequent disability.

Venous sinus thrombosis

This usually results from spread of infection from the middle ear, mastoid or air sinuses. It may be associated with cerebral abscess. Venous sinus thrombosis also occurs in association with pregnancy and may result from a head injury associated with skull fracture. Anticoagulants are contraindicated because of the risk of haemorrhage. Treatment is that of the cause, and steroids may be helpful in reducing the associated cerebral oedema.

Intracranial tumours

Any of the intracranial structures may give rise to tumour. The following list includes some of the common tumours:

meninges	meningioma
brain parenchyma	gliomas
cranial nerves	optic nerve glioma, neurofibromas (acoustic and trigeminal)
endocrine	pituitary and pineal
congenital	craniopharyngioma, chordoma
blood vessels	angioma, haemangioblastoma
granulomas	TB, sarcoid and syphilis
metastatic tumours	usually from lung or breast

In adults the most common neoplasms are supratentorial gliomas and metastatic tumours. In children, posterior fossa tumours are more common and they are usually medulloblastomas or astrocytomas.

Clinical features

The presentation of an intracranial tumour depends very much on its location and speed of growth. About 5 per cent of tumours present with fits or may initially be diagnosed as strokes. The majority of supratentorial tumours present with steadily progressive neurological deficit. A tumour in the frontal lobe may present with personality changes and dementia. If slightly more posterior, it may present with a slowly progressive hemiplegia and there may be speech involvement if it affects the dominant hemisphere. The earliest features of a temporal lobe tumour are facial weakness, slight drift of the outstretched arm and an upper quadrantic hemianopia. Parietal lesions often cause hemianopia and may be associated with receptive speech difficulty in the dominant hemisphere or difficulties with spatial orientation in the non-dominant hemisphere.

Epilepsy may be the earliest symptom, and this implies involvement of the cortex. In some very slowly growing tumours, such as meningiomas, the epilepsy may precede the development of other focal signs by many years.

Posterior fossa tumours usually present in a slightly different way. There is comparatively little space in the posterior fossa, so that a relatively small tumour quickly obstructs CSF pathways; headache, vomiting and papilloedema may occur early and there may be signs of brain-stem compression.

Investigation

A CT brain scan, MRI, plain skull films and cerebral angiography may all be required to determine the precise location and likely nature of an intracranial tumour.

Treatment

Treatment of intracranial tumours depends entirely on their nature and their situation. An attempt should be made to remove benign tumours, such as pituitary adenomas, acoustic neuromas and meningiomas, except where to do so would leave unacceptable deficit. Malignant gliomas are, on the whole, not removable, although if confined to the anterior part of the frontal lobe or the anterior part of the temporal lobe, it may be possible to carry out a radical resection. Otherwise, the nature of the tumour should be determined by biopsy and consideration given to the possibility of X-ray therapy. Metastatic tumours, if solitary and near the surface, can often be removed entirely. Chemotherapy has so far proved disappointing. Many cerebral tumours, particularly metastases and meningiomas, are associated with extensive white-matter oedema. This can be effectively treated with betamethasone (16 mg a day initially) and this treatment will often result in a dramatic improvement in the patient's condition.

Disseminated sclerosis (multiple sclerosis)

In this condition patches of demyelination occur at different times scattered throughout the central nervous system. These 'plaques' evolve and resolve to give the characteristic episodes of neurological dysfunction, from which there may be complete clinical recovery, although pathologically they leave small scars in the white matter.

Aetiology

The cause is unknown. There are features which suggest an immunological mechanism perhaps with a slow virus, and these two possibilities are not mutually incompatible. In addition there is evidence that the composition of myelin in patients with multiple sclerosis is slightly different from normal subjects.

Epidemiology

The disease seems to be much more common in temperate climates and is comparatively rare in equatorial countries. There is some evidence that migration from a high-risk area to a low-risk area or vice versa only changes the risk for an individual if this migration takes place before adolescence. These geographical features have been disputed.

About 60 per cent of patients have their first attack between the ages of 20 and 40, and a first attack below the age of 15 or over the age of 50 is rare. In the UK women are more affected than men in a ratio of 2:1.

Clinical features

The signs and symptoms of disseminated sclerosis depend entirely on the site of the lesions but it is confined to the central nervous system. Although cranial nerve palsies occur, lower motor neurone signs in the limbs do not. Unilateral retrobulbar neuritis is often an early feature with the rapid progression of visual impairment, usually due to a central scotoma, associated with pain on eye movement. An afferent pupillary defect is a characteristic feature (see page 202).

Vision may remain unchanged for days or a few weeks and then gradually improve. The disc may show swelling (papillitis) initially and later optic atrophy. Involvement of cerebellar pathways in the brain stem is common and results in nystagmus, internuclear ophthalmoplegia, dysarthria, ataxia and disequilibrium. Spinal cord involvement is also common with involvement of the pyramidal tracts and posterior columns. Sphincter disturbance is an early feature with spinal cord involvement.

These features usually evolve over a few days, last a few weeks and resolve over weeks or months. There may be complete remission of all signs and symptoms after the first episode and recurrence may not occur for many years. Often recovery is incomplete if the relapses are frequent, causing increasing permanent disability. It is not possible to predict the outcome of the disease in the early stages, but the state of the patient five years after the first attack is some guide to prognosis. In some patients, particularly the young, the disease shows wide fluctuations between exacerbations and remissions whereas others, particularly the older patients, may show a very slow progressive course over many years without obvious remissions.

Diagnosis

The diagnosis depends on the demonstration of multiple lesions within the nervous system and documented evidence of multiple lesions in time (definite multiple sclerosis). The demonstration of a single focal lesion for which no other cause can be found, with a history suggestive of other lesions, is usually designated 'probable multiple sclerosis', whereas a single lesion without any evidence of other lesions, but no alternative diagnosis, may be called 'possible multiple sclerosis'. It is, of course, necessary to exclude focal lesion due to some other cause. This difficulty often occurs with a slowly progressive spinal-cord lesion in middle age and no other features. A compressive lesion must be excluded by myelography.

Investigation

Analysis of the CSF may show a slightly raised CSF protein with a disproportionate increase in the amount of the immunoglobulin IgG. This is usually expressed as the IgG/albumin ratio. A more accurate test compares the relative amount of IgG to albumin in CSF to the same measurement in the blood and, by this means, it can be demonstrated that the immunoglobulin is produced on the brain side of the blood–brain barrier. The abnormal IgG is oligoclonal and this can be demonstrated by immunoelectrophoresis.

In patients with a single focal lesion both clinically and historically, additional focal lesions within the nervous system may be demonstrated by measurement of central conduction velocities:

Visual evoked responses. The patient is asked to look at a black and white checkerboard pattern, which flashes black and white alternately. This produces a time-locked response in the visual cortex which can be recorded by surface electrodes. The amplitude is much less than that of the EEG so that an averager is required. Delayed conduction from one eye compared with the other or to normal values indicates a lesion of the optic nerve on that side. A similar technique can be used to measure central conduction velocities in the auditory system (auditory evoked responses and crossed acoustic response) and in the sensory system (somatosensory evoked responses).

Magnetic resonance imaging is a particularly sensitive technique for showing the multiple periventricular plaques in multiple sclerosis.

Treatment

There is no specific treatment which influences the course of the disease. There is some evidence that a short course of high-dose steroids given during the acute attack induces a remission earlier and with less deficit than might otherwise have occurred. This is presumably by an effect on the oedema associated with an evolving plaque. There is no case for continued treatment with steroids.

Neuromyelitis optica (Devic's disease)

This condition is closely related to disseminated sclerosis but it tends to develop at an earlier age, usually affecting adolescents. The clinical picture is that of bilateral retrobulbar neuritis occurring either simultaneously or consecutively and associated with a transverse myelitis which results in a spastic paraplegia or quadriplegia. The pathological changes are similar to disseminated sclerosis. Recovery is often poor but relapses are rare. The treatment is with steroids.

Hereditary spinocerebellar degenerations

Any part of the neuraxis may be affected by genetically determined degenerative processes. The most common parts of the nervous system to be involved are the cerebellum, the spinal cord and the peripheral nerves. The extent to which these structures are involved varies from family to family but tends to breed true within a family. Although there is a continuum from a pure cerebellar degeneration to pure peripheral nerve involvement, some combinations of signs are much commoner than others and these were recognized early; an eponymous nomenclature has continued.

Friedreich's ataxia

This is the commonest form of this group of degenerative disorders and is the result of degeneration in the cerebellum, posterior and lateral columns of the cord and less severe involvement of the optic nerves and peripheral nerves. The onset is usually in the first or second decade with unsteadiness of gain followed by clumsiness of the hands. The cerebellar degeneration results in nystagmus, dysarthria and ataxia. Spinal cord involvement results in pyramidal weakness of the legs with extensor plantar responses, but the knee and ankle reflexes are usually absent because of the associated peripheral neuropathy. The condition is associated with pes cavus, which may be found in unaffected members of the family, and there may be cardiac changes.

Hereditary motor and sensory neuropathy

This condition (*peroneal muscular atrophy*, or *Charcot–Marie–Tooth disease*) is characterized by pes cavus with wasting and weakness of the muscles which begins in the peronei and progresses proximally, later involving the hands. The wasting seldom progresses above mid-thigh to give an 'inverted champagne bottle' appearance to the legs. It is a degenerative disease predominantly of the peripheral nerves, but there is evidence of anterior horn cell involvement and sometimes of cord involvement. There are two principal types, one presenting in the first decade (dominant and demyelinating; HMSN type 1) and the other in the fifth or sixth decade (dominant and axonal; HMSN type 2).

Hypertrophic interstitial neuropathy

This condition (*Dejerine–Sottas disease*) is inherited as an autosomal dominant and affects peripheral nerves with marked thickening due to Schwann cell proliferation. There is marked slowing of peripheral conduction. The disease is slowly progressive, usually presenting in adolescence. If it starts in the first decade marked kyphoscoliotic deformities may develop. The CSF protein is always raised because the roots are consistently involved.

Neurofibromatosis

Von Recklinghausen's disease is a congenital ectodermal abnormality inherited as an autosomal dominant. Both the central and peripheral nervous system may be involved with multiple neurofibromas. The most striking feature is multiple tumours of the cutaneous nerves, which present as subcutaneous nodules of varying size; they may be pedunculated. Patchy cutaneous pigmentation is almost invariably present; these too may vary in size from a few millimetres to several centimetres. They are usually described as 'café au lait' spots and there should be more than five. Phacomas may be found in the retina and there are often congenital abnormalities of the skeleton. The condition may be confined to the peripheral nervous system. Axillary freckling is said to be a reliable marker of central envolvement.

Neurofibromas of the cranial nerves, particularly of V, VIII and IX, may occur in association or as an isolated occurrence. Similarly, isolated neurofibromas of spinal roots may occur and these give rise to wasting, weakness and pain in the myotome affected as well as causing a characteristic enlargement of the intervertebral foramen; the tumour assuming a dumb-bell appearance on either side of the foramen, cord compression often occurs. Central nervous system neurofibromas are almost invariably associated with a markedly elevated CSF protein.

Complications. There is a high incidence of glioma, ependymoma and meningioma in association with neurofibromatosis. Occasionally, a neurofibroma may become sarcomatous.

Deficiency states (See Chapter 9)

Vitamin B₁ deficiency

Thiamine deficiency may present as a peripheral neuropathy (beri-beri) or as one of two forms of encephalopathy (Korsakoff's psychosis and Wernicke's encephalopathy).

1 Beri-beri

This presents with pain and paraesthesia in the hands and feet, followed later by weakness. Examination shows wasting and weakness of the small hand muscles and the feet, absent reflexes and 'glove and stocking' cutaneous sensory loss. If there is associated cardiac failure with oedema, the condition is known as wet beri-beri.

2 Korsakoff's psychosis

This is often associated with polyneuritis. The syndrome

is characterized by confusion, disorientation and striking loss of recent memory with a tendency to confabulate.

3 Wernicke's encephalopathy

This too may be associated with Korsakoff's psychosis and polyneuritis. The characteristic features are vertigo, nystagmus, ocular palsies, ataxia and drowsiness.

These clinical manifestations of thiamine deficiency are usually associated with chronic alcoholism but may be due to malnutrition. Wernicke's encephalopathy is a rare complication of hyperemesis gravidarum.

The treatment is with large doses of thiamine, which may be given intravenously at first. Since thiamine deficiency is often associated with deficiency of other vitamins, it is usual to give a preparation containing other vitamins of the B complex and vitamin C (Parentrovite Forte).

Vitamin B$_{12}$ deficiency (see also page 360)

Deficiency of vitamin B$_{12}$ may give rise to a macrocytic anaemia, subacute combined degeneration of the cord associated with a mild peripheral neuropathy, dementia, and optic atrophy.

The normal serum B$_{12}$ level is above 350 ng/l. Macrocytosis may develop at levels below this but neurological complications are rare if the level exceeds 100. Neurological complications are virtually unknown in the presence of a normal blood picture.

Subacute combined degeneration of the cord is so called because of the combined involvement of the posterior and lateral columns of the cord. This gives rise to impairment of touch, vibration and joint position sense, together with pyramidal tract signs, which always involve the legs first. Patients complain of paraesthesia in the hands and feet, followed by increasing numbness and sensory ataxia. The knee and ankle joints are absent because of the associated peripheral neuropathy but the plantar responses are extensor. Mental symptoms may accompany this condition but may rarely appear alone. Optic atrophy occurs in about 5 per cent of cases.

Treatment is by intramuscular injection of hydroxycobalamin 1 mg 6 doses over two weeks and then at increasing intervals to a maintenance dose of 1 mg every three months. This treatment must be continued for life.

Non-metastatic neurological complications of carcinoma

Any part of the neuraxis may degenerate in the presence of a carcinoma elsewhere, usually an oat-cell carcinoma of the lung. It is possible that the carcinoma produces a substance toxic to parts of the nervous system. The commonest manifestation is a mixed motor and sensory polyneuropathy, but dementia, cerebellar atrophy and myelopathy may also occur. These conditions may occur in association with myeloma and the lymphomas.

Further reading

Aids to the Examination of the Peripheral Nervous System (1986) Baillière Tindall, London.

Rowland, L.P. (1984) *Merritt's Textbook of Neurology*, 7th edn. Lee and Febiger, Philadelphia.

Walton, J.N., (1977) *Brain's Diseases of the Nervous System*, 8th edn., Oxford University Press, Oxford.

Walton, J.N., (1981) *Disorders of Voluntary Muscle*, 4th edn., Churchill Livingstone, London.

6
Disorders of Joints and Connective Tissues

Introduction and definitions

Rheumatic diseases constitute a heterogeneous group of conditions affecting joints, muscles and ligaments and causing much suffering in the community through pain, stiffness and loss of mobility. Although acute episodes and life-threatening complications may be seen in certain of the conditions under consideration, the bulk of the problems encountered are less spectacular in their presentation and give rise to prolonged discomfort and disability without seriously impairing the general health of the patient. A wide spectrum of disease is seen in this group, including hereditary, inflammatory (both acute and chronic; infective and non-infective), metabolic, traumatic, degenerative, as well as neoplastic, neuropathic and psychogenic disorders. The aetiology and patho-genesis is in many cases unknown or poorly understood.

Treatment is aimed at suppressing inflammation, reducing the disease activity and preserving and restoring the function of the locomotor system by physical therapy or surgical intervention or by adapting the environment to suit the patient's limited capabilities. Few of the diseases are amenable to eradication by medical means, but fortunately there is, in many cases, a strong tendency towards spontaneous recovery or remission. Twenty-three per cent of the work of a general practitioner involves rheumatic disorders. The importance of rheuma-tology in the medical curriculum is thus self-evident.

The terms rheumatism, fibrositis and lumbago have imprecise meanings and are best avoided. The following terms have more precise definitions and are in common usage:

Ankylosis: complete loss of joint movement

Arthralgia: pain in a joint
Arthritis: inflammation in a joint
Arthropathy: any lesion affecting a joint
Bursitis: inflammation in a bursa
Chondritis: inflammation in cartilage
Cruralgia: pain in the distribution of the femoral nerve
Effusion: presence of an excess of synovial fluid within a joint
Enthesopathy: inflammatory lesion at the point of insertion of a tendon or a ligament in bone
Monarthritis: inflammation in a single joint
Myalgia: pain in a muscle
Myositis: inflammation in a muscle
Oligoarthritis: inflammation in two, three or four joints
Osteitis: inflammation in a bone
Osteoarthritis, osteoarthrosis: degeneration in a peripheral joint
Polyarthritis: inflammation in five or more joints
Sciatica: pain in the distribution of the sciatic nerve
Spondarthritis: inflammation in the spine and peripheral joints
Spondylitis: inflammation in the spinal joints
Spondylosis: degeneration in the spinal joints
Synovitis: inflammation of synovial membrane
Tendonitis: inflammation of a tendon
Tenosynovitis: inflammation in a tendon sheath

Assessment of the arthritic patient

Symptoms

The clinical history provides important clues to the diagnosis of rheumatic diseases, and so the time devoted to a careful history-taking is well spent. Aspects such as mode of onset, duration, aggravating and relieving factors, response to treatment, effects on ability to function normally in the home and at work, are all essential for a complete understanding of the patient's condition. Important and relevant information can be gleaned by enquiry of the patient's past medical, family and occupational histories. Of particular importance from the diagnostic point of view, in both the acute and chronic rheumatic diseases, is the pattern of progression of the ailment, whether it follows a self-limiting, recurrent, acute or chronic course.

The principal symptoms of arthritis are pain, stiffness, swelling and limitation of movement.

Pain

Pain is the most frequent symptom of musculoskeletal disease. It is a complex symptom, difficult to define and difficult to measure. Being a subjective phenomenon its perception is strongly influenced by a patient's emotional state.

The site of the pain (whether it is felt in joint, muscle, bone or ligament) is often indicative of the anatomical site of the lesion. The exception to this is so-called referred pain (e.g. hip joint pain referred to the knee region, shoulder joint pain referred to the insertion of deltoid, and sciatica and cruralgia seen in intervertebral disc prolapse). The nature of the pain and the effect of movement may be helpful. Aching around and within a joint suggests an arthropathy, whereas a burning or lancinating nature suggests a pain of nerve origin. An 'excruciating' pain in someone able to function normally suggests symptom-amplification of emotional origin. Pain due to inflammatory joint disease is usually present both at rest and with movement, whereas pain of degenerative or mechanical origin is often present only on movement.

Stiffness

True stiffness implies the need to apply additional effort to overcome resistance to movement. Prolonged stiffness after a period of mobility (usually early-morning stiffness on waking or less commonly vesperal stiffness) is the hallmark of inflammatory joint disease, its duration (e.g. from half an hour to all day) being directly proportional to the severity of the inflammatory process. By contrast, in osteoarthritis stiffness (known here as articular gelling) lasts only a few moments.

Swelling

Although strictly speaking joint swelling is a physical sign (see below), it may also be a presenting symptom and cause the patient to seek medical advice.

Limitation of movement

Diminution of range of movement is a cardinal feature of joint disease and may render the patient incapable of performing normally because of reduced flexibility. Patients with hip disease complain of difficulty with putting on socks or mounting on to a bus platform; patients with spinal disease notice difficulty in getting in and out of the car and in reversing; loss of knee extension leads to difficulties in walking.

Signs

Physical signs in joint disease can be broadly categorized into those determined by the presence of inflammation within joints and those features, largely mechanical in nature, which result from damage to the joints. Since joint damage may result from the effects of inflammation, the two sets of features are by no means mutually exclusive.

Signs of inflammation

Because the synovial joints (with the notable exception of the hips and spinal joints) are so accessible to inspection and palpation, the cardinal signs of inflammation can be readily recognized. Redness of the overlying skin and swelling can be observed, while tenderness and heat are detected by manual palpation. Loss of function is translated to limitation of active and passive movement, and inhibition of strength of movement by pain. An important sign of inflammation is the detection of an effusion (synovial fluid exudate) within the joint cavity by means of careful palpation for fluctuation.

Signs of mechanical dysfunction

These include crepitus, loss of range of movement, deformity and instability.

1 Crepitus

A fine crepitus on passive movement is the clinical hallmark of the osteoarthritic joint, being caused by movement between roughened surfaces. A coarser form of crepitus is seen in any condition where the articular cartilage has been damaged by disease (e.g. in rheumatoid arthritis). Loud clicks emanating from a joint are usually of no pathological significance and, provided they are painless, may be ignored.

2 Loss of range of movement

This can arise when a joint is distended by thickened synovium and by an effusion, the sheer bulk impeding movement by its very presence. When articular cartilage is eroded by disease, the extremes of ranges of movement are initially lost. As the condition progresses, so the range decreases progressively until ankylosis occurs. The sudden complete loss of movement is known as 'locking'. This occurs when a 'loose body' (for example, a detached fragment of cartilage or torn meniscus) becomes impacted in the joint.

3 Deformity

This refers to any malalignment of articulating bones which is liable to occur when joint surfaces are severely damaged, or sometimes where supporting structures (e.g. ligaments, tendons or muscles) are weakened or ruptured. The presence of deformities greatly reduces the efficiency and effectiveness of movement, whether it be in the upper limb where hand and wrist involvement drastically reduce hand function or in the lower limbs where locomotion may be severely impaired. Specific deformities are discussed under the sections relating to individual diseases.

4 Instability

Loss of the normal joint stability may also arise from damage to joint surfaces or supporting structures. It, too, can have a disastrous effect on function; for example, a strong hand grip depends on normal wrist joint stability, and standing relies on stability of the knee joint. Inflammatory joint diseases such as rheumatoid arthritis can cause irreversible damage, not only to articular cartilage and bone, but also to intra- and extra-articular ligaments whose prime function is to maintain stability. Joint laxity and instability may arise from an inherent weakness of collagen, as in the *hypermobility syndrome*.

The recognition of joint abnormalities can only be determined by appreciation of the normal anatomy and range of motion of individual joints. Such familiarity derives from the incorporation of the examination of joints into the routine clinical examination of all patients.

The vertebral column poses particular problems because it is a composite structure of 25 interarticulating vertebral segments which also articulate with the skull (via the atlanto-occipital joints), the thoracic cage (via the costovertebral joints) and the pelvis (via the sacroiliac joints). Because of the inaccessibility of the spinal articular structures, the examination is limited to (a) elicitation of tenderness by deep palpation over individual intervertebral joints; (b) observation of spinal posture—exag-

geration or diminution of normal lordotic or kyphotic (or the presence of abnormal (e.g. scoliotic) curves; and (c) observation of restriction (painful or otherwise) of normal movements pertaining to the region in question. Thus, for the cervical spine the movements tested are rotation to the left and right, flexion, extension and lateral flexion to the left and right; for the dorsal spine, rotation of the trunk to the left and to the right; and for the lumbar region flexion and extension and lateral flexion to the left and right. An integral part of the examination of the spine involves a complete neurological examination of the upper and lower limbs, since the spinal cord and the nerve roots which constitute the brachial, lumbar and sacral plexuses are very vulnerable to pressure from degenerative changes in the intervertebral discs, especially disc prolapse and osteophyte formation. Evidence for tension of the L2/3/4 roots and the L5/S1 roots may be obtained by performing the femoral nerve stretch tests and the straight leg raise combined with the sciatic nerve stretch test respectively.

No consideration of the locomotor system can be complete without full examination of the other systems and an assessment of the patient as a whole. Features such as the presence of rheumatoid nodules or tophi are helpful in confirming rheumatoid arthritis and gout respectively. Other features such as psoriasis, uveitis, genitourinary or inflammatory bowel diseases should be sought. Many rheumatic diseases have characteristic clinical features so that clinical diagnosis is often not difficult.

Diagnostic aids in rheumatology

The following diagnostic tests are helpful in difficult cases and as confirmation of the clinical diagnosis.

The *ESR* serves to distinguish inflammatory from degenerative and mechanical joint disease. The test for *rheumatoid factor* (latex fixation test and sheep cell agglutination test) are positive in two-thirds of patients with rheumatoid arthritis but also in a substantial number of patients with systemic lupus erythematosus (SLE) and in 5 per cent of the normal population. *Antinuclear factor* is positive in most patients with SLE but in substantial numbers of patients with rheumatoid arthritis and scleroderma. The pattern of immunofluorescent staining varies from disease to disease. Whilst the homogeneous pattern may be seen in all the connective tissue diseases as well as the drug-induced lupus erythematosus, the speckled pattern is particularly seen in the sera of patients with SLE, RA, systemic sclerosis and Sjogren's syndrome. The *DNA-binding test* is more specific for SLE. *Plasma urate* is raised in primary and secondary gout.

X-rays can provide diagnostic pointers to rheumatoid arthritis, (periarticular osteoporosis, joint space narrowing and erosion of cortical surface of articulating bone), osteoarthritis (periarticular osteosclerosis, joint space narrowing with osteophyte formation), ankylosing spondylitis (with sacroiliitis, syndesmophyte formation leading to bony ankylosis), gout (presence of bony tophi) and pseudogout (chondrocalcinosis articularis). Contrast radiology is used as *arthrography* (in the diagnosis of ruptured Baker's cyst and ruptured rotator cuff lesions) and in *radiculography* or *myelography* in the investigation of disc prolapse and other spinal lesions. The use of these techniques is currently complemented by newer imaging methods such as computerized tomography and magnetic resonance imaging.

Synovial fluid analysis should be undertaken whenever the diagnosis is uncertain and a joint effusion is detected. Bacteriological examination by *Gram stain* and *culture* are of paramount importance in patients suspected of having infective arthritis, and positive evidence of gout and pseudogout is obtained by the recognition of crystals of sodium urate and calcium pyrophosphate respectively by polarizing microscopy. *Anthroscopy* provides the opportunity (as yet only in the knee joint) of inspecting the inside of the joint and observing morbid anatomy, whilst synovial biopsy undertaken during arthroscopy or by closed needle biopsy can provide useful histological information on the underlying pathology.

No assessment of the chronic arthritic patient could be complete without a consideration of his capacity to undertake the basic tasks of daily living and his capacity for return to work, preferably undertaken by an occupational therapist.

Rheumatoid arthritis (rheumatoid disease)

Rheumatoid arthritis is the most common form of chronic inflamatory disease affecting synovial joints. It should be seen, however, in a larger context as a multisystem disease of connective tissue which produces systemic manifestations in viscera as well as the locomotor system.

Aetiology and pathology

The precise aetiology is still unknown. There is a distinct familial tendency, and an important recent discovery is a significant association (70% RA, 28% controls) between occurrence of the disease and an inherited tissue antigen DR4. The presence of an auto antibody, rheumatoid factor (which may be of the IgM or IgG class) in approximately 70 per cent of sufferers and the occasional identification of circulating immune complexes has led to the theory that the disease has an 'autoimmune' pathogenesis. The current prevailing view is that these features of autoimmunity are almost certainly epiphenomena triggered off by a virus or other infective agent yet to be isolated. The resultant synovial inflammatory response is characterized by hyperplasia, increased vascularity and a dense infiltration of lymphocytes and plasma cells, sometimes aggregated into follicles. This granulation tissue, commonly known as pannus, releases enzymes including collagenase, a neutral protease and lysosomal cathepsin D capable of destroying cartilage, ligament and bone. The process may result in destruction of the joint with subluxation and instability, ultimately leading to fibrous and, occasionally, bony ankylosis. A characteristic feature is the formation of the rheumatoid nodule over the ulnar aspect of the forearm (Fig. 6.1) and other points of pressure. Histologically, these are examples of a 'pallisading granuloma' with a central zone of connective tissue necrosis surrounded by radiating histiocytes and a peripheral zone with small round-cell infiltration.

The non-articular manifestations of the disease are explained on the basis of an arteritis occasioned by the deposition of immune complexes. This usually takes the form of a mild endarteritis, but occasionally a more serious necrotizing arteritis is seen. Secondary amyloid deposition may also occur in a small percentage (5–19 per cent) of patients with rheumatoid arthritis which, with the falling prevalence of chronic sepsis, constitutes the major cause of secondary amyloid today.

Epidemiology

Rheumatoid arthritis may affect all ethnic and geographical groups but it is certainly more common and more severe in temperate than in tropical climates. In the UK the prevalence of adult rheumatoid disease is in the order of 1 per cent with an annual incidence of new cases of approximately 0.02 per cent. The comparable figures for chronic juvenile arthritis are 0.06 and 0.006 per cent a year respectively. The adult disease is seen in between 3 and 8 per cent of first-degree relatives of patients with the disease. There is evidence to suggest that life expectancy is reduced, particularly in those patients in whom the disease starts before the age of 45 years and those with more severe disease at the time of first diagnosis. Women are affected three times more often than men.

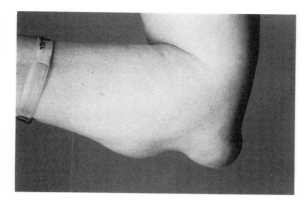

Figure 6.1 *Rheumatoid nodule over the olecranon.*

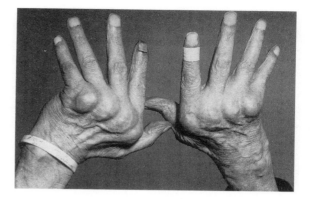

Figure 6.2 *Severe ulnar drift and subluxation of the meta-carpophalangeal joints in rheumatoid arthritis. Note the nail-fold lesions on both ring fingers and left index.*

Clinical features

The disease usually commences with articular symptoms, namely pain, swelling and stiffness in one or more synovial joints. The onset is usually insidious but may be acute, particularly in the aged. Classically, the joints favoured are the proximal interphalangeal joints, and metacarpophalangeal joints of the hands (the distal interphalangeal joints are usually not affected), the wrists, elbows, shoulders, hips, knees, ankles, tarsal joints and metatarsophalangeal joints. In the spine the cervical region is the only area commonly involved. Occasionally one encounters arthritis of the temporomandibular joints, the sternoclavicular joints, and even the cricoarytenoid joint may also be affected.

A typical feature of all inflammatory arthritides is the early-morning stiffness experienced by the patient on rising. The affected joints are tender, swollen and often warm and an effusion may be detected. In the hands the soft tissue swelling produces a spindling of the fingers with increased sweating of the skin and visible muscle atrophy. Involvement of weight-bearing joints causes difficulty in standing, walking and negotiating stairs. Occasionally, the disease commences in one solitary joint or two or three simultaenously, whence it may spread to become a widespread polyarthritis.

As the disease progresses unchecked, deformities commonly develop. These are seen as the characteristic ulnar deviation and eventually subluxation (Fig. 6.2) of the metacarpophalangeal joints, the 'swan-neck' or 'boutonniere' deformities of the fingers, fixed flexion deformities of the wrists, hip, knee and ankle, valgus deformity of the knee, hind foot and big toe and subluxation of the metatarsophalangeal joints. Subluxation of the cervical spine may occur in approximately 25 per cent of the rheumatoid arthritis patients, either at the atlantoaxial

joint (C1/C2) (Fig. 6.3) or lower down. This may cause compression of the cervical cord, but fortunately tetraparesis from this is surprisingly uncommon. Cricoarytenoid involvement when present may give rise to hoarseness, laryngeal discomfort or even stridor.

A common feature of knee involvement is the development of a *Baker's cyst*. This arises when synovial fluid under pressure is forced from the knee joint into a communicating bursa which enlarges to produce a palpable and often painful swelling in the popliteal fossa or upper calf. While often asymptomatic, a Baker's cyst may rupture its contents into the tissues of the calf (Fig. 6.4)

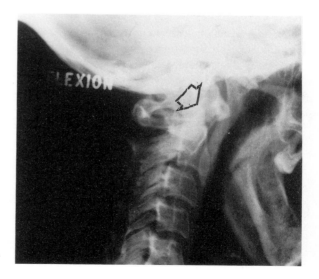

Figure 6.3 *Atlantoaxial subluxation in rheumatoid arthritis. Note the posterior movement of the ondontoid peg in relation to the anterior arch of the axis in this lateral cervical spine X-ray taken in flexion.*

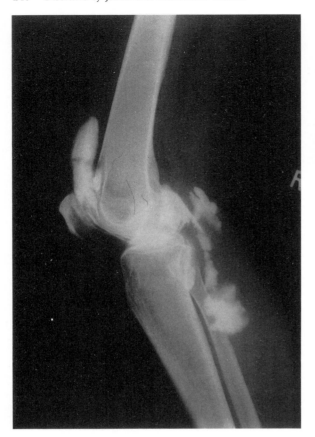

Figure 6.4   *Contrast arthrogram showing a popliteal cyst (Baker's cyst) that has ruptured its contents into the calf.*

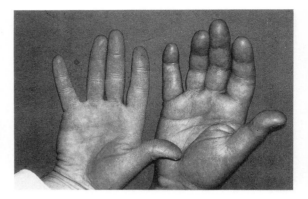

Figure 6.5   *Swelling of the fingers due to flexor tenosynovitis in rheumatoid arthritis on the right: normal hand on the left for comparison.*

Subcutaneous rheumatoid nodules, most commonly seen over the ulnar border of the forearm and olecranon (Fig. 6.1), over the sacrum, the fingers and in large tendons, notably the Achilles, occur in one third of patients. Although unsightly and occasionally liable to infection, these are painless and cause little trouble. Their presence, however, is of diagnostic and prognostic significance, in that it helps to establish the precise diagnosis and implies a liability to more destructive joint disease and vasculitis. Patients with nodules are invariably seropositive with a high titre of rheumatoid factor.

to produce a painful, oedematous lower extremity with a positive Homan's sign, thereby mimicking a deep-vein thrombosis. Rheumatoid synovitis also commonly affects tendon sheaths and bursae, producing soft tissue swelling seen over the dorsum of the hand, the flexor aspect of the fingers (Fig. 6.5), the olecranon, the deltoid region and the malleoli. Synovial swelling may give rise to compression of peripheral nerves (in particular, the median nerve at the wrist), causing carpal tunnel syndrome. Rheumatoid arthritis may be complicated by pyogenic joint infection, either blood-borne or introduced at the time of an intra-articular injection through faulty technique. Suspicion of this is aroused when a single joint appears to be more actively inflamed than the remainder.

Extra-articular manifestations. Weight loss, lethargy, anorexia, pyrexia and symptoms of anaemia may be seen in varying degrees of severity and exemplify the systemic nature of the condition. Reactive depression not infrequently results from the pain, disability and frustration that ensues.

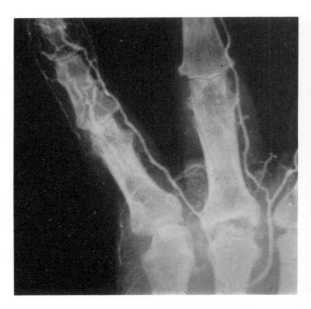

Figure 6.6   *Arteriogram showing occlusion of the ulnar digital arteries of the 4th and 5th digits due to rheumatoid digital vasculitis. Note the severe erosive changes at the metacarpophalangeal and proximal interphalangeal joints.*

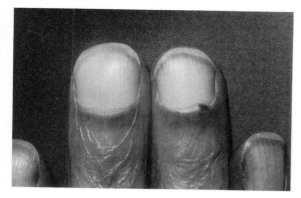

Figure 6.7 *Close-up view of a nail-fold lesion seen in the ring finger. This 'micro-infarct' is the result of digital arterial occulusion due to arteritis.*

Visceral involvement may occur as a result of nodule formation, arteritis or amyloid deposition, as seen in Table 6.1.

The term *'Felty's syndrome'* is used to describe the triad of rheumatoidarthritis, splenomegaly and neutropenia ($<2 \times 10^9$/l). Although it may occur early in the course of rheumatoid arthritis, the common presentation is in severe destructive disease of long duration. Infections are common but their incidence does not correlate with the degree of neutropenia. Other features include skin pigmentation, chronic leg ulceration and occasionally nodular degenerative hepatic hyperplasia.

Diagnosis

The erythrocyte sedimentation rate is raised whilst the disease remains active. Recently, it has been suggested that measurement of acute-phase proteins (e.g. C-reactive protein) may be a more reliable index of disease activity. A normochromic, normocytic anaemia is a feature of the active disease, but a superimposed iron deficiency pattern should raise the suspicion of gastrointestinal blood loss, possibly the result of drug treatment.

As previously mentioned, the antiglobulin rheumatoid factor is present in approximately 60 per cent of patients with established rheumatoid disease. The tests commonly in use include the Rose–Waaler test in which sheep red cells coated with gammaglobulin agglutinate in the presence of a patient's serum are used, or the latex fixation test in which similarly-coated polystyrene particles are used. The latter is more sensitive but is less specific, being positive in a variety of other conditions

Table 6.1 Extra-articular manifestations of rheumatoid arthritis

Lesion	Site	Clinical features	Complications
Rheumatoid nodule	Subcutaneous tendon		
	Pleura	Effusion	Bronchopleural fistula
	lung	Asymptomatic	
	Pericardium	Effusion	Tamponade; constriction
	Myocardium	Myocarditis	Cardiac failure
	Endocardium	Valvulitis	
	Sclera	Scleritis	Scleromalacia perforans
Endarteritis	Digital arteries (small-calibre $<15\,\mu$m diameter: Fig. 6.6)	Raynaud's phenomenon; sensory neuropathy	Digital 'nail-fold' infarcts (Fig. 6.7)
	Eye	Episceritis	
Necrotising arteritis	Large arteries	Necrotic skin ulcers; sensorimotor neuropathy	Rupture/occlusion of mesenteric or other visceral arteries (life-threatening)
Amyloid deposition	Bowel; liver; kidney; spleen	Proteinuria; nephrotic syndrome	Irreversible renal failure
'Rheumatoid lung'	Lung parenchyma	Fibrosing alveolitis; Caplan's syndrome (in mine-workers)	Respiratory failure
Sjogren's syndrome	Lachrymal and salivary glands	Dry eyes (kerato-conjunctivitis sicca); dry mouth (xerostomia)	Keratitis; corneal ulcer lymphoma
Felty's syndrome	Haemopoietic system; spleen	Splenomegaly; neutropenia; (thrombocytopenia 1/3)	Infections

including bacterial endocarditis, tuberculosis and cirrhosis. The titre of rheumatoid factor tends to parallel the activity of the disease, rising with exacerbations and falling with remissions. In some patients the test is negative at the onset, later becoming positive as the condition progresses. Subsequently, when the disease becomes totally inactive, it may return to a negative state. A high titre is associated with the possible development of nodules and arteritic manifestations. Rheumatoid factor is invariably negative in the so-called seronegative arthropathies (see below) but may be positive in SLE, scleroderma and Sjögren's syndrome. A positive antinuclear factor test and a positive LE cell preparation may be seen in up to 20 per cent of patients with rheumatoid arthritis, and this occasionally causes diagnostic confusion. Such patients, however, follow the pattern of rheumatoid disease rather than SLE. Plasma electrophoresis frequently reveals an increase in the alpha-2 and gammaglobulin fractions during the active phase of the disease.

Radiography is helpful in monitoring the progress of the disease. Early features include juxta-articular osteoporosis, later leading to erosion of the articular surface and loss of joint space. Finally, total destruction of a joint may be seen with or without bony ankylosis.

Synovial fluid analysis generally reveals a loss of the normal viscosity, and a cellular exudate (predominantly polymorphonuclear leucocytes) containing anything between 5 and 60 billion (10^9) per litre. Synovial biopsy, performed when the diagnosis is in doubt, may reveal the characteristic synovial reaction referred to above.

Treatment

Since the aetiological agent is unknown, it is not yet possible to eradicate the disease by chemotherapeutic means. Much, however, can be done to mitigate the effects of the disease. The principal aims of treatment are:

1 to control the synovitis, thereby relieving symptoms and reducing the likelihood of erosions. This is achieved by rest, anti-inflammatory drugs, disease-modifying drugs and, where single joints are involved, by intra-articular steroid injections, and where these fail by surgical or radio-isotope synovectomy.
2 to prevent deformities by splinting inflamed joints, which would otherwise develop serious flexion contractures of the hand, wrist, knee or ankle.
3 where irreversible damage has occurred to a joint, to improve joint and muscle function by physiotherapeutic means—exercises, appropriate surgical appli-

cances (splints, collar, caliper, corset etc.)—and surgical means where necessary (prosthetic joint replacement).

Acute exacerbations respond to a short period of joint immobilization by splinting in the case of a single joint, or by a short period (one week) of bed-rest in the presence of a polyarthritis. The latter must be carefully supervised since bed-rest carries certain risks (bed sores, deep-vein thrombosis, contractures, muscle atrophy and pneumonia) especially in the elderly or debilitated. Light resting splints are essential when joints of the hand, wrist, knee or ankle are involved if serious deformity is to be avoided. A cervical collar is helpful if the cervical spine is affected. Isometric exercises at this stage help to prevent muscle atrophy. The most actively inflamed joints may be aspirated and injected with corticosteroid (e.g. hydrocortisone acetate 25–50 mg, methylprednisolone acetate 20–40 mg or triamcinolone hexacetonide 5–20 mg), the dose depending on the size of the joint. The effect of these injections is often dramatic. The duration of benefit varies and is often prolonged, particularly with the longer-acting preparations.

Non-steroidal anti-inflammatory drugs

These drugs (NSAIDs) are also administered at this stage, and will continue to be required for as long as the synovitis remains active—in most cases over a period of several years or even decades. It is essential, therefore, to choose the best drug for each individual patient, which is a process of trial and error. Many NSAIDs are currently available.

1 Aspirin

Potent, and still widely used, this drug is liable to cause tinnitus, deafness, and overt or occult gastrointestinal bleeding in therapeutic doses. These side-effects and the large numbers of tablets required reduces its acceptability and thereby patient compliance. Alternative formulations including enteric-coated and microencapsulated forms, aloxiprin, choline magnesium trisalicylate, diflunisal, salsalate, and benorylate (an ester of aspirin with paracetamol) have proved more acceptable than soluble aspirin.

2 Indomethacin

This, too, is potent and liable to cause headache and dizziness in many patients. Long-term use may give rise to prepyloric gastric ulceration. The dose is 25–50 mg three times daily. A sustained-release oral preparation (75 mg) and a suppository (100 mg) is available for night use and helps to control morning stiffness. Sulindac is a chemically related preparation which has fewer side-effects.

3 Phenylbutazone

This is pyrazole, which may cause fluid retention, gastric ulceration and bone-marrow depression, particularly with long-term use. It is, therefore, suitable only for short-term use for acute exacerbations. In the UK this drug is only available for hospital-treated patients with ankylosing spondylitis. The chemically related preparation aza-propazone is less toxic.

4 Propionic acid derivatives

These are ibuprofen (400–600 mg t.d.s.), naproxen (250 mg in the morning, 500 mg at night), ketoprofen (50 mg t.d.s.), fenoprofen (300–600 mg t.d.s.), flurbiprofen (50 mg q.d.s.) and fenbufen (600–900 mg once daily).

5 Aryl-acetic acid derivatives

These are diclofenac and tiaprofenic acid.

6 Miscellaneous

These are tolmetin, a pyrole derivative, piroxicam (20 mg once daily), an oxicam derivative, and etodolac.

By and large, all the drugs listed in groups 4–6 have been shown in clinical trials to be comparable in terms of efficacy with the older drugs (groups 1–3). They are undoubtedly better tolerated, although rashes occur. Gastric intolerance is common and occasionally gastric haemorrhage may be seen. They should be used with extreme caution in the elderly, patients suffering from known peptic ulceration and those on anticoagulants, and they should all be avoided in pregnancy. All the newer preparations are more expensive than the earlier ones. With few exceptions their mode of action is believed to be inhibition of prostaglandin synthetase. Their use is applicable in other forms of inflammatory joint disease, including acute gout. They may also be helpful in degenerative joint disease and soft tissue lesions when symptoms merit their use. NSAIDs should be avoided in the presence of seriously impaired renal function.

Disease-modifying agents in rheumatoid disease

These drugs (DMARDs) are introduced as second-line drugs where NSAIDs have failed to control joint inflammation and/or where erosions have developed on X-ray. They include gold salts, d-penicillamine, sulpha-salazine, chloroquine, immunosuppressive and immuno-potentiating drugs, and corticosteroids.

1 Gold

Injections of sodium aurothiomalate are given by weekly intramuscular injections of 50 mg (after a test dose of 10 mg) until a total of 1 g has been given. If by the end of that time a favourable response is seen, treatment is continued indefinitely on a monthly basis, provided that side-effects are not forthcoming. Skin reactions are common and may be severe. Temporary suspension of the injections is recommended. Many patients, however, are subsequently able to resume the course. Proteinuria should be looked for at each attendance and injections are not given if it is present. Gold nephropathy is a rare complication which may lead to nephrotic syndrome. Gold should be withdrawn, but even so, it may take a year before the kidney recovers. Of greatest importance is the liability to bone-marrow depression which may lead to serious (even fatal) aplastic anaemia. Fortunately, this is rare but thrombocytopenia alone is more common. These haematological complications can only be prevented by careful and regular monitoring of blood and platelet counts, preferably before each injection. With these precautions gold salts have proved themselves over a half century to be a useful and effective means of suppressing rheumatoid synovitis. Gold-induced remissions are accompanied by an improvement in systemic features. Its mode of action is still uncertain.

2 D-penicillamine

This drug has been introduced for the treatment of rheumatoid arthritis in the past two decades and has been shown in trials to be equivalent to gold in its efficacy, though similar and serious side-effects do occur. These include rashes, proteinuria (with nephrotic syndrome), loss of taste (which is transient), abdominal symptoms and thrombocytopenia (rarely aplastic anaemia). Like gold its effect does not become apparent until 3–6 months after starting treatment. It has the advantage of being administered orally.

3 Sulphasalazine

Thus drug, widely used in the treatment of inflammatory bowel disease, was originally introduced 40 years ago for the treatment of rheumatoid arthritis. However, it fell from favour and only recently with the successful conclusion of controlled comparative studies has its use been re-established. It is given orally in a dose of 0.5 g per day rising by monthly increments of 0.5 g to a maintenance dose of between 2 and 3 g per day. Although generally well-tolerated, it can cause rashes, methaemo-globinaemia and occasionally bone-marrow depression. It is degraded in the intestine to its two components 5-aminosalicyclic acid and sulphapyridine. Whereas the former is not absorbed and is the active ingredient for colitis, it has been shown that the sulphapyridine which is absorbed is responsible for the improvement in RA. It is also responsible for most of the adverse effects.

4 Chloroquine

This antimalarial drug was introduced in the 1950s for

rheumatoid arthritis. It has somewhat fallen out of favour owing to its propensity for causing retinal damage. It should only be used if facilities are available for an ophthalmological examination at six-monthly intervals.

5 Immunosuppressive drugs

These include azathioprine, methotrexate, chlorambucil and cyclophosphamide and are mainly used to treat the serious arteritic complications. This is because of their tendency to serious side-effects, including bone-marrow depression.

6 Corticosteroids

Oral corticosteroids are now rarely used in the treatment of rheumatoid arthritis owing to the cumulative side-effects: osteoporosis, skin atrophy, peptic ulceration, steroid myopathy, steroid cataracts and suppression of the hypophyseal–pituitary–adrenal axis. If they are to be used at all, it should be a very minimal dose (e.g. 5–7.5 mg of prednisolone daily). It has been shown that alternate-day therapy is less harmful, particularly in children where suppression of growth is an additional hazard. Pulse steroid IV 1 g prednisolone is advocated for the treatment of severe RA with arteritis.

Synovectomy

Persistent refractory inflammation in a single joint may be treated by synovectomy—removal of the synovial membrane—by either medical or surgical means. In either case, relief of pain and stiffness and restoration of movement is achieved, although relapse may occur subsequently. Medical synovectomy is obtained by the intra-articular injection of a radio-isotope (e.g. Yttrium 90) in colloidal form. The isotope is taken up by the synovial cells and the membrane is thereby ablated by the ionizing radiation (beta particles). This form of treatment is reserved for patients over the age of 45, because of the (largely theoretical) risk of oncogenesis.

Surgical synovectomy is the surgical excision of the synovial membrane as far as this is possible, and it is most widely used in the knee and small finger joints. Postoperative stiffness of the joint is a hazard, which usually responds to manipulation under anaesthetic and vigorous physiotherapy.

Other surgical measures

Total joint destruction may be treated either by arthrodesis (still widely practised in the wrist, big toe and thumb joints), or total joint replacement in those joints where a satisfactory prosthesis is available. This is most successful in the hip joint where the Charnley type of low-friction arthoplasty (metal on plastic) is the most widely used. Many total knee protheses are now available and prostheses are available for the shoulder, elbow, ankle, and the MCP and PIP joints of the hands. In other joints attempts at joint replacement have been less successful. The main problems of joint replacement are inadequate facilities for carrying out all the operations that need to be undertaken, and the complications of injection and/or loosening of the prosthesis which may require it to be removed. Subluxation of the cervical spine which causes cord compression requires cervical fusion.

Rehabilitation

Total management of the patient with rheumatoid arthritis requires a team approach in which specialist medical and nursing skills are supplemented by those of the trained physiotherapist, occupational therapist and medical social worker. Careful assessment of the patient's ability to cope with daily living, together with monitoring of progress, enables realistic goals to be set for the patient to return to as full and as active a life as possible. Skills lost as a result of the ravages of the disease may be restored partly by retraining and partly by adapting the environment to the needs of the handicapped patient. Both home and work environments need to be considered, and it is essential that the patient, his family and employer be put into the picture in order to achieve an optimal result.

The seronegative spondarthritides

This group of chronic arthritic conditions is characterized by the absence of rheumatoid factor in the serum, the absence of nodules, a largely asymmetrical distribution of peripheral joint involvement, and a tendency towards bilateral sacroiliitis progressing, in some cases, to a picture of ankylosing spondylitis. The presence of spinal disease is commonly associated with the tissue antigen HLA B27. Despite this important hereditary factor the precise aetiological agent responsible for these diseases is as yet unknown.

Ankylosing spondylitis
Aetiology and pathology

This disease predominantly affects young men and has a prevalence of approximately 1 per 1000 of the population. Recent epidemiological studies suggest that it

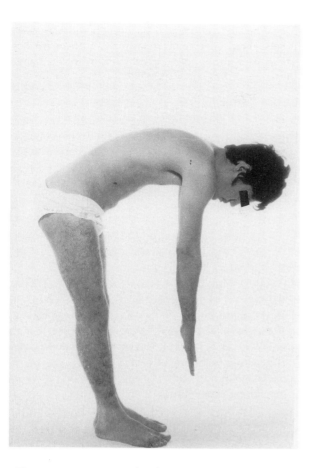

Figure 6.8 *Loss of spinal mobility in ankylosing spondylitis.*

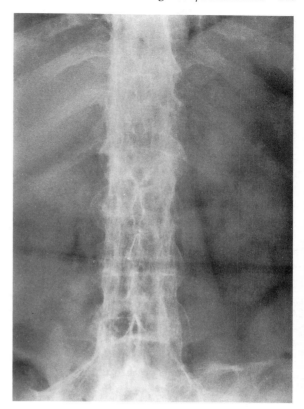

Figure 6.9 *The 'bamboo spine' of ankylosing spondylitis.*

may be considerably more common than this. This condition has a predilection for synovial joints of the vertebral column commencing in the sacroiliac joints and spreading cranially. Larger peripheral joints may also be affected. In conclusion HLA B27 is present in 90–95 per cent of cases compared with 5–10 per cent in the normal population. Recent evidence suggests that *Klebsiella pneumoniae* may be an important pathogen in this disease, but this is as yet unconfirmed. Although the synovial histopathological reaction is similar to that seen in rheumatoid arthritis, the tendency is for bony ankylosis to occur. Syndesmophytes or bony bridges form between adjacent vertebrae and ultimately the facet joints, intervertebral discs and ligaments ossify, giving rise to the classical radiological appearance of the 'bamboo spine.'

Clinical features

Persistent low back pain with morning stiffness in the young adult male is the classical presentation. Impercept-

ible progressive loss of spinal movement occurs, with flattening of the lumbar spine, dorsal kyphosis and a compensatory cervical hyperlordosis (Fig. 6.8). Loss of chest expansion results from costovertebral joint involvement. As the spinal deformity develops the patient tends to adopt a hyperextension of the hips in order to maintain his centre of gravity. Symptoms may be so mild that the condition remains undiagnosed until advanced or it may be ascribed in error to intervertebral disc disease or psychogenic backache. On occasion the pain may be severe, particularly at night, waking the patient in the early hours. Pain and limitation of movement in the hip joints and shoulder and/or effusions in the knees indicate peripheral joint involvement which adds to the disability imposed by an increasingly rigid spine. Enthesopathies (tender lesions at the site of tendinous insertions, for example, plantar fasciitis) are common, and alternating sciatic pain may occur as well as discomfort around the thoracic cage.

A tendency to recurrent, acute iritis occurs in 20 per cent of cases. A normochromic normocytic anaemia is common during active phases of the disease, which may be aggravated by gastrointestinal blood loss caused by

NSAIDs. Amyloid deposition (see above) is said to occur in 6 per cent of patients coming to necropsy. Rarely, cardiac involvement with conduction defects (e.g. complete heart block) and/or aortic regurgitation occur from aortitis. A bilateral upper lobe fibrosis of the lungs has been reported in this condition.

Diagnosis

The diagnosis is based on the clinical history and examination and is confirmed by the radiological appearance of the spine, notably the sacroiliac joints (blurring of the joint margins, sclerosis, erosion and ultimately ankylosis) and the vertebral bodies (formation of syndesmophytes, squaring of the vertebrae and ultimately the appearance of the 'bamboo spine' (Fig. 6.9)). The sedimentation rate and C-reactive protein are raised while the disease remains active.

A quantitative radionuclide scintiscan is sometimes helpful in detecting sacroiliitis before the radiological changes have become established. Because ankylosing spondylitis can occur in subjects who do not carry the tissue antigen HLA B27, performing this test is of no value in establishing a diagnosis of AS. It is sometimes useful in excluding it.

Treatment

The aim is to relieve pain and stiffness by the application of non-steroidal anti-inflammatory drugs, which permit the patient to take part in vigorous physiotherapy necessary to restore and maintain the spinal mobility and to prevent flexion deformity of the spine. The patient is encouraged to lie prone as much as possible and to practise mobilizing exercises daily for the rest of his life.

Evidence to date suggests that the DMARDs (see page 243) are ineffective, corticosteroids are contraindicated owing to the risk of osteoporosis, and deep X-ray therapy (formerly used widely to relieve pain and stiffness) is now no longer used owing to the increased risk of leukaemia. Total hip replacement is indicated in the presence of advanced hip-joint destruction, and spinal osteotomy is occasionally used in the presence of severe spinal deformity. Acute iritis is treated along conventional lines by local corticosteroid drops and mydriatics.

Psoriatic arthritis

Aetiology

Arthritis occurs some six to ten times more frequently in psoriatic patients than in controls. Psoriatic arthritis has been estimated to occur in 0.1 per cent of the population. It is slightly more common in males than in females. There is a strong genetic component with a raised frequency of B27, Cw6 and DR7.

Clinical features

Arthritis associated with psoriasis may take one of the following forms:

1 A widespread polyarthritis typically involving the distal interphalangeal joints (Fig. 6.10), the interphalangeal joint of the thumb and great toe as well as larger joints.
2 A severe mutilating arthritis affecting the hands, causing widespread osteolysis as well as total destruction of the small finger joints.
3 A polyarthritis which, from the point of view of distribution, is indistinguishable from that seen in rheumatoid arthritis. This is the most common variety. It does, however, pursue a more benign course, though erosions do occur. Rheumatoid nodules and rheumatoid factor are, of course, absent.
4 Sacroiliitis progressing in many cases to a picture of ankylosing spondylitis.

Treatment

The general principles are similar to those adopted for rheumatoid arthritis. Because of the more benign nature of the condition, drug treatment is usually limited to the NSAIDs. In more severe cases gold injections and methotrexate may be effective, but d-pencillamine is ineffective and oral corticosteroids are rarely indicated.

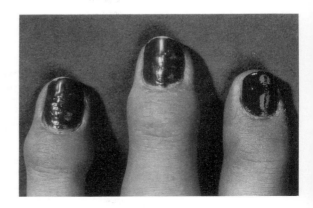

Figure 6.10 *Distal interphalangeal joint involvement in psoriatic arthropathy. Note the characteristic pitting of the nails.*

Reactive arthritis

Aetiology

This term denotes the development of arthritis in a patient suffering from an infective process elsewhere in the body (usually in the gastrointestinal or genital tracts), but without evidence of infection in the joint itself. It occurs almost exclusively in patients showing the tissue antigen HLA B27 who develop enteric infection with *Salmonella*, *Shigella*, *Yersinia* or *Campylobacter* organisms. It may also occur as sexually acquired reactive arthritis (SARA), and there is evidence to suggest that the offending organism here may be *Chlamydia trachomatis*, though this remains to be confirmed.

Reiter's syndrome

This was originally described as a triad of urethritis, conjunctivitis and arthritis, but it often presents additional features including balanitis circinata or sicca, keratoderma blennorrhagica, uveitis, aortitis, sacroiliitis and ankylosing spondylitis. It has long been known that Reiter's syndrome may complicate sexually acquired non-specific urethritis or dysentery, but living micro-organisms have never been isolated from the affected joints. For this reason Reiter's syndrome is now classified as a form of reactive arthritis.

Acute rheumatic fever can be considered as a form of reactive arthritis and is considered on page 39.

Other arthritides associated with bowel disease

An inflammatory polyarthritis may occur in patients suffering from ulcerative colitis (see page 163), Crohn's disease (page 161) and Whipple's disease (page 159). This tends to be a recurrent, acute or persistent affection of large, predominantly lower, limb joints. By and large, the activity of the arthritis mirrors that of the underlying intestinal disease. In addition some 18 per cent of patients suffering from inflammatory bowel disease will develop sacroiliitis, approximately one half of whom proceed to the full picture of ankylosing spondylitis. In these circumstances the activity and progression of the spinal disease appears to bear no temporal relationship to the activity of the underlying bowel condition.

Arthritis is also a feature in about 15 per cent of patients suffering from the multi-system disease that follows intestinal bypass surgery used as a treatment for obesity. The cause of the arthritis is believed to be due to immune complex deposition. Bacterial antigens of intestinal origin have been implicated.

Behçet's syndrome

A subacute or chronic, usually non-destructive, arthritis with a predilection for knee joint involvement, but with occasional involvement of the axial skeleton, is seen in association with buccal and genital ulceration, erythema nodosum, meningoencephalitis and uveitis in Behçet's syndrome. Skin, mucosal and joint symptoms respond to high-dose corticosteroids, uveitis to chlorambucil.

Inflammatory disorders of connective tissue

The group of diseases included under this heading (formerly referred to as the collagen diseases) include systemic lupus erythematosus (SLE), polyarteritis nodosa, dermatomyositis and polymyositis, and scleroderma (systemic sclerosis). The members of this group have a number of features in common, namely, abnormal immunological reactivity, multi-system involvement, a (variable) therapeutic response to corticosteroids, and a usually unremittent course. Overlap syndromes do occur.

Systemic lupus erythematosus (SLE)

(see also page 273).

Aetiology

This is a multi-system disease with protean manifestations. It is nine times more common in women than in men, with an onset during the child-bearing years, though occasional onset during childhood or advanced age occurs. It appears to be much more common in negroes than caucasians and a familial tendency is seen. The aetiology is unknown.

Pathology

Widespread fibrinoid deposition (containing gamma-globulin and fibrin, together with complement) is seen throughout the body, notably in relation to small arterioles and capillaries, in connective tissue and in serous membranes. These changes are almost certainly due to the deposition of immune complexes which, particularly in the kidney, is an important pathogenic mechanism. A wide variety of humoral antibodies is encountered in the serum. These include antinuclear antibodies directed against a variety of nuclear constituents, native double- and single-stranded DNA, DNA-histone (detected in the SLE cell preparation), double-stranded nuclear ribonucleoprotein (RNP), two other RNP antigens, SS-A (previously called Ro) and SS-B (previously called La) and Sm antigen. In addition, both IgG and IgM rheumatoid factors and a biological false-positive test for syphilis (BFP) are found in approximately one-third of patients. Serum complement levels (C3, C4 and total haemolytic complement) are lowered, particularly in the presence of renal involvement, and cryoglobulins and antibodies directed against erythrocytes (detected by the Coombs test), leucocytes, lymphocytes and platelets are widely seen. Circulating anticoagulants are found in up to 10 per cent of patients. In addition, there is also evidence of impaired cellular immunity in SLE resulting from an impairment of suppressor T-lymphocyte activity. A possible viral aetiology responsible for the immunological abnormalities is likely, but as yet no viral agent has been identified. An SLE-like illness occurs in some patients treated with hydralazine, penicillamine, procainamide, practolol, isoniazid and anticonvulsant drugs. In patients so afflicted renal involvement is absent and complete recovery is seen on withdrawal of the offending drug.

Clinical features

(See Table 6.2).

1 General
Fever, malaise, anorexia and weight loss are common.

Table 6.2 System involvement in SLE (based on four large series totalling 365 patients)

	Per cent
Facial erythema ('butterfly rash')	40–65
Discoid lupus	20–30
Raynaud's phenomenon	20–44
Alopecia	40–70
Photosensitivity	17–41
Oral or nasopharyngeal ulceration	15–36
Arthritis without deformity	86–100
LE cells	48–92
Chronic biological false-positive test for syphilis	8–26
Proteinuria > 3.5 g/day	16–25
Cellular casts	16–48
Pleurisy and/or pericarditis	30–60
Psychosis and/or convulsions	16–20
Haemolytic anaemia	14–16
Leucopenia < 4.0×10^9 per litre	40–54
Thrombocytopenia < 100×10^9 per litre	11–14

2 Skin
The classical rash of SLE is the erythema seen typically in the butterfly region of the cheeks and bridge of the nose but also areas exposed to ultraviolet light to which the skin in this condition is particularly sensitive. Other skin lesions include discoid lupus, urticaria, periungual erythema and cutaneous vasculitis. Alopecia is a frequent feature limited to SLE within this group of conditions.

3 Joints
A symmetrical peripheral polyarthritis affecting predominantly small finger joints and reminiscent of rheumatoid arthritis is a common finding. Ulnar deviation of the fingers may occur, but erosions are characteristically absent. Subcutaneous nodules are uncommon.

4 Tenosynovitis
This may occur in the hands, and aseptic necrosis of the femoral head (osteonecrosis) is a common finding even in the absence of corticosteroid treatment.

5 Respiratory system
Pleurisy with effusion is common, and parenchymal pulmonary involvement (pneumonitis) may be seen. Diffuse pulmonary fibrosis is less common.

6 Cardiovascular system
Raynaud's phenomenon may be a presenting symptom. Pericarditis with effusion, myocarditis and verrucose (*Libman–Sacks*) endocarditis may all occur. Cardiac failure, arrhythmias and conduction defects.

7 Kidney
Renal involvement occurs in most patients, although in only half is it clinically significant. Four pathological types of lupus nephritis have been defined: focal proliferative (mild), diffuse proliferative (severe), membranous, and mesangial (minimal). Presentation is with proteinuria which may be heavy and lead to nephrotic syndrome and be associated with hypertension and renal failure. Clues to the prognosis may be gleaned from renal biopsy, examined by immunofluorescence, light and electron microscopy.

8 Haemopoietic and reticuloendothelial systems
Anaemia (usually normocytic but in 10 per cent of patients haemolytic), neutropenia and thrombocytopenia are common events and may be severe. Hepatosplenomegaly and lymphadenopathy are commonly seen. Thrombotic complications occur in association with the presence of anti-cardiolipin antibodies.

9 Gastrointestinal tract
Sjögren's syndrome may be present, and abdominal pain and diarrhoea occasionally occur owing to intestinal arteritis, pancreatitis or peritonism. Significant involvement of the liver does not occur, and the formerly styled 'lupoid hepatitis', thought to be a feature of SLE, is now

termed 'chronic active hepatitis' and considered to be a separate entity.

10 Central nervous system

Brain involvement is now known to be one of the most common features, presenting as a neuropsychiatric disorder (e.g. depressive state, convulsions, hemiplegia, cranial and peripheral nerve lesions, cerebellar disorder or aseptic meningitis). Transverse myelitis may also occur. Conventional neurological investigations (angiography, brain and CT scanning) are generally unhelpful. EEG may show a non-specific diffuse abnormality. By contrast, oxygen scanning appears to be a promising marker, although not widely available.

11 Eye

Retinal haemorrhages and exudates are common but major ocular disturbances are rare.

12 Pregnancy

Post-partum exacerbations are not uncommon in SLE. Spontaneous abortions are common. Congenital heart-block is seen in infants born of mothers with SLE, especially those carrying serum anti-Ro (SS-A) antibodies.

Diagnosis

This is based on the above-mentioned clinical features. The LE cell preparation has been largely replaced by the antinuclear antibody immunofluorescent test, which is positive in virtually all cases, though it is not specific for the disease (see above). The DNA binding test for double-stranded (native) DNA is a more specific indicator of SLE, though it may be negative during inactive phases of the disease. It may therefore be used as an index of disease activity, and in this context is a more reliable pointer than the sedimentation rate which is often markedly elevated in this condition.

Prognosis

There has been a remarkable improvement in the prognosis of this disease in recent years, due in part to the wider (and earlier) recognition of this condition, and in part to the greater restraint in the uses of corticosteroids for treatment. The five-year survival has virtually doubled in the last 25 years and is now over 90 per cent. Severe renal and neurological complications carry the poorest prognosis.

Treatment

NSAIDs are valuable in the treatment of the articular complaints, while antimalarials are also capable of sup-pressing the disease, particularly in those patients with skin and joint involvement. Severe manifestations are treated by oral corticosteroids, sometimes supplemented by immunosuppressive drugs (e.g. azathioprine or cyclo-phosphamide). These drugs undoubtedly carry a morbidity and mortality in their own right and should be used with extreme caution and prudence. Recent evidence suggests that low-dose prednisolone (7.5 mg daily) is a more satisfactory treatment than high-dose (over 30 mg daily) even for mild renal and brain involve-ment. The use of large-dose pulse steroid treatment (e.g. 1 g prednisolone IV) is currently being evaluated.

Polyarteritis nodosa (PAN) (see page 274)

This disorder is characterized by a necrotizing arteritis of small and medium-sized vessels, thought to be due to the deposition of as yet unidentified immune complexes. Hepatitis-associated antigen has been found in the serum and in the lesions of patients with polyarteritis, which suggests that serum hepatitis virus may be participating in the pathogenesis. The arteritic lesions are widely dis-seminated through the body and may lead to aneurysm formation, rupture and haemorrhage, thrombosis, and ultimately recanalization. A rare variant of PAN is Wegener's granulomatosis, a locally destructive granuloma affecting the nasal passages and upper and lower respiratory tract associated with glomeruloneph-ritis.

Clinical features

Males predominate with an incidence rising with age. Features include fever, weight loss, hypertension, tachy-cardia, gangrene on the extremities, asthma, pneumonitis, an acute abdomen (due to mesenteric arteritis), proteinu-ria and renal failure, arthralgia and myalgia, cutaneous vasculitis and peripheral neuropathy of the mononeuritis multiplex type. In addition, focal brain and spinal-cord involvement and ocular vascular accidents complete the truly protein nature of the disease.

Diagnosis

There are no specific laboratory tests for PAN. Serologi-cal tests such as the ANA and rheumatoid factor are usually negative. Confirmation is usually obtained his-tologically by muscle, skin, kidney or nerve biopsy. Hepatic or renal arteriography may reveal multiple small neurysms which are said to be diagnostic of this condition (Fig. 6.11).

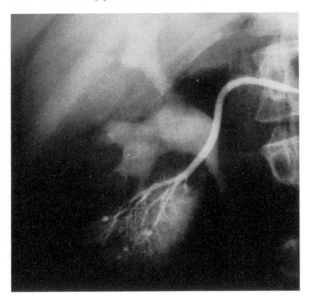

Figure 6.11   *Renal arteriogram in a patient suffering from polyarteritis nodosa, showing the presence of multiple aneurysms.*

Prognosis

This depends on the distribution of organ involvement. The five-year survival rate is 50–60 per cent with steroid treatment, compared with less than 15 per cent in untreated cases.

Treatment

High-dose corticosteroids (prednisolone 40–50 mg daily) are generally recommended initially with a view to slowly reducing and eventually withdrawing the drug in the light of the subsequent progress. Use of the immunosuppressive drugs (e.g. cyclophosphamide or azathioprine 2 mg/kg/day) may be helpful as steroid-sparing agents.

Giant cell (temporal) arteritis

Pathology and aetiology

This is a granulomatous form of arteritis affecting predominantly the branches of the external carotid artery, notably the temporal and facial arteries, and certain branches, notably the ophthalmic, of the internal carotid artery. Only occasionally are arteries emanating from the aorta (e.g. coronary arteries) involved. A possible immunological mechnism has been suggested by the finding of increased cellular immune responses by lymphocytes from patients with this condition to constituents of the arterial wall. The condition is predominantly seen in middle and old age. No consistent relationship has been observed with HLA A, B or C antigens, although an association with DR4 has been recorded.

Clinical features

The common presentation is with pain in the head and face due to ischaemia, and intermittent claudication of the muscles of mastication has been reported. The temporal arteries are characteristically thickened, tender and pulseless and the overlying scalp may be reddened and occasionally frankly gangrenous. Other modes of presentation include sudden visual failure owing to ophthalmic artery thrombosis, polymyalgia rheumatica (see page 259), pyrexia of unknown origin, anaemia, or high ESR for no obvious reason.

Diagnosis

The sedimentation rate is invariably elevated, often markedly so. Since the arteritis may be distributed patchily, the temporal arteries may be normal on palpation, and where doubt exists it is prudent to perform a temporal artery biopsy. The characteristic features are thickening of the media with infiltration by inflammatory cells, including giant cells, and intimal proliferation leading to gross narrowing of the lumen. The condition should be suspected in particular in elderly patients suffering from (often vague) headaches or rheumatic symptoms in the presence of a raised ESR.

Treatment

Oral corticosteroid treatment is indicated as soon as the diagnosis is made in order to prevent blindness, since this is irreversible. Prednisolone (40–60 mg a day) may be required to bring the condition under control, the dose being tapered in response to the fall in the sedimentation rate. Long-term surveillance is essential if relapse is to be avoided. The condition may remain active for months or years.

Other forms of necrotizing arteritis

Rheumatoid vasculitis

See page 241. Manifestations of necrotizing arteritis indistinguishable from those seen in polyarteritis nodosa are encountered in rheumatoid disease which enters a 'polyarteritic' or 'malignant' phase.

Hypersensitivity angiitis

In this group of conditions, small blood vessels are infiltrated with polymorphonuclear leucocytes with destruction of the vessel wall. Such changes are seen in Henoch–Schönlein purpura, cryoglobulinaemia, serum sickness, hypocomplementemic vasculitis as well as vasculitis seen in association with Sjögren's syndrome, hypergamma-globulinaemic purpura, chronic active hepatitis, ulcerative colitis and primary biliary cirrhosis.

Churg–Strauss vasculitis

The association of vasculitis with asthma, eosinophilia and extravascular granulomas is known as Churg–Strauss vasculitis. It is a rare syndrome, more common in males. The cause is unknown. Small granulomas with eosinophilic centres are seen in the small arteries and veins. Vasculitis and granulomas are seen similarly through the viscera including liver, spleen, kidney, heart and lymph nodes. The treatment of choice is high-dose corticosteroids.

Lymphomatoid granulomatosis

This is a rare disease of unknown aetiology. There is widespread evidence of vasculitic infiltration about the major viscera, and a high proportion progress to malignant lymphoma.

Takayasu's disease

In this condition (otherwise known as 'pulseless disease'), which affects mainly children and young women, the aorta and branches are involved in an arteritic process which leads to thickening of the arterial wall and progresses to occlusion. The media is infiltrated with lymphocytes and plasma cells and the intima is proliferated. It is common in Japanese subjects who show an association with HLA Bw 52, implying an important hereditary component. In its early stages the disease may be reversed by treatment with corticosteroids.

Erythema nodosum

This term is given to the presence of raised, red, tender lumps on the surfaces of the lower legs which are thought to represent a hypersensitivity reaction to a variety of agents, including infection (e.g. tuberculosis, streptococ-

cus, yersinia, leptospirosis, psittacosis, certain mycotic infections), drugs (e.g. halides, oral contraceptives and sulphonamides) and unknown agents (e.g. sarcoidosis, ulcerative colitis and Crohn's disease). There is a self-limiting symmetrical arthritis notably affecting the knees and ankles. Treatment is with NSAIDs. Occasional courses of corticosteroids may be required. Essentially the management is that of the underlying condition.

Subacute non-migratory panniculitis

This is a variant of erythema nodosum and occurs primarily in caucasian females between the ages of 50 and 60. Individual lesions spread to considerable size and show central clearing. The aetiology is unknown and the prognosis is excellent. Treatment is symptomatic.

Scleroderma (systemic sclerosis, SS)

This uncommon condition is characterized by an excessive deposition of collagen in the dermis and in the viscera (notably the gastrointestinal tract), together with a small-vessel arteritis involving, in particular, the extremities.

Aetiology

The cause is unknown, but it is relatively more common among miners. The finding of antinuclear antibodies and other features of altered immunity in approximately 50 per cent of patients suggests a possible immunological pathogenetic mechanism.

Clinical features

It is three times more common in women than in men. The onset is often insidious and Raynaud's phenomenon may antedate other symptoms by several years. Pain and stiffness in the small joints and tendon sheaths is a common early symptom. Gradually the skin of the distal extremities becomes thickened, tethered, and rigid, inhibiting movement. This process gradually extends proximally and may envelop the whole body. Puckering of the mouth leads to a characteristic appearance. Calcinotic nodules appear over the fingertips and pressure areas. Telangiectasia are seen on the skin of the extremities, face and on the tongue (Fig. 6.12). Joint and tendon-sheath involvement causes pain and additional stiffness and flexion deformities of the fingers. A palpable crepitus is a feature of tenosynovitis of the wrist. Tapering of the fingers is due to osteolysis occasioned by

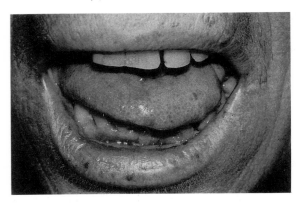

Figure 6.12 *Puckering of the mouth in a patient suffering from systemic sclerosis. Note the presence of telangiectasia on the tongue and lips.*

ischaemia. Muscle involvement also commonly occurs, although this may be mild.

Gastrointestinal involvement occurs in 70 per cent of patients. The most common manifestation is in the oesophagus, where there is loss of peristalsis, acid reflux and stricture formation, resulting in dysphagia, which may be severe. Small-bowel involvement gives rise to malabsorption, which may be aggravated by bacterial overgrowth. A rare complication is the presence of collections of gas in the intestinal wall (pneumatosis intestinalis). Coexistent primary biliary cirrhosis or chronic active hepatitis may be seen. Colonic involvement is common but usually asymptomatic. Occasionally distension or perforation may occur.

Pulmonary fibrosis is common, although it may be asymptomatic in the initial stages. In the heart, pericarditis and myocardial fibrosis may be present. A variety of ECG changes is seen, including arrhythmias and heart block. Frank renal involvement tends to lead to a rapidly progressive spiral of hypertension and renal failure. Central nervous system involvement does not occur but trigeminal neuropathy has been described. Sjögren's syndrome may occur in association with scleroderma.

Diagnosis

The ESR is raised in two-thirds of patients, while one-third give a positive test for rheumatoid factor. Antinuclear antibody is present in over 50 per cent. Characteristic changes in the skin biopsy include increased dermal collagen, a thinning of the epidermis and a loss of the normal appendages.

Prognosis

In the absence of major organ involvement, scleroderma may pursue a relatively benign though usually progress-ive course. Over 70 per cent survive for five years. In the presence of lung but no heart or kidney involvement, or heart but no kidney involvement, the corresponding figures are 50 and 30 per cent. Renal involvement usually imposes a survival of less than one year. 'Diffuse scleroderma' (i.e. widespread skin involvement including the trunk) is usually associated with major organ involvement and a poorer prognosis, whereas the CREST syndrome (calcinosis, Raynaud's, oesophageal, sclerodactyly and telangiectasia) carries a more favourable outlook. It has recently been shown that anticentromere antibodies are common in this subgroup.

Treatment

There is no really effective treatment for this disorder. D-penicillamine has been used and may be helpful with regard to the skin condition if instituted early.

Corticosteroids are of little benefit except in relieving the rheumatic symptoms, which are probably better treated by NSAIDs. Raynaud's phenomenon and digital ischaemia have been treated by intra-arterial reserpine and a variety of other vasoactive drugs (e.g. nifedipine) but with limited success. The use of infusions of commercially available prostacyclin is currently under investigation. Cervical sympathectomy, plasmaphoresis and hyperbaric oxygen give only limited and transient relief. Cardiac, pulmonary, renal and gastrointestinal symptoms are treated on their own merits along conventional lines.

Variants of scleroderma

Eosinophilic fasciitis. In this condition, which affects mainly young males, thickening of the skin occurs in the extremities in the absence of Raynaud's phenomenon. Visceral abnormality does not occur, but eosinophilia (up to 50 per cent of granulocytes) is seen with hypergammaglobulinaemia and elevated immunoglobulin levels. Biopsy of the skin shows a mononuclear infiltration, often with eosinophils in evidence, which affects the deep fascia which is densely fibrosed.

Scleredema. This is a rare self-limiting condition which follows bacterial infection. It, too, is not associated with Raynaud's phenomenon or visceral involvement and carries a good prognosis.

Toxic-oil syndrome. Scleroderma-like skin changes were seen in the chronic phase of the epidemic of poisoning which occurred in Spain in 1981 resulting from the adulteration of rapeseed oil. Severe repiratory symptoms and muscle weakness, fatal in many cases, were also seen. A noteworthy feature was an increase in the haplotype of HLA DR 3–4.

Scleroderma-like changes are also seen in *graft-versus-host* disease and in *vinyl chloride poisoning*.

Morphoea. This is a localized form of scleroderma of the skin which only rarely progresses to systemic sclerosis.

Dermatomyositis and polymyositis (see page 211)

Clinical features

These are inflammatory disorders of striated muscle of unknown aetiology, which present with weakness of the limbs and trunk, respiratory difficulties, dysphagia and diplopia. The term dermatomyositis denotes an additional skin involvement, notably the heliotrope eruption around the eyelids, periungal erythema, an inflammatory oedema of the skin causing induration and later atrophy, collodion patches and subcutaneous calcinosis (Fig. 6.13). Other features include Raynaud's phenomenon, arthralgia and arthritis, cardiac failure, and occasionally pulmonary fibrosis. An association between malignancy and both dermatomyositis and polymyositis is generally accepted (incidence 15–20 per cent in dermatomyositis, 2–3 per cent in polymyositis). Carcinoma of the lung, prostate, uterus, ovary, breast and large bowel are the most common tumours. There is a juvenile form without this association with malignancy.

Diagnosis

This is confirmed by typical EMG changes and on muscle

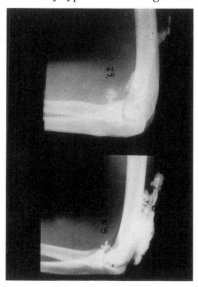

Figure 6.13 *Subcutaneous calcinosis in a patient suffering from dermatomyositis. Note the partial disappearance of the subcutaneous calcinotic deposits which has occurred spontaneously over a three-year period.*

biopsy by histological evidence of degeneration of muscle fibres, regeneration and chronic inflammatory infiltration. The serum creatine phosphokinase is elevated. The ESR may be mildly elevated or normal in the presence of active disease, and serological tests are unhelpful.

Treatment

Oral corticosteroids (prednisolone 40–60 mg—occasionally more—daily initially) are used to suppress the disease and are usually effective. The addition of methotrexate, azathioprine or cyclophosphamide may be helpful in resistant cases. During acute phases the patient is treated with bed-rest with appropriate splinting to avoid contractures and deformities. Even in the absence of an associated malignancy the prognosis may be poor, particularly in older subjects with heart or lung complications. Overall the five-year survival rate is 70 per cent.

Overlap syndromes

Not infrequently, clinical features of two or more of the inflammatory disorders of connective tissue are seen in the same patient, causing diagnostic difficulty. A particular subset, called 'mixed connective tissue disease' (MCTD), has been identified by the presence in the serum of antibodies to extractable nuclear antigen (ribonucleoprotein (RNP) component). The original claims that MCTD is responsive to steroids and carried a better prognosis have not been borne out.

Metabolic arthritis, gout, pseudogout and ochronosis

Acute synovitis may be provoked by the liberation into the joint cavity of microcrystals—monosodium urate monohydrate in the case of gout and calcium pyrophosphate dihydrate in pseudogout.

Gout

Aetiology

The concentration of urate in plasma and body fluids represents a fine balance between production and excretion. Owing to the limited solubility of urate, its accumulation (recognized as hyperuricaemia—plasma urate in excess of 0.5 mmol/l) leads to precipitation of crystals, particularly in joints, subcutaneous tissues and in the renal collecting system. This may arise as a result of increased *de novo* purine synthesis, from excessive intake of high purine foods, or from excessive catabolism of nucleoproteins as occurs in the myeloproliferative disorders, leukemia, myeloma and polycythaemia rubra vera (secondary hyperuricaemia), particularly when these conditions are treated by cytotoxic agents. Failure of the kidney to excrete urate, as in renal failure, or tubular retention of urate, as occurs with certain drugs (e.g. oral diuretics and pyrazinamide), also results in accumulation.

Gout is rare in the first two decades of life. The peak age of onset is in the fifth decade in males who constitute 90 per cent of gout sufferers. Gout is unusual in females before the menopause and for this reason the peak age of onset in females is in the sixth decade.

Only in very rare instances (for example, in the Lesch–Nyhan syndrome) can the increased *de novo* synthesis be ascribed to an hereditary enzyme deficiency (hypoxanthine-guanine-phosphoribosyl transferase (-HGPRTase) in the case of the Lesch–Nyhan syndrome). Gout occurs in approximately one-third of patients with hyperuricaemia, the risk increasing with the height of the urate level. Gouty subjects tend to be obese, hypertensive and regular drinkers of alcohol. There is also an association with hyperlipidaemia and coronary artery disease. There is a strong familial tendency; the pattern of inheritance suggests a multifactorial aetiology. Other conditions in which hyperuricaemia is seen include chronic lead poisoning, toxaemia of pregnancy, starvation, hyperparathyroidism, hypothyroidism, Down's syndrome and glycogen storage disease. Urate deposits are seen as tophi in and around joints and bursae, in cartilage such as the pinnae, over bony prominences and (rarely) in the kidney. Renal changes are those of hypertension with nephrosclerosis and interstitial nephritis. Urate calculi may be seen in 8 per cent of patients.

Clinical features

Intense self-limiting attacks of acute arthritis favouring the first metatarsophalangeal joints (but occurring in others too) is the classical presentation of gout. The joint is hot, swollen and tender with reddened overlying skin. The attacks may be associated with pyrexia, leucocytosis and an elevated sedimentation rate. Spontaneous remission (if the attack has not been aborted by medical treatment) occurs within a week in most patients, though a migratory polyarthritis is sometimes seen. The natural history is for recurrent acute attacks to occur with increasing frequency, and eventually a chronic deforming arthropathy may result from tophus formation. Tophi may discharge releasing a chalky material, composed of urate crystals, and readily identified as such by microscopic examination or chemical analysis. Despite hyper-

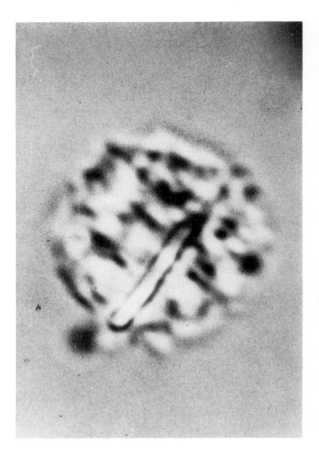

Figure 6.14   *Intraleucocytic polymorph containing needle-shaped urate crystal—diagnostic of classical (urate) gout as seen on polarizing microscopy.*

tension, proteinuria and mild renal impairment gout does not usually reduce longevity.

Diagnosis

Clinical diagnosis is confirmed by the finding of hyperuricaemia and the identification of urate crystals, seen on polarizing microscopy as negatively birefringent needles within synovial fluid polymorphs (Fig. 6.14). X-rays are normal in the early stages, but eventually punched-out areas caused by the tophi are seen in relation to the chronically affected joints (Fig. 6.15).

Treatment

Acute gouty episodes respond to oral colchicine (0.5 mg 4-hourly until relief or diarrhoea ensues) or full doses of indomethacin. The newer NSAIDs (e.g. naproxen, fenoprofen, ibuprofen or piroxicam) constitute a malignant disease. The usual daily dose is 300 mg but it is adjusted in response to serum urate level. Smaller doses are required in patients with renal failure. Asymptomatic hyperuricaemia does not generally require treatment.

Pseudogout (pyrophosphate arthropathy)

Aetiology

This disorder is principally seen in elderly subjects and is rarely encountered in early life. It occurs as a result of calcium pyrophosphate dihydrate ($CaP_2O_7 \cdot 2H_2O$) crystal deposition in cartilage (*chondrocalcinosis*) which in most patients appears to be a feature of ageing of cartilage. In a few patients it is a manifestation of a metabolic disorder (for example, hyperparathyroidism or haemochromatosis). A familial variety has been recorded.

Clinical features

Recurrent acute episodes of arthritis occur predominantly in the larger joints (knee, wrist, etc.) resembling urate gout, and following a similarly self-limiting course. The average duration of attack is nine days. Precipitating factors include trauma, surgical operations or other acute illnesses. Occasionally polyarticular involvement occurs and a destructive arthropathy resembling either rheumatoid or osteoarthritis may be seen.

Diagnosis

The sedimentation rate may be elevated during an attack, but other blood investigations are normal (except when there is an associated metabolic disorder). Plain radiographs will reveal fine stippling of chondrocalcinosis seen in the fibrocartilagenous menisci of the knee or wrist joints—or as a fine line within the articular cartilage of involved joints. Chondrocalcinosis is a common finding in elderly subjects, only a small percentage of whom suffer from pseudogout. It should not be assumed, therefore, that the presence of chondrocalcinosis is pathognomonic of pseudogout. Confirmation of this diagnosis can only be made satisfactorily by identifying the intraleucocytic crystals of calcium pyrophosphate on polarizing microscopic examination of synovial fluid aspirated from an affected joint. These crystals (unlike those of gout) are oblong in shape and are weakly positively birefringent.

Treatment

Acute attacks are treated by resting the affected joint and by the administration of NSAIDs. An intra-articular

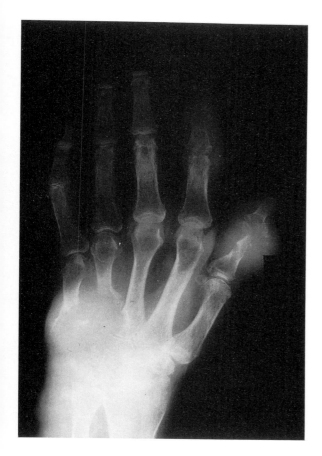

Figure 6.15   *Severe tophaceous gout. Note the destructive changes affecting the interphalangeal joint of the thumb, the distal interphalangeal joint and distal phalanyx of the finger and the bases of the 4th and 5th metacarpal bones and adjacent carpals. These changes are due to the deposition of urate crystals (tophi).*

promising and better-tolerated alternative. An intra-articular steroid injection often aborts an attack. Systemic steroids are reserved only for the most intractable cases. In the face of recurrent acute attacks it is justified to institute hypouricaemic drugs—probenecid or sulphin-pyrazone, which are uricosuric agents promoting the excretion or urate, or allopurinol which is a xanthine-oxidase inhibitor which curtails urate synthesis by blocking the last stage of the pathway. All these drugs require to be taken indefinitely and patient compliance may be a problem. Their institution may result in a temporary exacerbation of acute attacks during the first few months and it is wise, therefore, to cover this period by the concurrent administration of an anti-inflammatory drug. Allopurinol is the drug of choice in the presence of renal failure, renal stones or overproduction of uric acid, particularly when cytotoxic drugs are used to treat steroid injection is helpful in aborting an attack. There is no known means whereby the deposited articular calcification can be removed or recurrence prevented. Even treatment of an associated metabolic disorder (for example, removing a parathyroid adenoma in hyperparathyroidism or venesection in haemochromatosis) fails to halt the (albeit slow) progression of the chondrocalcinosis.

Hydroxyapatite arthropathy

Another crystal capable of inciting an inflammatory reaction in and around joints is hydroxyapatite. Examples of this phenomenon include calcific tendinitis of the shoulder (see below), and a particularly destructive form of arthropathy known as the 'Milwaukee shoulder' associated with the presence of large quantities of collagenase and neutral proteinase within the synovial fluid. The role of hydroxyapatite crystals in the pathogenesis of inflammation in osteoarthritis generally remains controversial.

Ochronosis

This inborn error of metabolism is due to an absence of the enzyme homogentisic acid oxidase, which results in deposition in connective tissues, notably cartilage, of polymerized homogentisic acid. The resultant premature degeneration of cartilage results in destructive changes in the intervertebral discs and larger peripheral joints. The disc spaces become extremely narrowed, with sclerosis of vertebral plates. The result is a severe loss of spinal movement. In the peripheral joints the features are those of severe osteoarthritis. The condition is diagnosed by the detection of homogentisic acid in the urine, which classically turns black on standing or when alkali is added.

Infective arthritis

Invasion of a synovial joint by pathogenic micro-organisms occurs in a wide variety of infections caused by viruses, bacteria and fungi. For practical purposes, the most important infections are those due to pyogenic bacteria, including the *Staphylococcus*, *Streptococcus*, *Gonococcus*, *Meningococcus*, *Pneumococcus*, *E. coli*, *Salmonella*, *Haemophilus*, *Brucella* and *M. tuberculosis*.

Spread to the joint is usually via the blood stream, though direct invasion may occur from adjacent osteomyelitis, or when organisms are inadvertently introduced

into the joint during an aspiration procedure or a surgical operation. Predisposing factors include the presence of debilitating illness (diabetes, alcoholism, uraemia, malignant disease) or treatment with steroids or immunosuppressive agents.

Virus infections

A symmetrical self-limiting polyarthritis occurs in rubella at about the time that the rash develops, and it is particularly common in young, adult female subjects suffering from this condition. A similar complication is seen after rubella immunization with live attenuated virus. Acute polyarthritis may occur in human parvovirus infection, accompanied by fever, rash and lymphodenopathy. Arthritis is occasionally seen in other virus conditions including mumps, chickenpox, smallpox, infectious mononucleosis and infective hepatitis. In some of these conditions the arthritis is due to the presence of live virus within the joint, while in others it appears to be due to the deposition of immune complexes.

Bacterial arthritis

Involvement of one or more joints may arise in the presence of bacteraemia in the course of an infection from a wide variety of bacteria (see above). A focus of infection elsewhere in the body would be an important clue to this diagnosis. However, any patient with an acute monarthritis should be suspected of suffering from bacterial arthritis, particularly in the presence of unexplained fever, until proved otherwise. Bacterial endocarditis may present with this manifestation. Rheumatoid arthritis sufferers are particularly prone to secondary bacterial joint infection.

The only way to confirm (or exclude) this diagnosis with certainty is to obtain a sample of synovial fluid by aspiration of the affected joint and submit it to full bacteriological examination, including Gram staining of the smear and culture. This procedure has the added advantage of permitting antibiotic sensitivity testing to be undertaken and correct therapy to be instituted. Undiagnosed (and therefore untreated) bacterial arthritis may rapidly lead to total destruction of the joint—a tragedy in a condition so readily amenable to treatment. In gonococcal arthritis a febrile illness is seen, particularly in female subjects presenting with fever and oligoarthritis, or migratory polyarthritis, and tenosynovitis in association with a widespread skin eruption composed of macules, petechiae, vesicles or pustules.

Though arthralgia is a common event in brucellosis (see page 428), a true arthritis, usually monarticular, and favouring the hip or knee joint is seen. Spondylitis may also occur. Tuberculous infection (see page 108) frequently occurs in bone, notably the spine, where it may give rise to serious destructive changes and compression of the spinal cord. Peripheral joint involvement may also occur, particularly in the knee or hip with pain and gradual loss of mobility. Severe destructive changes are seen on X-ray. Other manifestations include tenosynovitis, particularly involving the flexor tendon sheaths at the wrist, and tuberculous dactylitis which presents as a painless swelling in relation to a metatarsal or metacarpal bone.

Treatment of infective arthritis

Rational treatment will depend on identifying the precise aetiological agent involved, and no amount of effort should be spared to this end. It is important to emphasize that where bacteriological culture is concerned appropriate examinations should be carried out expeditiously and before antibiotic treatment is instituted, otherwise negative cultures will result, confusing the issue. For reasons already stated, bacterial arthritis is a medical emergency and needs to be handled as such. Therapy with antibiotics such as erythromycin and fucidin given intravenously is instituted as soon as synovial fluid and blood have been sent to the laboratory for culture pending the result of antibiotic sensitivity testing. The joint should be treated by splinting and anti-inflammatory analgesic drugs prescribed as appropriate. Full parenteral antibiotic therapy obviates the need for intra-articular installation of antibiotics, though daily aspiration of the joint should be performed to remove accumulated purulent exudate. As the bacterial inflammation subsides the joint may be gently mobilized, though antibiotic therapy should be continued for 6–12 weeks depending on the severity of the condition. Surgical drainage is performed for bacterial arthritis only when medical treatment fails. Tuberculous infection in bone and joint (which can only be confirmed by histological and bacteriological examination of biopsy material) is treated by anti-tuberculous drugs in combination for a period of not less than 18 months.

Degenerative joint diseases (osteoarthritis, spondylosis)

Aetiology

These common conditions result from degeneration of cartilage, both articular cartilage in synovial joints and fibro-cartilage in the intervertebral discs. The prevalence increases sharply with advancing age; but other factors, notably previous fracture in relation to a joint, recurrent dislocation, occupational over-use, previous joint or spinal diseases whether congenital or acquired, are important. Hereditary factors may also play an important aetiological role. Epidemic forms due to unidentified environmental agents also occur (e.g. Kashin–Beck disease in Siberia and China and Mseleni disease in South Africa).

Where five or more joints are involved the term 'generalized osteoarthrosis (GOA)' is used. One particular variety, nodal GOA, in which Heberden's nodes are a common feature, shows a strong hereditary tendency, tending to present chiefly in females at around the time of the menopause.

Pathology

The primary event in osteoarthritis is believed to be a break-up in the articular cartilage where a reduction in the proteoglycan content is seen. Together with the size of the proteoglycan aggregates there is increased proteoglycan synthesis, but this is believed to be compensatory response to the degradation of cartilage by enzymatic breakdown of proteoglycans by neutral proteinases and collagenase.

Clinical features

Osteoarthritis is suspected in any middle-aged or elderly patient who presents with pain, stiffness and deformity of one or more joints in the absence of symptoms and signs of inflammation. Commonly involved joints are the distal interphalangeal and proximal interphalangeal joint of the hands (with bony deformities known as the Heberden and Bouchard node respectively, Fig. 6.16), the first carpometacarpal joint at the base of the thumb, ankle and metatarsophalangeal joint of the great toe. Hip involvement causes a limp and difficulty in climbing stairs, and examination reveals limitation of passive movement, notably rotation. Knee involvement gives rise to pain on walking and difficulty with stairs and may be recognized by crepitus on passive movement, deformity (genu varum) and loss of joint range, both flexion and extension. Quadriceps wasting is usually evident and an effusion may be present, though this is usually small. A Baker's cyst may be seen (see page 239). Cervical spondylosis may cause local pain and restriction of movement of the neck; pain, paraesthesiae and weakness in the upper limb due to cervical nerve-root compression by osteophytes, (rarely) cord compression known as cervical

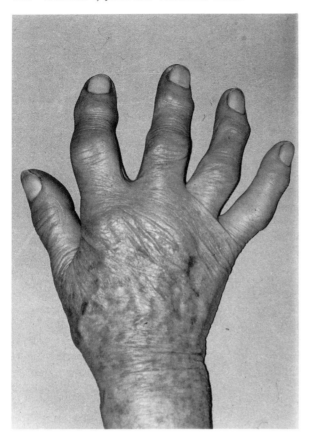

Figure 6.16 *Polyarticular (generalized) osteoarthritis with bony swelling and deformity affecting the distal and proximal interphalangeal joints of the hand. Because of its polyarticular pattern, this condition is commonly misdiagnosed as rheumatoid arthritis.*

myelopathy; or brain-stem ischaemia due to vertebral artery compression. Dorsal spine involvement is usually asymptomatic but may give rise to local pain or referred pain radiating around the side of the chest.

The lumbar spine is particularly vulnerable to acute and chronic trauma occasioned by lifting, bending, etc. Prolapse of a lumbar interverterbal disc is a common disorder affecting adults of both sexes. Herniation of the nucleus pulposus through a rent in the annulus fibrosis may compress one or more nerve roots constituting the cauda equina. The clinical picture is one of acute lumbar pain after strenous activity, inability to move the spine followed by pain down the leg in the distribution of either the femoral nerve (cruralgia) or sciatic nerve (sciatica). Signs of femoral or sciatic nerve tension (femoral nerve stretch test and reduced straight leg raising test respectively) and an associated neurological

deficit may be present, and cauda equina compression may occur. Causes of acute lumbar pain in the absence of evidence of nerve-root compression include a central disc prolapse; facet joint dysfunction; muscle and ligamentous injury; vertebral fracture due to trauma or secondary to infective metabolic or neoplastic disease of the bones; spondyloysis or sponylolisthesis; as well as visceral causes. Chronic low back pain is a serious problem both in human and economic terms. Any of the above-mentioned cases may participate and there may be a strong psychogenic element. The syndrome of 'intermittent claudication of the cauda equina' in which symptoms of lumbar nerve-root compression are brought on by exercise has now been accepted as being due to further reduction in the capacity of the vertebral canal of those with a congenitally small canal acquired pathology (spinal stenosis).

Diagnosis

This is usually made on clinical grounds. Evidence of systemic disease is absent and blood tests are usually normal. Radiological appearances are characteristic and include narrowing of the joint space, subchrondral sclerosis and loss of the normal joint contour and the presence of osteophytes. Such changes may, however, be present in asymptomatic individuals, and undue importance should not be placed on their finding in the absence of appropriate clinical features. In spondylosis confirmatory evidence of cord and/or nerve root compression may be found using contrast radiculography, myelography or computerized tomography.

Treatment

There is no known way of halting the progress of this condition. Fortunately, it is often asymptomatic and patients may be tided over painful episodes by short courses of NSAIDs coupled with physiotherapy in the form of heat and exercises, hydrotherapy or gentle manipulation. Intra-articular injections of corticosteroids are generally not indicated except in the presence of a joint effusion. Compression of nerve roots should be treated by immobilization—with a collar in the case of cervical spine or with bed-rest in an acute lumbar intervertebral disc prolapse.

Most episodes of acute low back pain (including that associated with acute disc prolapse) respond to a short period of complete bed-rest lasting from a few days to a week. Patients should lie on a firm mattress or should use a board under a poorly supported mattress. Some patients prefer to lie directly on the floor! The patient is allowed up to use the toilet but should remain flat at other times. With this regime, the majority of disc lesions will remit. However, patients with persistent referred pain with or without neurological signs may benefit from epidural corticosteroid injections or failing that discectomy. Pre-operative investigations would include the performance of either a radiculogram using a water-soluble contrast medium, a C.T. scan or magnetic resonance imaging of the lower lumbar region. Worsening neurological signs, in particular, evidence of an acute cauda equina compression with difficulty in micturition and defaecation, need urgent neurosurgical consultation and possible urgent decompression.

Advanced osteoarthritis affecting the hip or knee joint may be satisfactorily treated by total joint replacement.

Non-articular rheumatic disorders

Polymyalgia rheumatica

This condition of elderly patients presents with muscle pain and stiffness predominantly affecting the muscles of the shoulder and the pelvic girdle and the proximal limb muscles. Muscle weakness and tenderness are not seen, though occasionally synovitis of central joints (e.g. the sternoclavicular joint) may be present. Some patients also experience malaise, weight loss and anaemia and a proportion show features of temporal (cranial) arteritis (see page 250). Tests for rheumatoid and antinuclear factor are usually absent, although an increase in the gamma globulins may be present and the immuno-globulin levels may be raised. The ESR is strikingly elevated, which is a hallmark of the condition. Another characteristic feature is the dramatic response to oral corticosteroid medication, response being evident within hours of starting. The usual dose is between 10 and 20 mg of prednisolone daily until such time as the ESR falls to within normal limits, whereupon the dose may be tapered accordingly. Because of the close relationship between this condition and temporal arteritis (with the attendant risk of retinal artery occlusion) it is important that this condition be recognized and adequately treated without delay and careful follow-up instituted. Because of the rather non-specific nature of the symptoms, alternative diagnoses—including myeloma, carcinomatosis and polymyositis—should be borne in mind. A temporal artery biopsy, a muscle biopsy, a creatine phosphokinase estimation and an EMG are helpful in this regard.

Soft tissue lesions

Under this heading are included a group of common, benign, though troublesome conditions seen in clinical practice that may mimic arthritis and cause diagnostic difficulties for the unwary. For convenience they may be divided into five main categories.

1 Enthesopathies

These may be either acute traumatic episodes or chronic over-use injuries affecting sites of attachment of ligaments, tendons or fascial bands. Common examples include lateral epicondylitis ('*tennis elbow*'), medial epicondylitis ('*golfer's elbow*') and *plantar fasciitis*.

2 Periarthritis

(including capsulitis and periarticular tendonitis). These lesions affect predominantly the shoulder joint which, being a shallow ball and socket, depends to a considerable extent for its stability on the complex of muscles, tendons and joint capsules known collectively as the rotator cuff. Four syndromes are commonly described within this entity: tendonitis of supraspinatus, infraspinatus, sub-scapularis or long head of biceps—identified by a painful arc of movement when the affected muscle is moved; subacromial bursitis with tenderness over the site of the bursa; acute calcific tendonitis associated with a brisk inflammatory reaction due to crystals of hydroxyapatite reminiscent in its ferocity of acute gout and distinguished by the presence of calcific material seen on X-ray; and adhesive capsulitis ('*frozen shoulder*') in which gross restriction of movement in the shoulder joint is apparent in all directions, though pain is variable. Adhesive capsulitis is commonly seen after pleurisy, myocardial infarction, hemiplegia and certain operations in the region, notably mastectomy. An extension of this condition is known as the shoulder/hand syndrome in which the hand becomes diffusely swollen and tender followed by progressive atrophy of the muscle, bone and skin with severe contractures and deformities. It is believed to be due to a reflex neurovasuclar dystrophy (algodystrophy).

3 Entrapment neuropathy

The carpal tunnel syndrome is the most commonly seen variety.

4 Bursitis

Excessive friction between bone and overlying moving soft tissues may give rise to bursitis. Commonly affected sites include olecranon bursitis, prepatella bursitis and preachilles bursitis.

5 Tenosynovitis

Inflammation of synovium of the tendon sheaths occurs in a wide variety of conditions of over-use, particularly involving the long flexor tendons of the fingers or the extensor and abductor tendons of the thumb. Blocking of the movement of the tendon within the sheath may result in 'triggering'. This condition is known as stenosing tenosynovitis or de Quervains's disease.

For a more detailed description of the conditions mentioned in this section the reader is referred to standard rheumatological and orthopaedic texts. The majority of the conditions listed are amenable to treatment, which may be on the basis of local corticosteroid injections, physiotherapeutic techniques or minor surgical procedures. Drug treatment has little part to play in the management of these conditions.

Psychogenic rheumatism

This term is used to denote a condition whereby rheumatic-type symptoms manifest an underlying psychological disorder such as depression, hysteria, anxiety or compensation neurosis. Arthralgia and low back pain in the absence of clinical signs of organic disease are characteristic features of this condition.

Tietze's syndrome (costal chondritis)

In this obscure condition pain and tenderness are observed in the costochondral junctions. It is usually self-limiting, but occasionally local infiltrations of corticosteroids are required which may be helpful.

Heritable disorders of connective tissue

These are multi-system disorders resulting from the inheritance of abnormalities in either the fibrous proteins (collagen and elastin) or the ground substance (glycosaminoglycans).

The disorders of fibrous proteins share a common feature, namely, generalized laxity of ligaments, resulting in hypermobility of joints which may result in articular symptoms. They include *Marfan's syndrome* (see page 340) (long, slender extremities, arachnodactyly, high arched palate, dislocation of the lens and dilation of the ascending aorta); *homocystinuria* (due to a deficiency of the enzyme cystathionine synthetase and similar to Marfan's syndrome with the additional features of thrombosis in medium-size arteries, osteoporosis and mental handicap); *Ehlers–Danlos syndrome* (characterized by hyperextensible (Fig. 6.17) and fragile skin, a tendency

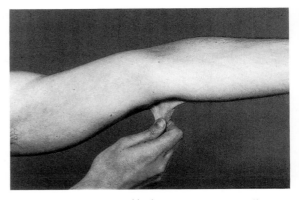

Figure 6.17 *Hyperextensible skin seen in a patient suffering from the Ehlers Danlos syndrome. Note that the elbow joint shows hyperextension (hypermobility).*

to bruising and rupture of arteries); and *osteogenesis imperfecta* see page 340 (fragilitas ossium), in which a marked tendency to fracture of bone and a blue appearance of the sclera of the eye are the most characteristic features.

With the exception of homocystinuria which is inherited as a recessive, all these conditions are inherited as a dominant gene. The term 'hypermobility syndrome' denotes generalized laxity of ligaments in otherwise healthy subjects. It, too, may be an hereditary disorder (albeit mild) of connective tissue. Hypermobility, irrespective of the cause, may result in synovitis of the joints, recurrent dislocation and possibly premature osteoarthritis.

The disorders of ground substance comprise the mucopolysaccharidoses, a group of eleven diseases with differing manifestations (including the Hurler, Hunter, Scheie, Sanfilippo, Morquio and Maroteaux–Lamy syndromes). Patients manifest a variety of features including dwarfism, stiff joints, clouding of the cornea, aortic regurgitation, hepatosplenomegaly and mental handicap. Excessive quantities of mucopolysaccharides are found in the urine. In a number of these conditions the underlying enzyme defect has been identified.

Miscellaneous rheumatic conditions

1 Sarcoidosis (see page 125)
In early sarcoid the arthropathy of erythema nodosum may be seen. Later in the disease sarcoid granulomata may appear in the synovial membrane or bone, causing synovitis and destructive arthropathy respectively.

2 Familial Mediterranean fever
Episodic arthritis of short duration with spontaneous remission is common, and a chronic, destructive arthritis

has also been reported. The episodes of arthritis respond to colchicine.

3 Hyperlipidaemias (see page 327)

A migratory polyarthritis is seen in type II, whilst in type IV an episodic arthopathy is reported.

4 Hypogammaglobulinaemia

An arthropathy similar to rheumatoid arthritis is seen, although destructive changes are rare.

5 Haemophilia and Christmas disease (see page 387)

In these bleeding diatheses recurrent haemarthroses give rise to acute episodes of joint pain and swelling and eventually to severe destructive changes, deformity and fibrous ankylosis.

6 Leukaemia (see page 375)

Arthralgia, arthritis and bone pain are frequent symptoms in acute leukaemia, whilst in chronia leukaemia symmetrical arthritis of larger joints results from infiltration of articular structures. Secondary gout may also occur in these conditions.

7 Sickle cell disease (see page 366)

In this condition bone infarction, arthralgia or synovitis may occur during crises.

8 Pigmented villonodular synovitis

This granulomatous condition of synovium may affect joint tendon sheath or bursa. It presents as a painless swelling of a single joint, usually of the knee, leading to erosion and cyst formation. Treatment is by synovectomy.

9 Hypertrophic (pulmonary) Ostoarthropathy

This is a combination of finger clubbing with painful, tender swelling of ankles and wrists with characteristic periosteal new bone formation seen radiologically. Joint effusions may occur. It is associated with intrathoracic or intra-abdominal pathology, usually infective or neoplastic.

10 Avascular necrosis of bone (Osteonecrosis)

The femoral head is the most commonly affected site, though the humeral head and femoral condyles may be affected. It is seen in trauma, sickle cell disease, caisson disease, high-dose corticosteroid therapy, SLE and alcoholism.

11 Neuropathic (Charcot's) joints (see page 223)

This is a severe form of destructive arthropathy seen in certain neurological diseases with loss of pain sensation. The common causes are tabes dorsalis, syringomyelia, diabetes mellitus with peripheral neuropathy and congenital indifference to pain.

Juvenile chronic arthritis

Many patients carry their chronic rheumatic disease into adult life from childhood. It is for this reason that a note on juvenile chronic arthritis is out of place in a volume devoted to adult medicine. It is now known that several clinical and pathological entities fall within this broad title and the use of the term 'Still's disease' to cover them all is no longer tenable. Rheumatic fever is not included and is dealt with separately (see page 39). The following entities have been delineated.

1 Seropositive (adult-like) juvenile rheumatoid arthritis

This variety is very similar to the adult one with IgM rheumatoid factor, nodules and erosive disease.

2 Juvenile ankylosing spondylitis

This presents in childhood as a peripheral arthropathy, and only in the late teens do the classical features of ankylosing spondylitis develop with spinal involvement. These patients are almost exclusively HLA B27 positive and have a tendency to recurrent acute iritis.

3 Juvenile chronic arthritis (Still's disease)

This comprises three entities:

(a) There is systemic onset, with fever, lymphadenopathy, splenomegaly and pericarditis, which may all precede the polyarthritis and cause diagnostic confusion.

(b) Pauciarticular disease, as its name implies, commences in a small number of joints (1–4). Although the articular disease may not be very severe there is a real danger of severe eye problems following chronic iritis, which may be insidious in its onset and pass undetected. The antinuclear factor is commonly positive.

(c) Polyarticular disease develops in five or more joints, particularly in the knees and wrists. Small finger joints may also be involved, including the distal IP joints. The cervical spine may also be involved.

4 Other

The following are uncommon childhood ailments and their clinical presentation follows the general pattern of adult disease (see above):

Juvenile scleroderma
Juvenile dermatomyositis
Juvenile systemic lupus erythematosus
Juvenile psoriatic arthritis
Polyarthritis associated with ulcerative colitis and regional enteritis

Further reading

Gibson, T. (1986) *Rheumatic Diseases—An Introduction for Medical Students*, Butterworth, London.

Reports on Rheumatic Diseases (1983) *Collected Reports*, The Arthritis and Rheumatism Council for Research, London.

Scott, J.T., ed. (1984) *Copeman's Textbook of the Rheumatic Diseases*, 6th edn. Churchill Livingstone, Edinburgh.

7
Kidney Disorders

Introduction

Renal medicine, which is a combination of science and practical bedside treatment, has completely changed with the development of effective and safe methods of treating patients with endstage renal failure. Our understanding of the disease processes leading to renal failure has correspondingly increased. The purpose of this chapter is to provide an outline of renal disease and its treatment. For this, an understanding of the anatomy and structure of the kidney is essential.

Anatomy of the kidney

The upper pole of the human kidney lies next to the twelfth thoracic vertebra and the lower pole lies next to the third lumbar vertebra. The average adult kidney is approximately 110 mm in length and weighs 150 g. It is normally supplied by a single renal artery which arises from the aorta. Occasionally there are aberrant arteries from the superior mesenteric or suprarenal arteries, and accessory arteries, usually to the lower pole, may arise from the aorta.

There are several clinically significant abnormalities. Bilateral agenesis is rare, but unilateral agenesis occurs in approximately 1 in 1000 people. Hypoplasia is rare. Extra kidneys have been described and are generally small and ectopic in position. Fusion of the kidneys usually occurs at the lower pole to form a horseshoe kidney in approximately 0.25 per cent of individuals.

Structure of the kidney

Nephrons

These are the functional units of the kidney. There are approximately 1.2 million nephrons in each human kidney. Each nephron consists of a glomerulus filtering into the proximal convoluted tubule, which leads into the loop of Henle. This dips into the medulla before turning back on itself to form the distal convoluted tubule, which drains into the collecting duct.

There are two types of nephron: the outer cortical nephrons have short loops of Henle, whereas the inner juxtamedullary nephrons have long loops.

Glomeruli

A glomerulus (Fig. 7.1) consists of a capillary network which provides approximately one square metre of ultrafiltration surface. The endothelial cells of the glomerular capillaries abut on to a three-layered basement membrane. This basement membrane is negatively charged and the passage of molecules through the membrane is dependent on both their size and charge. The epithelial cells of the glomerulus come into contact with the outer layer of the glomerular basement membrane via trabeculae, called foot processes. Proteinuria is associated with the fusion of these foot processes. The glomerular capillaries are further supported by a series of specialized cells (mesangial cells) which have phagocytic properties, secrete their own supporting

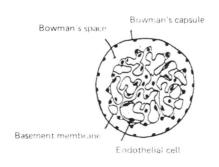

Figure 7.1 *A normal glomerulus.*

matrix (the mesangial matrix) and are probably responsible for the synthesis of the glomerular basement membrane. The glomerular capillaries originate from the afferent arteriole which enters the glomerulus at the hilus before reforming to make the efferent arteriole.

Proximal convoluted tubules (PCTs)

The lumen of a PCT remains patent under normal circumstances, collapsing when the PCT becomes ischaemic. It is lined by a columnar epithelium whose brush border projects into the PCT lumen, providing a large surface area for reabsorption of glomerular filtrate. The PCT becomes the thin, descending loop of Henle when the nephron passes from the cortex into the medulla.

There are several different types of epithelial cells which line the loop of Henle and are responsible for concentrating the urine by active transport and counter-current mechanisms. The thick ascending loop of Henle becomes the distal convoluted tubule.

Distal convoluted tubules (DCTs)

The epithelial cells lining the initial segment of a DCT are very important in active transport of NaCl and are impermeable to water. Potassium secretion takes place further along the DCT before it becomes the collecting duct.

Collecting ducts

There are two types of epithelial cell lining the collecting duct which are responsible for the secretion of hydrogen, potassium and ammonium and the reabsorption of bicarbonate.

The interstitium

The nephrons within the kidney are supported by a framework of interstitial matrix and cells. These cells, in addition to their structural functions, express HLA antigens and may secrete prostaglandins.

Glomerular and tubular function

The kidney receives 20 per cent of the cardiac output and produces an ultrafiltrate by passive diffusion across the glomerular basement membrane. This is dependent on the difference between capillary hydrostatic and plasma oncotic pressures. In the proximal and distal convoluted tubules various constituents of the glomerular filtrate are selectively reabsorbed by active and passive mechanisms, keeping the composition of body fluids constant. Various metabolites and hydrogen ions are excreted. The final filtrate of unwanted water, electrolytes, acid and metabolites passes into the collecting ducts and is excreted as urine. The kidney also has certain endocrine functions, including the production of erythropoietin, renin and 1,25-dihydroxycholecalciferol.

Assessment of function

Although there are a number of specialized tests to measure renal filtration and reabsorption, only a few are useful in clinical practice. These tests are simple and can be performed quickly and reliably.

Urinalysis

This is an important and frequently forgotten investigation. The common causes of proteinuria, haematuria and pyuria are shown in Table 7.1.

The most common and best way of detecting proteinuria and haematuria is the dipstick (Labstix) test, which is a colourimetric method using a variety of indicators.

Table 7.1 Common causes of proteinuria, haematuria and pyuria

Proteinuria
Orthostatic (proteinuria on standing)
Exercise
Febrile illnesses
Heart failure
Primary glomerular disease (e.g. minimal change
  nephropathy, focal segmental glomerulosclerosis)
Multisystem diseases (e.g. SLE, polyarteritis)
Interstial nephritis
Amyloid
Multiple myeloma
Pregnancy

Haematuria
Glomerular disease
Renal cysts, polycystic kidney disease
Benign and malignant tumours of kidney, ureter, bladder,
  urethra
Exercise
Trauma
Bleeding diatheses

Pyuria
Urinary tract infection
Calculi
Analgesic nephropathy
Chemical cystitis (e.g. cyclophosphamide)
Glomerular disease

1 Proteinuria

This is detected by indicators, methyl red and bromophenol blue, which turn green on exposure to as little as 150 mg/l of protein in the urine. Normal adults excrete 100–150 mg/l of protein, which may give a weak positive result and does not usually indicate significant renal pathology. The test is most sensitive for albumin, and does not detect Bence–Jones protein. False-positive results may occur with alkaline urine during infection with urea-splitting organisms.

2 Haematuria

This is defined as the presence of more than 500–1000 red cells per millilitre of urine. The Labstix test detects small amounts of haemoglobin released from lysed red cells. Urine microscopy is necessary as false positives may occur because of free haemoglobin and myoglobin filtered from the plasma into the urine. The Labstix test does not detect other causes of red urine, such as drugs (e.g. phenindione) and food products (e.g. beetroot).

Urine microscopy

A fresh urine specimen should be collected and examined for the presence of white and red cells. In a non-centrifuged specimen, more than ten white cells per cubic millilitre is abnormal. The presence of any number of red cells in unspun urine is abnormal. Phase-contrast microscopy may be used to distinguish the dysmorphic red cells produced by glomerular bleeding from the undistorted cells that are found when the bleeding is of lower urinary tract origin. Bacteria may be seen in infected urine and their presence confirmed by Gram staining and culture.

Casts are formed in the lumen of the distal convoluted tubule and collecting ducts. They have a cylindrical structure composed of Tamm–Horsfall proteins secreted by the distal tubule. A variety of casts exist, made up of cells and debris which can be identified in centrifuged urine. Hyaline casts often occur in normal subjects, particularly after exercise or treatment with diuretics. Epithelial casts occur in acute tubular necrosis. White cell casts are found in acute pyelonephritis, and red cell casts are pathognomic of glomerular disease.

Plasma urea and creatinine

Although the plasma urea is routinely measured as a test of renal function, it is unreliable and insensitive as values are affected by protein intake and catabolism, hydration, liver function and gastrointestinal bleeding. A 70 per cent reduction in renal function is needed to cause any increase in urea levels.

In contrast to urea, creatinine production remains constant until the development of endstage renal failure, anorexia and loss of muscle mass. However, certain situations affect the plasma creatinine: creatinine production is greater in men than in women, lower in children and the elderly, and in patients with chronic wasting disorders. Creatinine estimations may be influenced by cooked meat intake and drugs which interfere with tubular secretion, such as aspirin and co-trimoxazole. Creatinine is also excreted into the tubules in endstage renal failure. The plasma creatinine only rises above the upper limit of normal when the GFR (see below) has halved. Despite these problems, the plasma creatinine is the most reliable and convenient method of monitoring renal function.

Glomerular filtration rate (GFR)

The GFR is determined by the net filtration pressure and the permeability of the glomerular basement membrane. It is an extremely sensitive method of assessing early changes in renal function.

The GFR can be estimated by calculating the clearance of agents which are freely filtered through the glomerulus and not excreted or reabsorbed in the tubules. Creatinine clearance (for example) is calculated using the following formula:

$$\text{Creatinine clearance (ml/minute)}$$
$$=$$
$$\frac{\text{urine volume (ml/minute)} \times \text{urine creatinine concentration (mmol/l)}}{\text{plasma creatinine concentration (mmol/l)}}$$

Various substances are used to estimate the GFR, including inulin, radio-isotopes and creatinine. Inulin is the best physiological agent and gives an accurate result. However, the test is time-consuming and the results not always reproducible, and so the test is reserved for research purposes. A radio-isotope such as ^{51}Cr-labelled ethylene diamine tetra-acetic acid (EDTA) is commonly used to measure the GFR. This is given as a single injection followed by repeated, timed blood samples and the test is not dependent on an accurate 24-hour urine collection. This avoids uncertainties of bladder emptying and measurements of urine flow. Results compare favourably with inulin but are unreliable in the presence of gross oedema, and cannot be used in pregnancy and young children. Creatinine clearance is the most widely used method in clinical practice. It is measured using a 24-hour urine collection and a single plasma sample taken during the collection period. Although an accurate measure of renal function may be obtained, unreliable collection of urine results in errors and low reproducibility ($\pm$ 25 per cent). Tubular secretion of creatinine in endstage renal failure may cause the GFR to be overestimated.

Tubular function

In chronic renal disease and isolated distal tubular damage the kidney loses its ability to concentrate urine. This can be investigated by measuring the osmolality in random early-morning urine samples, which normally exceeds 550 mOsmol/kg. Failure to achieve this level requires overnight fluid-deprivation tests to confirm impaired concentrating ability. Diabetes insipidus may be distinguished from a primary renal cause using 20 μg of desmopressin intranasally. This should increase urinary osmolality over the following eight hours.

Renal acidosis is caused by reduced bicarbonate reabsorption and impaired distal tubular secretion of hydrogen ions. The latter occurs in distal tubular acidosis and is confirmed if the urinary pH is over 5.3 in the presence of a systemic acidosis. This can be achieved by giving patients ammonium chloride (100 mg/kg) and monitoring the urinary pH over the following eight hours.

Water homeostasis

Approximately 65 per cent of the average adult male and 55 per cent of the average adult female is water; 70 per cent is extracellular and 30 per cent intracellular. The extracellular space is further divided into intravascular and interstitial spaces, with ions and water passing freely between these compartments. The plasma volume is maintained by proteins confined to the intravascular space. Changes in the major intracellular cation (potassium) and extracellular cation (sodium) control the passage of water between their respective compartments.

Normally, total body water is maintained by balancing the intake with the combined losses from skin, lungs, gut and kidneys. This is achieved by haemodynamic and hormonal mechanisms which regulate the renal excretion of water. Water loss from the skin and lungs normally amounts to 900 ml in 24 hours, but can be much higher with heavy exercise and fever. Approximately 300 ml of fluid are lost from the gut daily, but this can increase considerably with vomiting and diarrhoea. Water intake and thirst are controlled by receptors in the hypothalamus which respond to changes in intracellular hydration, extracellular volume and plasma angiotensin-2 levels. These receptors control thirst and the release of antidiuretic hormone which has a major role in the control of urine volume. It is synthesized in the anterior hypothalamus, and secretory granules travel to the posterior pituitary where it is released into the circulation in response to osmotic and neurogenic stimuli. Eighty-five per cent of water filtered by the glomerulus is reabsorbed passively in the proximal tubule, whilst the remainder passes to the distal tubule where further reabsorption occurs under the control of ADH.

1 Dehydration

Isolated dehydration is rare except in hospital where debilitated or comatose patients may be given insufficient fluid. More commonly it results from excessive gastrointestinal losses, or sweating in hot climates and febrile illnesses. Renal causes include diabetes insipidus, either cranial or nephrogenic, and losses resulting from a solute diuresis and in uncontrolled diabetes mellitus.

Pure water deficiency results in shrinkage of both intra- and extracellular spaces, resulting in a hyperosmolar state, thirst, and in severe cases confusion and coma. Treatment should consist of gradual correction of the hyperosmolar state with isotonic or hypotonic intravenous fluids. If fluid depletion is corrected too rapidly there is a risk of cerebral oedema.

2 Overhydration

This occurs as a result of excessive intravenous fluid replacement, impaired renal function or rarely inappropriate ADH secretion. It is easily treated by reduction in intravenous fluid replacement, the appropriate use of diuretics and, if necessary, dialysis or haemofiltration. The syndrome of *inappropriate ADH secretion* is rare and caused by malignant tumours, chest infections and intracerebral disturbances. The treatment of inappropriate ADH secretion involves treatment of the underlying cause, water restriction, and the use of demethylchlortetracycline or lithium carbonate which antagonize the effects of ADH.

Sodium homeostasis

Sodium is the major cation in the extracellular space. Plasma concentrations are maintained by the kidney despite a variable and often excessive dietary intake. Normally little sodium is lost from the bowel, but skin losses may be considerable in hot, dry climates.

Regulation of the plasma sodium is controlled by various mechanisms, including the renin–angiotensin–aldosterone system, and natriuretic peptide which impairs tubular reabsorption of sodium.

Eighty per cent of sodium is reabsorbed in the proximal convoluted tubule. The remainder is reabsorbed in the ascending limb of the loop of Henle and distal tubule. This is controlled by aldosterone which is produced in response to a fall in blood volume or renal blood flow.

1 Hyponatraemia

This is usually the result of excess water without any sodium deficit. Excessive sodium losses may result from vomiting, diarrhoea and gastrointestinal fistulae. Failure to conserve sodium follows prolonged diuretic use, tubulointerstitial diseases such as analgesic nephropathy, chronic pyelonephritis, relief of urinary obstruction, and recovery from acute tubular necrosis. Sodium depletion causes a reduction in the extracellular fluid volume with hypotension and peripheral vasoconstriction. Hyponatremia due to excess water is simply remedied by water restriction. Treatment of true sodium depletion is with sodium replacement, using either isotonic saline or dietary salt.

2 Hypernatraemia

Increased plasma sodium levels are most commonly due to water depletion and a true excess is always iatrogenic. This occurs with inadvertant use of saline enemas, emetics, and hypertonic saline and sodium bicarbonate infusions. Symptoms include lethargy, drowsiness and coma. Treatment is by water repletion and removal of underlying iatrogenic causes.

Potassium homeostasis

Ninety-eight per cent of the total body potassium is in the intracellular space, and so plasma potassium measurements may be misleading. Dietary intake varies between 80 and 150 mmol daily and the kidney is the major route of excretion. Potassium is almost completely reabsorbed in the proximal tubule, and is subsequently excreted by the distal tubule in competition with hydrogen ions.

1 Hypokalaemia

The most important causes (Table 7.2) are excessive loss from the gut and kidneys.

Marked potassium depletion causes muscle weakness and wasting which may progress to paralysis. In addition, paralytic ileus, cardiac failure and arrhythmias may develop. Hypokalaemia may cause a nephrogenic diabetes insipidus and a fall in glomerular filtration rate. Hypokalaemia should be corrected using oral or intravenous preparations of potassium chloride, with careful monitoring of plasma potassium levels.

2 Hyperkalaemia

The common causes are shown in Table 7.3. Patients are often asymptomatic but may have increasing muscle weakness and paralysis. ECG abnormalities include loss of P waves, widening of the QRS complex, slurring of the

Table 7.2 Causes of hypokalaemia

Intracellular shifts
Alkalosis
Periodic paralysis

Kidney
Diuretics
Solute diuresis (glucose, urea, saline)
Aldosteronism (primary and secondary)
Cushing's syndrome
Bartter's syndrome
Magnesium depletion
Renal tubular acidosis

Gut
Pyloric stenosis
Ileostomy
Fistulae
Purgative abuse
Villous adenoma of the rectum

ST segment and tall peaked T waves. Hyperkalaemia can be temporarily lowered using injections of dextrose and insulin, and sodium bicarbonate especially if patients are acidotic. However, these effects will only last approximately 2–3 hours, and therefore in renal failure urgent dialysis is the correct treatment. Arrhythmias may be temporarily prevented with intravenous calcium and it should be given while awaiting definitive treatment.

Magnesium balance

Magnesium is primarily an intracellular cation which is regulated by the kidney. Disturbances in magnesium usually occur with other electrolyte changes or with chronic diuretic therapy.

1 Hypomagnesaemia

The blood level (normal range 0.7–1.1 mmol/l) may be an unreliable guide to magnesium deficiency since it is prin-

Table 7.3 Causes of hyperkalaemia

Excessive intake
Impaired renal excretion
Acute and chronic renal failure
Potassium-sparing diuretics
Adrenal insufficiency
Renal tubular disorders

Intracellular shifts
Acidosis
Crush injuries, burns, rhabdomyolysis
Hyperkalaemic periodic paralysis
Succinyl cholinee
Digoxin poisoning

cipally intracellular. The main causes are:

(a) decreased intake (parenteral feeding)
(b) poor absorption
(c) urine loss (diuretic therapy; diabetic ketoacidosis; renal tubular acidosis)
(d) loss from the gut (prolonged vomiting; diarrhoea)
(e) acute pancreatitis

The clinical features are muscular weakness, tetany, cardiac arrhythmias, confusion and convulsions. The ECG abnormalities are similar to hypocalcaemia. The management involves treating the underlying cause and replacing magnesium intravenously. In some circumstances (such as in patients who have been on chronic diuretic therapy and who have arrhythmias) the replacement should be on the clinical suspicion rather than reliance on the blood levels.

2 Hypermagnesaemia

This is generally restricted to patients with chronic renal failure given magnesium in the form of laxatives or antacids. Clinical features are neurological depression and arrhythmias. The treatment is withdrawal of the cause and intravenous calcium gluconate or dialysis if necessary.

Acid–base balance

The kidney is the principal organ maintaining the acid–base balance by reabsorbing filtered bicarbonate, acidifying urinary buffers and excreting ammonia.

Of the four standard types of acid–base abnormality, respiratory acidosis and respiratory alkalosis relate to increases and decreases in arterial carbon dioxide levels for which there will be a slower compensation by way of renal excretion of hydrogen ions.

1 Respiratory acidosis

This occurs when carbon dioxide excretion is reduced because alveolar ventilation drops, as occurs in severe chronic bronchitis and emphysema (see page 118) and when there is depression of respiration through drugs or muscular weakness.

2 Respiratory alkalosis

This is an indication of hyperventilation, voluntarily or driven by a respiratory stimulant such as salicylate (see page 507).

3 Metabolic acidosis

This occurs when there is excessive production or ingestion of acid, or reduced excretion. It also occurs when there is a loss of bicarbonate from the renal tubules or from the gastrointestinal tract. The common causes of a metabolic acidosis are:

(a) ingestion of acids (e.g. aspirin, ammonium chloride)
(b) increased acid production (e.g. diabetic ketoacidosis)
(c) lactic acidosis type A (hypoxia; shock; poor tissue perfusion)
(d) lactic acidosis type B (metformin; liver failure)
(e) renal tubular acidosis
(f) acute and chronic renal failure
(g) gastrointestinal bicarbonate loss (e.g. diarrhoea; fistulae).

Metabolic acidosis usually leads to hyperventilation to remove carbon dioxide and compensate for the acidosis. The treatment involves correcting the underlying cause when possible, fluid replacement as necessary and, in some circumstances such as lactic acidosis, administration of bicarbonate.

4 Metabolic alkalosis

This occurs when there is loss of potassium or chloride, the common causes being diuretic therapy, prolonged vomiting, increased aldosterone production and excess intake of liquorice or carbenoxolone. Removing the cause and replacement of potassium as necessary is generally adequate treatment.

Hormones

Erythropoietin is produced in the kidney, although the exact site of synthesis is unknown. It regulates erythropoiesis, and its deficiency in endstage renal failure contributes to the anaemia of chronic renal failure. Overproduction may occur in certain renal cystic disorders, causing erythrocytosis.

Renin is an enzyme produced by the juxtaglomerular apparatus of the kidney. It is responsible for splitting angiotensin-1 from its glycoprotein precursor and the release of aldosterone. It is thought to be important in the control of blood volume and hypertension.

In the normal kidney the vitamin D metabolite 25-hydroxycholecalciferol is converted to 1,25-dihydroxycholecalciferol. This is impaired in renal failure, causing reduced intestinal absorption of calcium, retarded skeletal growth and renal osteodystrophy.

Imaging of the kidney

Enormous improvements in diagnostic imaging of the kidney and urinary tract have occurred. In addition radiologists have largely taken over the drainage of obstructed kidneys and the removal of stones using percutaneous ultrasound or X-ray-guided techniques.

Radiography of the kidneys and urinary tract

Straight radiographs of the kidneys, ureters and bladder are useful in establishing renal size and outline and in detecting renal calcification and radio-opaque caculi. However, this may be limited by gas and faeces within overlying bowel.

Intravenous urography (IVU)

This technique depends on the excretion of radio-opaque, iodine-containing compounds into the ureters and bladder by the kidneys. X-ray films are taken in rapid sequence following intravenous injection of the contrast agent. This method provides useful information as to renal size, outline, position, excretory ability and the presence or absence of obstruction. The ureters and bladder can be visualized and this technique was the baseline imaging investigation of the urinary tract until the advent of ultrasound. Occasionally anaphylactic reactions to the contrast agent may occur and, despite the use of non-nephrotoxic agents, acute renal impairment may follow the examination, particularly in patients with diabetes mellitus or myeloma.

Renal arteriography and venography

With the recognition that atherosclerotic renal artery stenosis is a cause of renal impairment and hypertension in middle age, percutaneous transfemoral renal arteriography is becoming an increasingly important investigation. In addition, many of these stenoses may be successfully dilated by balloon angioplasty. Renal arteriography is also useful in the diagnosis and assessment of renal tumours as they often have abnormal vascular anatomy. Renal venography is rarely indicated, usually to demonstrate renal venous thrombosis in patients with the nephrotic syndrome.

Computer-assisted tomography and magnetic resonance imaging

CT and MRI scans of the kidney and urinary tract are at present particularly useful in the diagnosis, assessment and management of tumours. These techniques are being further developed and may provide useful information on renal parenchymatous disease and blood flow.

Ultrasonography

Because high-quality ultrasound equipment and radiologists familiar with the use of this technique are readily available, ultrasonography is now the initial baseline method of imaging the kidneys and urinary tract. Ultrasound is particularly useful in the management of patients with renal failure who are unable to excrete intravenous contrast, providing rapid data on renal size, position and obstruction.

Radionuclide examinations

Radio-isotopes are particularly useful in assessing renal perfusion and the glomerular filtration rate. In addition, dimercaptosuccinic acid (DMSA) labelled with technetium binds to protein and gives a measure of the mass of renal cortex. Diethylene triáminepenta-acetic acid (DTPA) is also labelled with technetium but is filtered by the glomeruli. DTPA scans provide information on renal blood flow and comparative function of the two kidneys.

Inherited diseases

Adult polycystic disease

Inherited as an autosomal dominant, this disease occurs with a frequency of 1 in 500. A genetic marker for this disease has recently been found on the short arm of chromosome 16. The kidneys are usually enlarged with multiple cysts of varying sizes throughout the renal substance. The cysts are filled with clear fluid or blood. As the cysts enlarge normal parenchyma becomes distorted and compressed. One-third of patients also have hepatic cysts, and occasionally pancreatic, splenic, uterine, ovarian and pulmonary cysts. There is an association with subarachnoid haemorrhage due to the increased incidence of berry aneurysms of the cerebral arteries.

Clinical features

The clinical presentation of this disorder is variable. Patients can develop renal impairment at any age, but more commonly in the third and fourth decades. There may be abdominal pain, haematuria, urinary tract infection, or hypertension.

On examination the kidneys are usually enlarged and the diagnosis is confirmed using ultrasonography. However, in early disease computerized tomography is a more sensitive diagnostic tool:

Treatment

There is no treatment to halt the progression of renal failure, but the rate of deterioration may be slowed by treating associated hypertension, urinary tract infection and hypovolaemia.

Infantile polycystic disease

This is a rare autosomal recessive condition. It frequently presents at birth, or soon after with bilaterally enlarged kidneys and renal failure. There may be hepatic cysts and progressive hepatic fibrosis.

Alport's syndrome

This form of heriditary nephritis is frequently associated with high-frequency hearing loss. In most families it is transmitted as an X-linked trait and males are more severely affected than females. Men often develop renal failure before the age of 20 years, while women have intermittent haematuria or develop renal insufficiency later. The major renal defect is in the glomerular basement membrane which on electron microscopy is split and lamellated.

Clinical features

Patients present with haematuria, hypertension and progressive renal impairment. In 15 per cent of patients there are ocular abnormalities, including cataracts, keratoconus, myopia and nystagmus.

Glomerulonephritis

Introduction and classification

Glomerulonephritis is a term used to describe immune-mediated glomerular injury. Although glomerulonephritis is the most common cause of endstage renal failure in the West, relatively little is known about its pathogenesis in humans. Even more unfortunate is the fact that most forms have no specific, effective treatment.

The classification of glomerulonephritis is often confusing. The outline below is primarily clinical, with an attempt to fit the clinical syndromes with their histopathological and pathogenic features.

Clinical syndromes

The essential features of glomerular injury are proteinuria, haematuria, reduced GFR and impaired salt and water excretion leading to oedema, hypertension and renal failure.

1 Acute glomerulonephritis (sometimes referred to as the nephritic syndrome)
This describes the abrupt onset of the features of glomerular injury described above. The term 'rapidly progressive glomerulonephritis' (RPGN) is used when the glomerulonephritis is particularly aggressive and associated with acute renal impairment.

2 Chronic glomerulonephritis
This is a term used to describe the gradual deterioration of renal function following glomerular injury leading to endstage renal failure.

3 Nephrotic syndrome
This is a term used to describe the triad of oedema, proteinuria (usually greater than 3.5 g/day) and hypoalbumenaemia (less than 35.0 g/l in the West).

4 Persistent proteinuria
Many patients have persistent proteinuria (usually less than 2.0 g/day) and/or haematuria with no symptoms. Occasionally the haematuria may be macroscopic. Many of these patients are hypertensive and a small proportion go on to develop endstage renal failure.

Pathogenic mechanisms in glomerular injury

Immunologically mediated glomerular injury is dependent on a combination of specific immune mechanisms, and environmental and genetic factors.

1 Immune mechanisms

(a) Antibody directed against glomerular basement membrane antigens. These cause an acute, severe inflammatory reaction (e.g. Goodpasture's syndrome).

(b) Circulating antibody–antigen immune complexes deposited within the glomerular mesangium and basement membrane. These result in inflammation (e.g. SLE, post-streptococcal nephritis).

(c) *In situ* formation of immune complexes; circulating 1 gG binding to trapped or fixed antigens within the glomerular basement membrane forming deposits (e.g. idiopathic membranous nephropathy). The precise role of these deposits is unclear in the mediation of glomerular injury.

2 Environmental factors

(a) Infections. There is very good evidence in animal models that chronic infections are complicated by immune-complex mediated nephritis. In humans there is little direct evidence that infections cause glomerulonephritis other than the post-streptococcal type. Other organisms associated with post-infectious nephritis include staphylococci,

Salmonella typhi, hepatitis B, mumps, *Candida albicans* and *Plasmodium malariae*.

(b) Toxins and drugs. There is good evidence linking exposure to various hydrocarbons in petrol and model airplane glue with Goodpasture's syndrome. Captopril, penicillamine and gold are associated with the development of membranous nephropathy.

(c) Poor living conditions and social deprivation. The incidence of post-streptococcal glomerulonephritis has dramatically declined in the West with improvements in living conditions and ready access to antibiotics. Post-infectious nephritis is particularly common in the Third World.

3 Genetic factors

(a) Associations with HLA antigens. Several forms of glomerulonephritis are associated with certain HLA antigens. Examples include Goodpasture's syndrome and DR 2, membranous nephropathy and DR 3 and DR 4. The pathogenic role of these HLA antigens is unknown.

(b) Associations with congenital complement deficiencies. The solubilization of immune complexes and their removal from the circulation is complement dependent. Approximately 50 per cent of patients with C2 or C4 deficiency develop various forms of glomerulonephritis.

(c) Non-specific genetic factors. There is an increased familial incidence of certain forms of glomerulonephritis such as minimal-change nephropathy and SLE.

Investigations

Proteinuria and haematuria are the hallmarks of glomerulonephritis and are simply detected, as described above, by stix testing. Twenty-four-hour urinary protein excretion and renal function as determined by plasma creatinine and GFR measurement are mandatory baseline investigations. C3 and C4 levels, titres of anti-double-stranded DNA antibody, anti-glomerular basement membrane antibody and anti-neutrophil antibody, as well as plasma levels of IgG, IgA and IgM, are important investigations in the assessment of patients with glomerulonephritis.

Percutaneous renal biopsy is essential for the diagnosis of most forms of glomerulonephritis. In experienced hands, fewer than 1 per cent of biopsies are associated with significant haemorrhage and should be performed in centres where immunofluorescence or peroxidase and electron microscopic facilities are available. Their interpretation is also specialized and requires both pathological and nephrological input. In general there are only two contraindications to renal biopsy. The first is an uncontrollable bleeding diathesis, and the second is a single functioning kidney. There is no point in biopsying the small, shrunken kidneys of endstage renal failure as the procedure is difficult and dangerous, and the results are unhelpful as the fibrotic and sclerotic changes are non-specific.

Primary forms of glomerulonephritis

Clinically, glomerulonephritis can be classified into *primary* and *secondary* glomerular diseases. The histopathological features of these two groups may be similar and this is the source of much confusion.

Primary forms are where the immunological injury is restricted to the kidney. Any systemic consequence of the disease (e.g. oedema) is a result of the glomerular injury.

Acute glomerulonephritis

Post-infectious glomerulonephritis is the most common acute form. Group A, b-haemolytic streptococcal infections used to be the most common cause of this form of nephritis. However, this is now relatively rare in the developed world and other bacterial, viral and parasitic causes are probably more common.

Children and young adults are most often affected, and the illness is characterized by a latent period of 10–20 days from the onset of the infection to the development of nephritis. Clinically there is an abrupt onset of varying amounts of proteinuria, haematuria which may be macroscopic, oedema, hypertension and renal failure. The diagnosis is made by percutaneous renal biopsy which shows proliferation of both mesangial and capillary endothelial cells. Polymorphs may also be found within the glomeruli, and if the nephritis is severe these infiltrating cells will spill over into Bowman's space to form a crescent. IgG and C3 are often deposited in both the mesangium and capillary walls. In a few cases these deposits have been shown to contain the appropriate bacterial or viral antigens. Complement levels, usually C3, are low and rising titres of antibody to the infecting agent can be demonstrated.

Treatment is symptomatic. Antibiotics should be used to treat any remaining infection. Anti-hypertensives and diuretics are sometimes required. Occasionally patients, particularly those with a crescentic nephritis, may develop acute renal failure requiring dialysis. Immunosuppressive treatment is of unproven value. Most patients, especially children, make a spontaneous recovery, although the proteinuria and haematuria may take months to resolve. A small proportion of patients, particularly those with severe clinical and histological disease, have been shown to develop endstage renal failure.

Minimal change nephropathy

Eighty per cent of children and 20 per cent of adults with the nephrotic syndrome will have minimal change nephropathy. The disease is characterized by the development of massive proteinura, oedema and hypovolaemia. Hypertension, haematuria and renal impairment are uncommon and their presence should stimulate the search for another cause of the nephrotic syndrome. Boys are more commonly affected.

The onset of proteinuria may follow a viral or bacterial infection. Rare cases have been described in association with allergic phenomena, such as hay fever. Removal of the antigen or desensitization results in remission and re-exposure in relapse.

Renal biopsy is essentially normal by light microscopy (hence the term minimal change), and electron microscopy shows glomerular epithelial cell foot process fusion which is common to all causes of the nephrotic syndrome. There are no significant glomerular immune deposits.

Treatment is with high-dose corticosteroids; most children lose their proteinuria within a fortnight and adults within six weeks of steroid therapy. Minimal change does not progress to endstage renal failure, although 50 per cent of patients will have further episodes or relapses of their nephrotic syndrome. Serious, multiple relapsing patients may benefit from a six-week course of cyclophosphamide or chlorambucil. Fifty per cent of these patients will go into long-term remission, whereas the remainder will continue to relapse. Cytotoxic therapy should not be undertaken lightly, particularly in young people, as there is a high incidence of gonadal dysfunction following treatment.

Because of its response to immunosuppressive therapy and the relationship to exposure and removal of specific antigens, minimal change is thought to have an immunological pathogenesis. Renal biopsy, because of the high incidence of minimal change in children, is not justified unless the nephrotic syndrome is resistant to steroids or atypical in presentation. All adults with the nephrotic syndrome should undergo renal biopsy.

Complications of the nephrotic syndrome

Since minimal change nephropathy is the most common cause of the nephrotic syndrome, it is appropriate to review its complications and their management at this stage. All patients with the nephrotic syndrome, irrespective of the cause, may develop the following problems.

1 Hypovolaemia and renal impairment

Hypoalbumenaemia lowers the plasma oncotic pressure, resulting in hypovolaemia, interstitial oedema, reduced renal blood flow and renal impairment. This situation may be further worsened by the injudicious use of diuretics. The plasma albumen and circulating volume of hypoalbumenaemic and hypovolaemic nephrotics should be corrected by intravenous albumen infusions, with central venous pressure monitoring if necessary. Diuretics to reduce oedema should be withheld until the patient's circulating volume has been restored.

2 Increased susceptibility to infection

Nephrotic patients are particularly prone to serious infection with encapsulated bacteria such as the pneumococcus, haemophilus or klebsiella. This is because these patients are unable to produce optimal antibody and T cell responses to foreign antigens. Nephrotic patients with infections should therefore receive aggressive treatment with antibiotics.

3 Thromboembolic disease

Nephrotic patients are hypercoaguable with low levels of anti-thrombin III, impaired fibrinolysis, increased platelet aggregability and plasma viscosity, resulting in an increased incidence of renal venous thrombosis and pulmonary emboli. Nephrotic patients who are admitted to hospital and require bed-rest should receive prophylactic heparin. Any patient whose proteinuria increases or renal function deteriorates should be suspected of having developed a renal venous thrombosis. The only sure way of diagnosing this complication is renal venous venography.

4 Hyperlipidaemia (see page 327)

Most nephrotics have elevated levels of plasma cholesterol, phospholipids and triglycerides. The cause and significance of this is uncertain.

Focal glomerular sclerosis

Approximately 10 and 15 per cent of children and adults respectively with the nephrotic syndrome have focal glomerular sclerosis on renal biopsy. Most patients present with proteinuria (often of nephrotic proportions), haematuria, hypertension and renal impairment. Approximately 60 per cent of patients will develop endstage renal failure within ten years, particularly those who have persisting nephrotic proteinuria. Renal biopsy reveals areas of glomerular segmental sclerosis with an increase in mesangial matrix and hyalinosis. These changes may initially be subtle and restricted to the juxtamedullary glomeruli.

The pathogenesis of this disease is unknown. Heroin addicts, patients with AIDS and some patients with reflux nephropathy who develop the nephrotic syndrome have this lesion on renal biopsy. Occasionally patients with minimal change nephropathy may go on to develop focal glomerular sclerosis, and some authorities believe that the two conditions represent different ends of the same spectrum.

Treatment is symptomatic with diuretics and antihypertensives. Only 15 per cent of patients respond to immunosuppressive therapy with steroids and cyclophosphamide. A few patients have been successfully treated with cyclosporin. Unfortunately the disease often recurs in patients who have been successfully transplanted, resulting in massive proteinuria and allograft failure.

Membranous nephropathy

Thirty per cent of adults with the nephrotic syndrome will have membranous nephropathy on renal biopsy. It is rare in children in the West. Approximately 75 per cent of patients with membranous nephropathy present with the nephrotic syndrome, whereas the remainder have non-nephrotic proteinuria. Most patients have microscopic haematuria and will become hypertensive. Twenty-five per cent of patients will go into remission, 25 per cent will have persistent proteinuria, and the remainder will develop endstage renal failure within 10–15 years. Fifty per cent of patients will have an underlying cause or associated condition (Table 7.4) treatment of which may result in remission, making a careful search for these conditions doubly important.

The group of patients without an underlying cause are referred to as having idiopathic membranous nephropathy.

The characteristic renal histological feature of this disease is the presence of immune deposits between the glomerular basement membrane and epithelium, which on light microscopy with silver stains may have a spike or hump-like appearance. The deposits contain IgG and C3. The presence of other immunoglobulins and complement components is suggestive of SLE. Patients with idiopathic membranous nephropathy do not have excessive amounts of circulating immune complexes, and it is thought that these deposits represent the combination of antibody and antigen within the glomerular basement membrane; so-called *in situ* complex formation.

Treatment of the secondary forms of membranous nephropathy involves the treatment of the underlying condition. For example, the successful removal of an underlying tumour will result in remission of the nephrotic syndrome; recurrence is associated with its return. Treatment of the idiopathic form is controversial. Some authorities advocate the use of steroids and other immunosuppressive agents. There is little controlled trial data to suggest that this form of treatment is effective, particularly as the disease has a tendency to remit spontaneously. The disease may recur or occur *de novo* in a transplanted kidney.

Table 7.4 Causes and associated disorders of membranous nephropathy

Connective tissue disorders
Systemic lupus erythematosus
Mixed connective tissue disease
Sjögren's syndrome

Drugs
Gold
Penicillamine
Mercury

Malignancy
Bronchus
Bowel

Infections
Malaria
Schistosomiasis
Hepatitis B

Mesangiocapillary glomerulonephritis (MCGN)

Sometimes referred to as membranoproliferative glomerulonephritis, this disease primarily affects patients under the age of 30 and accounts for approximately 10–15 per cent of all cases of the nephrotic syndrome. Like membranous nephropathy it may be associated (Table 7.4) with infections or systemic diseases such as SLE.

There are two important idiopathic forms of the disease, types I and II, based on histological appearance. MCGN presents with proteinuria (nephrotic range in 50 per cent of cases), haematuria and renal impairment.

Approximately 70 per cent of patients have low levels of C3. Sixty per cent of patients with type II MCGN and 10 per cent of patients with type I have an IgG auto-antibody, termed the C3 nephritic factor, which prevents the inhibition of C3 convertase. As a result C3 is constantly degraded and the patients become hypo-complementaemic.

Approximately 60 per cent of patients develop endstage renal failure within ten years, particularly those with heavy proteinuria and hypertension at presentation. Patients with type II MCGN are said to have a worse prognosis.

The characteristic renal histological lesion in type I MCGN is proliferation of both mesangial cells and matrix together with capillary wall thickening; hence the term MCGN. Type II MCGN, or dense-deposit disease, is characterized by the presence of dense non-immuno-globulin deposits within the glomerular basement membrane as well as the other features of type I disease described above.

The pathogenesis of MCGN is unknown. Type II MCGN may occur in individuals with partial lipody-strophy. The basis of this association is unknown.

There is no satisfactory treatment for MCGN other than any possible underlying cause (Table 7.4). MCGN, particularly type II, may recur in the transplanted kidney, causing the nephrotic syndrome and allograft failure.

IgA nephropathy

This (Berger's disease) is an increasingly common cause of both macro- and microscopic haematuria in the developed world. It occurs usually in males between the ages of 10 and 50. Bouts of haematuria with loin pain and dysuria are frequently associated with upper respiratory or other viral infections. Proteinuria is mild and only of nephrotic proportion in 10 per cent of patients. Most patients become hypertensive. Approximately 50 per cent of patients have elevated circulating levels of polymeric IgA. Only 15 per cent of patients, particularly those with bad hypertension, develop endstage renal failure.

The characteristic renal histological finding is of mesangial polymeric IgA deposits. Focal and segmental sclerosis often occurs. Occasionally these patients may present with an acute crescentic nephritis, and it is said that if patients are biopsied during an attack of macros-copic haematuria, crescents will be found.

The pathogenesis is unknown. Patients with alcoholic cirrhosis have mesangial IgA deposits because it is thought that their Von Kupffer cells are unable to remove gut-derived IgA complexes. Whether a similar mechanism is involved in IgA nephropathy is uncertain.

Similarly there is no specific treatment. Mesangial IgA deposits have recurred in transplants without any short-term significance.

Glomerulonephritis as part of a systemic disease

In this group of diseases immunological glomerular damage occurs as a part of a systemic disease. The main features of these diseases are discussed elsewhere in this book and only their renal aspects will be reviewed in this chapter.

Systemic lupus erythematosus (see also page 247)

Approximately 40 per cent of patients will have clinical renal involvement at presentation. However, nearly all patients with SLE have histological evidence of renal involvement despite the absence of clinical signs.

SLE is a disease of women, particularly non-caucasoids. Renally the disease may present with proteinuria, haematuria, hypertension and renal impairment, together with other non-renal manifestations, usually arthritis and skin involvement. Occasionally it may present as the nephrotic syndrome or even as acute renal failure with few non-renal features. Most patients will have raised levels of anti-nuclear factor, anti-double-stranded DNA antibodies and low levels of C3 and C4. Occasionally patients will have no positive serological markers at the onset of the disease, but go on to develop them.

Renal biopsy shows a variety of histopathological abnormalities, ranging from minimal change to an acute crescentic nephritis. The histological hallmark of SLE is the presence of immune complexes containing IgG, IgA and IgM together with several different complement components (C1, C1q, C3, C4) within the mesangium and capillary wall.

SLE is considered to be the classical immune-complex-mediated disease. The mechanisms by which these complexes cause damage in the kidney is, however, uncertain.

Treatment of the renal disease is based on the clinical and histopathological severity of the disease. High-dose steroids and immunosuppressive agents such as azathio-prine and cyclophosphamide are used to treat diffuse proliferative forms of the disease, whereas steroids alone are used to treat the milder forms. Plasma exchange and high-dose intravenous methyl prednisolone are used in patients with very severe renal SLE, particularly those with acute renal failure. The role of anticoagulants and drugs to reduce platelet aggregation is unproven.

The management of patients with SLE in remission can be difficult. Overall, levels of anti-double-stranded DNA antibody and complement are of limited use in assessing disease severity and response to treatment. However, in individual patients these immunological parameters may be of value and can predict relapses and remissions.

The prognosis of renal SLE has greatly improved over recent years with the prompt use of immunosuppressive agents and better medical management. SLE is a rare cause of endstage renal failure and most deaths are due to cerebritis, coronary artery disease or therapy-related infection. Interestingly, SLE rarely recurs in the transplanted kidney.

Polyarteritis and Wegener's granulomatosus

There are two forms of polyarteritis, which is a term describing inflammation of muscular arteries. The first is the classical form, polyarteritis nodosa, (see page 249) which affects medium-sized arteries. The second form is called microscopic polyarteritis because it affects smaller vessels and is much commoner in the kidney. Wegener's granulomatosus (see page 99) is also a vasculitic disease, pathologically producing necrotizing granulomas with a predeliction for the upper respiratory tract.

Microscopic polyarteritis and Wegener's granulomatosus characteristically affect middle-aged men with a prodrome of malaise, arthralgia, fever and cutaneous vasculitis lesions. Patients with Wegener's granulommatosus may also have a bloody nasal discharge or haemoptysis. Renally the patients have non-nephrotic proteinuria, haematuria, hypertension and renal impairment, often presenting as acute renal failure. The ESR is usually more than 50 mm/hour, and a leucocytosis and eosinophilia are common. Renal biopsy shows characteristic necrotizing glomerular lesions, often with crescent formation. Occasionally involvement of vessels larger than glomerular capillaries may occur, and interstitial necrotizing granulomas may be found in patients with Wegener's granulomatosus.

The pathogenesis of the disease is essentially unknown. Polyarteritis has been described in association with various infections, including hepatitis B, following penicillin and sulphonamide treatment and leukaemia and other neoplasms. Recently raised levels of an anti-neutrophil cytoplasmic antibody have been found in patients with these two forms of vasculitis. There is some evidence to suggest that this antibody reacts with vascular endothelium and that its levels parallel disease activity.

Treatment, particularly of those patients with acute renal failure, should be aggressive with high-dose steroids, cyclophosphamide and plasma exchange. Milder forms of these diseases respond well to steroids alone. Some patients have a single episode of vasculitis and can be rapidly weaned off immunosuppressive therapy, whereas the others have a continuing disease process which, if not carefully monitored and treated, ends in endstage renal failure. If patients with endstage renal failure are transplanted in the presence of active disease, it will recur in the allograft.

Henoch Schönlein Purpura (see also page 385)

This is another form of multi-system vasculitis more common in children, occasionally following infection or drugs. Renal involvement results in proteinuria (which is nephrotic in up to 50 per cent of cases), haematuria, hypertension and varying degrees of renal impairment. Skin rashes, joint and abdominal pains are common. The renal biopsy shows mesangial matrix and cell proliferation and deposits of IgA which may be difficult to distinguish from IgA nephropathy. The pathogenesis is unknown.

There is no specific treatment and most patients make a spontaneous recovery. A few patients, particularly adults, have recurrent episodes and may go on to develop endstage renal failure.

Goodpasture's syndrome

In this rare form of glomerulonephritis, an auto-antibody direct against a type IV collagen glycoprotein antigen in the glomerular and pulmonary alveolar membranes causes a severe glomerulonephritis and pulmonary haemorrhage. The disease usually occurs in young people and can be associated with glue sniffing and exposure to other hydrocarbons. However, the disease may occur at any age and usually presents with oligoanuric acute renal failure and inappropriately severe anaemia due to intra-alveolar haemorrhage.

Renal biopsy usually shows an acute crescentic glomerulonephritis with linear deposits of IgG along the basement membrane. The diagnosis can be further confirmed by the detection of circulating anti-glomerular basement membrane antibody, titres of which are a good index of disease activity and response to treatment. Lung involvement is variable, but may be life-threatening.

Most patients are HLA DR2 positive.

Treatment is aimed at the removal of antibody by plasma exchange and the prevention of its resynthesis by steroids and cyclophosphamide. Early, aggressive therapy prevents the development of endstage renal failure. Transplantation in the presence of residual antibody results in recurrence of the disease and should be avoided until the antibody has been undetectable for at least a year.

Bacterial endocarditis (see page 41)

Glomerulonephritis associated with bacterial endocarditis is well recognized, occurring more frequently in patients who present late or in whom the diagnosis is missed. Non-nephrotic proteinuria, haematuria and renal impairment, together with hypocomplementaemia and raised titres of rheumatoid factors, are the hallmarks of this complication of endocarditis.

Renal biopsy shows most frequently focal and segmental proliferative lesions with mesangial deposits of IgG, IgM and C3. Occasionally patients may have a diffuse proliferative crescentic nephritis.

Successful treatment of the endocarditis results in recovery of the renal lesion. Patients with endocarditis may also develop renal impairment as a result of renal embolization or drug therapy.

Other systemic diseases affecting the kidney

Diabetes mellitus (see page 314)

Between 20 and 30 per cent of the patients on most endstage renal failure programmes in countries where health care is not rationed have diabetic nephropathy. In the UK where endstage renal failure facilities are limited, fewer patients with diabetic nephropathy are treated. Up to 50 per cent of juvenile onset diabetics will develop endstage renal failure within 10–30 years of the start of their disease, and this is the most common cause of their death.

Clinical features

The disease starts with an increase in GFR (up to 200 ml/minute), microalbumenuria (above 100 mg/day), large kidneys and glomerular and tubular basement membrane thickening on renal biopsy. As the disease progresses the patients become hypertensive, nephrotic and develop increasing renal impairment. These changes are associated with the appearance of other diabetic complications such as retinopathy, peripheral and autonomic neuropathy, and peripheral vascular disease. In the kidney the basement membrane thickening progresses with the development of mesangial hyaline nodules, called Kimmelstiel–Wilson lesions, and progressive glomerular sclerosis. The cause of these microvascular changes is uncertain. Poor metabolic control, hypertension, smoking and genetic factors are all probably contributory but not necessarily causative.

Endstage renal failure occurs within 3–4 years of the onset of heavy proteinuria.

Treatment

At present, other than careful control of hypertension, improvement of diabetic control and possibly the institution of a low-protein diet, there is no specific treatment to prevent endstage renal failure. Continuous ambulatory peritoneal dialysis and transplantation are the preferred forms of endstage renal failure therapy. Haemodialysis may be difficult owing to problems with vascular access and heparin-induced intraocular haemorrhage. Mortality is approximately 25 per cent greater than for other patients with endstage renal failure and is mainly due to cardiac and cerebrovascular disease.

Diabetics have a higher incidence of urinary infections and may develop obstruction as a result of papillary necrosis.

Light-chain nephropathy and myeloma (see page 381)

The deposition of immunoglobulin light chains within the glomerular and tubular basement membranes is associated with the development of proteinuria, which may be of nephrotic proportions, and progressive renal impairment. There is no specific treatment and, in particular, cytotoxic therapy is of little use. Patients with myeloma may present with acute renal failure caused by hypercalcaemia, tubular obstruction by immunoglobulin, hyperuricaemia following chemotherapy and, rarely, amyloidosis or glomerulonephritis. Treatment should be directed at the cause of the renal failure. Patients with myeloma presenting with renal failure often do badly, despite dialysis.

Amyloidosis (see page 342)

The glomerular mesangium, capillaries and tubular basement membranes are common sites of amyloid deposition. Patients with amyloid characteristically present with the nephrotic syndrome and renal impairment. Other organs, such as the heart, liver and adrenals, are often also involved. There is no specific therapy and once endstage renal failure has developed treatment is supportive with dialysis or transplantation. These patients often do surprisingly well.

The kidneys in hypertension (see page 65)

In essential hypertension some changes occur in the renal arterioles but there is not usually a significant effect on renal function. In accelerated or malignant hypertension severe renal damage can, however, occur rapidly. Damage to the vessel walls leads to fibrinoid necrosis of the arterioles. Fibrin deposition within the lumen of arterioles and capillaries can lead to damage to circulating red cells and platelets, producing a microangiopathic haemolytic anaemia. In severe hypertension, protein, casts and red cells may appear in the urine as renal function deteriorates. Careful blood pressure control is essential in maintaining good renal function. Treatment should be initiated before significant renal impairment occurs.

In 10–15 per cent of cases of hypertension there is an underlying renal cause for the hypertension. Hypertension is seen sooner and more frequently with cortical problems rather than interstitial disease. It occurs most often with glomerulonephritis, pyelonephritis and polycystic disease or unilateral renal disease.

Unilateral renal disease and hypertension

A small proportion of patients with hypertension have demonstrable unilateral renal disease which may be pyelonephritis, hydronephrosis or stenosis of the renal artery. Renal artery stenosis is usually due to fibrous hyperplasia when it occurs in young patients and to atheroma in the older group.

Clinical features

Suspicion should be aroused if the patient is young (under 40) with severe hypertension of rapid onset and with a negative family history. Physical examination is unhelpful except that a murmur may be heard over the affected renal artery.

Unilateral renal ischaemia as a cause of hypertension is very rare and the most useful screening test is an intravenous pyelogram which will show:

1 a smaller kidney on the affected side;
2 delayed appearance of the contrast medium in the

ischaemic kidney; this will require X-rays taken minutes after the injection of the contrast medium;
3 ultimately a denser shadow on the affected side because the contrast medium is more concentrated by the ischaemic kidney.

Digital subtraction angiography provides an alternative screening process. If investigations suggest unilateral renal disease which might be ischaemic, the next step is to confirm the presence of stenosis by arteriography. Even the presence of a stenosis, however, does not necessarily imply that the kidney is ischaemic. *Divided renal function studies*, for which the urine is collected from each kidney separately, are rarely required.

Treatment

The correct management is very difficult, for no test shows without doubt which patient will derive benefit from correction of the stenosis. Renal vein renin levels from the affected abnormal kidneys, when compared with the level in the peripheral blood, provide the best prediction of successful relief. If there is unequivocal evidence of unilateral renal artery stenosis and the other kidney is normal, there is about a 50 per cent change of relieving the hypertension by nephrectomy or by some plastic operation on the stenosed renal artery. Balloon angioplasty is the least invasive way of opening up a stenosed renal artery.

Interstitial nephritis

Interstitial nephritis is a term used to describe inflammation of the renal interstitium. The most common cause of interstitial nephritis is pyelonephritis and urinary tract infection. Systemic diseases such as SLE may involve the interstitium. Drugs, either by an immunological process or a direct toxic action, are a common cause of interstitial nephritis.

Infections of the kidney and urinary tract

The urinary tract is the most common site of bacterial infection. Approximately 20 per cent of all Gram-negative septicaemias arise from the urinary tract.

Pathogenesis

Escherichia coli, *Proteus mirabilis*, *Klebsiella aerogenes* and *Streptococcus faecalis*, which originate from the bowel, are the most common bacterial causes. Renal tuberculosis is now rare in the UK.

Factors which predispose to urinary infection include instrumentation of the urinary tract, particularly bladder catheterization, the presence of stones or necrosed papillae, urinary obstruction and anatomical abnormalities. Immunosuppressed patients, diabetics and recipients of renal transplants are more prone to urinary infections and their septicaemic complications. Urinary infections are more common in women than men because they have shorter urethras.

The nature of the infecting organism is an important clue to its aetiology. For example, proteus infections are often associated with stones or foreign bodies. Staphlococcal infections in young women, so called 'honeymoon cystitis', often follow sexual activity.

Clinical features

Symptoms consist of dysuria, frequency (referred to often as 'cystitis'), suprapubic discomfort and foul-smelling urine. The patient may be systemically unwell with a fever and suprapubic tenderness. The urine usually contains white cells and at least 100 000 organisms per millilitre. Small amounts of protein and blood, which occasionally can be macroscopic. are frequently found. The presence of large amounts of protein is indicative of glomerular disease and should not be solely attributed to the urinary infection. Fewer than 100 000 bacteria per millilitre of urine, particularly if they are of the same species, may indicate a significant infection. Pyuria in the absence of a positive bacterial culture (so-called 'sterile pyuria') may be due to tuberculosis, and so cultures of early-morning urine should be performed.

Treatment

In general, young women do not need further investigation if the infection is related to sexual activity and should

be advised to drink and empty their bladders after intercourse. Recurrent infections, urinary infections in children and men should be investigated for an underlying cause with intravenous urography and an assessment of renal function. A 'clean catch' sample should be sent to the laboratory for culture and the patient treated with the appropriate antibiotics (Table 7.5). The prescription of multiple courses of antibiotics without culture and investigation is bad medicine.

Prostatitis, urethritis, epididymitis and orchitis will not be considered here.

Pyelonephritis

Pyelonephritis is an infection of the pelvicalyceal system and kidney. It is a serious disorder for it can lead to chronic pyelonephritis particularly if recurrent attacks occur in early childhood and, if bilateral, can cause end-stage renal failure. It may occur *de novo* or be secondary to some lesion (often obstructive) in the urinary tract.

Acute pyelonephritis

This is usually due to infection by *E. coli*. The onset is abrupt with loin pain, shivering, fever and malaise. There may or may not be frequency and dysuria. Examination shows tenderness in the affected loin. There is pyuria, bacteriuria and sometimes bacteraemia. Underlying causes should be excluded by ultrasound or urography.

Treatment with antibiotics should be started immediately after a urine sample has been obtained for culture. In mild cases trimethoprim orally is satisfactory but in those who are seriously ill or vomiting gentamicin or cefuroxime i.v. are indicated (see Table 7.5). A high fluid intake is required either orally or by infusion if necessary. Follow-up observation with urine cultures is advisable.

Table 7.5 Antibiotics commonly used in renal infections

Acute cystitis	Trimethoprim 200 mg 12 hourly orally	Not if GFR < 30 ml/minute
	Amoxycillin 250 mg 8 hourly orally	Resistant strains common in some areas
	Nitrofurantoin 100 mg 6 hourly orally	Not in renal failure
		Taken with food
Prophylaxis	Trimethoprim 100 mg at night	
Acute pyelonephritis	Trimethoprim 200 mg 12 hourly orally	Mild cases
	Cefuroxime 750 mg 8 hourly i.v.	
	Ampicillin 500 mg 6 hourly i.v.	
	Gentamicin 60–80 mg 8 hourly i.v.	Less in renal impairment
		Blood level control of dose

The regimen should be modified in the light of response and cultures.

Pyelonephritis in childhood

Repeated attacks of pyelonephritis in early life can lead to permanent damage to one or both kidneys. This is often due to congenital vesico-ureteric reflux which allows organisms to be washed back into the kidney, causing infection with renal scarring and failure of the kidney to develop. Most damage occurs before two years and is more common in girls.

Management. When a child presents with frequency and dysuria the presence of infection should be confirmed by urinary culture. If infection is present it should be treated with a course of trimethoprim followed by an ultrasound or pyelogram and possibly a micturating cystogram. If the urinary tract is structurally normal further infections should be treated as they arise. If reflux is present, prophylaxis is required and the child should be given trimethoprim 2.5 mg/kg as a single nightly dose continued until the reflux, which is usually self-limiting, disappears. Rarely, surgical correction is required.

Chronic pyelonephritis

This is a term used to describe renal damage from repeated bacterial infections. It may affect one or both kidneys and is the second most common cause of end-stage renal failure in the UK.

Patients with chronic pyelonephritis often present with chronic renal failure, preceded by hypertension and pro-teinuria. There may be a history of recurrent episodes of acute infection. Urography or ultrasound shows small, scarred kidneys and scars are related to the calyces.

Treatment. Symptomatic renal infections should be treated with the appropriate antibiotic (see above) but complicated regimens to try to eradicate the infection do not alter the course of the disease. Hypertension, if present, should be controlled and a low protein diet may delay the onset of end-stage renal failure. These patients usually do well with dialysis or transplantation if this becomes necessary.

Drug-induced interstitial nephritis

Non-steroidal inflammatory agents and antibiotics such as methicillin cause an acute, allergic interstitial nephritis in certain, susceptible individuals. They often present with acute renal failure. Examination of the urine reveals moderate proteinuria and haematuria and occasionally the presence of eosinophils. Renal biopsy is diagnostic. Histologically, the interstitium is infiltrated by cytotoxic T cells, macrophages and eosinophils. Treatment with high-dose steroids is generally successful.

Cadmium, lead, irradiation, uric acid deposition and other drugs directly damage the kidney, producing an interstitial nephritis.

Analgesic nephropathy

The consumption of large quantities (kilograms over several years) of analgesics, classically phenacetin, leads to the development of a chronic interstitial nephritis and endstage renal failure. There is reasonable evidence to suggest that paracetamol, aspirin and the non-steroidal anti-inflammatory agents taken in sufficient quantities over long periods of time may have similar results.

Generally, the patients present with endstage renal failure, are often female and have a long history of ill-health with headache and backache. Occasionally papillary necrosis may cause bilateral ureteric obstruction and acute renal failure. Treatment of endstage renal failure is complicated by a high incidence of uroepithelial malignancy and a reluctance to stop taking analgesics.

Disorders of tubular function

A small number of patients will be encountered who appear to have disorders of tubular function without much evidence of glomerular disease. In many of these patients the disorder is congenital, but in others it is the result of various forms of renal disease, particularly chronic pyelonephritis. These disorders may be simple or multiple and may affect nearly every aspect of tubular function. Three such disorders are mentioned here.

Fanconi's syndromes

1 Lignac–Fanconi syndrome (cystinosis)

This is an inherited metabolic disorder of childhood. There are widespread deposits of cystine throughout the body together with tubular renal defects. Death is usually due to renal failure, which may be associated with renal rickets.

2 Adult Fanconi syndrome

This is a disorder of both proximal and distal tubules. It may occur as an idiopathic inherited disorder or be secondary to poisoning by heavy metals or some antibiotics.

There is a failure by the tubules to reabsorb phosphate, amino acids, glucose, bicarbonate and uric acid which are excreted in the urine. This form of Fanconi's syndrome usually presents in adult life as renal osteodystrophy and carries a relatively good prognosis.

Renal tubular acidosis

In this condition there is a failure by the kidneys to produce an acid urine (below pH 6.0). The reduced excretion of hydrogen ions results in:

1 systemic acidosis;
2 low plasma phosphate;
3 hypokalaemia (if distal tubule is involved);
4 hypercalcuria.

Several varieties have been described.

Type I (*distal tubular*) can occur as a self-limiting disorder of infancy or be found in adults due to an inherited defect or secondary to renal disease such as pyelonephritis. *Type II* (*proximal tubular*) may be an isolated phenomenon, usually developing in childhood, or it may be part of multiple proximal tubular defects as in the adult Fanconi's syndrome.

Clinical features

In *infants*, renal tubular acidosis is characterized by failure to thrive, dehydration and vomiting.

In *adults*, the main symptoms are osteomalacia of the skeleton and calcification of the kidney, which may ultimately lead to chronic renal failure.

Treatment

The acidosis should be corrected if possible by giving bicarbonate and citrates, and the calcium deficiency, if present, should be replaced.

Amino-acidurias

Amino acids are normally almost completely reabsorbed in the proximal renal tubule. They appear in the urine in two circumstances: *overflow amino-aciduria*, when because of an abnormality of amino acid metabolism some amino acid (or amino acids) is produced in excess; and amino-aciduria due to *failure of reabsorption*. This occurs in the multiple proximal tubular defect of the Fanconi syndrome, and when all amino acids are present in the urine (*generalized amino-aciduria*). There are a number of rare conditions in which specific renal tubular transport mechanisms for amino acids are defective, but the only clinically important condition is *cystinuria*. Cystine is insoluble in all but very alkaline urine, and in about 5 per cent of cystinurics this leads to recurrent formation of renal stones which are only faintly opaque. Symptoms usually develop in early adult life.

Medullary sponge kidney

In medullary sponge kidney (cystic disease of the renal pyramids) cysts of varying size are found in the pyramids, and they communicate with the collecting tubules, which are dilated. The cysts often contain stones. The condition may be generalized, or affect one kidney, or part of one kidney. Renal function is not affected except secondarily by infection or stones.

Patients present with urinary infection, haematuria and stones. The diagnosis is radiological and is best shown on pyelography.

Acute renal failure

Acute renal failure is defined as a rapid deterioration of renal function which is often reversible, depending on the cause. Traditionally acute renal failure is divided into pre-renal, renal, or post-renal. Although this is often too simple and there may be overlap, the classification is still useful. *Pre-renal causes* of renal failure result from reduced renal blood flow, such as in hypovolaemia and a low cardiac output state. The pathological end-point of these processes is acute tubular necrosis. *Renal* causes of acute renal failure are those associated with an intrinsic renal

Table 7.6 Causes of renal hypoperfusion associated with acute renal failure

Hypovolaemia
Vomiting, diarrhoea, intestinal fistulae
Haemorrhage (post-partum, gastrointestinal, surgical)
Inadequate replacement of fluids
Inappropriate use of diuretics
Nephrotic syndrome
Burns

Low cardiac output states
Myocardial infarction
Severe valve dysfunction
Cardiac tamponade
Pulmonary embolism
Cardiomyopathy
Septicaemia
Pancreatitis and hepatic failure

Drugs
Non-steroidal anti-inflammatory agents
Vasoconstrictors (e.g. adrenaline and high doses of dopamine)
Possibly aminoglycosides and Cyclosporin A

Renal artery occlusion
Emboli, resulting from infective endocarditis or after
    myocardial infarction
Aortic aneurysm with involvement or dissection of renal
    arteries
Captopril therapy in presence of renal artery stenosis

problem, such as rapidly progressive glomerulonephritis. *Post-renal* acute renal failure is primarily due to obstruction of the urinary tract.

Pre-renal acute renal failure

Causes

The major causes of impaired renal blood flow are listed in Table 7.6. It does not include causes of damage to the intrarenal vascular endothelium, such as the haemolytic uraemic syndrome. However, septicaemia, endotoxaemia and disseminated intravascular coagulation, which share common pathogenic mechanisms, are included.

1 Hypovolaemia
This is a common cause of acute renal failure which is usually iatrogenic and occurs mainly in hospital. It often follows incorrect assessment of the patient's circulating volume and the inappropriate use of diuretics. Certain groups of patients, such as the elderly and those with the nephrotic syndrome, are particularly intolerant of fluid depletion. Haemorrhage, trauma and burns are now less common causes of acute renal failure owing to treatment with intravenous fluids prior to the patient's arrival at hospital.

2 Low cardiac output states
Impaired renal function or renal failure frequently occur with cardiogenic shock after myocardial infarction, worsening the prognosis. Patients with severe cardiac failure, due either to valvular or myocardial dysfunction, may have impaired renal function which is exacerbated by the excessive use of diuretics. Pulmonary embolism is a rare cause of acute renal failure since patients usually fail to survive long enough when pulmonary arterial obstruction is severe enough to compromise cardiac output.

3 Septicaemia
This is a common cause of renal failure. It has a high mortality owing to the involvement of other systems. Renal failure results from the release of endotoxins which are components of bacterial cell walls. These cause intense vasoconstriction, endothelial damage, disseminated intravascular coagulation and complement activation.

4 Pancreatitis and hepatic failure
Severe pancreatitis causes hypovolaemia and release of vasoactive substances which reduce renal blood flow. In hepatic failure reduced renal blood flow may be due to hypovolaemia, septicaemia, or the syndrome of hepatorenal failure. The cause of this syndrome is uncertain, but it may result from impaired Von Kupffer cell function allowing endotoxins from the gut into the systemic circulation. Renal failure rarely recovers unless liver function improves.

5 Drugs
These can either be the primary cause of reduced renal blood flow, or further compromise pre-existing renal hypoperfusion. Non-steroidal anti-inflammatory agents reduce renal blood flow by inhibiting prostaglandin synthetase. They also cause an interstitial nephritis, or rarely the nephrotic syndrome. Aminoglycoside nephrotoxicity may also be partially mediated by the inhibition of prostaglandin synthesis. Adrenaline and high doses of dopamine are powerful vasoconstrictors often used in low-output cardiac states. They further reduce renal blood flow and may cause renal failure.

6 Renal artery occlusion
Embolization of the renal arteries is a rare cause of acute renal failure in bacterial endocarditis and after myocardial infarction. Aortic aneurysms may reduce renal blood flow by involvement of the renal arteries, or cholesterol embolization during investigation or surgery. Renal blood flow in renal artery stenosis is angiotensin-II dependent, and the use of angiotensin-II converting enzyme antagonists may severely reduce renal blood flow.

Frequently there is more than one cause, such as septicaemia, hypovolaemia and the inappropriate use of an aminoglycoside. Multivariate analysis of the causes of acute renal failure has shown that 62 per cent of patients have more than one insult.

Pathophysiology

Although there have been many studies in animal models and humans, the exact pathophysiology of this form of renal failure is still uncertain. Initially, renal vasoconstriction occurs with increased tubular reabsorption of sodium and water. Later, glomerular filtration is impaired owing to afferent arteriolar vasoconstriction and altered glomerular capillary permeability. There is tubular ischaemia, damage, and finally necrosis. Cellular debris may cause tubular obstruction with backflow of filtrate in the tubules. In addition, certain substances involved in the regulation of glomerular filtration, including renin/angiotensin and prostaglandins, may play a role in increasing renal vasoconstriction. If renal blood flow is restored before significant tubular damage develops, this syndrome may be reversed. Otherwise there is a decline in renal function, with acute renal failure.

Pathology

The kidneys are large and oedematous. Histologically the glomeruli and vessels appear normal, but the proximal

Table 7.7 Renal causes of acute renal failure

Glomerulonephritis
Polyarteritis nodosa, Wegener's granulomatosis
Goodpasture's syndrome
Systemic lupus erythematosus
IgA nephropathy
Post-infectious glomerulonephritis
Henoch–Schönlein purpura
Infective endocarditis

Interstitial nephritis
Drugs, including non-steroidal anti-inflammatory agents,
   penicillins, rifampicin, cephalosporins, sulphonamides,
   thiazide and loop diuretics, allopurinol and phenytoin
Acute pyelonephritis
Malignant lymphoma

Small vessel damage
Haemolytic uraemic syndrome
Disseminated intravascular coagulation
Scleroderma
Malignant hypertension

Endogenous nephrotoxins
Rhabdomyolysis and haemolysis
Myeloma and paraproteinaemia

and distal tubules show varying degrees of vacuolization, flattening and necrosis. The interstitium is oedematous and there is an inflammatory cell infiltrate. Occasionally, when this process is particularly severe, the glomeruli are affected as well as the tubules. Because glomeruli are cortical structures, and unlike the tubules do not have the capacity for regeneration, this syndrome is called acute cortical necrosis and is irreversible. It occurs with severe or prolonged renal ischaemia, such as post-partum haemorrhage or severe sepsis. As treatment of these events has improved, acute cortical necrosis has become much less common with an incidence of between 5 and 10 per cent in episodes of acute tubular necrosis.

Renal causes of acute renal failure

These include parenchymal renal disease, small vessel damage, and certain endogenous nephrotoxins, as listed in Table 7.7.

Glomerulonephritis, interstitial nephritis and causes of small vessel damage are described elsewhere in this chapter. However, they are important causes of acute renal failure which are often reversible if diagnosed early and treated appropriately.

1 Accelerated hypertension
There is fibrinoid necrosis of renal arterioles secondary to the physical effects of the rate and degree of rise of arterial pressure. This results in acute renal failure, which may partially recover weeks or months after control of blood pressure.

2 Rhabdomyolysis
There are many causes of muscle damage with myoglobinuria and renal failure. These include crush injuries and trauma, myositis, prolonged convulsions, severe exercise including marathon running, alcohol and drug abuse. There may be muscle pain, tenderness and swelling, but these are not always obvious.

Clinical features

Acute renal failure may present with oliguria, disorders of fluid balance or frank uraemia. It can also present with symptoms and signs of any underlying cause, or be discovered on routine biochemical investigation.

1 Urine output in acute renal failure
Oliguria, which is defined in adults as a urine output of less than 700 ml in 24 hours, is the most common pattern. Some patients, with polyuria, continue to pass normal or increased volumes of urine with renal failure, and have quicker recovery of renal function. Anuria is uncommon and is usually due to obstruction or a rapidly progressive glomerulonephritis.

2 Hypovolaemia and fluid overload
Signs of salt and water depletion include tachycardia, hypotension, a low central venous pressure and peripheral vasoconstriction. Subjective signs such as skin turgor and ocular tension are of little value. Fluid overload may present with hypertension, elevation of the central venous pressure, peripheral and pulmonary oedema. Daily body weights are helpful but often unavailable, while fluid balance charts are frequently misleading unless very carefully monitored.

3 Uraemia
Ideally renal failure is diagnosed before uraemic symptoms develop. These include anorexia, nausea, vomiting and diarrhoea, confusion and coma.

4 Underlying causes
There are often extrarenal manifestations suggesting the cause of renal failure. These include signs of cardiac and hepatic disease, pancreatitis or the presence of an aortic aneurysm. Previous drug prescription cards must be checked for nephrotoxic drugs, and sepsis must always be excluded. Causes of intrinsic renal disease may be detected by the presence of a cutaneous vasculitis, as in SLE, polyarteritis nodosa and Henoch Schönlein purpura. There may be features of scleroderma, or muscle damage and swelling as in rhabdomyolysis.

5 Acute on chronic renal failure
There may have been pre-existing renal disease, and so details of past medical records, hypertension and urine testing should be checked.

Investigations

1 Haematology

The haemoglobin is initially normal, unlike chronic renal failure, but falls rapidly as renal function fails. Patients with Goodpasture's syndrome are often particularly anaemic because of pulmonary haemorrhage. Blood films should be examined for red cell fragmentation and loss of platelets, indicating intravascular haemolysis.

2 Biochemistry

(a) Plasma urea and creatinine. These rise with loss of renal function. Urea often increases disproportionately owing to protein catabolism.

(b) Plasma potassium. Hyperkalaemia is a life-threatening complication, especially in catabolic states such as burns, sepsis, starvation and rhabdomyolysis. It is often asymptomatic but may cause muscular weakness and paralysis. Characteristic ECG changes occur and are often swiftly followed by potentially fatal cardiac arrythmias. Metabolic acidosis is common and will exacerebate hyperkalaemia.

(c) Plasma calcium and phosphate. Hypocalcaemia and hyperphosphataemia occur early in acute renal failure. They are asymptomatic unless calcium falls sufficiently to cause tetany and fits. Hypercalcaemia may suggest multiple myeloma, and skeletal X-rays, bone marrow and protein electrophoresis should be performed.

(d) Other investigations. In rhabdomyolysis there are high levels of plasma creatine phosphokinase, with marked hypocalcaemia and hyperphosphataemia. Plasma creatinine levels are often disproportionately increased to the plasma urea.

Liver function should be checked and serum amylase measured to exclude pancreatitis. Echocardiography should be performed to look for evidence of cardiac disease and endocarditis. The presence of haematuria and proteinuria on testing the urine may indicate glomerular disease. Serum complement, immunoglobulin levels, and titres of antibodies directed against double-stranded DNA (SLE), glomerular basement membrane (Goodpasture's syndrome) and neutrophil cytoplasm (Wegener's granulamatosis, arteritis) should be measured.

Sepsis must be excluded by taking blood, urine and other body fluid samples for culture. If aminoglycosides have been used, levels must be measured.

2 Radiology

The investigation of choice is ultrasonography to assess renal size and exclude obstruction. There is no role for intravenous pyelography, which is uninformative and nephrotoxic.

3 Renal biopsy

This is an important investigation as renal causes of acute renal failure are often missed until too late. Any patient with acute renal failure in whom the diagnosis is not clear-cut should have a kidney biopsied.

Management

If renal failure is not yet established, then any underlying cause must be treated and factors compromising renal function corrected.

1 Treatment of reduced renal blood flow

Oliguria may be reversed by the rapid restoration of the circulating volume by colloid or blood, with central venous or pulmonary capillary wedge pressure monitoring.

Certain drugs are used to improve renal blood flow. Dopamine in low dosage (2–3 μg/kg/minute IV) causes renal vasodilatation and often increases urine output. This may help reverse renal ischaemia and allow tubular damage to recover. Frusemide is also used to increase renal blood flow and urine output, often in combination with dopamine. Large doses are required and its exact mechanism of action is uncertain. Failure to respond within 24 hours usually indicates established renal failure, and the drug should be discontinued to avoid causing ototoxicity. Mannitol has no advantages over frusemide and can cause pulmonary oedema and haemolysis.

2 Treatment of underlying disease

Any underlying disorder causing renal failure must be treated appropriately to hasten renal recovery. Nephrotoxic drugs should be discontinued and sepsis treated aggressively.

3 Treatment of established renal failure (dialysis)

Once preventative measures have failed, renal failure must be treated with dialysis. Often patients have multiorgan failure and require full intensive care support.

Studies have shown that early and frequent dialysis improves patient survival. Indications for dialysis depend on the level of catabolism and the clinical situation, but include:

(a) plasma potassium above 6.0 mmol/l;

(b) plasma urea above 30 mmol/l, creatinine above 500 μmol/l;

(c) severe acidosis;

(d) fluid overload;

(e) need for parenteral nutrition.

Haemodialysis is the method of choice with better clearance and control of hypercatabolic states. Improved techniques, including the use of bicarbonate rather than acetate dialysis, enable most patients to tolerate the haemodynamic disturbance. An important development has been the use of continuous arteriovenous haemofiltration.

Patients in acute renal failure often require large volumes of fluid in the form of parenteral nutrition, blood products and drugs. Until recently this was only possible by removing fluid on dialysis and was often poorly tolerated. The use of continuous haemofiltration allows fluid to be easily removed and replaced between dialysis sessions. Satisfactory access, such as an arteriovenous shunt, is essential, and anticoagulation must be kept to a minimum to avoid bleeding.

Peritoneal dialysis is often not possible owing to recent intra-abdominal surgery, and is complicated by leaks and peritonitis. It is usually reserved for situations where haemodialysis is unavailable.

4 General care

Patients require high levels of medical and nursing care. Fluid balance must be carefully monitored and regular laboratory investigations carried out. Adequate nutrition and calories are essential to control catabolism, and can be given enterally or parenterally. Patients need 2000–4000 calories daily, as well as essential vitamins and trace elements. Hypophosphataemia often occurs and must be corrected.

Complications

Renal failure can often be successfully treated with dialysis until renal recovery occurs. However, complications are common and account for the high mortality.

1 Hyperkalaemia

Catabolic patients are especially at risk of hyperkalaemia, and so plasma potassium levels should be regularly checked during each day. Care should be taken that potassium is not given inadvertently in feeding regimes. Hyperkalaemia is an indication for urgent dialysis and should not be treated by conservative measures such as ion-exchange resins.

2 Fluid overload

This is a common complication resulting in pulmonary oedema. Fluid must be removed urgently using dialysis and ultrafiltration, or continuous haemofiltration.

3 Sepsis

This is the commonest cause of death in acute renal failure and must be suspected with any sudden deterioration in a patient's condition. Cultures should be taken and broad-spectrum antibiotics started without delay. In-dwelling lines should be changed and cultured. Atypical bacterial and fungal infections should be considered.

4 Gastrointestinal haemorrhage

In the past this was a common cause of mortality which has been greatly reduced with the use of prophylactic H_2 receptor antagonists and antacids.

5 Clotting disorders

These often require correction using fresh-frozen plasma and platelet transfusions. DDAVP may be used during bleeding to increase circulating levels of factor VIII.

6 Cardiovascular and respiratory complications

These include myocardial infarction, cardiac arrhythmias and tamponade, cardiac and respiratory failure.

7 Drugs in acute renal failure

Many drugs excreted by the kidney must be given in reduced dosage in renal failure. The pharmacokinetics of these drugs must be checked and, if possible, levels measured. Drugs precipitating renal failure or known to reduce renal blood flow should be avoided. A useful table on prescribing in renal impairment can be found in the British National Formulary.

Clinical course

In acute tubular necrosis the duration of oliguria varies from a few hours to weeks or even months, with an average of 10–14 days. Failure to recover may suggest continuing renal hypoperfusion, acute cortical necrosis or undiagnosed intrinsic renal disease. As renal recovery occurs there may be a diuresis and hypovolaemia must be avoided. Renal function may continue to improve for weeks and usually patients regain function comparable with normal health. In acute cortical necrosis most patients are left with severe renal impairment or require long-term dialysis.

The clinical course of acute renal failure resulting from 'renal causes' depends on the underlying disease and its response to treatment. Often patient survival depends on the incidence of complications such as sepsis.

Prognosis

Despite improvements in medical care, acute renal failure still has a 50 per cent mortality. This is partially attributable to an increase in the age of patients and the incidence of multi-organ failure. Although there are no reliable prognostic indicators, patients who develop renal failure from surgical causes or who have multi-organ failure tend to have a higher mortality, approaching 90 per cent.

Post-renal failure

Urinary tract obstruction is an important cause of acute renal failure and must always be excluded as it is often

Table 7.8 Causes of urinary tract obstruction

Intraluminal
Calculus
Papillary tissue (diabetes, analgesic abuse, sickle cell disease)
Blood clot
Tumour of renal pelvis, ureter, bladder

Intramural
Pelviureteric dysfunction (congenital, 10 per cent bilateral)
Ureterovesical dysfunction
Neurogenic bladder
Congenital bladder neck obstruction
Tumours
Infection-granuloma (tuberculosis, ureteritis cystica)
Stricture (radiation, calculus, gonococcal, after instrumentation)
Urethral valves

Pressure from outside
Pelviureteric compression (bands, aberrant vessels)
Tumours (retroperitoneal, colonic)
Inflammatory (Crohn's disease, diverticulitis, aortic aneurysm)
Retroperitoneal fibrosis
Accidental ligation of ureter
Prostatic obstruction
Tumours in pelvis (carcinoma cervix, uterus, prostate)
Phimosis

reversible. The obstruction may be partial or complete and can present as acute or chronic renal failure. This is a common disorder which has been found in 3.8 per cent of routine autopsies. It is more common in women between the ages of 20 and 60 years, and men over the age of 60.

Actiology

The cause may lie within the lumen or the wall, or may come from pressure outside the urinary tract (Table 7.8).

Renal calculi commonly occur in young men in their second and third decades, and they consist of calcium oxalate. Renal failure is more frequently due to intraluminal obstruction when there is a solitary kidney.

In children the commonest site of obstruction is at the pelviureteric junction owing to hypertrophy of longitudinal smooth muscle fibres. Causes of a neurogenic bladder may be congenital as in spina bifida, or acquired by trauma or multiple sclerosis.

The commonest cause of obstructive uropathy in females is pelvic malignancy, and in males over the age of 60 years benign and malignant disease of the prostate.

Retroperitoneal fibrosis occurs equally in both sexes between the ages of 7 and 85 years, but occurs predominantly if the fifth and sixth decades. The middle and lower third of the ureters are embedded in dense fibrous tissue and pulled towards the midline. The condition is pro-

gressive and may involve the aorta, vena cava and psoas muscles. The aetiology is unknown, but it may be associated with retroperitoneal lymphoma, aortic aneurysms, autoimmune disease and exposure to drugs such as practolol and methysergide.

Pathophysiology

In obstructive uropathy there is a progressive rise in intraluminal pressure and dilatation proximal to the site of obstruction. As the intraluminal pressure increases the glomerular filtration rate falls. The degree of renal damage depends on the duration and severity of the obstruction. Superimposed infection causes further damage.

Clinical features

These may be related to obstruction, the underlying cause or renal failure.

In acute obstruction loin pain is severe and fluctuating. In chronic obstruction there is discomfort in the loin exacerabated by the ingestion of large volumes of fluid and diuretic therapy. Complete bilateral obstruction, or unilateral obstruction with a single functioning kidney, causes anuria. In partial obstruction normal or increased volumes of urine are often passed. Enlarged kidneys may be palpable on abdominal examination. Rectal and vaginal examinations are essential.

Investigation

Obstruction must be excluded in any patient with unexplained renal failure. The most reliable and convenient method is ultrasonography.

Treatment

The aim is to relieve the obstruction and treat the underlying cause. The use of nephrostomies, ureteric stents and urinary catheters often allows relief of the obstruction and recovery of renal function prior to any definitive treatment. After relief of the obstruction there is often a diuresis, with heavy sodium losses which need replacing. The degree of renal recovery depends on the duration and severity of obstruction. Retroperitoneal fibrosis can be treated with corticosteroids or surgically by ureterolysis.

Chronic renal failure

This is defined as the progressive and irreversible impairment of renal function.

Endstage renal failure is a term used to describe the requirement for dialysis or transplantation, or death from chronic renal failure.

The incidence of endstage renal failure is approximately 100 new patients per million of the population each year in the UK, and is more common with increasing age. The incidence of chronic renal failure varies in different countries, being more common in the Third World.

Pathophysiology

As renal function declines there is a loss of functioning nephrons and a fall in glomerular filtration rate. Initially patients are asymptomatic with normal plasma biochemistry, owing to the considerable reserves in renal function. As the GFR falls below 50 ml/minute, biochemical abnormalities develop which only become symptomatic as the GFR falls below 30 ml/minute. Finally as the GFR falls to 10 ml/minute life-sustaining renal excretory and homeostatic functions fail and patients reach endstage renal failure.

The underlying cause of renal failure determines the primary mechanism of damage to the kidney. However, the subsequent loss of nephrons can cause hyperperfusion and hyperfiltration in the remaining intact nephrons. This causes progressive nephron destruction independent of the original cause and leads to glomerulosclerosis.

When the GFR falls to approximately 30 ml/minute the kidneys are unable to concentrate urine, causing polyuria, nocturia and thirst. This is more common in tubulointerstitial diseases such as pyelonephritis, interstitial nephritis and analgesic nephropathy. Further deterioration in renal function causes fluid overload with hypertension, peripheral and pulmonary oedema.

Body sodium balance is maintained as the renal function deteriorates by increasing the fraction of filtered sodium excreted. When the GFR falls below 10 ml/minute this mechanism is insufficient, causing an increase in body sodium and extracellular fluid volume. Patients can continue to excrete a normal intake of potassium until the GFR falls to 10 ml/minute. However, rapid hyperkalaemia may develop with a sudden reduction in residual GFR, excess dietary intake such as chocolate and fruit, and catabolic states including sepsis and surgery.

1 Urea and metabolites

As the GFR falls below 30 ml/minute there is a progressive rise in plasma levels of urea and creatinine. In advanced renal failure the rate of rise in plasma creatinine may fall owing to loss of muscle mass. In addition many other toxic metabolites accumulate owing to impaired excretion. These include sulphates, guanidines, uric acid, cAMP, amines from the gut, phenols, and a large number of unidentified substances with molecular weights between 500 and 5000 daltons. The role of many of these substances in chronic renal failure is unknown and they are not routinely measured.

2 Acid–base

Normally the kidney maintains acid–base haemostasis by reabsorption of filtered bicarbonate and excretion of hydrogen ions. Compensatory mechanisms prevent the development of acidosis until the GFR falls below 10–20 ml/minute. Then the net acid production exceeds the excretory capacity of the remaining nephrons, and impaired tubular function causes reduced bicarbonate regeneration and ammonia synthesis. Acidosis may occur earlier in renal disease involving the tubules and interstitium.

3 Calcium and phosphate

In chronic renal failure plasma calcium levels are determined by the secretion of parathyroid hormone and 1,25-dihydroxycholecalciferol. As the GFR falls below 30 ml/minute, hyperphosphataemia and hypocalcaemia develop.

4 Endocrine

The kidney secretes certain hormones, including erythropoietin and 1,25-dihydroxycholecalciferol as previously described. As the renal function deteriorates, production of these hormones falls, causing anaemia and renal osteodystrophy.

Causes of chronic renal failure

Nearly any disease that affects the kidney may cause chronic renal failure and only the most common are listed in Table 7.9. The frequency with which these disorders cause renal failure varies greatly, depending on patient age, sex and country of origin.

Clinical features

Chronic renal failure is an insidious disorder which, in up to 30 per cent of cases, presents late, with advanced renal failure. Early renal impairment is asymptomatic, but may be discovered because of the underlying cause or on routine investigation. Patients complain of polyuria, nocturia and thirst. Gastrointestinal symptoms such as

Table 7.9 Common causes of chronic renal failure

Glomerulonephritis
Chronic pyelonephritis
Adult polycystic kidney disease
Hypertension
Diabetes mellitus
Analgesic nephropathy
Amyloidosis
Obstruction
Multiple myeloma

anorexia, nausea and vomiting are common, and pruritis, malaise and lethargy are universal.

On examination patients are usually anaemic and pigmented and may exhibit the features of their underlying disease. Patients should be asked about urinary tract infections occurring in childhood and pregnancy, hypertension and urinary abnormalities at routine medical and employment examinations. A careful drug, environmental and family history should be obtained.

Investigations

1 Haematology

A normochromic, normocytic anaemia occurs early in most forms of chronic renal failure; patients with polycystic disease usually maintain their haemoglobin levels. Iron deficiency may be caused by the increased incidence of peptic ulceration and menorrhagia associated with chronic renal failure.

2 Biochemistry

In chronic renal failure there is a rise in plasma urea, creatinine, potassium, uric acid and phosphate as renal function deteriorates. A compensated metabolic acidosis develops, and the plasma calcium falls with a rise in plasma alkaline phosphatase owing to the development of renal bone disease. Hypercalcaemia may suggest multiple myeloma or primary hyperparathyroidism.

Rarely, metabolic disorders such as gout, oxalosis and cystinosis need to be considered as causes of renal failure.

3 Immunology

The presence of anti-double-stranded DNA, anti-neutrophil cytoplasmic and anti-glomerular basement membrane antibodies should be sought. Although SLE, polyarteritis and Goodpasture's syndrome usually present as acute renal failure, they can have a slower and more insidious course. Hypocomplementaemia is associated with SLE, mesangiocapillary glomerulonephritis and post-infectious nephritis. Paraprotein bands and hypogammaglobulinaemia are suggestive of myeloma.

4 Urine

The urine should be examined for blood, protein and casts.

5 Renal imaging

The renal size should be determined by ultrasonography. Small, shrunken kidneys are found in many renal disorders such as chronic glomerulonephritis. In diabetes mellitus and amyloid, the kidneys are of normal size. Ultrasound is also reliable in the diagnosis of polycystic kidney disease and chronic obstruction. Renal arteriography is indicated in the diagnosis of renal artery stenosis.

6 Renal biopsy

This is an important investigation provided the kidneys are of reasonable size and the diagnosis not obvious (e.g. in polycystic disease). A histological diagnosis may reveal a treatable disease, give prognostic information and indicate whether the disease may reoccur in the transplant. There is no point in biopsying small, shrunken kidneys as the procedure is uninformative and dangerous.

Treatment of chronic renal failure

The management of chronic renal failure should be directed as follows:

1 reversal of the underlying disease (e.g. immunosuppressive treatment for SLE);
2 management of associated hypertension, fluid overload and intercurrent infection;
3 reversal of glomerular hyperfiltration;
4 preparation for dialysis or transplantation;
5 treatment of complications of renal failure, such as renal bone disease, with 1-alphacalcidol.

There is good evidence in animals and emerging evidence in humans to show that the reduction of the raised intraglomerular pressure associated with the loss of nephrons in chronic renal failure reduces continuing glomerular damage. This may be achieved by a low-protein diet or possibly the use of certain anti-hypertensive agents such as captopril.

Management of endstage renal failure

Prior to the development of dialysis and transplantation, the treatment of patients with endstage renal failure was restricted to diet and fluid restriction, prolonging a miserable life for a short period of time.

Most patients with endstage renal failure are suitable for renal replacement therapy.

The three forms of treatment are haemodialysis,

continuous ambulatory peritoneal dialysis (CAPD), and transplantation. There is considerable variation between different countries and centres as to which of these treatments patients are likely to receive.

1 Haemodialysis

This depends on the passage of fluid and solutes across a semipermeable membrane such as Cuprophane. Patients should commence dialysis before they develop terminal uraemia, and early referral of patients with chronic renal failure allows them to be prepared psychologically, and to be provided with the necessary vascular access. There are various forms of vascular access.

(a) Arteriovenous Cimino fistula. This is the best form of access for long-term haemodialysis. A fistula is formed in the arm between a suitable artery and vein, which matures over three to four weeks. Blood flow exceeds 300 ml/minute, and during dialysis the fistula is cannulated with 13 to 16 gauge needles.

(b) Arteriovenous Scribner shunt. This was a commonly used form of access which is now reserved for acute dialysis. Teflon vessel tips are placed in an artery and adjacent vein. These are connected with silastic tubing which can be separated during dialysis. The disadvantage of this method are frequent thrombosis and infection.

(c) In-dwelling central venous cannulae. These are used temporarily in acute dialysis, or more permanently in patients where the formation of an arteriovenous fistula is impossible. The major complications are infection and thrombosis of the catheter, which frequently require it to be replaced.

In most patients haemodialysis is performed three times per week for 4–6 hours. The duration of dialysis is determined by the size of the patient, the dialyser used, the plasma biochemistry and the presence of any residual renal function. Patients may receive haemodialysis in a hospital dialysis unit or be trained to dialyse at home.

2 Peritoneal dialysis

The peritoneal membrane is semipermeable, and sterile dialysis fluid is infused via a special catheter into the peritoneal space. Solutes, water and metabolites diffuse across the peritoneal membrane and are removed when the dialysate is drained out.

The two treatment regimes in widespread use are CAPD and intermittent peritoneal dialysis. In CAPD, the catheter is flexible and has a Dacron cuff to reduce the incidence of infections and leaks. Patients quickly learn the technique and continue their daily life while fluid is present in the intraperitoneal space. This form of treatment offers greatest freedom with dietary and fluid intake, as well as less interruption of work and family life. The major complication is peritonitis. It is now established as an important form of treatment of endstage renal failure and is used as a holding therapy prior to transplantation.

3 Transplantation

The development of improved immunosuppression and medical care has resulted in renal transplantation becoming the treatment of choice in endstage renal failure. Experienced renal units are now able to achieve one-year patient and allograft survivals of 80 and 90 per cent respectively using cadaver allografts.

Patients with active infection or malignancy should not be transplanted as this may be exacerbated by immunosuppression. Transplantation may be performed at any age. Children under the age of five years are technically difficult to transplant. Patients over the age of 65 have a higher mortality and transplantation in this age group should be reserved for the very fit elderly patient.

Certain renal diseases recur in the transplanted kidney. These include anti-glomerular basement membrane disease and other forms of rapidly progressive glomerulonephritis, focal glomerulosclerosis, mesangiocapillary glomerulonephritis (types I and II), membranous nephropathy and IgA nephropathy. Most of these diseases recur slowly and do not preclude transplantation, but patients with rapidly progressive glomerulonephritis should only receive an allograft when their disease is quiescent.

Human leucocyte antigens (HLA) are responsible for the induction of the allograft rejection response. These antigens are products of genes on the short arm of chromosome 6. The most important antigens in transplantation are the class I (A, B, C) and class II (Dr). The combination of these antigens is referred to as the patient's tissue type. Knowledge of this is important in assessing potential donors, as allograft and patient survival is improved when the HLA antigens of the donor and recipient are similar. However, the benefit of matching HLA antigens has been reduced since the development of cyclosporin.

Before proceeding with a transplant, serum from the recipient is mixed with lymphocytes from the donor in a lymphocytotoxicity test. This procedure, referred to as the *crossmatch*, detects the presence of anti-HLA antibodies against the donor antigens. If a patient is transplanted across a positive crossmatch there is usually immediate destruction of the graft, called hyperacute rejection.

Cadaveric and live-related transplantation. Most renal

transplants are obtained from cadavers, but live related transplantation is still common in some centres where there are few cadaveric grafts available. It is important that the donor is well and has no pre-existing renal disease.

Immunosuppression. This is needed to modify the immune response and prevent graft loss from rejection. For many years prednisolone and azathioprine were the main immunosuppressive agents. However, the first-line treatment is now cyclosporin, usually in conjunction with prednisolone. This has significantly improved patient and allograft survival. Cyclosporin inhibits the proliferation of T helper lymphocytes and interleukin-2 production. Cyclosporin is nephrotoxic and therefore must be used with care.

Complications of transplantation

1 Rejection
This can be divided into hyperacute, acute and chronic rejection. Hyperacute rejection results from pre-existing anti-HLA antibodies causing immediate destruction of the allograft. This should not occur with a negative crossmatch. Acute rejection is most common in the first two weeks after transplantation but can occur over the following weeks. Chronic rejection occurs more than three months after transplantation and causes a progressive deterioration in graft function.

2 Infection
The most common sites of infection are in the urinary and respiratory tracts. They may result from bacterial, viral and protozoal infections. Bacterial causes are the most common in the early post-transplant period, while cytomegalovirus and pneumocystis carinii start to occur in the second month.

3 Malignancy
Immunosuppressed patients have a higher incidence of malignancy. Most common are skin tumours, lymphomas, and disease of the cervix, uterus, bladder, kidney, breast or colon. Growth of the tumour may decline after stopping immunosuppression.

4 Other complications
These include cyclosporin nephrotoxicity, obstruction and renal artery stenosis.

The kidneys in pregnancy

In pregnancy the glomerular filtration rate and renal blood flow are both increased owing to a combination of cardiovascular, fluid volume and endocrine changes. There is also dilatation of the calyces, renal pelvis and ureters and hypertrophy of ureteral smooth muscle.

Routine urinary screening has shown that 4–7% per cent of *pregnant women have a significant bacteriuria* (< 100 000 organisms/ml) although they may be symptomless. About 40 per cent of these will develop overt *urinary infection* as pregnancy progresses. Infection may be associated with an increased incidence of prematurity, toxaemia and foetal abnormalities.

Treatment. Asymptomatic bacteriuria or mild cystitis is treated with amoxycillin 250 mg orally three times daily for a week. If the patent is pencillin-sensitive or if resistant strains of *E. coli* are a local problem a short course of nitrofurantoin is probably safe. She should be observed for recurrence throughout the rest of her pregnancy.

Severely ill patients with pyelonephritis should be treated as quickly as possible as miscarriage is a risk. Dehydration should be avoided by infusion if necessary and cefuroxime or ampicillin i.v. (see Table 7.5) should be given for a few days. If the patient does not respond, a switch can be made to gentamicin (although this carries a theoretical risk of fetus ototoxicity). When the infection has been controlled oral treatment should be continued for a further ten days. It may be necessary to determine whether there is an obstructive lesion in the urinary tract and for this an ultrasound scan in invaluable.

Acute renal failure has markedly decreased during the last two decades with improvements in perinatal care and liberalized abortion laws. Common causes of acute renal failure include pre-eclampsia/eclampsia, ante-partum haemorrhage, prolonged intrauterine death, amniotic fluid embolism and (now less commonly) septic abortion. There is a high incidence of acute cortical necrosis, ranging from 5 to 30 per cent. Patients should receive haemodialysis, and renal recovery depends on the degree of cortical necrosis.

Pregnancy is rare in chronic renal failure, but some women have had successful pregnancies whilst on maintenance haemodialysis. There is a high risk of premature birth and retarded fetal growth. Women who receive renal transplants usually have restored ovulation and menstruation. Many transplanted women have had successful pregnancies, but there may be deterioration in graft function either during or after the pregnancy. There is also an increased risk of pre-eclampsia, urinary tract infection, premature birth and minor congenital abnormalities.

Further reading

Brenner, B.M. and Rector, F.L. (1981) *The Kidney*. W.B. Saunders, Philadelphia.

Weatherall, D.J., Ledingham, J.G. and Warrell, D.A. (1987) *The Oxford Textbook of Medicine*, 2nd edn. Oxford University Press.

8

Endocrine Disorders

Introduction

Endocrine secretions, acting in one sense as another nervous system, coordinate and control a wide variety of functions. As in the nervous system, positive and negative feedback are crucial, and this feedback is exerted either by hormones themselves or by the metabolic effects of hormones. Top-level control, in the hypothalamus, integrates both these forms of feedback and the signals related to the subject's environment, such as dark or light, sleep or wakening, stress and excitement. The network of endocrine control is also held together by influences between the different hormone 'channels', both at hypothalamic–pituitary level and at the periphery where hormones act. Table 8.1 outlines the principal control mechanisms of the pituitary gland.

The variety of levels at which modulation or feedback can occur deserves emphasis. Some hypothalamic factors act on tissue other than the pituitary; for example, LHRH influences the mood (a cerebral effect) and the uterus, and somatostatin occurs in high concentration in the islet cells of the pancreas and the wall of the gut. Pituitary hormones may act directly on tissue receptors (e.g. prolactin on milk-producing cells), on 'non-endocrine' tissues to release secondary 'hormones' (e.g. GH on the liver to release somatomedin), or on other endocrine glands (e.g. TSH on the thyroid). The hormones secreted by target glands in their turn activate receptors which usually elicit the cellular response through a mechanism involving a second messenger, in many cases cyclic-AMP, as shown in Fig. 8.1. The 'adrenergic' effects of thyroid hormones are a result of interaction at this sort of level, and it is likely that local factors such as prostaglandins also act here. Within the pancreatic islet the various cell types and their products, including insulin, glucagon and somatostatin, operate and interact as a functional metabolic unit.

The nervous and endocrine systems also share evolutionary origins in primitive chemical mediators, and even in man the borderline between the two systems is often academic. The 'posterior pituitary' hormones oxytocin and vasopressin (ADH, page 311) are synthesized in the hypothalamus and secreted down axons of the nerve fibres, to be released in the posterior lobe. Adrenaline at the nerve endings is a neurotransmitter; adrenaline released from the adrenal medulla is a hormone. Hormones of the gut and pancreas, responsive particularly to stimuli from the gut and to levels of various substrates in the blood, are strongly influenced by autonomic nervous signals and themselves influence the gastrointestinal response to the vagus nerve.

Thyroid disorders

Goitre

A goitre is an enlarged thyroid gland. If it occurs in the absence of thyrotoxicosis it is a *non-toxic* goitre. The term *simple goitre* is used for the diffuse non-toxic goitre that is not uncommon in adolescent girls; it usually resolves spontaneously. In the context of thyroid disease the word *toxic* means thyrotoxic, in other words a thyroid condition accompanied by the disorder of function known as thyrotoxicosis. This is defined and discussed in more detail below.

Iodine deficiency is a potent cause of non-toxic goitre, and goitre is or was endemic in certain areas where the levels of iodine in the drinking water are low or the iodine is diverted from the thyroid gland by pollutants, fluorine or other factors. Endemic goitre has been eliminated in many areas by iodination of table salt. For reasons unknown, endemic goitre is much more frequent in

Table 8.1 Anterior pituitary and hypothalamic hormones and factors

Anterior pituitary hormone		Hypothalamic hormone
ACTH (adrenocorticotrophic hormone) and, as byproducts, α and β liptrophins and MSH	released by	CRF (corticotrophin releasing factor); the negative feedback here is through cortisol
FSH (follicle stimulating hormone), which in the male stimulates spermatogenesis	released by	LHRH (LH and FSH releasing hormone, or LRH), a decapeptide; the negative feedback here is through gonadal hormones
LH (luteinizing hormone), which in the male stimulates interstitial Leydig cells to produce testosterone	released by	
GH (growth hormone, somatotrophin), which stimulates production of somatomedin (sulphation factor) by the liver	released by	GHRH (growth hormone releasing hormone), the dominant control
	inhibited by	GHRIH (growth hormone release inhibitory hormone, somatostatin) which also inhibits TSH release and several pancreatic hormones
TSH (thyroid stimulating hormone, thyrotrophin)	released by	TRH (thyrotrophin releasing hormone), a tripeptide, the dominant control
	inhibited by	GHRIH (and by the thyroid hormones)
Prolactin	inhibited by	Dopamine, the dominant control, thus allowing marked increase in prolactin secretion if control is 'impaired'
	released by	TRH; a prolactin releasing factor other than TRH may exist

women than men. The incorporation of iodine into thyroid hormone may also be blocked by anti-thyroid drugs, phenylbutazone, sulphonylureas or PAS (which are therefore goitrogens), or by congenital deficiencies of

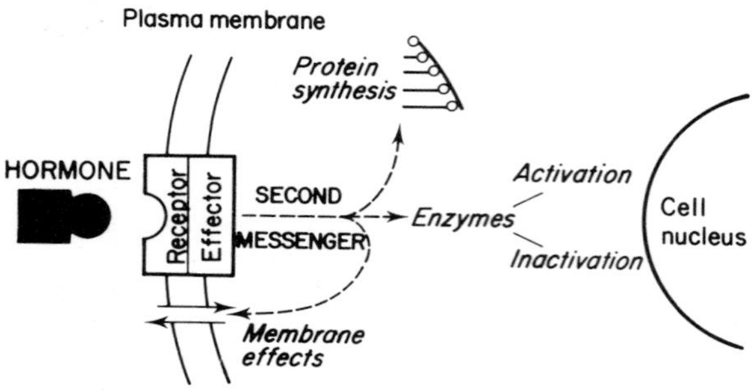

Figure 8.1 *Typical scheme of peptide hormone action. Note the many points at which the effect of the hormone could be modified.*

the enzymes involved in thyroid hormone synthesis, resulting in so-called *goitrous cretinism.*

Thyrotoxicosis

This is the clinical state associated with raised circulating levels of free tri-iodothyronine (T3) and usually thyroxine (T4). The metabolic rate is increased, and the patient's resting state may mirror that of an athlete after a run —hot, flushed, sweaty, with a fast pulse. In adults it is due to one of two disorders: either *Graves' disease*, which would classically be accompanied by a *diffuse toxic goitre;* or *toxic nodular goitre.*

Clinical features

1 Behaviour

There is nervousness and irritability; inability to relax or stay still and visible hyperkinesia; shaking and fine tremor; rarely, psychotic states. Conversely, in some older persons, there is apathy and depression.

2 Hypermetabolism

There is weight loss with increased appetite; warm, moist skin (with or without fever); and diminished tolerance of warm temperatures.

3 Muscles

There is general weakness and fatigue; muscle weakness and sometimes myopathy, especially of proximal muscles; dyspnoea on exertion.

4 Eyes

A staring appearance results as eyelid retraction widens the palpebral fissure. When the patient looks up and then down a rim of white sclera appears over the cornea (so-called 'lid-lag').

5 Bowels

Diarrhoea (increased frequency and/or looseness) is common; nausea and vomiting, but rarely.

6 Cardiovascular

There are palpitations, tachycardia persisting during sleep or occurring in paroxysms, and atrial fibrillation; angina and high-output state with flow murmurs, bounding pulse, and sometimes heart failure.

Osteoporosis or *myasthenia gravis* may occur.

Graves' disease

In this condition the goitre is usually diffuse and there are changes outside the thyroid gland which are *not* a direct consequence of elevated levels of T3 and T4, as if some unknown factor was acting both on the thyroid and on those other tissues. Many years ago it was shown that pituitary TSH was not the factor, and indeed the concentrations of TSH are suppressed to low or undetectable levels in all forms of thyrotoxicosis. The factor appears to be an IgG immunoglobulin, or a group of such immunoglobulins. The plasma of most patients with Graves' disease contains immunoglobulins, of which some stimulate *mouse* thyroid tissue at a slow rate in the TSH bioassay system (LATS, long-acting thyroid stimulator), some fail to stimulate but share binding properties with LATS (LATS-protector), some bind specifically to *human* thyroid membranes and can be displaced by TSH (TDA, thyrotrophin-displacing activity), and some activate adenylate cyclase in *human* thyroid preparations (HTS, human thyroid stimulator; TSI, thyroid-stimulating immunoglobulin). The values obtained by the various systems vary within the same plasma; this might be explained by the existence of a large variety of potentially stimulating immunoglobulins, some binding very

specifically to human receptors and some non-specifically (so as to include the mouse receptor), some being biologically active in activating the receptor and some not.

Features specific to Graves' disease

The disorder particularly affects women aged between 20 and 40, but the age range is wide and men are sometimes affected. One-third of patients remit spontaneously within one or two years.

The thyroid is diffusely enlarged (Fig. 8.2), but if the condition occurs in a previously lumpy gland (with previous non-toxic nodules) then one may find what is *clinically* a 'toxic nodular goitre'. It is important to distinguish this descriptive term, literally 'a clinically nodular goitre in a thyrotoxic patient', from the aetiologically distinct disorder described below.

A systolic bruit is sometimes audible over the gland.

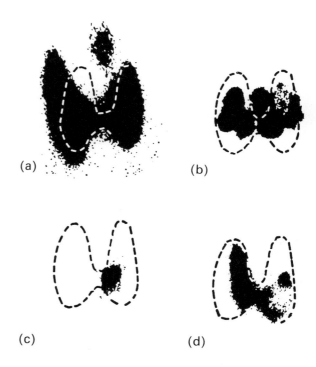

(a) (b) (c) (d)

Figure 8.2 *Typical thyroid isotope scans. The dashed line indicates the outline of a 'normal' thyroid gland, which is of course variable. (a) Graves' disease, diffuse toxic goitre with obviously active left pyramidal lobe. (b) Multinodular toxic goitre, with several adenomata (nodules). (c) Autonomous toxic nodule in left lobe, suppressing the remainder of the gland. (d) 'Cold nodule' —the white area of low uptake within the left lobe. As 10 per cent are malignant lesions, surgery is indicated unless an ultrasonic scan suggests that it is cystic and needle aspiration of the cyst confirms its benign nature.*

Exophthalmos (protrusion of the eyeball) may aggravate the staring appearance associated with both forms of thyrotoxicosis. Infiltration of the extraocular muscles may occur, with consequent diplopia and/or paralysis of upward gaze. In severe cases, conjunctival irritation, chemosis (inflammation of the eyelids) and even corneal ulceration may occur. *Malignant exophthalmos* is the progression of these changes to a condition of raised intraocular pressure, with pain, fall in visual acuity and a risk of permanent damage to the optic nerve. Guanethidine eye drops and systemic steroids at high doses may reduce the intraocular pressure; but if sight is seriously threatened then surgical decompression may be

necessary. In *ophthalmic Graves' disease* the eye changes occur in the absence of thyrotoxicosis, levels of T4 and T3 being normal. About half these patients progress eventually to thyrotoxicosis.

Pretibial myxoedema (mucopolysaccharide infiltration under the skin of the shin) and *thyroid acropachy* (a form of finger clubbing which is secondary to periosteal new bone formation and soft tissue thickening) are rare but pathognomonic signs of Graves' disease.

Toxic nodular goitre

A disorder which is essentially 'local' in origin, the toxic nodule is an actively secreting thyroid adenoma which

Table 8.2 Thyroid function tests*

Abbreviation	What does it measure?	Normal range	Comment
FT4	Free unbound T4	8–22 pmol/l	Low in hypothyroidism
FT3	Free unbound T3	3–10 pmol/l	High in thyrotoxicosis
T4	Total T4 including bound T4	70–190 nmol/l	Increased by increased TBG[†]
T3 (RIA)	Total triiodothyronine, by radio-immunoassay	1.2–3.0 nmol/l	Particularly valuable in diagnosing thyrotoxicosis (T4 may be normal)
TBG	Thyroid binding globulin	12–28 µg/ml	See footnote[†]
T3 resin uptake	Binding sites on TBG occupied by T3 or T4[†]	90–120% of normal	Decreased by increased TBG[†]
FTI	Free thyroxine as an index, 'T4 × T3 resin'	70–180 nmol/l	Not significantly affected by TBG; correlates with free unbound T4[†]
ETR	Effective (i.e. free) thyroid ratio: T4 available in the presence of the patient's plasma	90–110% of normal	*In vitro* test—gives same information as FTI but in one test
TSH	Hypothalamic–pituitary function, or the degree of suppression by T4 and T3 secreted autonomously	Approx. 1–3 mU/l (varies with assay) (see Fig. 8.3)	Low in pituitary failure; high in 1° hypothyroidism; response to TRH 200 µg increased in 1° hypothyroidism, suppressed in thyrotoxicosis, diminished in hypopituitarism
Scan (^{99}Tc or ^{131}I)	Localization of trapping of I (if ^{131}I, also rate of total uptake)	Symmetrical, each lobe approx. 2.5 cm × 4.0 cm (see Fig. 8.2)	May suggest size and location (e.g. retrosternal) of gland, or nature of disease

*This is a selection of the most useful tests of thyroid function. Tests now superseded by improved methods, or appropriate only in very special circumstances, are omitted from this list.

[†]Both thyroxine (T4) and triiodothyronine (T3) are largely in bound form in the plasma, the main carrier protein being 'thyroid binding globulin' (TBG). The *total* concentration of T4 and T3 is therefore increased when the TBG level is increased (as during pregnancy and treatment with oestrogens), and decreased when TBG is decreased. The physiologically important levels are those of the *free* unbound hormones (FT4, FT3) but these are more difficult to measure directly. The T3 resin uptake is valuable in overcoming this difficulty because the test actually 'reads' the number of binding sites on the patient's TBG which are *not* occupied by T4, or T3; the *more* such *unoccupied* sites there are, the *lower* the 'reading' of thyroid hormone concentration. With an *increase* in the number of *unoccupied* binding sites, the T3 resin uptake will give a falsely *low* estimate of the effective free concentration of thyroid hormones. The free thyroxine index (FTI), a product of T4 × T3 resin uptake, combines the bias in each direction to produce a reading that is less affected by the TBG concentration than either measurement alone.

Notes on drug interference with test results:
By displacement of T4 and T3 from TBG, salicylates and other non-steroidal anti-inflammatory drugs may lower total T4 and T3 while free levels—and the TSH—remain normal. Phenytoin may also have this effect but additionally shares with phenobarbitone a hepatic enzyme induction which increases the rate of clearance of T4; the TSH may rise slightly and those with limited thyroid reserve may be made hypothyroid. Amiodarone and lithium may also cause hypothyroidism.

has become autonomous (independent of control by the pituitary). Early in its development the levels of T4 and T3 will be normal but not influenced by changes in circulating TSH. The patient usually presents when T4 and T3 are elevated, with features of thyrotoxicosis, and by this time the TSH levels are suppressed by the high thyroid hormone concentrations, with a consequent 'suppression' of the normal thyroid tissue around the adenoma (see Fig. 8.2). On palpation, such a thyroid gland may feel lumpy, one or more nodules enlarging part or parts of the gland. The nodule may be immersed in the gland and any goitre may seem clinically 'diffuse'.

Because this form of thyrotoxicosis affects an older age group than Graves' disease, and the eye signs are less noticeable, its presentation is often more subtle. Thus many older patients present with cardiac or bowel symptoms, unexplained weight loss, or myopathy, and they may be lethargic or depressed rather than overactive and anxious (*apathetic thyrotoxicosis*).

Investigation and diagnosis of thyrotoxicosis

Tests of thyroid function are summarized in Table 8.2. The serum T3 (tri-iodothyronine, not the resin uptake) is a more reliable index than T4 in diagnosing thyrotoxicosis because the T4 is normal in some patients with thyrotoxicosis. Suppression of TSH, measured before and after injection of TRH (see Fig. 8.3), is the most sensitive indicator of excessive or autonomous thyroid activity; but the test will only be necessary in borderline cases, particularly as more sensitive and precise measurements of basal TSH become widely available. Over-secretion of TSH by pituitary tumours is extremely rare.

Treatment of thyrotoxicosis

The fact that Graves' disease may remit spontaneously, and that in this condition surgical or radio-iodine therapy which restores normal thyroid function is accompanied by the later emergence of hypothyroidism in about 3 per cent of patients per year of follow-up, argues for a trial of drug therapy in such patients. In contrast, the toxic 'hot nodule' will not remit spontaneously and so merits definitive treatment as soon as convenient. Having temporarily suppressed any iodine uptake by the normal thyroid tissue, a hot nodule will take up virtually the whole of a dose of therapeutic radio-iodine, leaving the normal thyroid to resume normal function. But these comments and the following are in the nature of general guidance, the actual choice of treatment being tailored to the clinical state, age and circumstances of each patient.

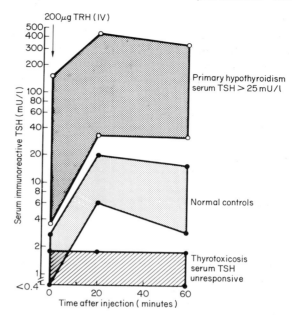

Figure 8.3 *The TRH stimulation test: an illustrative range of responses. Exact values vary with the assay with sensitive methods the lower limit for normal controls is around 1 mU/l.*

1 Surgery (thyroidectomy)

This is appropriate in these situations:
  (a) significant possibility of carcinoma;
  (b) very large goitres;
  (c) pressure symptoms whatever the apparent size of the goitre (e.g. deviation or compression of the trachea, or dysphagia);
  (d) alternative methods of treatment refused or impossible (e.g. allergies to anti-thyroid drugs, or radio-iodine contraindicated).

Patients must be rendered euthyroid by carbimazole and iodine aqueous solution (Lugol's iodine) before operation, and the use of propanolol considered.

2 Radio-iodine

In most cases this is the standard method of definitive therapy, either at the time of diagnosis or after an appropriate trial of anti-thyroid drugs. The full effect of the radiation will not be seen for several months, during which time anti-thyroid drugs should be prescribed. It is contraindicated in patients who are, or may be, pregnant and those in younger age groups. Although the theoretically increased risk of subsequent thyroid cancer has not been substantiated, there are some who argue against applying radiation to fertile subjects.

3 Anti-thyroid drugs

The drugs in common use are carbimazole (40 mg daily, reducing to 5–15 mg daily) and propylthiouracil (100 mg q.d.s., reducing to 50 mg daily). Carbimazole is the less toxic but even so causes skin rashes in 3 per cent, neutropenia in 1–2 per cent and agranulocytosis in about 0.5 per cent of cases. Several weeks will elapse before the clinical improvement is complete. At the end of one or two years of treatment of Graves' thyrotoxicosis the drug may be discontinued and the TSH response to TRH measured (Fig. 8.3). If this is normal then remission has probably occurred and no further treatment is necessary, but prolonged follow-up is advisable.

4 Propranolol

This acts peripherally to relieve those toxic symptoms due to sympathetic overactivity. Although the levels of T3 are slightly diminished, the blocking effect is largely independent of thyroid hormone concentrations. It may be of special value in three situations:

(a) for rapid control of cardiac effects of T4 and T3;
(b) for symptomatic relief while investigations proceed;
(c) for rapid preparation of the thyrotoxic patient and the thyrotoxic gland for thyroidectomy, as a fast-acting supplement to iodine aqueous solution and carbimazole.

5 Thyroxine

At a dose of 0.1–0.2 mg daily this is sometimes prescribed during or after anti-thyroid treatments to protect the patient from iatrogenic hypothroidism. It will always be required where an ablative dose of radio-iodine is employed as standard therapy for Graves' disease.

Treatment of thyrotoxicosis in pregnancy is best managed with carbimazole, using the minimum dose which will keep the Free Thyroxine or Free Thyroxine Index (Table 8.2) just inside the normal range. The baby may be born with maternal thyroid stimulator in the circulation, causing *neonatal thyrotoxicosis*; this needs immediate and careful control by those with special experience, so delivery should be arranged in an appropriate centre. As carbimazole is excreted in breast milk, the baby must not be breast-fed.

Thyroid crisis

Also known as thyroid 'storm', this consists of an acute exacerbation of thyrotoxicity, with especially marked hyperpyrexia and tachycardia. It can occur after thyroid surgery (or occasionally radio-iodine therapy) but is rare since patients have been rendered scrupulously euthyroid before surgery. Treatment may include physical cooling (*not* aspirin which may unbind even more T3 and T4), iodine aqueous solution, carbimazole, propranolol and hydrocortisone.

Thyroiditis

Autoimmune thyroiditis (Hashimoto's disease)

A diffuse firm goitre develops, usually insidiously but sometimes in a subacute manner with pain and tenderness, characteristically in a middle-aged woman. Lymphocytic infiltration of the gland and auto-antibodies to thyroglobulin and thyroid microsomes are to be expected. Early in the disease mild thyrotoxicosis may transiently occur, but 20 per cent present with, and many more progress to, overt hypothyroidism. Other autoimmune disorders may be associated with this disease and with those cases of Graves' disease and 'primary' myxoedema who exhibit thyroid auto-antibodies.

Subacute thyroiditis (De Quervain's disease)

Although mild cases occur, the thyroid generally becomes acutely enlarged, firm, tender and painful, in a patient who is unwell and feverish. Transient hypothyroidism may be noted. There is often a history of recent respiratory infection, and the aetiology is thought to be viral. If the symptoms are not relieved by simple anti-inflammatory analgesics, prednisolone or low-dose radiotherapy may be necessary. Rarely thyroid abscess can mimic this disorder.

Woody thyroiditis (Riedel's disease)

The thyroid gland becomes hard as a result of intensive and locally invasive fibrosis (analogous to retroperitoneal fibrosis). It is rare, non-metastatic and can only be treated by resection. Thyroid function may be normal or, in the advanced case, slightly diminished.

Hypothyroidism

In the infant, thyroid deficiency produces *cretinism*, evident by slowing of growth, mental and physical retardation, a characteristic appearance and a hoarse cry. The adult form of the disease was first described by Sir William Gull in 1874; its name, *myxoedema*, derives from the mucoprotein thickening of subcutaneous tissue which is found in severe cases.

Clinical features

1 Myxoedema

As mentioned above, this is a boggy non-pitting oedema

which may be diffuse but is especially noticeable around the eyes and on the hands and feet.

2 Skin

This is cool, dry and coarse in texture, pale or faintly yellow in colour (aggravated by the anaemia which is often present). The hair is also dry, coarse and thin, with particular loss of the outer third of eyebrows.

3 Slowness

There is slowness of thought, of action, of speech, of relaxation of the muscle after a reflex has been elicited (particularly at the ankle). The pulse is slow and constipation may be a feature. The mental state may exhibit memory loss, dementia, depression or psychosis (so-called 'myxoedema madness').

4 Hypometabolism

There is poor appetite yet mild weight gain and diminished tolerance of the cold. Hypothermia may occur, even to the point of coma in a severe case.

5 Voice

This may become hoarse as the vocal cords thicken.

6 Cardiovascular

One-third of patients show systolic hypertension until treated. Some have angina and/or palpitations, which are not always relieved by treatment of the hypothyroidism; some are dyspnoeic on exertion; intermittent claudication has been reported. Pericardial and pleural effusions occur.

7 Menorrhagia

This is a common complaint.

Investigation and diagnosis

Tests of thyroid function are summarized in Table 8.2. Non-specific findings may include a normochromic normocytic or macrocytic anaemia, a raised plasma cholesterol, low-voltage waves on the ECG, flattening of the glucose tolerance curve, and elevation of muscle enzymes. In doubtful cases an elevated TSH may provide valuable confirmation of the diagnosis (see Fig. 8.3).

Hypothyroidism may be the result of the following:

1 Primary failure of the thyroid gland

Even in those without a convincing history of Hashimoto's disease there is a high frequency of thyroid auto-antibodies, suggesting an autoimmune aetiology. Defects in thyroidal enzymes, and thus thyroid hormone synthesis, occur; they are rare and are usually discovered in early childhood in the form of *goitrous cretinism*. The latter accompanied by congenital deafness constitutes *Pendred's syndrome*.

2 External factors affecting the thyroid

Previous treatment for thyrotoxicosis is the commonest single cause of hypothyroidism. Severe iodine deficiency within the thyroid, associated with trapping or blocking of iodine, is a rare cause, usually presenting with a goitre.

The anti-arrhythmic drug amiodarone lowers T3 and T4 levels by interference in thyroid hormone metabolism; rebound thyrotoxicosis may occur if the drug is stopped abruptly. Lithium and phenobarbitone may also cause hypothyroidism, while other drugs alter binding to TBG (see Table 8.2).

3 Secondary failure, due to low TSH levels

This usually occurs as part of a panhypopituitary state, which is discussed on page 310. TRH is a very potent stimulus to TSH secretion and a TSH response to TRH may persist even in the presence of a pituitary lesion; the hypothyroidism in such cases is presumed to reflect a low average level of pituitary drive.

Treatment

Whatever the cause of the hypothyroidism, most patients need to be treated by gradual restoration of normal thyroid hormone levels using oral thyroxine, commencing with $50\,\mu g$ daily increasing over several weeks to 150 or $200\,\mu g$, at which dose level most hormone activity may precipitate angina or left ventricular failure, especially in the old. The adequacy and effectiveness of treatment is best assessed on clinical grounds, and confirmed by finding the dose of thyroxine at which T4 and/or TSH levels in the normal range are restored. The patient must clearly understand the lifetime nature of the medication.

In external and secondary types of myxoedema the primary cause must be remedied where possible.

Myxoedema coma

Especially in the cold of winter, the hypothyroid condition of an elderly patient may progress to such a degree that bradycardia, shallow breathing, hypoxia, carbon dioxide retention, hypoglycaemia, hyponatraemia and hypothermia all contribute to a lapse into coma (see hypothermia, page 516). The patient is cold to the touch, with depression of central and peripheral body temperatures, *often below the range of the standard clinical thermometer*, so that the severity of the problem is not recognized. Over half the patients die, so care must be intensive but not hasty—vigorous rewarming must be avoided, the gentle action of warm blankets being safer. Rapid-acting rapidly metabolized liothyronine ($20\,\mu g$ 8-hourly) and hydrocortisone ($100\,mg$ 8-hourly) should be administered intravenously, and the ECG and body functions closely monitored. As for any patient in coma and in shock, or on the brink of it, the airway, oxygenation and circulation must be maintained by appropriate means.

Thyroid carcinomas

Papillary, follicular and anaplastic tumours arise in the follicular epithelium of the thyroid, whereas the medullary carcinoma has a quite distinct origin in the parafollicular or C cells.

Papillary carcinoma

This tumour is the most common thyroid malignancy, occurring in the second and third decades and in later life. The solitary nodule in the thyroid gland may be unobtrusive and asymptomatic, and the first clinical sign may be an enlargement of the local lymph nodes, by which time more extensive metastasis may have occurred. These tumours usually take up iodine but much less avidly than normal thyroid, so they appear as a 'cold' nodule on a thyroid scan (see Fig. 8.2) and solid or semi-solid on ultrasound examination. Any such nodule deserves excision: evidence of recent increase in size or of frank malignancy calls for total thyroidectomy and total excision of nodes or tissue involved. Some weeks later, if malignancy is confirmed, a large ablative dose of radio-iodine is administered, and a whole-body iodine scan is carried out. Tumour tissue (in the absence of the thyroid gland) now takes up the radio-iodine, both displaying the extent of any local or distant metastases and receiving treatment by irradiation. Because the tumours are TSH-responsive in their rate of growth, thyroxine is administered from this point onwards so as to completely suppress TSH secretion. At intervals of 3–6 months, the ablative and diagnostic radio-iodine scan is repeated, after a brief pause in the thyroxine suppression to allow TSH levels to rise and stimulate iodine uptake by any surviving thyroid tissue. Apart from these pauses, thyroxine should be continued for life.

Follicular carcinoma

Histologically and functionally this tumour is closest to normal thyroid tissue. It tends to metastasize through the blood stream earlier than the papillary form, so it may be first identified through its distant metastases or by the finding of a stony hard nodule, which becomes subsequently locally invasive. The uptake of iodine may be similar to that of the thyroid gland, or even excessive, with the production of thyrotoxicosis. Management is along the lines of that for papillary carcinoma.

Anaplastic carcinoma

The rapid painful enlargement of a 'cold' nodule may indicate the presence of this highly malignant form, which is fortunately less common than the related papillary and follicular carcinomas. Anaplastic tumours rarely concentrate radio-iodine, so following surgery consideration should be given to external radiotherapy. If there should be a recurrence, cytotoxic therapy may be useful.

Medullary carcinoma

This C-cell tumour, which accounts for between 5 and 10 per cent of all thyroid carcinomas, secretes calcitonin. Even so, it usually presents clinically as a malignant tumour of the thyroid, often with regional lymph-node involvement, sometimes with early extensive blood-borne metastases. The tumour carries a worse prognosis than papillary or follicular carcinomas, even if total thyroidectomy, neck dissection and radiotherapy are instituted promptly. It is therefore especially valuable to have high calcitonin levels, basal or stimulated by alcohol, as a 'marker' for the tumour. Furthermore, like many tissues thought to be of neural crest origin, these tumours often demonstrate avid uptake of meta-iodobenzyl guanidine (MIBG), the basis of an isotope scan. Although the scan has been documented principally as a diagnostic measure, its therapeutic potential is now being explored.

Medullary carcinoma may occur sporadically but it tends to be familial, with an autosomal dominant pattern. In the familial cases there is a particular association with *multiple endocrine adenomatosis* (MEA) *syndromes*, both MEA type II-A (with phaeochromocytoma and hyperparathyroidism) and MEA type II-B (with phaeochromocytoma and mucosal neuromas). Relatives of an affected patient should therefore be screened for raised calcitonin levels; if such an elevation is found and confirmed, total thyroidectomy is appropriate before the cancer becomes clinically overt.

Adrenal disorders

Cushing's syndrome

Excessive levels of glucocorticoids, if not the result of steroid treatment, arise from a disorder of the adrenal gland itself (about 20 per cent) or from an outside influence. The adrenal gland may harbour an adenoma or a carcinoma. The outside influence, which will induce adrenal hyperplasia, may take the form of an abnormally high level of ACTH from the pituitary—often driven by hypothalamic oversecretion of CRF (corticotrophin-releasing factor) or an ACTH-like peptide secreted by a non-pituitary tumour (*ectopic*). The disease that Harvey

Cushing described was that in which pituitary adenomas, usually small and basophilic, over-secrete ACTH.

Many of the clinical features of the syndrome reflect impaired protein synthesis or redistribution of fat.

Clinical features

1 Those related to the effects of cortisol

The face is typically plethoric and mooned as the skin gets thinner and adipose tissue rounds out the chin and cheeks; the supraclavicular notch may be filled, and posteriorly fat in the upper thoracid/lower cervical area produces the 'buffalo hump'. Obesity especially affects the trunk.

(a) Muscle. As wasting occurs the thin legs and arms contribute to the 'lemon-on-sticks' shape, and the patient suffers from fatigue and weakness, sometimes severe (steroid myopathy).

(b) Skin. This is thin and atrophic, so that purplish striae are seen.

(c) Vessels. Purpura, or easy bruising, is common. The blood pressure may be moderately raised. Polycythaemia may be a feature.

(d) Nervous system. Psychoses related to the condition are relieved as steroid levels return to normal.

(e) Bones. Osteoporosis leads to compression fractures of the vertebrae and thus spinal curvature, and pathological fractures of the ribs.

(f) Metabolic. Glucose tolerance is often impaired. The mineralocorticoid effects of cortisol and related compounds may result in a low serum potassium with alkalosis, but this is prominent only when very high levels of cortisol are circulating, and so more common in cases of ectopic ACTH production.

2 Androgenic effects (especially if an adrenal tumour is present)

In men there may be impotence, increasing baldness, and acne; in women, hirsutism (increased body and beard hair), recession of hair at the temples, menstrual irregularities or amenorrhoea, enlarged clitoris, and an increase in musculature.

3 Other effects

(a) Pituitary tumour. Most often this is a rather small basophil adenoma, which will produce no local signs.

(b) Adrenal tumour. Signs related to the tumour itself are unusual but an adenocarcinoma may metastasize.

(c) Ectopic tumour. At least 12 per cent of cases of adrenal hyperplasia are caused by secretion of an ACTH-like peptide by a tumour outside the pituitary. Typically the peptide level and therefore the adrenal output of cortisol is very high in such cases, the result being a severe Cushing's syndrome with hypokalaemic alkalosis and pigmentation. Oat-cell carcinoma of the bronchus, bronchial adenoma, carcinoid, thymic and pancreatic islet-cell tumours are especially associated with this picture. Anaemia rather than polycythaemia may then occur.

Investigation and diagnosis

Non-specific findings may include polycythaemia, a neutrophilia between 10 000 and 20 000, depressed lymphocyte and eosinophil counts, mild glucose in-

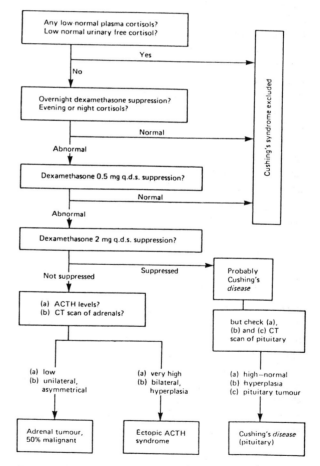

Figure 8.4 *Diagnostic flow-chart for suspected Cushing's syndrome.*

tolerance with or without a raised fasting blood glucose, and hypokalaemic alkalosis.

This is one of several endocrine disorders in which the diagnostic process divides into two quite separate phases: first, 'Is the hormonal function normal (physiological) or abnormal (autonomous)?' ... a *biochemical* question; second, 'Once an abnormality of function is proven, what is the source of abnormality?' ... a *pathological* and *anatomical* question. A basic scheme is shown in Fig. 8.4, the normal ranges are listed in Table 8.3, and specific tests are discussed below.

1 Plasma cortisol

This is often the most convenient measurement, and a low or low normal level virtually excludes Cushing's syndrome. The levels may be misleadingly high in the anxious or obese subject, or in patients with high levels of the carrier protein transcortin in the blood such as those who are on 'the pill' or pregnant. A useful screening test for outpatients requires blood samples at 9.00 a.m. and 6.00 p.m. on the first day and 9.00 a.m. on the second day; dexamethasone (2 mg) is taken by mouth at 11.00 p.m. on the first day. In Cushing's syndrome and in some stressed patients the normal diurnal variation is lost and the second 9.00 a.m. cortisol is not suppressed to less than 150 mmol/l as it should be in a normal subject. If the result of this study is not completely normal then further investigation is required.

2 Urinary free cortisol

This is unaffected by transcortin concentrations and accurately reflects the secretion rate of cortisol. It is diagnostically more precise than measurements of 17-hydroxycorticoids, and even more useful than plasma cortisol, provided the urine collection is accurately timed. It may be mildly elevated by illness or continued stress.

3 17-Oxogenic corticoids

These include not only cortisol but several precursors and a metabolite, cortilone. While it is a more sensitive test for abnormalities of steroid synthesis such as congenital adrenal hyperplasia (adrenogenital syndrome, p. 302), it is less generally useful because high levels occur in some

---

Table 8.3 Adrenal function tests

Plasma cortisol (nmol/l)

	09.00 h	*24.00 h*	*09.00 h after dexamethasone (2 mg) at 23.00 h of preceding evening*
Healthy non-stressed subjects	150–700	80–220	5–150
Cushing's syndrome	400–2400	400–2400	> 300

Response to tetracosactrin (Synacthen; 250 µg IM)

	0 min	*30 min*	*60 min*
Healthy non-stressed subjects	150–700	> 800	> 800
Adrenal insufficiency	30–150	30–400	30–400
Disuse atrophy (chronically low ACTH)	30–150	30–400	30–400

Response to insulin-induced hypoglycaemia: see Table 8.7

Plasma ACTH

Normal range 10–80 ng/l at 09.00 h
Less than 10 ng/l at 24.00 h

Urinary steroids (output per 24 hours)

	Male (normal)	*Female (normal)*	*Suppressed by dexamethasone (2 mg/day for 3–5 days)*
Free cortisol (nmol)	130–600	130–600	< 150
17-hydroxycorticoids (µmol)	11–45	11–30	< 9
17-oxogenic corticoids (µmol)	15–60	11–48	< 11
17-oxosteroids (µmol)	18–64	11–51	< 11
Pregnanetriol (µmol)	1–3	1–3	< 0.7

The normal ranges vary slightly between laboratories. The urinary output of steroids should be interpreted in the context of the patient's weight.

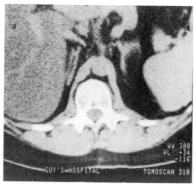
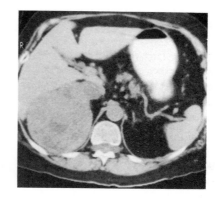

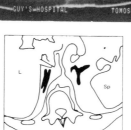
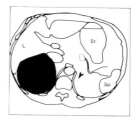

Figure 8.5 *CT scans of normal adrenal glands (on the left) and large adrenal tumour causing Cushing's syndrome (on the right). On the line diagram below each scan the adrenal tissue is shown by the solid black.*

hirsute patients with increased androgen production but normal cortisol levels.

4   17-Oxosteroids
These mainly reflect the androgenic steroid precursors. The latter are pathologically elevated in some patients with Cushing's syndrome, especially if associated with adrenal carcinoma when very high levels may occur, and in some patients with benign forms of hirsutism, including some with congenital adrenal hyperplasia (see page 302).

5   Dexamethasone suppression test
Urinary steroid excretion is suppressed in most normal or obese subjects by dexamethasone 0.5 mg q.d.s. and in most patients with adrenal hyperplasia due to pituitary ACTH by dexamethasone 2 mg q.d.s. (but not 0.5 mg q.d.s.); in most patients with adrenal tumours or an ectopic source of ACTH-like substance it cannot be suppressed even by the higher dose. However, the localization suggested by this test can be unreliable, and it is most useful in confirming the pathological nature of borderline hypercortisolism.

6   Plasma ACTH levels
These are depressed in the presence of adrenal carcinoma or adenoma, and modestly elevated in Cushing's syndrome of pituitary or hypothalamic origin. Most

ACTH assay systems give very high readings in most cases of *ectopic* peptide production.

7   Anatomical localization
Computerized tomographic (CT) scan of the suprarenal area will usually define the adrenal glands and/or an adrenal tumour (Fig. 8.5), while an isotope uptake adrenal scan employing labelled cholesterol will show the level of activity of one or both glands and/or tumour(s). The investigation of the adrenals may occasionally be taken further by arteriography or venography. *Bilateral* enlargement and active function favour hyperplasia secondary to an excess of ACTH, whereas *unilateral* 'suppression' as reflected by atrophy and loss of function, with marked enlargement and/or activity on the other side, suggest a primary adrenal tumour.

The search for the source of excess ACTH may require X-rays and CT scans of the pituitary gland and the chest, the latter because so many of the ectopic sources are bronchial or thymic. Selective venous sampling may suggest the source of the ACTH by the finding of an especially high concentration of ACTH in a particular vein. If the vein is draining from an area which includes a pituitary adenoma, then a preceding injection of CRF (corticotrophin-releasing factor) will markedly enhance the difference in ACTH concentrations compared with a simultaneous sample from a control vein.

Treatment

An adrenal tumour must be removed with the whole of the affected gland and the other gland must be carefully inspected. In the case of inoperable adrenal carcinoma, the excessive steroid synthesis may be controlled by the drug Mitotane, which is unfortunately too toxic to use in other situations. Any non-pituitary tumour secreting an ACTH-like peptide is resected.

When adrenal hyperplasia is secondary to pituitary overproduction of ACTH, the choice lies between pituitary ablation (by Yttrium implant or trans-sphenoidal hypophysectomy) and bilateral adrenalectomy with pituitary irradiation when indicated. The advantages of the latter approach are the immediate reduction in cortisol levels, the temporary maintenance of pituitary function and in particular fertility if that is appropriate, and the positive exclusion of an adrenal tumour. The disadvantage is the risk of developing *Nelson's syndrome* (in which an ACTH-secreting tumour of the pituitary produces generalized pigmentation and local signs of expansion) during the period before the pituitary gland is irradiated. Maintenance therapy with corticosteroids and other hormones will be necessary following some of these forms of treatment.

If eradication of tumour-producing ACTH is not possible, or the source of the ACTH cannot be identified, the drug Metopirone (metyrapone) may be valuable in diminishing cortisol synthesis. This will usually relieve symptoms but androgen levels will rise, a particular problem in female patients. The long-term objective is removal of the ACTH source.

Aldosteronism (Conn's syndrome)

In its *primary* form this is related to an adenoma or hyperplasia of the adrenal cortical zona glomerulosa, producing a raised level of aldosterone in plasma and urine and (to a variable degree) hypertension, low serum potassium, metabolic alkalosis, and thus polyuria, periodic paralysis and paraesthesias. The frequency of the condition is controversial, but between 1 and 5 per cent of hypertensive patients may have the condition. About 20 per cent of hypertensive patients exhibit low plasma renin, a result of suppression by high aldosterone in some and of unknown mechanisms in others. The condition is diagnosed by the finding of persisting high levels of aldosterone which cannot be suppressed by loading the patient with sodium, and low levels of renin which cannot be raised by sodium depletion. These tumours can be imaged by uptake of labelled cholesterol, but are often too small for a positive CT scan. In the future, MRI (magnetic resonance imaging) may prove helpful. Correction of hypertension and hypokalaemia may be initiated with spironolactone, but surgical excision of tumours is advised.

Aldosterone excess *secondary* to high renin and angiotensin levels is well documented in accelerated hypertension (see page 69), heart failure, cirrhosis of the liver, nephrotic syndrome, salt depletion and conditions of low blood volume.

Adrenal insufficiency (Addison's disease)

Atrophy of the glands occurs with prolonged administration of corticosteroids in pharmacological doses. Apart from this, the presence of auto-antibodies to adrenal tissue is the most common cause of deficient corticosteroid production. Tuberculous infiltration was once more common, and even now this aetiology may be betrayed by adrenal calcification and an appropriate history. Rare causes include carcinoma, various infiltrations, and haemorrhage in the gland in the course of meningococcal septicaemia (Waterhouse–Friderichsen syndrome, page 426). The circulating levels of ACTH are high in these conditions, which constitute true 'Addison's disease', but *secondary* adrenal insufficiency may occur with low ACTH levels in hypopituitary states (page 310). In patients with diminished adrenal reserve, *rifampicin* may cause insufficiency by induction of liver enzymes which increase the rate of metabolism of circulating cortisol and thus shorten its half-life.

Clinical features

1 Chronic insufficiency

Pigmentation is increased (an effect of ACTH), especially in skin creases, flexures, over the elbows and knuckles, in scars, on the gums and on the buccal mucosa.

Weakness, fatigue and lassitude will have been described and may be evident on examination.

Anorexia (apart from a specific craving for salt, which may be caused by the altered taste threshold in this disorder) is accompanied by weight loss and a decreased muscle mass. Nausea, vomiting and diarrhoea may also occur, and the patient may become clinically dehydrated.

A low blood pressure which falls further on standing may lead to dizziness and faintness.

Clinical features which, though important, occur less frequently, include the following: hypoglycaemia, hypothermia, vitiligo, hair loss, lymphadenopathy, asthma, rhinitis, and mental aberrations.

2 Acute insufficiency (Addisonian crisis)

This often occurs on a background of chronic deficiency, and it may therefore include any of the features described above, particularly severe hypotension, fever, profound weakness, nausea, vomiting and diarrhoea, progressing if untreated to coma. The coma may be complicated by hypoglycaemia or hypothermia. The precipitation of the crisis in a patient with chronic insufficiency may be provoked by some major stress (e.g. an infection, an accident, an operation), or by increased salt loss (e.g. in sweat).

Investigation and diagnosis

During the acute illness the patient is in danger of fatal collapse, so treatment should not be delayed. In the stress of any severe acute illness *other* than adrenal insufficiency the plasma corticosteroids will be elevated, so plasma cortisols on samples of blood taken on admission will confirm or refute the diagnosis of Addisonian crisis. The plasma ACTH, if available, indicates directly whether the condition is that of hypothalamic–pituitary failure or that of primary adrenal failure with consequent ACTH hypersecretion. The clinical clue to the level of ACTH is the degree of pigmentation, the pallor of chronic pituitary insufficiency contrasting with the 'tan' of chronic adrenal failure. It should be born in mind, however, that increased pigmentation may also occur in chronic renal failure, hepatic cirrhosis, malabsorption, haemochromatosis, collagen disorders, folate or B_{12} deficiency, acromegaly and chronic skin infestation.

If the situation is not acute, or if a loss of adrenal reserve rather than manifest insufficiency is suspected, the diagnostic tests fall into three groups:

1 Baseline measurements

Plasma cortisol or urinary free cortisol are persistently depressed in adrenal insufficiency (Table 8.3).

2 Response to ACTH

(For safety and convenience, in the form of the synthetic analogue tetracosactrin, Synacthen). This provides a test of adrenal function which is independent of the hypothalamic–pituitary axis. A normal response in the 'Synacthen test' indicates adequate function of adrenal cortical tissue. A poor response indicates *either* adrenal gland destruction *or* a state of disuse atrophy because ACTH secretion has been chronically low (e.g. hypopituitarism, or use of oral corticosteroid drugs). If the response is poor, a three-day course of intramuscular Synacthen-depot (2 mg daily) is followed by a second 60-minute Synacthen test. A marked improvement over the result of the first test suggests that disuse atrophy was the cause of the poor response; a persistently poor response points to primary adrenal disease.

3 Total response

If the adrenal gland is not primarily at fault, the response of the entire system, hypothalamus–(CRF)–pituitary–(ACTH)–adrenal–cortisol, can then be tested by inducing hypoglycaemia with soluble insulin (0.2 units/kg body weight intravenously). Hypoglycaemia should cause sharp rises in ACTH and plasma and urinary levels of cortisol. The 'Metopirone test' may precipitate acute adrenal crisis as it lowers cortisol levels even lower than they already are, and this method of testing the system should be avoided in cortisol-deficient patients.

Aldosterone secretion is usually reduced, as well as cortisol, and a considerable loss of sodium and water with shifts across cell membranes produces a low plasma sodium and chloride, a raised blood urea and often a high potassium, in a hypovolaemic patient. ADH secretion may be increased and aggravate the lowering of the plasma sodium. The blood sugar may be low.

Diagnostic procedures will include, where appropriate, a search for infective and neoplastic conditions which can destroy the adrenals. Only the autoimmune type of adrenal atrophy leaves adrenal medullary secretion intact, but it is not necessary to measure catecholamines in the average case.

Treatment

The acute Addisonian crisis requires immediate and generous infusion of normal saline and dextrose, to restore circulating volume and correct hypoglycaemia. Hydrocortisone sodium succinate (100 mg IV) is administered stat and 6-hourly or as required. Infections must be vigorously treated. The patient's blood pressure and salt–fluid status must be carefully followed.

The long-term treatment should be based on oral hydrocortisone (20–40 mg daily) and fludrocortisone (0.1–0.2 mg daily) to supplement the mineralocorticoid effect. In establishing the proper maintenance dose, these factors should apply: the patient's subjective response, the supine and erect blood pressure, the absence of oedema, plasma cortisol levels, and possibly the ACTH level. These patients are absolutely dependent on their steroid medication, which should be trebled in dose in the event of transient illness or stress and then gradually restored to normal levels. They must understand their condition and carry a card stating their situation, maintenance dose and procedure in the event of accident, and/or wear a Medic-Alert bracelet or necklace.

Virilization

This is the clinical state associated with excessive androgenic effect in the female. While commonly of adrenal or ovarian origin, an abnormal end-organ sensitivity to androgens may also be important in many patients. Hirsutism (increased body and facial hair) is marked, pubic hair becomes masculine in distribution, and recession of the hairline at the temples occurs. The voice becomes deep, muscles increase in size and the clitoris enlarges. In post-pubertal women there is amenorrhoea, reduced fertility and shrinkage of the breasts. This picture may be associated with:

1 *Adrenal tumours*, often with Cushingoid clinical features (see page 296); indicated by high levels of 17-oxosteroids in the urine, particularly if the tumour is an adrenal carcinoma, and high levels of free cortisol;
2 *Congenital adrenal hyperplasia* (see opposite);
3 *Arrhenoblastoma of the ovary* or *hilus cell tumours* (high plasma testosterone with normal urinary 17-oxosteroids).

Hirsutism with no major virilization, but often with menstrual irregularities and acne, is more common. Major causes include those of virilization and:

4 *Polycystic ovaries;*
5 *Mild androgen excess* (compensated partial enzyme defects along the pathways of synthesis of cortisol or oestrogens in the adrenal gland or ovary);
6 *Simple familial hirsutism* (diagnosed by family history) or *'constitutional'* hirsutism with no obvious cause. Certain races, families and individuals are naturally more hirsute than others, and the problem is often as much a cultural or social problem as it is hormonal.

Investigation and diagnosis

This is especially directed at the identification of patients with tumours. Both ACTH and the gonadotrophins stimulate the adrenal glands *and* the ovary to produce androgens, and in the absence of an obvious mass on examination (which will include a full gynaecological examination), localization of the source of the androgen can be difficult. Free testosterone is the most relevant hormone in this condition, but other specific androgens (such as androstenediol) are said to correlate highly with hirsutism, and sex hormone binding globulins (SHBG) levels are consistently low. 17-oxosteroids tend to be especially high in adrenal disorders. Ultrasound examination of the ovaries is usually required, and laparoscopy will be appropriate in doubtful cases.

Treatment

This is a condition in which it is particularly important to treat the patient and not just the 'disease'. Apart from those patients in whom a tumour can be identified and removed, the long-term response to treatment is generally disappointing. Tumours should be resected. Corticosteroids (for example, prednisolone 5 mg at night) and cyclical oestrogen therapy—separately or together—may be effective in reducing plasma testosterone levels. Cyproterone acetate, which blocks the effect of androgens on the androgen receptor, is used cyclically with low-dose oestrogens. Spironolactone has a similar action and may be effective when used with a combined 'pill'.

Congenital adrenal hyperplasia

In these disorders (adrenogenital syndromes) there are enzyme defects along the pathway of cortisol synthesis. In the absence of a feedback system the cortisol levels would fall markedly, but plasma cortisol is protected by a very efficient homeostatic mechanism, and indeed this hormone is the only major restraint on the secretion of CRF and hence ACTH. The result of the enzyme deficiency is therefore an increased ACTH drive, which has the effect of increasing the concentration of cortisol precursors 'proximal' to the 'block', so restoring towards normal the concentrations of substances 'distal' to the block (including cortisol itself). Some of the common levels of 'block' are illustrated in Fig. 8.6. In every case the accumulating precursor steroids have an androgenic effect overall, and in some syndromes potent mineralocorticoids are also formed in excess. While a common feature, valuable diagnostically, is the increased concentration of 17-OH-progesterone and hence urinary pregnanetriol, the presentation depends not only on the level of the 'block' but also on severity and age at presentation.

Clinical features

Typical clinical presentations include:

1 Perinatal and infantile. In the male, phallic enlargement and the 'infant Hercules' appearance (musculature over-developed). In the female, pseudohermaphroditism with genital abnormalities. In both sexes, early perfusion of epiphyses; adrenal insufficiency depends on severity of block.
2 Delayed female puberty, primary amenorrhoea.
3 C-21 hydroxylase partial block: high levels of 17-OH-

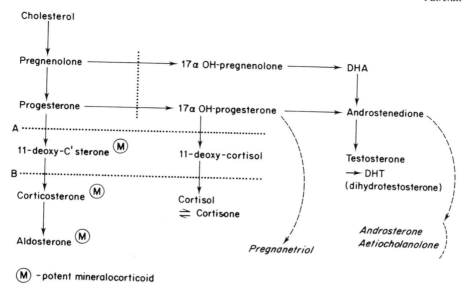

Figure 8.6 *Outline of adrenal steroid synthesis. The dotted lines indicate levels at which enzyme deficiencies may occur, acting as a block to synthesis and so causing accumulation of precursors 'above' the block. The upper horizontal line (A) indicates C-21 hydroxylase level; the lower (B) indicates C-11 hydroxylase level. The dashed lines indicate metabolites excreted in urine.*

progesterone etc. produce virilization, high levels of ACTH producing pigmentation.

4 C-11 hydroxylase partial block: as C-21 with the addition of hypertension, produced by high levels of 11-desoxycorticosterone (a potent mineralocorticoid).

5 Compensated enzyme deficiencies responsible for some cases of 'constitutional hirsutism'?

Treatment

Corticosteroids will abolish the excessive ACTH drive in these patients and restore normal androgen levels. If adrenal insufficiency is present this is treated as would be a case of Addison's disease (see page 300).

Phaeochromocytoma

This very rare tumour of the adrenal medulla is important as a curable cause of hypertension, and as a 'mimic' of anxiety neurosis, thyrotoxicosis and diabetes mellitus. About 10 per cent of the tumours are malignant and 10 per cent bilateral, and about the same proportion are associated with parathyroid adenomas or medullary carcinoma of the thyroid. The clinical features are related to the effects of excess adrenaline and/or noradrenaline.

Clinical features

Most patients are hypertensive and complain of headaches. The hypertension is usually constant, but there occurs sometimes a characteristic picture of paroxysmal hypertension, with concurrent headaches, nose bleeds, or pulmonary oedema. Palpitations with or without tachycardia are common. Increased perspiration is a frequent complaint. Tremor, weakness, weight loss, feeling of warmth, even psychosis, with an increased metabolic rate, may at first suggest thyrotoxicosis. Anorexia and constipation are not uncommon. Although few patients complain of postural symptoms, the blood pressure may drop sharply on standing.

Investigation and diagnosis

Tests currently in use include:

1 As a screening test: vanillyl-mandelic acid (VMA) in urine: normally less than 25 μmol in 24 hours (2.4 mmol/mol creatinine excreted); slightly higher in patients with hypertension, renal artery stenosis, or thyrotoxicosis, or those on tricyclic or related anti-depressant drugs; usually over 50 μmol in 24 hours (4.8 mmol/mol creatinine) in cases of phaeochromocytoma.

2 As definitive tests: adrenaline and noradrenaline in plasma and/or urine.

3 For localization (especially of second or secondary tumours): CT scans and isotope scans employing MIBG (meta-iodobenzyl guanidine).

Suppression and provocation tests, such as those

employing phentolamine or glucagon, are potentially dangerous and rarely indicated. Levels of blood glucose, free fatty acids and the haematocrit may be elevated. Calcium and calcitonin levels should be checked, to exclude parathyroid adenomas and medullary carcinoma of the thyroid.

Treatment

Radiological investigations and surgery should be preceded and covered by combined adrenergic blockade, anti-α (phenoxybenzamine by mouth or phentolamine intravenously) and anti-β (propranolol). During surgery both adrenal glands must be inspected. Following resection, precipitous falls in blood pressure may occur and rapid volume repletion and vasoconstrictor therapy may be necessary.

Reproductive hormone disorders

Menopause (female climacteric)

This can be regarded as physiological ovarian failure, leading to cessation of menstruation (menopause), sometimes preceded by menstrual irregularity. Episodes of 'hot flushes', with sweating and warmth, and symptoms of anxiety or depression may be prominent. LH and FSH levels are high. The psychological support of husband and physician is most important, with emphasis on the transient nature of the symptoms. If symptoms are severe then a combined or sequential low-dose preparation of oestrogen and a progestogen may be prescribed. Changes consequent upon the drop in oestrogen production include osteoporosis, which may become severe (see page 338), a rise in the risk of cardiovascular disease, a reduction in vaginal secretions (which may lead to vaginitis and dyspareunia), and some involution of the uterus and breasts.

Delayed puberty in the female

Regular menstruation normally commences between the ages of 10 and 16, with a mean of 12.9 years, the so-called *menarche*. The other major changes of puberty include breast development and nipple pigmentation, growth of pubic hair of increasingly coarse dark curled type, axillary hair growth, thickening of the vaginal epithelium and growth of the genitalia; the pelvis gradually becomes gynaecoid in shape and the subcutaneous fat assumes the typical female distribution. Delayed puberty may be physiological and/or familial, especially in the presence of

obesity. In *primary* ovarian failure the delay in fusion of the epiphyses eventually leads to overgrowth of the long bones, such that span exceeds height, and 'bone age' on X-ray may for a time be less than actual age.

Investigation and diagnosis

Any major disease, particularly thyroid disorders, diabetes, renal failure or chronic infection, may be contributory to such a delay. As discussed on page 302, the barrage of androgens secreted in congenital adrenal hyperplasia may impair female development. Beyond these possibilities, the main question is whether a primary ovarian defect or a failure of gonadotrophin secretion exists. If plasma and urinary FSH levels are low, the possible causes of hypopituitarism (see page 310) are pursued. Isolated gonadotrophin deficiency may be found, usually responsive to LHRH, suggesting that the basic problem may be LHRH failure; the line between such patients and 'late developers' is often indistinct and the initial treatment should be conservative. High levels of FSH are consistent with:

1 the first hint of puberty;
2 absence of ovaries, as in Turner's syndrome or testicular feminization;
3 damage to the ovaries by cysts, tumours, trauma, surgery or irradiation.

Turner's syndrome (gonadal dysgenesis)

The patients appear, act and think as women, but they have an XO or XO-mosaic karyotype and consequent dysgenesis of the testes. Having neither ovaries nor testes they develop into phenotypic females (as do all mammals lacking testosterone *in utero*, whatever their genetic sex). Secondary sexual characteristics and the normal menstrual cycle do not appear spontaneously.

They usually present as short women or girls, under 5 feet tall, who have failed to undergo sexual maturation. Numerous other clinical features occur but are variable in their expression, as might be expected from the variety of karyotypes found in the syndrome. The features may include; webbing of the neck, a short neck, increased carrying angle at the elbow (cubitus valgus), widely separated nipples, shield-like chest, coarctation of the aorta (20 per cent), abnormalities of the urinary tract (on investigation, 60 per cent), recurrent otitis media and sometimes deafness, lymphoedema (especially of the feet), hypoplastic nails and numerous pigmented naevi. Mild mental handicap with well-preserved verbal ability is not uncommon.

Ethinyloestradiol (0.02 mg daily) given cyclically with norethisterone (5 mg daily) on the last ten days of the cycle will induce menses and sexual characteristics without over-rapid fusion of the epiphyses. Higher doses of oestrogen will improve the rate of sexual development but may reduce the patient's final height.

Androgen resistance syndromes (testicular feminization)

Several syndromes exist but in the classical form most patients present as females, seeking medical advice because of primary amenorrhoea or infertility. They are genetic males with an XY karyotype, whose testes may be located in the abdomen, inguinal canal or 'labia'. Breasts and external genitalia are female in development with occasional slight enlargement of the clitoris, and only on investigation does it become apparent that the vagina ends blindly and there is no uterus. Testosterone production is normal in these patients, and the condition represents a diminished response to testosterone. There is diminished conversion of testosterone to the more active dihydrotestosterone and/or a deficiency of the appropriate receptors.

Amenorrhoea

The failure to initiate menstruation is termed by convention *primary* amenorrhoea and it is usually accompanied by the other deficiencies in sexual development discussed above ('delayed puberty in the female'). Mechanical factors obstructing menstrual flow may also require exclusion, and a gynaecological assessment is essential.

Secondary amenorrhoea implies the *cessation* of menstruation; the condition represents the end of a spectrum that runs from regular ovulatory menstruation, through regular menses that are often anovulatory, through irregular and/or infrequent cycles (*oligomenorrhoea*) that are all anovulatory, to amenorrhoea. Conditions that give rise to amenorrhoea may cause the lesser disorders in their early stages or milder forms. These various conditions are classified in Table 8.4.

Table 8.4 Scheme for main causes of secondary amenorrhoea

	Hormone lack	Hormone block
	DIMINISHED OR DISORDERED FUNCTION OF HYPOTHALAMUS AND/OR PITUITARY	HYPERPROLACTINAEMIA (see text for discussion)
Central	*Specific conditions*: Functional (any major physical or psychological stress) Anorexia neruosa Isolated LH, FSH deficiency Panhypopituitarism, idiopathic or secondary to … Pituitary tumour, trauma or infarct Pituitary irradiation or surgery	*Specific conditions*: Tumours, including Prolactinomas Drugs Hypothyroidsim Renal/hepatic failure, etc.
	Major hormonal findings: LH, FSH (basal, and/or after LHRH): low	*Major hormonal findings*: Prolactin, high LH, FSH: normal or slightly low
Peripheral	DIMINISHED FUNCTION OF OVARIES	EXCESS OF ANDROGENS OR THYROID HORMONES (see text regarding virilization and hirsutism)
	Specific conditions: Mild forms of ovarian dysgenesis or testicular feminisation (see text) Premature menopause (autoimmune?) Mumps oophoritis Ovarian irradiation or surgery	*Specific conditions*: Adrenal tumours Congenital adrenal hyperplasia Arrhenoblastoma of ovary Polycystic ovaries Thyrotoxicosis
	Major hormonal findings: OESTROGENS: LOW LH, FSH: HIGH	

Subfertility

The availability of new modes of investigation and successful treatment, both hormonal and surgical, has transformed this subject in recent years. Nevertheless, the enthusiasm of patients and doctors should be restrained, because a large proportion of couples who have failed to achieve conception after six months 'trying' will be successful without treatment within the following year or so. It is also important to confirm that 'trying' includes normal coitus of reasonable frequency, an assumption that proves to be untrue in a surprising number of cases.

In genuinely subfertile couples a reproductive problem of some sort will be found in 65–85 per cent of the women and about a third of the men, while in some a partial deficit is identified in both partners. The partners should be interviewed and examined independently in every instance. A cost-effective approach is then to:

1 follow any leads given by the history or physical signs;
2 check the sperm count on semen analysis;
3 establish the presence or absence of ovulation.

If a normal sperm count is confirmed and regular ovulation is occurring, further investigation should take place. This might include hysterosalpingography, laparoscopy, ovarian biopsy, and studies of 'mucous hostility' to the sperm (post-coital examination of the cervical mucus and *in vitro* studies).

Female subfertility

The occurrence of ovulation may be suggested by a history of transient mid-cycle ovarian pain, by a modest elevation of the basal body temperature during the luteal phase, by characteristic changes in the vaginal lining (hence 'serial smears') and the cervical mucus, or by more direct evidence of the hormonal changes illustrated in Fig. 8.7, such as a mid-luteal plasma progesterone exceeding 30 nmol/l. The absence of ovulation, or amenorrhoea, may be secondary to any of a large number of conditions, which have been listed under the heading of secondary amenorrhoea (see page 305). Prolactin is particularly important in subfertility, because even moderate elevation of prolactin may prevent ovulation or proper luteinization of the follicle.

Hyperprolactinaemia is corrected by removal of the cause, or use of bromocriptine, as discussed on page 310. Specific treatments of the other conditions listed are discussed in the relevant parts of the text. Ovulation may be provoked in some cases by the use of clomiphene, which blocks the oestrogen receptors of the hypothala-

mus, and induced in most cases by the programmed administration of human menopausal and human chorionic gonadotrophins or synthetic LHRH (LH- and FSH-releasing hormone).

Causes of female subfertility in the presence of ovulation include genital tract abnormalities such as blockage of the Fallopian tubes secondary to past or present infection, disease of the endometrium preventing implantation, and abnormalities of the cervical mucus or the sperm which impair penetration. Some of these are now treatable by specialist techniques.

Male subfertility

Although sperm counts as low as 10 million per millilitre have been associated with fertility, the normal range for fresh semen lies between 50 and 150 million per millilitre in at least 2 ml, of which at least 60 per cent of sperm are motile and normal in morphology. A low count (*oligospermia*) or total absence of motile sperm (*azoospermia*) may rarely be accompanied by impotence and signs of feminization, such as gynaecomastia and small soft testes, suggesting androgen deficiency or oestrogen excess. Usually the problem is confined to the germinal cells of the testis, and levels of testosterone and the oestrogens are within normal limits: a raised level of FSH is then a useful indicator of germinal cell failure or aplasia. Sometimes the process of spermatogenesis is normal but the delivery of sperm is obstructed by a lesion of the vas deferens, and this possibility needs consideration if the FSH level proves to be normal despite the occurrence of azoospermia. The more common specific causes to be considered are:

1 *With gynaecomastia*: Klinefelter's syndrome (described on page 308); testes damaged by trauma, surgery or irradiation or drugs; chronic liver disease (see page 187); androgen resistance syndromes (see page 305).
2 *Germinal cell failure or aplasia*: Idiopathic ('Sertoli cell only syndrome'); cryptorchidism (undescended testes); maturation arrest; mumps orchitis; cytotoxic drugs; varicocele; any chronic endocrine or debilitating disease.
3 *Hypothalamic/pituitary deficiency*: Hypogonadotrophic hypogonadism, either selectively (such as in Kallmann's syndrome, see below) or as one feature of panhypopituitarism.

Unless a particular hormonal deficiency can be identified and corrected, or a disorder such as obstruction of the vas or a varicocele put right surgically, treatment has little to offer. Traditional advice includes maintenance of a cool

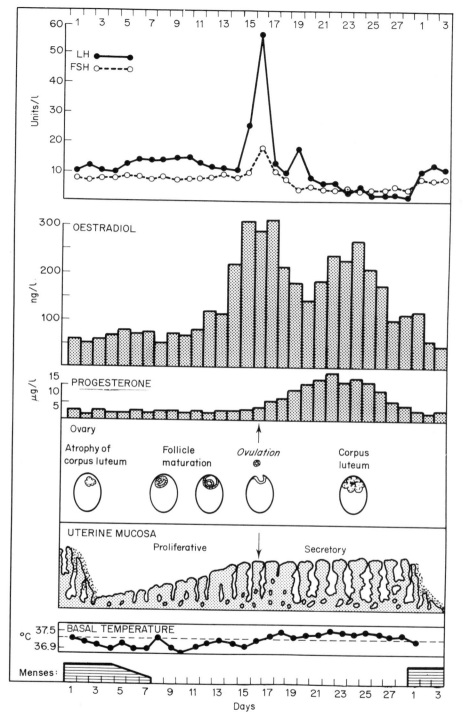

Figure 8.7 *Hormonal patterns during a normal menstrual cycle.*

scrotal environment, hence loose underwear and cold douches, and intermittent androgen therapy (such as mesterolone). Recent work supports the use of clomiphene for patients with the less severe degrees of oligospermia. The fertile effectiveness of a semen in which the sperm count is borderline can be enhanced by the use of artificial insemination, a fresh sample of the husband's semen being applied direct to or through the os of the uterine cervix (AIH), or *in vitro* fertilization of the ovum.

Delayed puberty in the male

In normal boys the earliest changes include enlargement of the testes and growth of coarse hairs in the pubic region. The scrotum develops rugal folds and darkens, the penis enlarges, axillary and then facial hair appears and the voice deepens. A mild degree of gynaecomastia is not uncommon. When the patient or his parents complain of 'delay' a family history of late puberty may be reassuring. In true gonadal failure the 'bone age' by X-ray falls behind actual age and—in the absence of epiphyseal fusion—the *eunuchoid* physique emerges, span exceeding height, ground to pubis exceeding pubis to crown.

Investigation and diagnosis

Any endocrine disorder or debilitating illness may delay puberty. When those are excluded, the diagnosis lies between a primary gonadal disease, with high levels of FSH and LH, and a hypothalamic–pituitary disorder, with low levels of gonadotrophins and bilaterally small soft testes (see hypopituitarism, page 310). An isolated deficiency of the hypothalamic factor LHRH may indicate *Kallmann's syndrome*; anosmia is a useful clue to the presence of this disorder.

The only cause of primary testicular failure to commonly affect puberty is *Klinefelter's syndrome*, in which very small firm testes are associated with variable degrees of eunuchoidism, gynaecomastia, impairment of intelligence, azoospermia, sterility and typically an XXY karyotype. Very rare versions of Turner's syndrome also occur in the phenotypic male.

Tumours of the testis or ovary

Tumours of the testes are rare (Table 8.5) but occur particularly in the 20–35 age group. If the tumour is

Table 8.5 Tumours of the testis

Type	Five-year mortality	Special features
Seminoma	10%	FSH frequently raised
Teratoma	30%	Spread by blood not lymph
Choriocarcinoma	100%	Raised HCG; gynaecomastia
Leydig cell (IC) tumours	± benign	Oestrogens or androgens

Table 8.6 Tumours of the ovary

Androgens secreted	Oestrogens secreted
Arrhenoblastoma Hilus cell tumour	Granulosa cell tumour Theca cell tumour Luteoma (and → progesterone) Teratoma, chorionepithelioma (and → HCG)

functional gonadotrophin secretion is suppressed and the other testis may be atrophied.

Most cysts and neoplasms of the ovary are non-secretory, but the tumours listed in Table 8.6 usually secrete hormones.

Pituitary hypersecretion

For discussions of hypersecretion of ACTH, ADH and prolactin refer to the appropriate page:

ACTH   page 296
ADH   page 313
prolactin   page 310

Tumours secreting TSH or gonadotrophins are exceedingly rare.

Growth hormone

The syndromes of growth hormone (GH) excess are usually related to an *eosinophil adenoma* of the pituitary, characteristically slow in growth and insidious in clinical presentation. Only in retrospect may it be realised that the disease has been active for 20 or more years before the patient presents.

Gigantism

This results from excessive GH effect before the epiphyses are fused, producing the features of acromegaly but in addition long limbs and abnormal height. The all-time record for height was held by a Robert Wadlow of Illinois, who died in 1940 at an authenticated height of 8 feet 11 inches; the better known case of Goliath is not well documented! These patients especially suffer from muscular weakness and arthritis. The total effects of the tumour may include hypothalamic irritation and so hyperphagia, and compression of the remaining pituitary and so hypogonadism.

Acromegaly

There are many clinical features of this disorder:

1. Headache; sometimes visual field defects, especially temporal; excessive tiredness.
2. Muscular aching; proximal muscle weakness.
3. Excessive sweating; skin thick, sebaceous, wrinkled.
4. Tingling in the fingers; carpal tunnel syndrome.
5. Progressive enlargement of hands and feet and head (perhaps noticed by change in size of gloves, shoes or hat); spadelike hands; soft and mushy grip; big feet; lips thick; nose bulbous; supraorbital ridges enlarged.
6. Dentures stop fitting; bite over-rides; teeth become separated as the mandible enlarges.
7. Arthritis and backache; kyphosis; enlarged vertebrae.
8. Loss of secondary sexual characteristics. In women: menstrual irregularities, amenorrhoea. In men: loss of libido, impotence.
9. Hoarseness of voice; larynx enlarges; vocal cords thicken.
10. A few patients have galactorrhoea, or uncinate fits, or rhinorrhoea.
11. Soft tissue enlargement may include thyroid (goitre), liver and spleen.
12. Excessive pigmentation is frequently present.

X-rays of the hands show increased soft-tissue thickness, tufting of the tips of the distal phalenges, increased width of phalanges and exostoses. Skull X-rays show an enlarged mandible, prominence of all the sinuses but notably the supraorbital, and in most cases enlargement of the sella. CT scan of the pituitary usually demonstrates the tumour (Fig. 8.8). The calcaneal skin pad may exceed 30 mm in thickness. Over 10 per cent of patients are frankly diabetic, and most have an impaired tolerance of glucose. Levels of GH in plasma are elevated even at rest and are not suppressed by oral glucose, the ultimate diagnostic test for this condition.

Treatment. Transphenoidal hypophysectomy, yttrium implantation and proton beam irradiation are effective treatments. Bromocriptine, and ergotamine derivatives with dopaminergic properties, will usually suppress high levels of GH, and are especially valuable for the occasional patient in whom pituitary 'ablation' fails to control the GH hypersecretion.

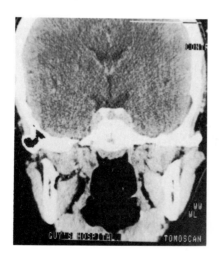

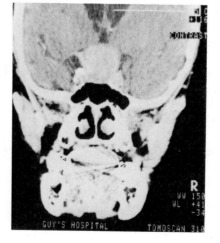

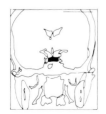

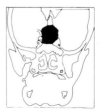

Figure 8.8 *CT scans of normal pituitary gland (on the left) and large non-functioning pituitary tumour (on the right). On the line diagram below each scan the pituitary tissue is shown by the solid black.*

Hyperprolactinaemia

The only effects of hyperprolactinaemia recognized as clinically important are: the stimulation of lactation, the inhibition of ovulation (with or without amenorrhoea), and the inhibition of spermatogenesis (with or without impotence). An elevated prolactin level may assume greater significance as a sign of some other pathology or disorder previously unsuspected:

1 Secretion of prolactin by a pituitary adenoma or micro-adenoma (e.g. a 'pure' *prolactinoma*, or an eosinophilic tumour also producing GH).
2 Interference by a tumour, trauma or inflammatory disease in the normal transmission of dopamine, the prolactin inhibitory hormone, between the hypothalamus and the pituitary, so 'releasing' the prolactin-secreting cells.
3 Pharmacological interference in the synthesis, release or activity of dopamine, with effects analogous to (2), by phenothiazines, methyldopa, reserpine, tricyclic antidepressants, opiates, oral contraceptives, chlordiazepoxide and perhaps diazepam.
4 Secretory response to increased levels of TRH, thyrotrophin-releasing hormone, such as occurs in the presence of hypothyroidism.
5 Prolactin levels raised by chronic renal failure, hyperparathyroidism or hepatic cirrhosis.

If the cause of the hyperprolactinaemia cannot be removed, corrected or identified, dopaminergic agents such as bromocriptine usually suppress prolactin levels to within the normal range.

Hypopituitary states

For purposes of discussion these can be classified as:

1 *Isolated hormone deficiencies* e.g. of TSH, ACTH or FSH. Pure growth hormone deficiency impairs growth in an otherwise normal person.
2 *Pituitary chromophobe adenoma* producing varying degrees of hypopituitarism and hypothalamic disorder.
3 *Panhypopituitarism*, juvenile and adult.

Pituitary chromophobe adenoma

Tumours of chromophobe histology often secrete prolactin and occasionally secrete ACTH (especially following adrenalectomy) or GH, but typically act as space-occupying lesions within the sella and then the brain.

Clinical features

The pressure within the sella may cause a classical 'bursting' bitemporal headache and radiologically visible expansion of the sella with erosion of the clinoid processes. The pressure on the optic chiasma causes loss of visual acuity, bitemporal hemianopia, and optic atrophy. Olfactory nerves may be involved with consequent anosmia. Signs of raised intracranial pressure may appear.

Local effects on the pituitary include progressive failure of most of the hormones of the anterior and posterior lobes, and the clinical picture may gradually move towards adult panhypopituitarims (see below).

Pressure on the hypothalamus may aggravate the pituitary failure, and also provoke characteristic hypothalamic features of weight gain, somnolence and polydipsia.

Investigation and diagnosis

For these and other tumours in the region of the sella turcica special investigations should include:

1 a combined pituitary test (see Table 8.7);
2 full visual testing including perimetry for visual fields;
3 skull X-rays;
4 computer tomography (CT scan) of the pituitary area (Fig. 8.8);
5 arteriography if an aneurysm must be excluded.

Treatment

Surgery and/or radiotherapy will be advised depending on the position and extent of the adenoma.

Panhypopituitarism

This condition may be congenital causing pituitary dwarfism with adult body proportions and combined failure of thyroid, adrenal and gonad function; this is rare and it is discussed fully in specialist and paediatric texts.

In the adult, panhypopituitarism (*Simmonds' disease*) may be caused by infiltration of the pituitary, by neoplasms or granulomas, by trauma or by infarction. The latter is the major cause, being especially associated with major haemorrhage at the time of parturition (*Sheehan's syndrome*).

Clinical features

1 History of ante- or post-partum haemorrhage.

Table 8.7 The combined pituitary test*

The following are injected intravenously at about 09.00 h:

1 *Soluble insulin*: 0.1 units/kg body weight in suspected hypopituitarism, 0.3 units/kg in conditions of insulin resistance, 0.2 units/kg otherwise. (The blood glucose must fall to 2.5 mmol/l or below for the test to be valid. It is necessary for a doctor to be present or immediately available throughout in case severe hypoglycaemia occurs and administration of glucose becomes necessary.)
2 *TRH*: 200 μg
3 *LRH*: 100 μg

Normal adult levels and responses (typical ranges)

Sample	GH (mu/l)	Cortisol (nmol/l)	TSH (mu/l)	Prolactin (mu/l)	LH (male) (u/l)	FSH (male) (u/l)	LH (female) (u/l)	FSH (female) (u/l)
Basal	1–10	150–170	1–3	< 500	3–10	1–8	3–10[†]	3–8[†]
30′			5–20	300–3000	8–35	15–11	8–25	4–11
60′	Peak exceeds 12	Peak exceeds 800	4–18	200–3000	6–35	1–11	6–20	6–12
90′								
120′								

*This is a combination of the insulin hypoglycaemia, TRH and LRH tests. In its complete form, the test measures the capacity of the anterior pituitary to secrete all the anterior pituitary hormones. In some patients a more selective test may be adequate.

The hypothalamic factors CRF (corticotrophin-releasing factor) and GHRF (growth-hormone-releasing factor) are sometimes employed in the detailed analysis of deficiencies, but mainly as research tools. In children exhibiting poor growth velocity the more relevant observation may be the nocturnal levels and patterns of GH secretion.

[†]Figures obtained in the follicular phase of the cycle. Levels are generally lower than this during the luteal phase, having risen to a peak at mid-cycle (see Fig. 8.5).

2 Failure of lactation and failure to resume menstruation (FSH, LH failure); uterus and vagina shrink; vaginal secretions reduced; secondary infertility.
3 Loss of libido; reduced pubic and axillary hair; impotence (FSH, LH and ACTH).
4 Mild adrenal deficiency may occur; depigmentation and pallor (ACTH).
5 Secondary myxoedema (TSH).
6 Skin characteristically soft, fine and wrinkled.
7 Hypoglycaemic episodes may occur (ACTH, GH).
8 Mineralocorticoid function is well maintained by the renin–angiotensin system.

Investigation and diagnosis

The several gland deficiencies should be quantitated by appropriate tests. Basal levels of anterior pituitary hormones may be low, but deficiencies will be more obvious under the conditions of a combined pituitary test (Table 8.7).

Treatment

Substitution by hydrocortisone (20–40 mg daily), regular androgens, and cyclical oestrogens are advisable. Thyroxine may be added gradually, when the adrenal insufficiency has been abolished. As the best treatment for the pituitary remnant is another pregnancy, a trial of gonadotrophins may be in order. Patients should take the same precautions as those with Addison's disease (see page 301).

Hypopituitary coma

This rare event, which should be prevented by good management, is dangerous in that it may involve the conjunction of hypoglycaemia, hypoadrenalism, hypothyroidism and hypothermia. The patient is treated specifically for these conditions and generally for shock.

Diabetes insipidus

This is a rare disease, characterized by the excretion of a large (10–20 litres in 24 hours) urinary volume and consequent great thirst. It is caused by either a deficiency of antidiuretic hormone from the posterior pituitary gland, or an inability of the distal renal tubule to respond to its action. Failure of secretion may occur when disease processes affect the region of the pituitary, for example tumours (ca. 50 per cent), inflammatory disease (ca. 25 per cent), vascular changes (ca. 10 per cent), trauma (ca. 10 per cent) and Hand–Schüller–Christian disease, histiocytosis, Langerhars cell histiocytosis (ca. 2–3 per cent).

Clinical features

The effect of the diuresis is to cause intense thirst. The condition should be suspected in all patients secreting over 4 litres of urine per 24 hours and drinking more than 5 litres per 24 hours. It must be differentiated from diabetes mellitus (glycosuria), terminal renal failure (proteinuria, uraemia) and hysterical overdrinking. Only the last is difficult to separate. The most useful confirmatory test is to deprive the patient of water for 8 hours. Normal subjects will achieve a urine concentration of at least 600 mOsmol/kg, whereas those with diabetes insipidus will achieve only a small rise in osmolality. This test requires care as it is possible to dehydrate the patient seriously: it should not be performed if the plasma osmolality is above 300 mOsmol/kg, and it must be terminated if the patient passes so much urine that body weight falls by more than 2 kg.

Treatment

The pitressin analogue desmopressin is given in a dose of 10–20 μg intranasally once or twice daily, or 2 μg intramuscularly daily. Some patients are helped by thiazide diuretics and chlorpropamide is sometimes of value. Cure can only be achieved by treating the cause.

Nephrogenic diabetes insipidus

This is almost always congenital, very rarely the result of destruction of the distal renal tubule in pyelonephritis. The congenital form is easily recognized by the family history, its early onset, male predominance, and failure to respond to desmopressin.

Prognosis is poor, but some sensitization to low levels of ADH may be achieved by use of thiazide diuretics, or chlorthalidone, or chlorpropamide (but not other sulphonylureas), or carbamazepine.

Hypothalamic deficiencies

Some typical pathological lesions leading to hypothalamic deficiencies are shown in Table 8.8.

Clinical features

Visual defects tend to occur early. In a small minority only, hyperphagia, weight changes, temperature disturbance and drowsiness occur.

Hyperprolactinaemia, with or without galactorrhoea,

Table 8.8 Pathological lesions causing hypothalamic deficiencies

Tumours
Craniopharyngioma (calcification visible on skull X-ray; common in children)
Chromophobe adenomas (early visual changes usually occur)

Granulomas
Sarcoidosis (look for disease elsewhere)
Tuberculosis (look for disease elsewhere)
Hand–Schüller–Christian disease (histiocytosis)

Trauma
Various kinds

may arise, and diabetes insipidus may occur in association with the anterior lobe hormone deficiencies (see page 310).

Pluriglandular disorders

These are disease states in which two or more endocrine glands are involved in the same patient.

Combined gland failures

1 Hypopituitary states (see page 310).
2 Autoimmune group (associated with HLA-DW3 and DW4):
   Hashimoto's, Graves', myxoedema
   Pernicious anaemia
   Addison's disease
   Insulin-dependent diabetes mellitus.

Combined gland hypersecretion

Multiple endocrine adenomatosis (MEA) may occur sporadically or as a familial disorder:
   Type I: especially pituitary, parathyroid and pancreatic adenomas
   Type IIA: parathyroid adenomas, phaeochromocytomas and medullary carcinoma of thyroid
   Type IIB: phaeochromocytomas, medullary carcinoma of the thyroid, and mucosal neuromas.

Endocrine functions of 'non-endocrine organs'

The kidney

The kidney is responsible for the secretion of at least three substances that are hormonal in character:

1 *Erythropoietin,* controlling red cell production.
2 *Renin,* controlling angiotensin production (see page 267).
3 *1-25-OH-vitamin D3* (see page 332).

The gastrointestinal tract

The gut wall secretes a number of identified peptides, such as pancreozymin-cholecystokinin, gastrin, secretin, gastric inhibitory polypeptide, vasoactive inhibitory polypeptide, enteroglucagon, pancreatic polypeptide, secretin, motilin, neurotensin, enkephalin, substance P, bombesin, somatostatin and probably many others.

Prostaglandins

These are modified long-chain fatty acids that are synthesized close to their site of action and are then very rapidly inactivated. They have powerful modulating influences on many processes, with effects in the inflammatory reaction, in pyrexia, in spontaneous abortion, gastric secretion, control of blood pressure, platelet aggregation and smooth muscle contractions.

Ectopic secretion of hormones

SIADH

This is the syndrome of inappropriate anti-diuretic-hormone (ADH) secretion. Excessive levels of ADH may be of pituitary origin, through hypothalamic pathways, and yet be truly pathological as in many cases of cerebral irritation or trauma, or compensatory to real or false 'volume signals' in various chest disorders, or in patients on ventilators. Malignant tumours, especially oat-cell lesions of the bronchus, may secrete such quantities of ADH as to produce an acute neurological disturbance, from confusion and nausea to fits, focal signs and coma. This reversible state is mainly caused by the possibly severe hyponatraemia, a dilutional effect seen also in the low blood urea concentration. (The dilutional changes distinguish this hyponatraemia from that seen in severe sodium depletion, when there will also be a tendency to hypovolaemia, hypotension, low CVP and tachycardia.)

Diagnosis

The urine osmolality in SIADH is inappropriately 'normal' (i.e. it is high *relative* to the *low* plasma osmolality: in a normal subject a fairly modest fall of plasma osmolality below the individual normal range will stimulate a marked diuresus and *very* low urine osmolalities.

Treatment

In management, removal of an ectopic source (or the bulk of it), water restriction, and the use of demeclocycline to block ADH effect on the renal tubules, may be helpful.

Other ectopic hormones

Many tumours arising in apparently non-endocrine tissues are found to contain or secrete peptide hormones or biochemically similar peptides. A wide variety of tumours and peptides have been associated, but the more common and important syndromes are described here.

1 Ectopic Cushing's
Very high levels of ACTH typically produce marked hypokalaemia and weakness: sources include oat-cell carcinoma of the bronchus, bronchial adenomas, thymomas, carcinoids, and carcinomas of the stomach, colon, gall-bladder and ovary.

2 Inappropriate ADH secretion
See above.

3 Hypercalcaemia
Non-metastatic, related to parathormone or other chemical factors: sources include squamous-cell carcinoma of the bronchus, hypernephroma, and carcinoma of the ovary (see page 332).

4 Polycythaemia
Secondary to erythropoietin secretion: sources include hypernephroma, fibromyoma of uterus, and stomach cancer.

Further reading

Refer to the list at the end of Chapter 9.

9
Metabolic Disorders

The line between endocrine and metabolic disorders is often indistinct and at times non-existent, as illustrated by the considerable discussion of hormones such as insulin and parathyroid hormone in this chapter. Yet the convention persists, perhaps reflecting the fact that the clinical disorders to be discussed are the product of the interactions with non-hormonal derangements of metabolism. Certainly they are of very considerable importance from the point of view of public health. Diabetes, atherosclerosis, obesity and bone disorders underlie a very large proportion of mortality and morbidity world-wide, but especially in developed countries.

Diabetes mellitus

The definition of diabetes mellitus has become much more complicated since the Egyptians of 1500 BC, and later Arataeus of Cappadocia, described a disease in which subjects lost weight, suffered extreme thirst, drank copiously and passed large quantities of urine to which 'ants were attracted by its sweetness'. To this clinical stereotype, now diffused by a wide range of clinical pictures, we could add the essential chemical criteria: the disease in its untreated state is identified by chronically raised blood glucose levels as a consequence of inadequate production and/or impaired effectiveness of insulin. This, then, is the middle ground of the *concept* of diabetes mellitus. We should recognize at one end of the spectrum there are patients who are virtually symptom-free but whose body chemistry is 'diabetic', while at the other end is a disease entity comprising late as well as immediate complications, with pathological associations (HLA, atherosclerosis, etc.) of considerable importance, let alone huge psychosocial impact.

The point having been made, Table 9.1 indicates the internationally agreed criteria for diagnosing or excluding diabetes, and the hinterland of 'impaired glucose tolerance' (IGT). The glucose tolerance test would be superfluous in a patient in whom a random blood or plasma glucose consistently exceeded 12 mmol/l; if a GTT is indicated then at least three days of normal carbohydrate intake and finally a 12–14 hour overnight fast immediately preceding the test are advised. On current evidence, those with IGT can be regarded as normally fit and healthy, but have a *slightly* increased risk of developing diabetes in the future.

Types of diabetes mellitus

Excluding those rare cases of diabetes in which pancreatectomy or severe pancreatitis has removed the bulk of islet cells, the diabetic population falls into two principal camps, insulin-dependent (IDDM) and non-insulin-dependent (NIDDM); there are, however, a few borderline stragglers. The main distinguishing features of the divide are summarized in Table 9.2.

The prevalence of NIDDM is five or six times greater than IDDM in most European countries, but there is an

Table 9.1 WHO diagnostic values (in mmol/l) for the 75 g oral glucose tolerance test (GTT). Intermediate values, or conflicting fasting and two-hour classification, would be regarded as 'impaired glucose tolerance' (IGT), *not* diabetes

Nature of samples	Within normal limits		Diabetes mellitus	
	Fasting	At 2 h	Fasting	At 2 h
Venous whole blood	< 6.7	< 6.7	⩾ 6.7	⩾ 10.0
Capillary whole blood	< 6.7	< 7.8	⩾ 6.7	⩾ 11.1
Venous plasma	< 7.8	< 7.8	⩾ 7.8	⩾ 11.1
Capillary plasma	< 7.8	< 8.9	⩾ 7.8	⩾ 12.2

Table 9.2 Types of diabetes mellitus

	I	II
Heredity	HLA-linked, DR3/4	Strongly familial, non-HLA
Islet cell antibodies at diagnosis	Frequent	Absent
DR-activated T cells	Often ++	Unchanged
C4 complement	Often ↓	Unchanged
Association with other autoimmune disorders	Yes	No
Viral associations (seasonality and animal models)	Yes	No
Age of onset	typically <25 yrs	typically >45 yrs
Sex: M:F	1:1	1:2
Habitus	Thin	Overweight
Presentation	Often acute	Usually subacute
Levels of plasma insulin	Absent or very low	Normal or increased
Ketosis-prone?	Yes	No
Insulin-dependent?	Yes	No
Nomenclature:		
traditional	Juvenile-onset	Maturity-onset
controversial	Type I	Type II
recommended	Insulin-dependent diabetes mellitus (IDDM)	Non-insulin-dependent diabetes mellitus (NIDDM)

extraordinary range of prevalence and incidence of both types across the world (Figs. 9.1 and 9.2).

Aetiology

1 Heredity

Table 9.2 indicates that the familial trait is quite distinct

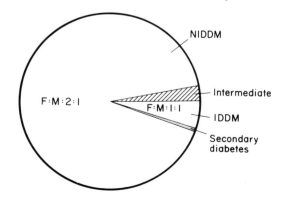

Figure 9.1 *Typical European distribution of the major types of diabetes. NIDDM = non-insulin dependent diabetes mellitus IDDM = insulin dependent diabetes mellitus.*

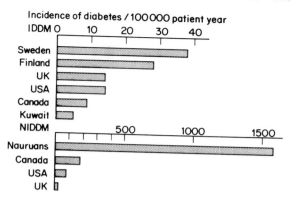

Figure 9.2 *Geographical/ethnic variation in the population incidence of IDDM and NIDDM. Note the difference in scales. The figures are illustrative rather than strictly comparable, as survey methods varied.*

between IDDM and NIDDM. There is *no* cross-risk; there is *no* linkage of NIDDM risk with HLA haplotypes, whereas those with neither DR3 nor DR4 virtually never get IDDM; the overall familial risk is nevertheless *higher* with NIDDM than IDDM. These risk figures are interesting for the light they throw on the importance of non-genetic, non-familial factors, and are also helpful for counselling diabetics who naturally become anxious for their relatives and especially their children (Table 9.3).

2 Mechanism

The variety of immune-related phenomena recorded in IDDM, its occasional epidemic and seasonal nature and other suggestive evidence supporting a role for viruses in the aetiology, and the existence of provocative animal models, together with the occasional finding of round cell infiltration consistent with autoimmune 'islet-cell-itis' at onset of IDDM, leads to a working hypothesis summarized in Fig. 9.3.

Table 9.3 Risks of developing diabetes mellitus

If this relative had the disorder indicated ...	this is the life-time risk of the 'susceptible' person developing the same disorder (as % risk)	
	IDDM	NIDDM
Identical twin	30–40	100
Non-identical sibling		
HLA not known: ?	5–10	10+
HLA Haplotypes: 2 identical	30–40	10+
1 identical	5–10	10+
0 identical	0–2	10+
Both parents	1–4	(?)
One parent	10–15	15

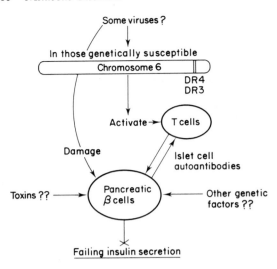

Figure 9.3 *Possible aetiological factors in insulin dependent diabetes mellitus.*

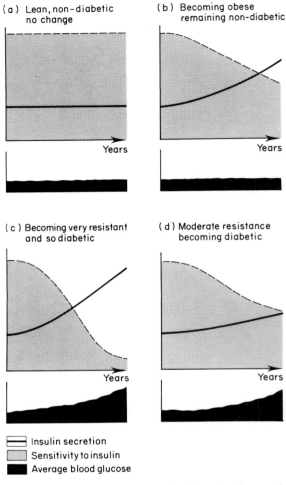

Figure 9.4 *NIDDM. Diagram of the relationships between the overall rates of insulin secretion and overall sensitivity to insulin and the development of NIDDM. The relative failure of the beta-cell in case D, compared to case C, would have implications for likely aetiology and likely modes of effective treatment.*

The constant end-point in IDDM, whatever the actual mechanisms, is absolute deficiency of insulin. In contrast, the absolute levels of insulin in the older patient with NIDDM are usually normal or even (in absolute terms) high. However, in relation to the coexisting hyperglycaemia, these NIDDM levels of insulin are just *not high enough*. Fig. 9.4 explores further this concept of *relative* deficiency (perhaps a limited reserve capacity) of insulin secretion in the face of insulin resistance.

3 'Secondary diabetes'

In most cases of NIDDM the only identifiable factors contributing significantly to 'insulin resistance' are obesity and hyperglucagonaemia; even then, the overlap with the non-diabetic population is such that a limited capacity of the beta cell has to be postulated as a contributory factor of major importance. The same caveat applies to virtually all the factors listed in Table 9.4; a vigorous beta-cell response would maintain homeostasis even in the face of considerable insulin resistance.

A more convincing 'secondary diabetes' is recognized when direct damage to, removal or impairment of action of the mass of beta cells is known to have occurred. Table 9.5 lists some mechanisms in this category.

4 Disorders associated but not causal

The disorders in which diabetes mellitus occurs more frequently than would be expected by chance include:

(a) the autoimmune endocrine disorders (DR3 and DR4 related);

Table 9.4 Causes of insulin resistance—hence sometimes diabetes or IGT

Obesity
Hyperglucagonaemia (rarely, glucagonoma)
Acromegaly
Steroid therapy/Cushing's syndrome
Phaeochromocytoma
Major stress (e.g. infarcts, burns)
Pregnancy: 'gestational diabetes'

Table 9.5 Secondary diabetes: beta-cell deficit

Severe malnutrition
Pancreatitis
Pancreatic damage or resection
Cystic fibrosis
Haemachromatosis
Drugs (e.g. thiazide diuretics)

(b) Turner's and Klinefelter's syndromes;
(c) Friedrich's ataxia (see page 233);
(d) dystrophia myotonica (see page 210).

Clinical features of moderate and relative insulin deficiency in NIDDM

The presence of some insulin, its persisting effect in controlling lipolysis and potassium efflux from cells, and some maintenance of its anabolic effect on protein, means that (with rare exceptions) patients in this state do *not* become ketotic, do *not* become hyperkalaemic or depleted, and do *not* exhibit gross wasting. The pathophysiology behind the clinical changes *does*, however, include:

1 Hyperglycaemia and glycosuria.
2 Impaired cell uptake of glucose and amino acids and protein synthesis.
3 Impaired cellular functions (e.g. defences against infection, wound healing).
4 Metabolic derangements in lipids, vessel walls, membrane, and tissues which are associated with the chronic complications.

Chronic and subacute

Weight will usually have been above-average, but most patients lose 5–10 kg in the weeks preceding symptomatic diagnosis.

Malaise may be obvious, or may be so subtle that patients only admit to it in retrospect.

Polyuria, nocturia and consequent *polydipsia* are secondary to the osmotic diuresis due to glycosuria; the pattern of drinking and micturition at night is more discriminatory than daytime habits.

Vulvitis in the female and *balanitis* in the male are very common examples of the several infections to which untreated patients are prone. The diminished resistance to infection is compounded by the favourable culture medium provided by the sugar-laden urine.

Tuberculous infection may be reactivated as immune resistance declines.

Chronic complications will occasionally become symptomatic *before* the hyperglycaemia has come to light. In most cases the disorder has been present without major symptoms for many years, and only a careful history will unearth the clues to the earlier onset.

Table 9.6 Factors possibly contributory to onset of hyperosmolar non-ketotic coma

NIDDM has become IDDM
Major intercurrent illness
Dehydration (impairing renal clearances)
Diuretics
Steroid therapy
Cimetidine
Phenytoin
Intravenous or intraperitoneal glucose solutions
Pancreatitis
Inadequate hypoglycaemic medication

Acute deterioration: hyperosmolar non-ketotic coma

Although uncontrolled NIDDM is eventually a most unpleasant state, and may be complicated by symptoms of neuropathy and vascular disease and their consequences, an acute exacerbation is very unusual unless additional provocative factors overstrain the system, or the patient's insulin secretory capacity has further declined and the therapeutic response has been inadequate. Table 9.6 summarizes possibly contributory factors.

Clinical features may include drowsiness, stupor, coma or fits; hypotension; hypothermia; gastroparesis and therefore dilatation, haematemesis, or ileus; neurological disturbance. All are reversible.

Biochemical characteristics include:
blood glucose in the range 20–200 mmol/l
pH normal; plasma negative for ketones
(Na^+), (K^+), urea: all concentrations raised
plasma osmolality above 300
(Plasma osmolality can be estimated roughly by $2(Na^+) + 2(K^+) + (blood glucose) + (urea)$.)

Treatment is discussed on page 324.

Clinical features of severe insulin deficiency in IDDM

The absolute or virtual absence of insulin in this condition, before treatment, unleashes some further pathophysiology, namely:

1 Uncontrolled lipolysis, hence increased production of FFA and ketones.
2 Protein catabolism, hence increased aminoacidaemia.
3 Consequent ketotic acidosis.
4 Intracellular potassium depletion, plasma hyperkalaemia.

5 Loss of protein body mass, impaired growth and healing.

Other than the non-ketotic coma, all the clinical features described in the preceding NIDDM section may and do occur in IDDM. A prolonged chronic or subacute stage is unusual, although recent research studies based on growth of identical twins one of whom becomes diabetic, and some prospective work in high-risk populations, suggest that for up to one year before the apparently abrupt acute presentation the disease process has been active.

Subacute and prodromal IDDM

Wasting and weakness may be extreme, and the children have usually ceased to grow by the time they present.

Symptoms and signs discussed above for the NIDDM may have been present and obvious to the patient for weeks or months; typically the final deterioration is accelerated (over a matter of days or just a few weeks), and many patients are still diagnosed in coma or just-precomatose states.

Acute deterioration: ketoacidosis and coma

In an ideal world of well-educated diabetics supported by first-class professional advice this condition would not occur, at least in the known diabetic. Yet it does, often because of silly errors such as reduction of insulin in the event of intercurrent illness (when *more* insulin may be needed), and the mortality remains significant. The likely provocative factors include: inadequate insulin therapy, accidental, misguided or intentional; major physical stress, especially infections but also infarcts, CVAs, etc; and induction of increased insulin resistance without appropriate adjustment in therapy.

Clinical features of ketoacidosis may include irritability, depression and lethargy, proceeding to confusion, stupor, coma and occasionally fits; nausea, vomiting and abdominal pain ('diabetic crisis') which may tempt the unwary towards a potentially and frequently disastrous laparotomy; cramps in muscles and paraesthesia related to acute mononeuritis; all this will have been preceded by at least a few days of prodromal and subacute symptoms as discussed above. On examination the patient displays Kussmaul-type 'air hunger' if very acidotic. The breath smells of acetone. The patient is typically very dry, hypotensive, and often tachycardic.

Biochemical characteristics include:

blood glucose in the range 18–40 mmol/l

pH low; plasma ketones high; PCO_2 low

(Na^+), (urea): concentrations raised

(K^+) in plasma: often high initially

total body K^+: depleted

Other findings often include leucocytosis and pyrexia, even in the absence of infection, but the latter must not be missed. There is a constant risk of cardiorespiratory arrest.

Treatment is discussed on page 324, and will usually require intensive care.

Lactic acidosis

This condition is not exclusive to diabetes but its presentation—an acute, severely acidotic illness in a known diabetic—may mimic ketoacidosis. It is unusual in British diabetics now that phenformin has been withdrawn, but can still occur under conditions of:

1 Impaired tissue perfusion: typically a patient in shock, secondary to circulatory failure or septicaemia.
2 Major disturbances in the lactate pyruvate ratio provoked by metformin, phenformin, alcohol, acute hypoglycaemia, leukemia, etc.; especially in the presence of hepatic or renal disease.

Clinical features may resemble those of ketoacidosis but the patient is less dehydrated and glucose levels may be low, high or normal. (The laboratory findings will thus confirm the low pH and PCO_2, and an abnormal anion gap above 10, often above 15: $(Na^+ + K^+) - (Cl^- + HCO_3^-)$; unexplained by any rise in ketones/ethanol/aspirin/etc.)

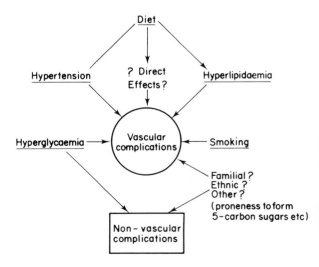

Figure 9.5 *Possible mechanisms of diabetic complications.*

Chronic complications of diabetes

There is a strong association between the overall degree and duration of hyperglycaemia and the development and severity of the late complications. In trials of intensive diabetic control, with multiple insulin injections or continuous subcutaneous insulin infusion, the maintenance of 'near-normoglycaemia' does limit and sometimes entirely reverse the markers of early tissue damage, so these are grounds for long-term optimism if practical means of extending this degree of control generally are perfected. Meanwhile the standard of control that we conventionally accept as 'good' actually reflects a far from physiological fluctuation of blood glucose, with major peaks and troughs despite the best efforts of the diabetic and his advisers; so it is not surprising that complications continue to be a problem.

Other factors must be important because, at the same degree of hyperglycaemia, some diabetics fare worse than others. These factors of vulnerability are not HLA-related, but there is some hint of a familial trend. Even modest elevations of the blood pressure compared with the ideal level may damage diabetic tissues. Possible interactions are summarized in Fig. 9.5.

The *pathology* of complications involves direct and complex metabolic derangements which damage tissues, and effects on large and small blood vessels, with important secondary damage, follow. Table 9.7 offers a useful conceptual framework of the principal complications, but should not be interpreted too literally.

Eye disease

Diabetes is the commonest cause of new blindness under the age of 65 in the UK; 10 per cent of those who have had the disease for 40 years or more are now blind, while many more have impaired vision. Much of the visual loss is preventable.

Cataracts occur earlier and with increased frequency, probably through repeated osmotic damage to the lens.

Transient refractive changes, with blurring of vision, are common when blood sugar levels are altered rapidly.

Retinopathy is a consequence of microvascular damage, partly ischaemic and partly related to secondary tissue damage, as illustrated in Fig. 9.6.

Optic atrophy, iritis, secondary glaucoma, or a lateral rectus muscle palsy through a neuropathy of the sixth cranial nerve may occasionally occur.

Neuropathy and the central nervous system

Acute neuritis or radiculitis, with pain, paraesthesia or numbness in the dermatome, and perhaps muscle pain and tenderness, may occur during severe hyperglycaemic crises, and largely resolve with re-establishment of control.

Mononeuritis, sometimes '*multiplex*', may occur in this acute form or as a chronic problem, presumably secondary to a vascular event in the vasa nervorum of that particular nerve or nerves.

The *peripheral neuropathy* most typical of diabetes is chronic, symmetrical, and most obvious at the extremities ('glove and stocking'). The longer the axon the more the cumulative effect of the diffuse disorder on the action potential, so symptoms and signs are usually first detectable in feet and ankles. Vibration sense and ankle reflexes are lost early. The 'cotton-wool' sensations and paraesthesia follow, then loss of pain sensation. The analgesia is no blessing for it allows joints to be damaged (Charcot's arthropathy) and ulcers to be caused by trauma with the patient unaware.

Diabetic amyotrophy is a rare lower-motor-neurone manifestation of diabetes, sometimes painful.

Autonomic neuropathy may cause a range of effects, as listed in Table 9.8. The loss of the adrenaline response allows some patients to become more readily hypoglycaemic, and reduces the early warning.

Renal disease (see page 275)

Nephropathy is an area in which scrupulous attention to control of blood *pressure* as well as blood *glucose* is probably of extreme importance. At the present time many long-term diabetics end up on dialysis or with transplants.

Table 9.7 Diabetic complications

Microvascular and basement membrane	Metabolic in tissues
retinopathy	cataract
mononeuritis	polyneuropathy*
nephropathy	arthropathies
dermopathy*	proneness to infection*
cardiomyopathy	hyperlipidaemia, thrombosis*
Macrovascular	*Gestational*
Coronary disease	fetal loss, etc.
cerebrovascular disease	maternal loss
peripheral vascular disease*	subfertility

*Important factors in diabetic foot problems, possibly leading to gangrene and amputations.

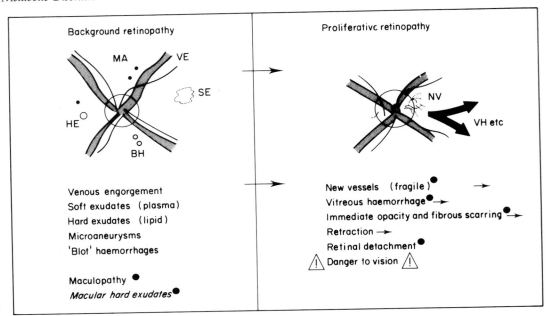

Figure 9.6   *Diabetic retinopathy. Urgent attention from an ophthalmologist, with a view to intervention by laser therapy, is indicated when background retinography is very severe, as soon as new vessels are seen, or at any observation marked ●. MA = microaneurysms, HE = hard exudates, SE = soft exudates, BH = blot haemorrhage, VE = torturous dilated view, NV = new vessels, VH = vitreous haemorrhage.*

Hyperlipidaemia

Excessive levels of total cholesterol, LDL-cholesterol and triglycerides occur with increased frequency in diabetes, and contribute to the premature occurrence of atherosclerosis and occasional incidence of *xanthomata* (see page 328). Familial and dietary factors are of particular importance, but good control of the diabetes is also relevant.

Heart and cerebrovascular disease

Coronary disease occurs earlier, and at a higher than average frequency, in the diabetic population, as part of the general proneness to atherosclerosis. Morbidity and mortality may be aggravated by coexisting

Table 9.8 Diabetic autonomic neuropathy

Gustatory sweating (autonomic imbalance)
Postural hypotension (unresponsive heart)
Respiratory arrest (unresponsive reflex?)
Impotence (neural and vascular)
Gastroparesis (dilatation)
Nocturnal diarrhoea (gut motility)
Rectal incontinence (sphincter impairment)
Impaired sweating (so dry skin)
Neurogenic bladder (loss of tone)

microvascular disease of the myocardium which is revealed histologically. 'Diabetic cardiomyopathy' also embraces neuropathic and metabolic disorders within the heart. An electrocardiogram should be checked routinely.

Strokes and transient ischaemic attacks are also more frequent in diabetics. Factors include atheroma in the main cerebral vessels, involvement of smaller arteries, and small vessel disease. During coma, diffuse intravascular coagulation may complicate recovery through cerebral damage.

Peripheral vascular disease

The combination of atheromatous occlusion with small vessel disease places the diabetic leg and foot in particular peril, and may make reconstructive relief rather difficult to achieve. Bruits may be audible and pulses diminished or absent. Ischaemia may be suggested by a history of intermittent claudication, chilblains or cold feet, and confirmed on examination by the low skin temperature, with poor hair, poor nail growth and poor healing of injuries or ulcers. Evidence of large and small vessel disease elsewhere will be relevant. At its worst, this may progress to deep ulceration and possible involvement of bone in an infective process. In an important minority, the foot or lower limb has to be amputated.

Infections

Polymorphic leucocyte *and* lymphocyte functions are impaired in diabetes; defences against bacterial infection and tissue reparative processes are further retarded by the poor tissue perfusion secondary to vascular disease. The frequent occurrence of boils, abscesses, skin crease infections, vaginitis and balanitis has been mentioned. Pulmonary (including tuberculous) and urinary tract infections occur more commonly, and osteomyelitis may complicate deep skin ulceration. The frequent recurrence or slow healing of infections should always arouse suspicion of diabetes.

Arthropathy

The anaesthesia of chronic neuropathy may allow joints to be unwittingly overstrained, abused and eventually disorganized, as originally described by Charcot. (the other classical causes for this state are tabes dorsalis and syringomyelia.) A more common, and less sinister, affliction of joints in diabetes is cheirarthropathy, a contracture which affects the small joint of the hand, and limits full extension: the patient is unable to flatten the palmar surfaces of the hands together.

The diabetic foot

The ranges of hazards to the diabetic leg and foot are summarized in Fig. 9.7. Most of the morbidity—and use of health resources—related to diabetes is the result of these foot complications and ensuing management.

Sex, conception and pregnancy

The neuropathetic and vascular changes that may cause impotence have been mentioned, but the usual range of non-diabetic causes should also be considered in each individual case.

There is some overall loss of fertility in sustained hyperglycaemia, and amenorrhoea or anovolatory menses may occur; but if the diabetes is mild or controlled then the reduction in fertility is slight.

Hyperglycaemia of the mother around the time of conception and early intrauterine development increase the risk of fetal malformation. Hyperglycaemia later in the pregnancy increases the risk of excessive fetal growth, hydramnios, placental insufficiency, prematurity and respiratory distress syndrome. These will all contribute to a higher fetal loss unless countered. Rigorous control virtually eliminates the excess risk. To achieve this the pregnant diabetic will need to monitor her blood glucose regularly and be supported by frequent supervision, ideally by a team including an obstetrician, a diabetologist and liaison nurse. Insulin requirements increase during pregnancy, especially in the third trimester, by as much as twofold.

Routine management of diabetes

The diabetic patient is in control

Diabetes is a way of life. It makes continuous demands on the patient, it is apparently lifelong, and its management is finally in the hands of the person with diabetes,

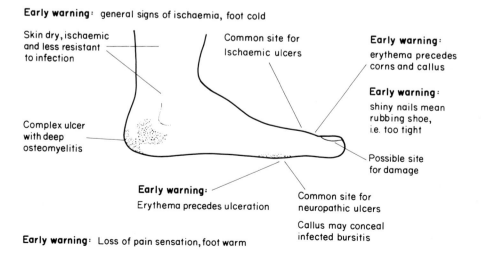

Early warning: general signs of ischaemia, foot cold

Skin dry, ischaemic and less resistant to infection

Common site for Ischaemic ulcers

Early warning: erythema precedes corns and callus

Early warning: shiny nails mean rubbing shoe, i.e. too tight

Complex ulcer with deep osteomyelitis

Possible site for damage

Early warning: Erythema precedes ulceration

Common site for neuropathic ulcers

Callus may conceal infected bursitis

Early warning: Loss of pain sensation, foot warm

Figure 9.7 *The diabetic foot.*

advised and supported by health professionals. The objective should be the reconciliation of optimum biochemical control with minimal disruption of normal living. This involves the education of the diabetic in his disorder and its control, and an imaginative partnership between diabetic and carers. Slavish 'compliance' to prescribed 'rules' is unnatural and difficult; the task is to help the diabetic assimilate the inconveniences of diabetes into a pattern of healthy living and a fulfilled lifestyle. To do this he needs a team, not a tyrant.

Measuring 'control': blood tests

As implied above, the aims include biochemical normality or something approaching it. Blood glucose can be measured directly from small drop samples usually obtained by pricking the finger. In day-to-day circumstances the drop is transferred to a small paper strip part of which has been coated with a glucose oxidase system: the colour change is read by eye against a standard range, or by a small portable meter. This can be done by the diabetic, and such 'home blood glucose monitoring' is generally accurate, informative and motivating. Measurements of urine glucose give an indication of fairly gross hyperglycaemia, by showing high levels when the renal threshold is being frequently exceeded, but are not helpful in achieving excellent control of blood glucose.

The process of glycosylation of proteins—and its relationship to mean glucose concentration—allows us to estimate the average glucose level over the time span represented within the half-life of the index proteins, currently haemoglobin (HBAlc) and serum proteins ('fructosamine'). Levels of the previous six to eight weeks are represented by the HbAlc concentration, and those of the previous two weeks or so by the fructosamine concentration; laboratories provide their own control values.

Diet, tablets or insulin?

Dietary advice is always relevant to management; in mild cases it may restore normal weight and normoglycaemia, in severe cases it underpins any other therapeutic measures. The choice between tablets and insulin can only be discussed in the context of the biochemical background (as discussed on page 315). Patients with evidence of absolute insulin deficiency, especially a history of ketosis, need exogenous insulin. Others who need insulin are listed in Table 9.9.

In some patients with relative insulin deficiency, having required insulin treatment, the daily requirement may decline to levels which justify a further trial of tablets

Table 9.9 Patients who require insulin for diabetic control

IDDM (patients with absolute insulin deficiency)
Those in whom maximum oral medication fails to achieve control (diet assumed)
Those unable to take tablets (acutely sick, etc.)
Pregnant patients
Patients undergoing surgery

replacing the insulin. This is rarely worth while if the daily exogenous insulin requirement exceeds 25 units.

Diet for the diabetic

Gradual but determined achievement and maintenance of weight within the normal range is an important target. In addition, the basic 'rules' are as follows:

1 Avoid foods containing large amounts of sugar.
2 Carefully restrict the amount of refined carbohydrates, dairy products and fats (remembering the associations with hyperlipidaemias).
3 There should be a good intake of fibre (e.g. in wholegrain cereals, fruit and vegetables).
4 Alcoholic beverages should be taken with caution; they are usually rich in calories, and particularly carbohydrate.
5 There should be scepticism regarding commercial 'diabetic' food and drink products, which are often expensive and high in calories although sucrose- and glucose-free.
6 The timing of meals and snacks must be considered in the context of any medication being used, especially insulin.
7 Variety and flexibility should be the long-term aims.

Dietitians have special expertise in this area, and will be particularly helpful in adapting these general rules to the personal needs of an individual.

Sulphonylureas and biguanides

Oral hypoglycaemic agents are required in non-insulin dependant patients whose diabetes cannot be controlled by diet alone. The *sulphonylureas* stimulate an augmented secretion of insulin, and may also increase peripheral sensitivity to insulin. Chlorpropamide and tolbutamide are long-established and cheap, but both may cause fluid retention; also, chlorpropamide is associated with flushing on imbibing alcohol, and occasional and dangerously prolonged hypoglycaemia. Of the newer short-acting agents, all of which may be effective where the original agents fail, glibenclamide is the most widely used. Glipizide is excreted via the liver, and is useful in patients with renal failure. Other useful sulphonylureas include glicazide, glibornuride and tolazamide.

Metformin, a *biguanide*, slows intestinal absorption and enhances the peripheral action of insulin on glucose uptake; it thus rarely causes hypoglycaemia and is associated with less weight gain than sulphonylureas. However, it is less potent than sulphonylureas, poorly tolerated by many patients (who complain of its gastrointestinal effects), and very occasionally it has been implicated in lactic acidosis (see page 318). It should certainly be avoided in any patients with a condition predisposing to lactate accumulation

Patients and doctors should be familiar with the likely peak and duration of action, the hazards, and interactions with other medications of whatever oral agent is being prescribed, and if necessary a formulary should be consulted.

Insulins

Diabetics inject their own insulin subcutaneously, and if they are going to achieve the best possible control then at least two (but sometimes three, four or even five) injections a day may be used. Depending on how rapidly the insulins are absorbed and cleared in a particular individual, many settle on *either* two injections daily each of which includes a mixture of short-acting soluble and intermediate-acting insulin, *or* a once-daily very-long-acting preparation with three injections (often by a portable 'pen' injection) of soluble insulin (see Table 9.10).

The actual distribution of units relates to the individual's pattern of overall diet, carbohydrate intake and physical activity on a typical day. The well-trained and confident diabetic will adjust dosage and timing, and his diet, in response to his activities and measurements of blood glucose. In the elderly some fineness of control can arguably be sacrificed, and a once-daily preparation may be regarded as adequate, particularly if the patient still has some endogenous secretory capacity to produce enough insulin to hold down his glucose through the night. In the UK the recommended insulins are all highly purified, neutral in pH and U100 (100 units per millilitre). *Bovine* is cheapest but most antigenic; *human* is least antigenic and increasingly the insulin of choice; but *porcine* is clinically equivalent.

Minimizing complications

As well as optimizing blood glucose, certain other aspects of self-care deserve emphasis.

Diabetics should avoid other vascular risk factors such as smoking, lack of exercise, excess fat, uncontrolled hypertension, and oestrogens. They should have regular medical checks to identify the earliest signs of complications, so that appropriate advice can be given or action taken (e.g. laser treatment of new retinal vessels to minimize the risks of subsequent vitreous haemorrhage and detachment).

Subjects should take particular care of the feet, avoiding pressure, trauma, infections or neglect of corns etc., any of which—especially in the foot with loss of pain sensation—may lead to ulceration, abscesses and gangrene. A chiropodist should be easily available.

Table 9.10 Insulin preparations: examples

Group	Type	Physical form	Onset, peak, duration*	Trade names
Short-acting	Soluble ('regular')	Neutral solution	0.5, 1–3, 7	Actrapid Humulin-S Velosulin
Intermediate-acting	Isophane	Suspension with protamine	1, 2–8, 20	Humulin–I Insulatard Protaphane
	Lente	Insulin–zinc suspension (amorphous + crystalline)	2, 6–4, 22	Monotard
Biphasic fixed mixtures	Mixtures	Soluble + isophane	0.5, 1–3, 4–8, 22 0.5, 1–3, 4–8, 22	Initard 50/50 Actraphane Mixtard 30/70 Humulin-M2
Long-acting	Ultra	Larger crystals in suspension	3, 6–16, 24 4, 12–30, 36	Humulin–Zn Ultratard

*Approximate time characteristics in hours. They may be prolonged in patients with insulin antibodies, in shock, coma or extreme cold.

Daily living

The diabetic will need advice on, for example, jobs, driving and insurance, all of which can be provided by the appropriate professionals and through the British Diabetic Association (10 Queen Anne Street, London W1M 0BD). Nurses associated with hospital departments but working in the community can help to keep up contact and improve control.

Management of diabetes in special situations

Hyperglycaemic coma

Whether *ketotic* or *non-ketotic hyperosmolar*, this is a dangerous state with a mortality of between 5 and 10 per cent, varying between centres. All the usual precautions in the care of the unconscious or semiconscious patient should be observed, and cardiovascular resuscitation may be required.

Insulin

Insulin by pump-controlled intravenous infusion (or hourly intramuscular injection) should be pure human and soluble, at a starting dose of 4–10 units/hour, after an initial priming injection of 20 units IV. The rate of infusion or injection can be adjusted on the basis of the blood glucose response, which should be closely monitored.

Fluid and electrolytes

Fluid replacement will be needed in large quantities: typically a litre of normal saline in the first half-hour, then a litre in the next hour, then a litre over two hours, then infused at the rate of a litre 8-hourly. Fluid overload should be avoided and is most likely in elderly patients and with renal or cardiac impairment. A central venous pressure line is necessary where there is any doubt. In extreme hyperosmolality, such as when sodium exceeds 150 mmol/l, half-normal saline may be preferred initially. Severe shock may call for plasma, blood and inotropic

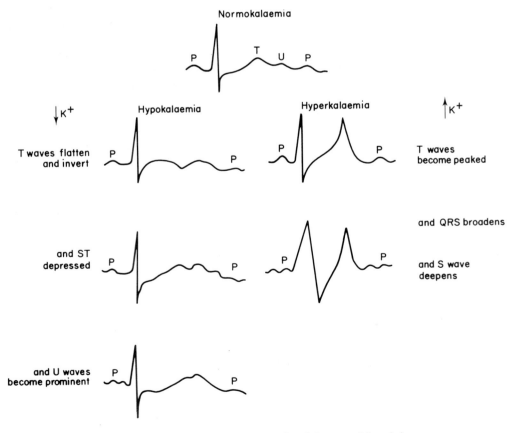

Figure 9.8 *The ECG changes of hypokalaemia and hyperkalaemia.*

agents. When the blood glucose approaches normal, 5% dextrose solution can be substituted for the saline, and subcutaneous insulin injections for the insulin pump.

Potassium concentrations in plasma may be initially elevated, concealing a total body potassium deficit. As insulin acts on tissues, potassium floods back into cells, and plasma levels may fall dangerously. Once insulin and fluids are being infused, set up an ECG to monitor the potassium status and measure plasma levels (Fig. 9.8). Most patients will require 20–40 mmol hourly (in the saline drip).

Bicarbonate is only appropriate in very severe acidosis, when the blood pH is less than 7. Complete correction is unnecessary and hazardous, and insulin and rehydration will achieve this normalization more safely.

Antibiotics

Infections that have provoked the crisis, and which may certainly complicate the clinical course, should be sought, identified and treated vigorously. The chest should be X-rayed and a urine sample examined in every case.

Complications

Thrombotic complications in major vessels, and disseminated through small vessels, may complicate recovery, and the use of low-dose heparin should be considered.

Renal function should be monitored closely, if necessary via catheter collection of urine hour by hour.

Intercurrent illness: 'sick day rules'

Stress-related 'resistance' to insulin, and the consequent increase in hepatic release of glucose, explains why insulin requirements in the sick patient will be the *same or even greater* than normal, *even if the patient is not eating*. One must maintain a generous fluid intake, an adequate caloric intake, and appropriate insulin, all monitored by regular blood glucose measurements. If necessary the patient should be admitted to hospital; those usually on tablets may need insulin injections; those on combinations of insulins may do better on a pump, as discussed in the previous section.

If major surgery is contemplated, control should be optimized before admission and certainly before the day of operation. The operation should be scheduled first on the list. If it is a morning list then no subcutaneous insulin is given, but early in the morning and at least one hour before surgery an intravenous infusion of 5% glucose (dextrose) containing 5 mmol of potassium in each 500 ml

is commenced at 100 ml/hour. Soluble insulin is infused at a rate of 2–6 units/hour, relating this to the patient's usual daily requirement (i.e. calculating from the number of units being administered over 24 hours).

If it is an afternoon list, half the usual morning dose is given at its usual time (about 10 units soluble if the patient is usually on tablets), then the same procedure followed. The insulin infusion rate can be adjusted during and following surgery on the basis of glucose levels estimated 1–2 hourly. When food and drink can again be taken normally, the patient's usual insulin regimen can be resumed; the intravenous infusion should not be stopped until the first injection has actually been given because the insulin is cleared from the circulation within minutes.

The diabetic *woman in labour* can similarly be managed with an insulin–dextrose infusion throughout.

Hypoglycaemia in the diabetic

In the diabetic a fall in blood sugar to symptomatic levels represents a temporary mismatch of insulin level to intestinal glucose uptake: a meal may have been missed or delayed, an injection dose mismeasured, unusual exertion undertaken, or an unusual degree of sensitivity to insulin experienced. The symptoms are related to activation of the sympathetic nervous system *and* the effects on central neurones of energy depletion (neuroglycopaenia). They vary from diabetic to diabetic, but remain fairly consistent within the individual (see Table 9.11).

The sympathetic symptoms are useful early-warning features. Unfortunately they may fade with tolerance, autonomic neuropathy or sympathetic-blocking medication.

Table 9.11 Clinical features of hypoglycaemia

Sympathetic
Tremulousness
Sweating
Hunger
Agitation
Rapid pulse

Neuroglycopaenia
Tingling of lips and tongue
Blurred vision
Light-headedness
Confusion, aggression
Stupor → coma
Cool skin
Fits
Retrograde amnesia
(Brain damage: rare)

Table 9.12 Causes of glycosuria

Diabetes mellitus/impaired glucose tolerance
Glycosuria of pregnancy
Fanconi's syndrome (with aminoaciduria)
Proximal renal tubule disorders
Chronic renal failure
Isolated deficit in glucose reabsorption (often familial)

Treatment

This can be as simple as persuading the diabetic to take sugar in some form. In the confused patient start with a glucagon injection, 1 mg into muscle, and in the stuporose or comatose patient commence an intravenous infusion of glucose, initially 20 ml of 50%. It must be remembered that the hypoglycaemia will often persist for an hour or many hours, so the treatment must be similarly sustained. For the ambulant patient a substantial snack may be appropriate, while for the more severe case continued observation for several hours is mandatory.

Renal glycosuria

Glycosuria in the presence of normal glucose tolerance is usually of little importance, but it may cause anxiety, but inappropriately diagnosed as diabetic, or provide a clue to an underlying renal problem (Table 9.12). The renal threshold for glucose, usually around 11 mmol/l in normal subjects, is lowered in normal pregnancy, and in the other non-diabetic conditions listed. The tubular deficits in reabsorption of glucose seem to be harmless, and no treatment or alteration in lifestyle need be suggested.

Whatever the circumstances, blood glucose values should be checked, and an oral glucose tolerance test performed in any doubtful case.

Hypoglycaemia

Clinical features

Symptoms usually become noticeable when the blood glucose has fallen to between 2.2 and 2.8 mmol/l, especially if falling rapidly, and if the subject has not been frequently exposed to such levels. The symptoms are listed in Table 9.11.

On examination in the early phase the patient is pale, cold, sweaty and the pulse is rapid. Later these signs may be less noticeable. Deep or prolonged hypoglycaemia may provoke epileptic fits, and may cause irreversible brain damage or death.

1 Reactive hypoglycaemia

This is noted as a biochemical phenomenon in some patients following partial gastrectomy, or in the very earliest stages of glucose intolerance, but the relevance to symptoms is doubtful. Controlled trials suggest that other mechanisms are responsible for the post-gastrectomy syndrome, and reports of benefit from high-protein small-snack regimens can be explained by a powerful placebo effect.

2 Fasting hypoglycaemia

This reflects an inability to switch off the metabolic pathways lowering glucose when the subject is already hypoglycaemic, or rarely an impaired ability to release glucose at an adequate rate when required. Some of the disorders will be apparent on very preliminary enquiry of the patient (Table 9.13).

Treatment

The cause should be identified and removed if possible. Immediate management of the hypoglycaemic crisis has been discussed above.

Insulinomas

These islet cell tumours may be especially insidious. Most are diagnosed after many months or even years of intermittent symptons, which have often been misinterpreted as functional or even psychotic. Many patients have learnt to avert their symptoms by frequent carbohydrate snacks, so they may be overweight. Most of the tumours are benign, and often small, so attempts to define or localize a tumour are often unsuccessful (although endoscopic ultrasonography offers some promise). The diagnosis may be spotted from a single

Table 9.13 Causes of fasting hypoglycaemia

Hypoglycaemic medication	Insulin/sulphonylurea: overdose, accidental or deliberate increased sensitivity missed meal or shock unusual exertion
Insulinoma	Islet cell tumour of the pancreas
Tumours	Secreting insulin-like substances (especially sarcomas)
Liver diseases	Glycogen storage disease (von Gierke's) Alcoholic cirrhosis Subacute necrosis
Other	Hypopituitary, hypoadrenal, hypothyroid Malabsorption syndromes Acute effect of alcohol, salicylates, anti-histamines

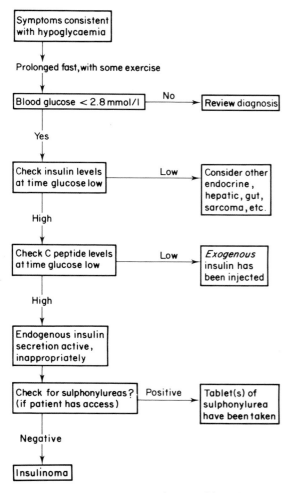

Figure 9.9 *Investigation of suspected hypoglycaemia.*

blood sample at the right moment, which may show a very low glucose reading but an inappropriately raised insulin reading (insulin should be virtually undetectable when the blood glucose is less than 2.5 mmol/l). However, there are some traps in the diagnosis, so an algorithm for the non-diabetic subject may be helpful (Fig. 9.9).

Treatment

The acute episode of hypoglycaemia can be treated as in the diabetic. While awaiting surgery, or following unsuccessful surgery, the rate of insulin secretion can usually be slowed by diazoxide tablets; unfortunately these and other beta-cell suppressants carry a toll of significant side-effects.

Surgical resection of the insulinoma, or even a subtotal pancreatectomy, will be necessary. The tumours are occasionally malignant and often locally invasive.

Atherosclerosis

This accounts for more deaths in Western societies than any other disorder. Coronary disease, strokes, visceral and peripheral vascular disease not only cripple and kill as primary disorders, but also complicate—often fatally—other illnesses or surgical procedures. The known risk factors include:

(a) familial and genetic;
(b) smoking;
(c) hypertension;
(d) physical inactivity;
(e) diabetes mellitus;
(f) atherogenic lipid profiles;
(g) alcohol;
(h) stress;

and most of these can be explained in terms of lipid and lipoprotein metabolism. However, effects on platelets, on vessel lumen, on collateral circulation, and on the physiology of the intima have all been established.

The evidence from animal models, and in human populations, encourages the belief that the atheromatous process is largely preventable and even reversible, provided that all the non-genetic factors are corrected and removed.

The hyperlipidaemias

These conditions are characterized by raised levels of cholesterol and/or triglyceride in plasma; an associated change in lipoprotein concentration is inevitably implied. Their primary importance in terms of the community's health derives from their considerable contribution to the aetiology of atherosclerosis, as discussed above, but the other clinical implications are not trivial:

1 Acute pancreatitis, or a more obscure abdominal pain, may occur. The discomfort and danger can be compounded by inappropriate laparotomy.
2 Other symptoms, xanthomata or arthralgia for example, can be troublesome.
3 Raised lipids may reflect an important underlying disease such as diabetes or nephrosis.
4 The very fact that these conditions are often both familial and reversible implies a special obligation to offer the patient and family appropriate advice and assistance.

Table 9.14 Characteristics of the various lipoproteins*

Lipoprotein	Density	Electro-phoretic mobility	Main lipid	Particle size (nm)	Pathways	Catabolism
CHYLO Chylomicron	< 1.006	0	Triglyceride	80–500	Intestine → Liver (50–100 g/day)	LPL
VLDL very-low density	< 1.006	+ + Pre-beta	Triglyceride	30–100	Liver → Periphery (triglyceride ↔ FFA) (10–30 g/day)	LPL
LDL low-density	1.006 − 1.063	+ Beta	Mixed, or cholesterol ester[†] only	20–25	Liver → periphery (cholesterol etc.) (1.5 g/day)	High affinity receptors Endocytosis + ACAT
HDL high-density	1.063 − 1.210	+ + + Alpha	Cholesterol ester	7–11	Cholesterol transfer between classes and tissues (LCAT)	?

Key to enzymes: LPL, liproprotein lipase; ACAT, acyl-CoA cholesterol acyltransferase; LCAT, lecithin cholesterol acyltransferase.
*It may be helpful to recall that fat is of low density and non-polar, especially relative to protein.
[†]More dense.

Table 9.15 WHO classification of hyperlipidaemias

Type	CHYL	VLDL	LDL	Triglyceride	Cholesterol	Clinical features, etc.
I	↑↑↑			↑↑	↑	Rare, mainly in children. *NO* atheroma. Due to LPL deficiency, Chylomicronaemia
IIa			↑		↑	Hypercholesterolaemia; atheroma; xanthelasma Nodular xanthomata on exterior surfaces. Deficient receptors to LDL. Often 2° to hypothyroidism, nephrosis, myeloma, or primary biliary cirrhosis
IIb	↑	↑	↑		↑	Combined hyperlipidaemia. Alcoholic excess may be associated. Similar to IIa (above) but complicated by obesity
III	↑	↑	↑↑		↑	Uncommon. Broad-band lipid spectrum; atheroma planar and tuberous xanthomata
IV		↑		↑		Hypertriglyceridaemia; eruptive xanthomata; hepatosplenomegaly; lipaemia retinalis. Often to diabetes, obesity, alcoholic excess or nephrosis
V	↑↑↑	↑		↑↑↑	↑↑	Uncommon. Mixed hyperlipidaemia. Similar to IV but complicated by pancreatitis, acute abdominal pain

The description of the various hyperlipidaemias is complicated by the fact that the convenient day-to-day measurements, total cholesterol and total triglyceride, do not express the complex distribution of these novelties between lipoproteinic particles of differing nature and pathogenetic potential. Table 9.14 represents a grossly simplified summary. The clinical patterns are also complex, and the international classification (Table 9.15) grew out of population and family studies by Fredrickson and others but is also employed to categorize a wide range of 'secondary' hyperlipidaemias. All are influenced by diet. Other major factors are indicated in the final column of Table 9.15. The clinical features correlate overall with the physicochemical criteria as outlined in Table 9.16.

1 Atherosclerosis
This has been especially well documented epidemiologically in relation to coronary disease.

2 Hepatosplenomegaly
This may be found when the disorders are severe and persistent.

3 Tuberous
Nodular or plaque-like yellowish deposits and *planer* (palmar surface) *xanthomata*. These occur only with very marked elevations of LDL, especially in type III disease.

4 Xanthelasma
Yellowish, flat lesions occur on the eyelids quite frequently, and nodular deposits on tendons and extensor surfaces occasionally, in moderate but sustained hypercholesterolaemia.

Table 9.16 Associations of lipoprotein and lipid classes with clinical consequences

Atherosclerosis	↑*LDL* or ↑VLDL or ↓HDL	↑*chol* or ↑TG
Hepatosplenomegaly	↑LDL or ↑VLDL	↑chol or ↑TG
Xanthomata		
tuberons and pla-nar	↑↑LDL	↑↑chol
xanthelasma and tendon	↑LDL	↑chol
eruptive	↑*chylo* or ↑↑VLDL	↑TG
Acute pancreatitis or abdominal pains	↑chylo or ↑VLDL	↑TG
Lipaemic retinalis	↑*chylo* or ↑VLDL	↑TG
Assay interference ('dilution', etc.)	↑chylo or ↑VLDL	↑TG

5 Eruptive xanthomate

Small, yellowish papules on an erythematous base reflect very high chylomicron concentrations. They resolve within weeks of effective lipid reduction.

6 Acute pancreatitis

There is significant risk of fatality, and episodic severe abdominal pain of uncertain origin. The condition can be missed by misinterpretation of the physical signs (and an apparently 'normal' amylase concentration: see below).

7 Lipaemia retinalis

A whitish cast to the venous circulation in the fundus is caused by light scattering by the high concentration of lipid droplets rich in VLDL. The serum in such patients will be overtly lipaemic in the test-tube.

8 Assay interference

'False' readings on laboratory tests can occur in all optically read methods (of which there are now many) or by the dilution of the plasma or serum sample by a major lipid component which distorts the normal range calculated for non-lipaemic plasma or serum (hence the apparently 'normal' amylase, pseudohyponatraemia, pseudohypokalaemia, etc.).

Treatment

The general rules are straightforward and universal, while specific medical remedies are more controversial.

1 Normalization of body weight

Continual prudence in total caloric intake is fundamental. The effect on hypertriglyceridaemia (for example, the type IV pattern) can be especially dramatic.

2 Specific reduction in total fat intake

This will benefit all patients. For those with marked chylomicronaemia, and any tendency to the abdominal complications, this component is critical. The use of medium-chain triglyceride can be helpful in these patients (e.g. types I and V).

3 Saturated fat

Within the reduced fat intake, the amount of saturated fat (or oil) should be minimal, and polyunsaturated oils and fats preferred. Foods rich in cholesterol should be avoided. The key dietary measures listed in Table 9.17 are targets to be approached with some discretion. If the hyperlipidaemia is relatively mild it may be possible to soften the advice; if the disorder is severe then patients may need time to gradually adjust their eating habits (and that of their families) towards the ideal. To encourage compliance, it is worth noting two points:

(a) The important change required is in the overall pattern. Freedom to *occasionally* eat 'outside' the rules will help preserve the individual's social life from a sentence of invalidism.

(b) Other interference with diet, such as changes in

Table 9.17 Dietary advice on hyperlipidaemia (and see text); these general rules are negotiable, and variable for special occasions

Don't …	Do …
Use butter, hard margarine or lard, or eat food rich in these (e.g. pastries and cakes from shops)	Use soft margarines marked 'polyunsaturated' for spreading or cooking
Eat fried food more than occasionally Use excess of dressings	When you do, use corn oil, sunflower or a little olive oil
Use cream or milk	Use skimmed milk, try coffee black, tea with lemon
Eat red meat in quantity Eat more than the occasional egg	Eat fish, chicken in preference Eat more vegetables and salad
Eat hard and cream cheeses	Try cottage cheese, etc.
Drink alcohol beyond the advised limit	Keep your weight within the agreed target range

overall carbohydrate or protein content, sucrose, fibre content, caffeine, vitamins, etc. are not justified by the available evidence, so these burdens should not be added needlessly.

4 Causative or aggravating medical disorders

Diabetes or renal problems, for example, should be controlled optimally.

5 Other risk factors for atherosclerosis

Smoking and hypertension, for example, should be tackled with vigour.

6 Chemotherapy

The medications of most value in patients in whom dietary measures prove inadequate are as follows:

(a) For *hypercholesterolaemia*: bile-sequestering agents such as cholestyramine or colestipol; with the addition if necessary of nicotinic acid or gemfibrozil (a congener of clofibrate but more effective in reducing LDL).

(b) For *hypertriglyceridaemia*: stimulators of lipolysis such as clofibrate, bezafibrate or gemfibrozil are usually effective, the last two (and newer) agents being possibly preferred as they show a lesser tendency to raise LDL cholesterol and a greater tendency to raise HDL (this rise being assumed but not proven to be a further protective factor against atherosclerosis).

(c) For *combined hyperlipaemia*: combinations of the bile-sequestering agents with nicotinic acid or one of the group, clofibrate, bezafibrate or gemfibrozil.

Obesity

The perception of obesity is subject to powerful cultural norms and the psychology of the individual, so for medical purposes the term is reserved for the degrees of fatness which are significantly above average for persons of that sex, age and height. In most research studies the excess above average is set at 20 per cent, though many young women apply criteria far more stringent. The indices that can be employed include:

(a) average weight-for-height tables;

(b) desirable weight-for-height tables (actuarial predictions of lowest morbidity/mortality);

(c) percentage of body mass which is adipose;

(d) skin-fold thickness measurements;

(e) weight:height ratio;

(f) body-mass index (weight:height^2 ratio);

(g) ponderal index (height:cube-root-of-weight ratio).

In formal evaluation of obesity it must be noted, too, that the lean body mass naturally declines with age, and

that the distribution of fat is dissimilar between men and women. Male fat distributes around the trunk, female more around the limbs and hips.

Does it matter?

Tables 9.18 and 9.19 suggest that it does, and the continuing interest of insurance companies indicates that as an overall predictor of mortality and morbidity this 'variable' is relevant. It is evident, too, that the extra load on a failing heart or arthritic joints must contribute to disability, and the surgeon and anaesthetist are faced with

Table 9.18 Mortality rates and body weight expressed as percentage deviation from the average

Men		Women	
Bodyweight	Mortality	Bodyweight	Mortality
−20	110	−20	100
−10	100	−10	95
−0	100	−0	100
+10	107	+20	108
+20	121	+20	123
+30	137	+30	138
+40	162	+40	162
+50	210	+50	200
+60	—	+60	—

Table 9.19 Disorders associated with obesity

Endocrine	Hypothyroidism (myxoedematous tissue)
	Cushing's syndrome (with truncal redistribution)
	Occasionally thyrotoxicosis (inc. appetite)
	Insulinoma (inc. intake plus inc. insulin)
	Stein-Leventhal syndrome (severe polycystic ovaries)
	Post-castration states
Neurological	Ventromedial hypothalamic lesions (tumours, trauma, infiltration)
Syndromes (hypothalamus?)	Prader–Willi syndrome (mental retardation, hypotonia, hypogonadism)
	Laurence–Moon–Biedl syndrome (mental retardation, hypogonadism, polydactyly)
	Fröhlich's syndrome (mental retardation, hypogonadism, short stature diabetes insipidus, poor visual acuity)
	And others
Psychological	Depressive illnesses
	Bulimia (self-induced vomiting)
	Subsequent to anorexia nervosa
Cardiac	Pickwickian syndrome (gross CCF, polycythaemia, cyanosis)

considerable extra difficulty when the patient on the operating table is obese. For many (but not all) obese individuals, their obesity is a constant psychological burden, damaging their self-esteem, confidence and social interactions.

Yet, there is a paradox: some extensive and thorough epidemiological studies employing multivariate analysis have suggested that *as an independent variable* obesity *per se* is of little significance. Obesity is strongly associated with several very powerful risk factors such as hyper-lipidaemia, hyperglycaemia, hypertension, hyperuricae-mia, lack of exercise and smoking. In the medical and social management of obesity the importance of these factors, and their correction, should be recognized.

Aetiology

With the exception only of the occasional hypothyroid patient and the rare patient with Cushing's syndrome, obesity in the human species is a disorder of *intake*. Most clinically obese patients have no identifiable disease or disturbance at all, and even in the vast majority of the disorders associated with obesity the excess weight is caused by a relative hyperphagia (Table 9.19). Although in certain animal species there have been identified some defects in thermogenesis, especially in the so-called 'brown fat cells', which limit the ability of these animals to 'burn off' calories, attempts to reproduce these findings in man have been unconvincing. Every good study of energy balance in human subjects has concluded that obese subjects, far from exhibiting low metabolic rates (basal or stimulated), have a tendency to rates somewhat higher than average 'lean' subjects, consistent with the extra 'work' involved in the operation of the heavier body mass. A similarly uniform finding has been that the obese have a generally impaired perception (sincere even if misguided) of their calorie intake, often underestimating their intake by anything from 20 to 200 per cent.

Treatment

Any associated disorders should be treated so far as possible, and the risk factors identified and treated on their own merits. To reduce weight patients must be helped to reduce their calorie intake to a level below expenditure. Basal metabolic rates in ambulant subjects are never less than 1200 calories, so weight-reducing diets of about 1000 calories daily are appropriate. The 'problem' is a lifetime adjustment, so crash diets—apart from hazards from severe metabolic disturbance and even cardiac arrest—are entirely inappropriate. The effects of crash diets are, as one might expect, transitory. The

difficulties in achieving long-term weight reduction are notorious, but some generally useful statements based on the experience of obesity clinics and slimming groups are offered:

1 This is absolutely a patient controlled problem, and the patient must be genuinely committed towards weight reduction.

2 The lifetime nature of the management means that eccentric and unbalanced diets are of limited usefulness, except as a starter to stimulate enthusiasm. The aim is the achievement of a healthy and enjoyable pattern of consumption which can fit into a normal socially active life-style.

3 The eating pattern will have more chance of permanence if it fits into the other important elements in that patient's life.

4 The motivation is far more likely to persist if it is *supported*, and compliance in most studies correlates almost directly with the regularity, frequency and intensity of the support. The support can be profess-ional or group (Weight Watchers and other similar groups and clubs), or family, or a mix of all these.

5 The targets should be initially modest, and therefore *achievable* within reasonable time: a few kilograms every quarter, perhaps, negotiating fresh targets closer to the ideal on each visit.

Medications aimed at decreasing appetite (for example, fenfluramine) may have a limited role in the initiation of new eating patterns; but there are problems with (psych-ological) dependence on 'the tablet' and a possible dis-traction from the lifetime concept discussed above. Although many patients try and fail, a proportion of patients do succeed in achieving long-term weight reduction. These successess, about one in three in most studies, justify the efforts made.

The *radical approaches* such as intestinal bypass procedures, gastric stapling, gastric balloons, wiring of the jaws, prolonged behavioural courses and surgical removal of excess adipose tissue, have not justified their dangers and expense when long-term results are reviewed. The time for cosmetic surgery may be at the conclusion of major weight loss (to remove excess skin folds, etc.), and it is then, too, that more attention can focus on regular exercise to achieve maximum overall *fitness*. As a means of losing weight, exercise has an insignificant role.

Bone and calcium metabolism

The connective tissue matrix of bone consists of collagen fibres in a polysaccharide ground substance. The turnover of this *osteoid*, its form and its mass, and hence those of whole bone, are influenced by those various factors affecting all other proteins, but more specifically by physical tension, use or disuse, and changes in mineralization. The osteoid is made rigid by the orderly deposition of mineral which consists mainly of crystalline bone salts of calcium, phosphate and carbonate. The mineralization of osteoid is partly a function of the chemical concentration—at the tissue surface—of calcium, phosphate and hydrogen ions, and the enzyme alkaline phosphatase, and partly a function of the pattern of activity of osteocytes. In the broadest terms, in bone, vitamin D acts especially on the chemical environment, while parathormone and calcitonin strongly influence the osteoclasts and osteoblasts.

Hormonal physiology

Parathyroid hormone (parathormone, PTH)

PTH is synthesized in the parathyroid glands, usually four in number but occasionally more, with one or more very occasionally retrosternal. A high-molecular-weight prohormone is cleaved to produce PTH and many N-terminal assays for PTH are plagued by the occurrence and cross-reactivity of molecular fragments of no biological significance. PTH itself is the dominant factor in calcium homeostatis, its secretion increasing when calcium levels fall, stimulating release from bone and calcium reabsorption by the kidney (Table 9.20).

Calcitonin

Calcitonin is secreted by parafollicular cells (C-cells) of the thyroid gland. When infused at high levels it diminishes plasma calcium by reducing the rate of osteoclastic resorption of bone and increasing urinary excretion. In many species it is an important hormone, but in human physiology it seems relatively insignificant. Raised levels of calcitonin are a useful marker of medullary cell (C-cell) carcinoma of the thyroid.

Vitamin D

This might have been 'hormone D' if the knowledge of its metabolism had unfolded earlier. Over 90 per cent of the parent hormone is synthesized in the skin, and the level of the critical highly active form $1,25(OH)_2D_3$ is directly influenced by the concentration of calcium ion and another hormone, PTH (Fig. 9.10). Vitamin D in its active form influences calcium and phosphate flux in bone, kidney and intestine.

Hypercalcaemia

In the patient without symptoms, primary hyperparathyroidism (see page 336) is by far the commonest cause. Most sick patients turn out to be suffering from some sort of malignancy (Tables 9.21 and 9.22). Any tendency to hypercalcaemia can be dramatically aggravated by dehydration, impaired renal function, or circumstances stimulating bone demineralization such as immobilization or fracture.

Table 9.20 Actions of calcium-regulating hormones

	Bone	Kidney	Intestines	Plasma
PTH	↑ Resorption of calcium and phosphate	↑ Resorption of calcium, but ↓ Resorption of phosphate (and bicarbonate), hence 'phosphaturic' ↑ Formation of $1,25(OH)D_3$ (see Fig. 9.10)	only via $1,25(OH)D_3$ (see kidney)	↑ Ca ↓ PO_4
Calcitonin	↓ Resorption of calcium and phosphate (significance?)	↓ Resorption of calcium and phosphate (significance?)	None	↓ Ca ↓ PO_4
$1,25(OH)_2D_3$ (and $25(OH)D_3$)	Facilitates calcium flux	↓ Resorption of calcium	↑ Absorption of calcium and phosphate	↑ Ca ↑ PO_4

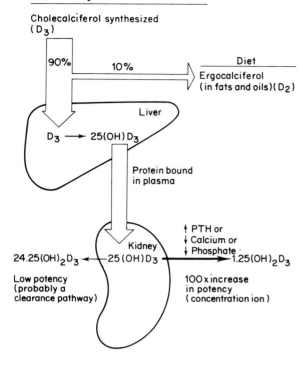

Skin : UV Light

Cholecalciferol synthesized
(D_3)

90%   10%

Diet
Ergocalciferol
(in fats and oils)(D_2)

Liver

$D_3 \longrightarrow 25(OH)D_3$

Protein bound
in plasma

Kidney

↑ PTH or
↓ Calcium or
↓ Phosphate

$24.25(OH)_2D_3 \longleftarrow 25(OH)D_3 \longrightarrow 1.25(OH)_2D_3$

Low potency
(probably a
clearance pathway)

100 × increase
in potency
(concentration ion)

Figure 9.10 *Vitamin D: main pathways.*

Clinical features of hypercalcaemia

1 Kidneys
Hypercalcaemia interferes with reabsorption of water by the renal tubules, producing polyuria and causing thirst. Eventually calcium may be deposited in the renal tubules, producing nephrocalcinosis and renal stones.

Table 9.21 Main causes of hypercalcaemia

Benign	Familial benign hypercalcaemia
Endocrine	Hyperparathyroidism (1° or 3°)
	Thyrotoxicosis
	Addison's disease
Vit. D/calcium	Excessive intake of vitamin D
	Milk–alkali syndrome (excess calcium)
	Sarcoidosis (excess production of $1,25(OH)_2D_3$)
Bone	Metastases, myeloma, etc.
	Non-metastatic hypercalcaemia of malignancy
	Paget's disease (with other factors)
Other factors	Thiazides, ion-exchange, resins, etc.
	Immobilization, fractures (Bed-rest and dehydration)

Table 9.22 Sources of malignancy in hypercalcaemia

	Typical proportion hypercalcaemic (%)
Myeloma	30
Lung (especially squamous cell)	5
Breast	5
Larynx, pharynx	5
Urogenital (especially female)	5
Oesophagus	5
Gastrointestinal tract	1

Mechanisms include:
  metastatic (with local factors)
  non-metastatic (PTH-like substances)
  non-metastatic non-PTH factors

2 Voluntary muscle
There is decreased neuromuscular excitability, which may lead to general muscular weakness.

3 Gastrointestinal tract
Decreased excitability also affects smooth muscle, causing constipation. Anorexia and vomiting are also common. Abdominal pain of a vague but persistent nature may occur in hyperparathyroidism (see below).

4 Malaise
Patients with hypercalcaemia may feel generally ill and depressed and may indeed be diagnosed as having some psychological disorder.

5 Deposits of calcium
These may occur at the junction of the cornea and sclera. The deposits have a granular gritty appearance and are associated with increased vascularity.

6 Bone
If bone is affected by the primary disease there may be pain and weakness, perhaps with fractures.

Marked hypercalcaemia produces confusion, coma, anuria and death, sometimes through cardiac arrest.

Treatment

If possible the specific cause should be removed or alleviated, but other general measures are useful as temporary expedients or to achieve symptomatic relief.

Rehydration is essential, and diuresis may be further encouraged by the combination of generous intravenous fluid infusion with normal saline and loop diuretics such as frusemide, taking care to avoid potassium depletion.

Steroids (400 mg daily of intravenously infused hydrocortisone or 40–60 mg daily of oral prednisolone) can be effective, especially in malignant conditions.

Intravenous *phosphate* or intravenous *mithramycin* in

Table 9.23 Hypocalcaemia: causes, real and apparent

Calcium ↓	Hypoparathyroidsim
	Pseudo-hypoparathyroidism
	Deficiency of dietary vitamin D and
	    sunlight (hence rickets and
	    osteomalacia)
	Failed absorption or activation of
	    vitamin D (malabsorption or renal
	    disease)
	Anticonvulsants (impaired vitamin D
	    metabolism)
	Acute pancreatitis

Protein ↓ (normal [Ca^{++}])	Nephrotic syndrome Hepatic cirrhosis Severe malnutrition
Alkalosis (normal total Ca)	Hyperventilation, lowering [Ca^{++}] Prolonged vomiting or gastric aspiration

malignant disease may be used briefly for severe hypercalcaemic crises, but toxic effects on the kidney and liver limit their value in the longer term. Oral phosphate reduces calcium absorption from the gastrointestinal tract.

Calcitonin has a limited role: the effect on levels of calcium in the blood may be delayed, and the injections may cause local pain and other side-effects.

Hypocalcaemia

The biologically active fraction of total plasma calcium is the free ion, but for technical reasons it is the total figure, dominated by the protein-bound fraction, that is reported. The 'free ion' will also be reduced in concentration by alkalosis, as occurs during hyperventilation: thus the symptoms and signs of tetany may be reproduced during *hyperventilation episodes*, and indeed constitute one of the diagnostic markers for such episodes. The clinical state of 'hypocalcaemia' thus includes true calcium deficits, disorders which affect plasma albumin, and alkalosis (Table 9.23).

Calcium is an ion of critical importance in numerous cell systems, but the acute clinical effects of free-ion hypocalcaemia, *tetany*, are mainly those of increased neuromuscular excitability, while the long-term effects are mainly ectodermal.

Clinical features

In *tetany* there may be peripheral paraesthesia, muscle cramps, epileptic fits, laryngeal spasm in children, occasionally acute hypertension, or psychosis, and the key physical signs, Chvostek's and Trousseau's.

Chvostek's sign is elicited by tapping over the facial nerves as it emerges from the parotid gland beneath the zygoma. A hemifacial twitch consistutes a positive response. Minor contractions confined to the angle of the lips should be ignored, but the combination of twitching of the eyelids *and* the lips is usually significant. *Trousseau's sign* is elicited by the application of a cuff to the arm and raising the pressure to above the patient's systolic blood pressure for three minutes, by which time the hands should have adopted the classical 'main d'accoucheur' position—wrist and metacarpophalangeal joints flexed and fingers extended.

The signs of *longstanding hypocalcaemia* may also include a dry, scaly skin; loss of eyelashes, sparse eyebrows, patchy alopecia, and scanty axillary and pubic hair; brittleness of nails; (in children) hypoplasia or aplasia of teeth; cataracts; calcification in the basal ganglia; rarely papilloedema; susceptibility to moniliasis probably due to immune deficiency; and cardiomegaly, with prolonged QT interval on the ECG.

Treatment

1 Acute emergency
A slow intravenous injection of 10–20 ml of 10% calcium gluconate solution should be instituted until symptoms are relieved or total plasma calcium reaches 1.9 mmol/l.
2 Long-term
The basis of management is physiological. A diet adequate in calories, protein and calcium and encouragement of healthy levels of exposure to sunlight should underpin any 'medical' intervention.
3 Medication
Dietary calcium can be supplemented and a vitamin D preparation administered carefully. To avoid overdosage, levels of calcium and phosphate should be monitored, frequently at first, and at intervals not exceeding six months even when the situation is apparently stable. For most patients simple vitamin D (cholecalciferol) is effective and safest, with doses rarely needing to exceed 2000 units daily. For anephric patients on dialysis and those with severe renal disease or other types of vitamin D resistance, the highly active preparations such as 1,25(OH)$_2$D$_3$ or 1(OH)D$_3$ are more appropriate: they are not dependent on renal metabolism, they act quickly and they are cleared more rapidly.

Hypervitaminosis D

This iatrogenic disorder should not occur at all. Apart from occasional food cranks, the risk arises only in those

Table 9.24 Causes of osteomalacia

Low dietary intake of ergocalciferol (D_2)*
Low rates of synthesis of cholecalciferol (sun-deprived)*
  pigmented skin in Northern climates
  heavily clothed skin
  both
Impaired absorption of D_2 and reabsorption of D_3
  malabsorption syndromes
  following major intestinal resections
  biliary fistulas
Impaired absorption or retention of calcium and/or phosphates
  phytates in flour (especially chapattis)*
  excessive aluminium hydroxide
  renal phosphate wasting in rare renal tubular disorders
Impaired activation of vitamin D_3 (hence low $1,25(OH)_2D_3$)
  renal disease (renal osteodystrophy)
  low PTH in hypoparathyroidism
  enzyme deficiency ('D-resistant rickets type I')
Resistance to $1,25(OH)_2D_3$ ('D-resistant rickets type II')
Anticonvulsants (especially phenytoin)
Other toxins

*These factors may especially coincide in certain ethnic groups (e.g. Asian women living in Britain but adhering to their cultural habits of life-style, diet and dress).

who are on very high levels of unsupervised prolonged courses of cholecalciferol or one of the highly active compounds. The clinical features include all those of hypercalcaemia, but nausea and vomiting may be prominent early symptoms.

Osteomalacia and rickets (vitamin D deficiency)

Osteomalacia represents failure of the organic matrix of bone, the osteoid, to mineralize normally. In children there are also abnormal patterns of bone modelling, epiphyseal growth and dentition, giving rise to rickets. The mechanisms listed in Table 9.24 are best reviewed against the background of the physiology of vitamin D.

Clinical features of osteomalacia

Early symptoms are fatigue, stiffness and skeletal pains followed by muscular weakness and hyporeflexia. The gait is waddling and there is marked adductor spasm. Climbing up stairs may be particularly difficult. Costochondral swelling is common, and there is striking spinal curvature and the pelvic outlet is narrowed. Pathological fractures may appear in the pelvis and long bones, and may be exquisitely painful. Occasionally the plasma calcium level is low enough to produce tetany.

Radiology. Pseudo-fractures (Milkman, Looser) are the most frequent defect. These are lines of increased translucency running in from the surface of the bone, commonly found in the upper ends of the humerus and femur and in the pubic rami. They are strips of decalcification occurring in relationship to arteries or in areas of stress. In severe cases the bones show generalized decalcification with deformity and fractions.

The *biochemical* changes are similar in rickets and osteomalacia (Table 9.25). The plasma calcium is usually a little low and occasionally considerably reduced. The plasma phosphate level is low but the alkaline phosphatase is frequently increased.

Clinical features of rickets

The earliest clinical symptoms are tiredness and muscular weakness. There is bone pain and pain on movement. Dentition is delayed and the teeth may be deformed and quickly become carious. Swelling and tenderness of the distal ends of the radius and ulna are common, and so is

Table 9.25 Biochemical changes in some metabolic bone diseases

	Ca^{++} 2.10–2.60 mmol/l	PO_4^{---} 0.60–1.40 mmol/l	Renal function	Alk. phos. 7–106 u/l	Urinary Ca^{++}
Normal					Men < 10 mmol/24 h Women < 8.5 mmol/24 h
Rickets/osteomalacia	N or ↓	N or ↓	N	↑ or N*	↓
Primary hyperparathyroidism with bone disease	↑	↓	N or ↓	N	↑ or N (urine PO_4^{---} ↑)
	↑	↓	N or ↓	↑	↑ or N (urine PO_4^{---} ↑)
Secondary hyperparathyroidism	N or ↓	N or ↑	↓	N or ↑	↓
Hypoparathyroidism	↓	↑	N	N	↓
Osteoporosis	N	N	N	N	N
Paget's disease of bone	N or ↑†	N	N	↑	N or ↑†

*Rarely if complicating malabsorption.
†If immobilized or dehydrated.
N = Normal.

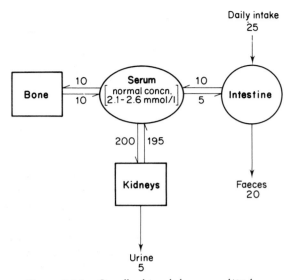

Figure 9.11 *Overall calcium balance, mmol/24 hours.*

the rickety rosary (costochondral swellings). Frontal and parietal bossing of the skull occurs and occipitoparietal flattening may result from the softness of the skull (craniotabes).

If the child can stand or walk, bowing of the legs may result from weight bearing, and kyphoscoliosis may appear.

Radiographs show widening and decreased density of the line of calcification next to the metaphysis, with irregularity and concavity of the metaphysis itself. In severe cases there may be rarefaction with deformities in the shaft of the bone.

Treatment

This depends on the cause (Table 9.24). For *simple dietary deficiency,* vitamin D (2000 units) or liq calciferol (BP) (1.0 ml; 3000 units) are sufficient. In *malabsorption,* doses of vitamin D up to 50 000 units daily by mouth may be required, or 20 000 units can be injected weekly. Treatment should be continued until healing occurs and a watch kept for vitamin D poisoning. In coeliac disease a gluten-free diet will frequently decrease the oral vitamin D requirements. Calcium is also required, and effervescent calcium tablets (Sando-Cal; 2.0 g daily) for an adult are satisfactory.

A few patients have the symptoms of rickets but do not respond to small doses of vitamin D. They are associated with disorders of the D3 receptor, the D3 enzyme system, or the renal tubule (see Table 9.24).

Phosphaturic rickets is *probably* due to a failure of the renal tubules to reabsorb phosphorus, and this defect may occur with renal tubular acidosis or Fanconi's syndrome.

(see page 278). The plasma calcium concentration is normal and the phosphate low. The bony lesions respond to 1,α-hydroxycholecalciferol (alfacalcidol) 1.0 μg daily, modified as necessary, and added sodium phosphate in the diet.

Primary hyperparathyroidism

This disorder is most commonly the consequence of a single parathyroid adenoma, but multiple adenomas and hyperplasia of all glands are nevertheless frequent. Carcinomas make up 1 per cent, but all carcinomas are secretory. Seventy per cent of patients are female.

Clinical features

In the UK most cases are detected on the basis of a chance finding of sustained hypercalcaemia, the patient being asymptomatic. The clinical features of more advanced disease may include all those of hypercalcaemia. Renal stones may be a presenting feature, and in one series of renal stones coming to operation parathyroid disease was present in 14 per cent. Silent renal disease, presenting as nephrocalcinosis or failure, or silent bone disease revealed by elevated alkaline phosphatase levels and a positive bone scan, may be uncovered during investigation.

Investigation

1 Plasma calcium and other biochemical criteria
The key to the diagnosis is sustained or recurrent significant levels of hypercalcaemia in the absence of another obvious cause. Allowance for total protein should be made in interpreting the calcium 'level'. Low levels of plasma phosphate, a raised plasma chloride and an elevated urinary calcium and phosphate loss are suggestive that primary hyperparathyroidism is the cause of the hypercalcaemia. The alkaline phosphatase is raised if there is bone disease, whether due to PTH or not (assuming it is not hepatic in origin). Any concomitant renal failure will tend to raise plasma phosphate and depress plasma calcium.

2 Excluding other causes
It is helpful to rule out sarcoidosis or malignancy as firmly as possible. If they are present a 10-day trial of steroids may markedly depress the calcium level, but 'false' responses do occur.

3 Identifying effects of excess PTH on bone
An isotopic bone scan may reveal a diffuse increase in metabolic activity (and exclude metastases from malignancy) even in the patient without symptoms in

bone. X-rays may reveal subperiosteal erosion, especially in the phalanges, or later in the disease much more dramatic changes: fuzzy trabeculae, patchy erosions and cysts, bowing or fractures in bones, even 'brown' tumours.

4 Identifying effects of excess PTH on the kidney
Phosphate excretion is stimulated, and this can be demonstrated as an increase relative to creatinine by the 'phosphate excretion index' and other special measurements. The 'calcium excretion index' will help identify those with benign familial hypercalcaemia, who suffer no ill-effects of their moderate sustained increase in calcium concentration.

5 Measuring PTH
The presence of elevated immunoreactive PTH in the presence of hypercalcaemia usually confirms parathyroid disease, but a non-parathyroid tumour can secrete a PTH-like factor. Any significant level of PTH secretion is 'inappropriate' when calcium levels are high, the properly assayed level being undetectable in such circumstances. Unfortunately most assays of PTH are rather imprecise.

6 Imaging of the parathyroid adenomas
This is sometimes achieved quite effectively by an isotope subtraction scan (thallium overall perfusion scan minus technetium thyroid scan), while the reliability of ultrasonic, CT and MRI scans in this context remains controversial.

Treatment

The indications for surgery in this condition are debatable: many patients remain symptom-free for many years, but some 30 per cent of those initially without symptoms progress to clinically apparent disease within five years. If the plasma calcium rarely exceeds 2.8 mmol/l and there are no obvious clinical consequences, then regular review may suffice. If symptoms of the disorder occur, or the glomerular filtration rate starts to decline, or an isotopic bone scan shows markedly increased bone turnover, or the calcium levels rise above 2.9 mmol/l, then it will usually be prudent to operate.

The surgery is assisted by preoperative localization of the lesion(s) by isotope thalium–technetium subtraction scan, and colouration of the glands peroperatively by methylene blue infusion. The possible multiple nature of the lesions, and the occasional retrosternal location of the adenoma, have to be considered. In a difficult case, multiple samples of appropriate veins for subsequent PTH assays can be useful in planning any subsequent operation.

Patients, especially those with bone disease, may drop their calcium sharply at operation, and short-acting potent forms such as $1(OH)D_3$ (perhaps 1 μg daily) can be given for as long as necessary, monitoring calcium levels daily and maintaining an adequate diuresis.

The short-term management of acute hypercalcaemia is discussed on page 333.

Secondary hyperparathyroidism and renal osteodystrophy

In conditions in which there is a tendency to hypocalcaemia (Table 9.23)—but especially in chronic renal disease where phosphate may be retained, and in malabsorption where the disorder may be very longstanding —PTH secretion is increased as the physiological mechanism of normalizing the plasma calcium, drawing on the reserves in bone. The result is osteomalacia with features in bone reminiscent of primary hyperparathyroidism. In these patients, however, the calcium levels are rarely abnormal and phosphate levels may be high (in renal disease) or low (in malabsorption).

Clinical features

In children, dwarfism with bone deformities similar to those found in rickets are the most prominent features. In adults the symptoms of chronic renal failure usually overshadow the bone lesions, although bone pain and fractures occasionally occur. The other feature is metastatic calcification which is occasionally palpable but is more frequently seen in radiographs. The *radiological* changes in the bones are complex and may be divided into:

1 Changes similar to rickets.
2 Changes similar to hyperparathyroidism, with subperiosteal absorption of bone often most marked in the phalanges.
3 Patchy osteosclerosis most marked in the skull. The vertebrae may show alternating bands of sclerosis and decalcification producing the 'rugger jersey' spine.
4 Metastatic calcification which may be widespread, both muscles and particularly blood vessels being affected.

Treatment

Bone symptoms can be controlled by giving 1,α-hydroxycholecalciferol (alfacalcidol) 1–2 μg daily together with calcium gluconate (5.0 g b.d.). The plasma calcium level must be estimated at least once a month and the dose modified accordingly.

Long-term management is less successful and the bone changes may progress in spite of continued treatment.

If metastatic calcification is a problem and the blood phosphate level is raised, phosphate absorption can be decreased by giving aluminium hydroxide orally.

Early treatment of this condition in the asymptomatic stage is now recommended using a vitamin D analogue, phosphate-binding drugs and calcium supplements.

Tertiary hyperparathyroidism

In a few patients who have had secondary hyperparathyroidism for many years, the secretion of PTH finally becomes autonomous. At surgery parathyroid adenomas or hyperplasia may be found. The condition might, of course, be the coincidence of primary hyperparathyroidism with a hypocalcaemic disorder, although some have argued that the relationship is causal. Patients are managed as if they had the primary disorder.

Hypoparathyroidism

This may be congenital (in which case there is often a familial trait) or autoimmune, but it is usually related to loss of all the parathyroid glands in the course of surgery on the thyroid gland or in the course of treating hyperparathyroidism. The symptoms are those of hypocalcaemia, and the differential diagnosis is outlined in Table 9.23.

In *pseudohypoparathyroidism* the PTH levels are high but the tissues are unresponsive. This can be demonstrated by injection of a test stimulus of PTH and failing to find the sharp rise in cyclic AMP output from the kidney which occurs in normals and those with PTH deficiency. In addition to the clinical features of hypoparathyroidism, these patients are short, thick-set, round-faced, with short metatarsals and metacarpals and fourth digits, and they are often mentally retarded. These clinical features occasionally occur with normal calcium levels (*pseudopseudohypoparathyroidism*).

Hypercalciuria

Chronic hypercalciuria may lead to nephrocalcinosis or renal stone formation, the risk of which is increased by high levels of oxalate, phosphate and uric acid in urine, by relative stasis (low urine volumes), or urinary tract infection. Hypercalciuria may be secondary to hypercalcaemia, especially the particularly chronic varieties such as primary hyperparathyroidism, but it also occurs in the presence of normal plasma calcium concentrations. This 'idiopathic hypercalciuria' is a disorder of excessive intestinal uptake of calcium, in many cases secondary to an unsuppressible high level of $1,25(OH)_2D_3$ produced by the kidneys. In this situation, PTH is suppressed. The treatment options include a high water intake of three to four litres daily, and a diet which lowers both calcium and phosphate intake and oxalate and uric acid production (low in protein, dairy products, etc.). Thiazide diuretics increase calcium reabsorption and hence diminish urinary levels, as oral phosphate and allopurinol may. Even the slightest urinary tract infection should be treated promptly.

Osteoporosis

This may be defined as an atrophy of bone; although the volume of the bone remains the same, its content of bone tissue decreases and the internal architecture of the trabeculae is severely disrupted. It affects equally both bone matrix and bone mineral, so there is no change in the quality of the bone substance.

Aetiology

Senile osteoporosis is a common disorder. Atrophy of the skeleton is part of the general process of ageing, and starts at about the age of twenty. In certain people atrophy progresses fast enough to produce symptoms which usually appear in late life. This occurs more commonly in women than in men. The main aetiological factors include androgen or oestrogen deficiency, vitamin D deficiency and low calcium intake (particularly in the elderly).

In *Cushing's syndrome* and *steroid administration* a negative nitrogen balance and failure to form bone matrix are important.

Hyperthyroidism and *hyperprolactinaemia* may be complicated by osteoporosis and are associated with increased loss of calcium in the urine.

Immobilization leads to osteoporosis and increased excretion of calcium in the urine, sometimes complicated by stone formation.

In *intestinal malabsorption*, osteoporosis may coexist with osteomalacia.

Rheumatoid arthritis is frequently associated with osteoporosis, especially in those treated with steroids.

Clinical features

The disease may be symptomless, or contribute to a fracture (e.g. of the neck of femur). Pains in the back, round the trunk or down the limbs may be aggravated by jarring or flexing the spine, but rarely have the characteristics of root pain. Sudden severe back pain suggests the collapse of a vertebra.

On examination, the spine is shortened so that height is lost and the distance from the ground to the iliac spine exceeds that from the iliac spine to the crown. Gross kyphosis is the rule and may decrease the vital capacity, but compression of the spinal cord is almost unknown. The consequent buckling of the trunk causes a characteristic transverse skin crease across the upper abdomen above the umbilicus. The infolded skin is keratinized, emphasizing that the changes are longstanding. Radiographs show rarefaction of the spine and biconcave (codfish) vertebrae. No typical biochemical changes are recognized and the alkaline phosphatase is normal.

Treatment

This consists of mobilizing the patient and the administration of hormones and calcium. Oestrogens will reduce the severity of the osteoporosis after the menopause. Their use is mandatory for those with symptoms or continuing major loss of bone mass, and arguably beneficial for many other post-menopausal women. To avoid endometrial hyperplasia and a possible cancer risk, the oestrogen should be accompanied by a cyclical progestagen to induce a monthly withdrawal bleed. This essential but inconvenient element of treatment is often unpopular with the patients. Several suitable sequential preparations are now marketed.

In men, norandrostenolone (Durabolin) 25 mg intramuscularly once weekly or norethandrolone (Nilevar) 10 mg three times daily have been used but are of doubtful value. A reasonably high protein diet and calcium 1.0 g daily (Sando-Cal three tablets daily is a useful preparation) are necessary to replace deficiencies. In older patients it is important to ensure that they are not vitamin D deficient. Relief of pain often occurs within a month or so, though it is rare for radiological improvement ever to be seen.

Paget's disease of bone (osteitis deformans)

Paget's disease usually affects a number of bones to greater or lesser degree, but some bones are completely spared. This is in distinction from osteomalacia and osteoporosis where the whole skeleton is affected, albeit unequally. Sometimes Paget's disease affects just one bone, particularly the tibia, femur, a clavicle, or a vertebra. It is rare before 40 and affects men more than women in

the proportion of 3:2. Occasionally it is familial. Aetiology is uncertain but a slow virus is suspected.

The bones in order of affection are the sacrum, pelvis, spinal column (from below upwards), femur, tibia, skull, fibula, clavicle, humerus, rib. The hands and feet are almost always spared. Clearly the distribution is to some extent governed by stress and strain; the part of the skull which is particularly affected is at the sites of origin of the temporal muscles.

Clinical features

The earliest symptom is pain, usually in the lower back, and often worse at night. Headaches are common, and there may be an unpleasant feeling of hotness from circulatory derangements. Deafness, often of nerve type, is common and the patient may have noticed an increase in the size of his head. The picture may be complicated by platybasia, and pathological fractures are common.

Examination of advanced cases shows enlargement of the head, kyphosis, shortening of the spine and bowing of the long bones, especially in the legs. The bones are highly vascular and act as an arteriovenous shunt. This causes tachycardia, wide pulse pressure with a collapsing pulse, and dilatation of the heart. The limbs and extremities are hot, and often a murmur can be heard over affected bones. *Congestive cardiac failure* of 'high output' type may supervene. In the earliest cases these signs are absent, but there is limitation of hip movement, especially rotation, by pain.

The *serum alkaline phosphatase* level is always raised, often to great heights (350–1000 u/litre). No other biochemical abnormality is found in the blood unless the patient is immobilized, when the serum calcium level rises. The changes in the bones are essentially the result of increased resorption, and are characterized by cystic fibrosis, in this respect resembling hyperparathyroidism. Radiography shows a typical picture; there is increase in total diameter of affected bones, with thickening and broadening of the cortex, and abnormal architecture of the cortex and cancellous bone. In some cases only the proximal part of a long bone is affected, and the area immediately beyond its distal extent is rarefied (*osteoporosis circumscripta*). The disease spreads distally, progressing about 1 cm every two years.

Complications

Pathological fractures are common, and generally heal well. *Deafness*, either from auditory nerve compression or otosclerosis, is ultimately the rule, and the optic nerve too may be compressed, causing *blindness*. Vertebrae may collapse and cause *spinal cord compression* and the effects of platybasia may be extreme. As more bone is involved so the tendency to *cardiac failure* increases. It is claimed that both hypertension and atheroma are more common than usual in Paget's disease; but the most serious (and least common) complication is the occurrence of *sarcomatous change* in the affected bone.

Treatment

There are several drugs that can be used to relieve bone pain and neurological complications.

Disodium etidronate stabilizes calcium phosphate crystals. The usual dose is 5–10 mg/kg daily orally. It may be successful when calcitonin fails and should relieve symptoms within six weeks. New diphosphonates with less damaging side-effects are now under investigation.

Calcitonin (100 i.u.) given subcutaneously daily for six months will usually relieve bone pain. It can also be used to control developing neurological lesions and promote healing of fractures.

Osteopetrosis (Albers–Schönberg's disease)

The outstanding feature is a great increase in bone density so that radiographically they warrant the description of 'marble bones'. The fetal form may be diagnosed radiographically *in utero*, and death always occurs shortly after birth. It is sporadic, whereas the juvenile and adult forms are familial and have Mendelian recessive characters.

Effects are produced by increase in size of bones, so as either to compress nerves (auditory, optic) or to encroach on the medullary cavity and to interfere with blood formation (anaemia initially, later leuco-erthroblastic anaemia, ultimately marrow aplasia). Extramedullary haematopoiesis causes hepatoplenomegaly and generalized lymphadenopathy. In *adults* the disease is relatively benign. About one-third of all cases sustain pathological fractures which heal badly; otherwise there are no symptoms or signs, and the diagnosis is made by chance radiography.

Osteogenesis imperfecta

This condition exists in two forms, *intrauterine* and *infantile*. The intrauterine form causes multiple fractures *in utero* and death either before or shortly after birth. The infantile form presents as pathological bone fragility,

resulting in frequent fractures. The bone changes are due to a defect on the connective tissue scaffolding of bone. The characteristic blue sclera may be absent in the most severe cases.

Achondroplasia

This disease appears in fetal life. The usual pattern of occurrence is of Mendelian dominance, but sometimes recessive characters appear. There is defective ossification of bones formed in cartilage, so the skull vault and spinal bones are normal, but the arms and legs are abnormally short, like those of a dachshund (a canine achondroplasic).

These are the typical circus dwarfs. The average height is about 4 feet; the trunk is normal but the arms and legs are short and the head misshapen. The vault appears large and the face is small with a sunken bridge to the nose. Musculature is well developed, and the hands rather small; the fingers are almost equal in length.

Many achondroplasics are stillborn, or die soon after birth. For those who survive the expectation of life is normal. No treatment is useful.

Other metabolic disorders

Marfan's syndrome

This is a hereditary disorder of connective tissue. The main manifestations, not all of which may occur, are the following.

1 Skeleton
The bones are elongated and thin and the span exceeds the height. The palate is high arched and the hands show arachnodactyly.

2 Cardiovascular system (see page 73)
There is necrosis of the elastic tissue of the aortic wall leading to aneurysm formation, dissecting aneurysm or aortic incompetence, sometimes with superimposed infective endocarditis.

3 The lens of the eye
This may be dislocated.

4 The urine
This may show increased excretion of hydroxyproline, a constituent of collagen.

Aortic aneurysm enlargement is slowed by beta blockade. Aneurysms require resection if they reach 6 cm diameter.

The porphyrias

These rare disorders are the result of specific enzyme

deficiencies on the synthetic pathway of haem: the feedback mechanism responds by increased activation of ALA-synthetase, hence an increased production of ALA (aminolaevolinic acid) and associated metabolites (porphyrins). Characteristic patterns of urinary and faecal excretion of ALA and various porphyrins are therefore diagnostic; in the less rare forms the urine may turn a dark red colour on standing.

Clinical features

1 Acute porphyrias

These are characteristically episodic. They may be provoked by medication, especially barbiturates or oestrogens, by intoxication with alcohol or lead, by severe infections or pregnancy. Severe abdominal colic with nausea and vomiting may mimic a surgical crisis. Fits, transient hypertension, polyneuritis with motor and sensory changes and sometimes pain may occur. Mental disturbance with hallucinations may obscure the picture.

2 Other porphyrias

Marked photosensitivity is the major feature. The porphyrins in tissue may also stimulate abnormal degrees of hirsutism, or in the congenital form discolour the teeth and bones. The colour may appear in urine as a 'port wine' appearance. In variegate porphyria, features of both acute and cutaneous may occur.

Alcohol and medications, as well as sunlight and trauma, may need to be excluded or minimized, there being no specific treatment yet available. A high carbohydrate intake seems to limit the acute episodes.

Hepatolenticular degeneration (Wilson's disease) (see also page 186)

Wilson's disease is characterized by the accumulation in many tissues of excess copper. Levels of serum copper and caeruloplasmin are low and urinary excretion of copper is increased, often with aminoaciduria. Copper deposited in Descemet's membrane gives rise to a golden-green ring at the limbus of the cornea; this Kayser–Fleischer ring may require slit-lamp examination for its presence to be firmly confirmed or excluded; it is pathognomonic.

Clinical features

These are secondary to copper deposition in the liver, basal ganglia and the lens, and usually become apparent between the ages of 15 and 30 years, slightly more commonly in males. In young children the effects of hepatic cirrhosis predominate. In adults, although hepatosplenomegaly often occurs and hepatic failure occasionally precedes significant neurological change, the typical picture is a movement disorder with tremor and rigidity. Cataracts may occur prematurely. Prognosis is often poor, death within 15 years being usual.

Treatment

Penicillamine (1–2 g daily) increases urinary excretion of copper and so the tissue levels. The clinical response may be marked. Dietary restriction of copper can also be helpful.

Carcinoid tumour (see also page 192)

The argentaffin cells of the gastrointestinal tract may give rise to tumours which appear histologically to be malignant but which clinically seem relatively benign; hence the name, carcin-oid.

The tumours secrete *serotonin* (5-hydroxytryptamine, 5HT) and other substances which stimulate smooth muscle. Normally these are detoxicated in the liver and probably the lungs, but if secondary hepatic carcinoid deposits have occurred, then high levels of 5HT appear in the blood. This causes widespread disturbance of smooth muscle. In the bowel, watery diarrhoea is provoked. There is generalized cutaneous suffusion, most marked in the face, and punctuated by attacks of vivid flushing, lasting for a minute or two and often precipitated by alcohol. Stimulation of the smooth muscle in the bronchi may cause asthmatic spasm, with persistent wheezing. A thick white layer of fibrous tissue is deposited on the endocardium of the right side of the heart, causing pulmonary and tricuspid stenosis and eventually leading to cardiac failure.

Some of the 5HT in the body is converted into 5 hydroxy-indole acetic acid (5HIAA), which is excreted in the urine and may be detected with Ehrlich's aldehyde reagent.

Treatment

This is unsatisfactory. It is justifiable to remove as much of the tumour as possible as this will reduce the production of 5HT and reduce the chance of subsequent metastasis. Intestinal symptoms can sometimes be controlled with methysergide which blocks the action of 5HT. Flushing may respond to a combination of an H_1 blocker (antihistamines) and an H_2 blocker (cimetidine), or other agents may be tried: for example, steroids, methyldopa, phenothiazimes or phenoxybenzamine. The course is variable, and patients may survive for ten years or more; the disease is usually fatal but trials of chemotherapy continue.

Amyloid disease

Amyloid is an abnormal protein which may accumulate in the tissues. Some amyloid is composed of light-chain residues from gammaglobulins. It may be secondary to longstanding inflammation (for example, rheumatoid arthritis or tuberculosis) when it is perireticular in distribution. It may also complicate myelomatosis (see page 381). Amyloidosis can also occur as a primary condition, although a number of these cases show a slight increase in plasma cells in the bone marrow. Amyloid also occurs locally in the thyroid in medullary carcinoma of the thyroid and in the brain in old age.

1 In secondary amyloidosis infiltration occurs in the liver, spleen, kidneys, small intestines, arteries and skin. The heart is spared. More rarely endocrine glands, such as the adrenals, are involved. The patient's already bad health grows worse, the skin takes on a waxy appearance, and diarrhoea and polyuria appear. Treatment is of the primary cause. There is some evidence that amyloidosis may be reversible in its early stages.
2 When it complicates myelomatosis the kidney is specially involved, and a nephrotic syndrome may result.
3 Primary amyloidosis affects men and women equally, and is occasionally familial. It occurs between 20 and 40, and may involve the heart, kidneys, muscles of swallowing and breathing, the peripheral nerves or the brain, the lymph nodes, liver and spleen, either singly or together. No treatment is very satisfactory but steroids are worthy of trial. Some intermediary forms with certain features of myeloma may respond to chemotherapy.

Further reading

Besser, G.M. and Cudworth, A.G. (1987) *Atlas of Clinical Endocrinology.* A comprehensive collection of clinical, radiological and pathological photographs illustrating a concise and intelligent text. A good book for visual reference or browsing.

Davidson, J.K. (1986) *Clinical Diabetes Mellitus.* Thieme, New York. An exhaustive reference book, with problem-oriented approach.

Edwards, C.R.W. (1986) *Endocrinology.* Heinemann, London. This is one of an Integrated Clinical Science Series and the approach is physiological, at the level of the clinical medicine student. Lucid text with good illustrations.

Greenspan, F.S. and Forsham, P.H. (1986) *Basic and Clinical Endocrinology.* Lange, Los Altos. An excellent postgraduate text, which is so clear and well-organized that the undergraduate will enjoy reading deeper into subject areas of particular interest.

Hall, R., Anderson, J., Smart, G.A. and Besser, M. (1981) *Fundamentals of Clinical Endocrinology,* 3rd edn. Pitman Medical, London.

Lee, J. and Laycock, J.F. (1983) *Essential Endocrinology.* Oxford Medical, Oxford. Excellent overall, this short text is weak on diabetes but strong on tests and investigation.

10
Disorders of Nutrition

Introduction

Appropriate nutrition plays an important role in many diseases. The aspects relevant to various renal, hepatic, cardiovascular and gastrointestinal disorders are dealt with mainly in their appropriate chapters. This chapter will deal with nutritional assessment, obesity and starvation, specific dietary deficiencies, vitamins and supplemental feeding.

Food intake varies a great deal between cultures and within communities. The necessary elements of the diet are calories, water, the essential amino acids, the essential fatty acids, some carbohydrate, various vitamins and elements. Generally these essential nutrients are provided in adequate quantities by any varied diet of sufficient quantity. However, when intake is strictly controlled, as with parenteral feeding, attention must be paid to specific supplementations. When taken in excess many constituents of the diet such as calories, fat and various vitamins produce their own problems.

The physical characteristics and preparation of the food are also of importance. Cereals and other substances may be deprived of some of their nutrient value by inappropriate preparation. Fibre in the diet may not have nutritive value of its own but will affect the absorption of other substances and alter the behaviour of the bowel. It has been suggested that these effects are important in the prevention of a number of conditions prevalent in Western society, including appendicitis, diverticular disease, carcinoma of the colon and haemorrhoids.

Recommended dietary intakes for adults in sedentary employment are 2500 kcal/day for men and 2000 for women, but 300 kcal/day less over 75 years.

The assessment of nutrition

One of the simplest methods of assessment, and of following changes, is by weighing. The scales must be accurate, and beam or lever balances are best for this purpose. Fluctuations of up to 1 kg occur in normal subjects even if care is taken to ensure the same quantity of clothing each time. Calorimetry suggests that, relating energy to weight change, 1 kg represents around 6000 kcal.

A brief dietary history should be part of the initial assessment of most patients. When dietary factors are felt to be important than a more detailed history is necessary. This is best done by asking either

(a) 'What do you eat on a typical day?'
or (b) 'What have you had to eat and drink over the last 24 hours?'
or (c) 'Write down everything you eat and drink over the next seven days'.

These methods depend on the honesty of the patient and the experience and knowledge of the interviewer. With practice and attention to detail they can provide reasonably accurate information. The contents of various foods can be obtained from standard food tables to produce a detailed analysis of the diet. Such analyses are only necessary usually in surveys and with specific sensitivities. A good idea of the general adequacy of the patient's diet can be obtained just from a careful description of a typical day. Recommended dietary amounts of some important nutrients are shown in Table 10.1.

Other methods of assessment of nutrition are measurement of mid-upperarm circumference, skinfold thickness and serum albumin.

Undernutrition

Most malnutrition world-wide is related to economic problems of food supply. In the Third World this is a considerable problem and has its most devastating effects

Table 10.1 Recommended daily intakes of essential nutrients

Nutrient	Recommended daily intake for young adult males
Energy	2500 kcal
Protein	63 g
Thiamine	1.0 mg
Riboflavin	1.6 mg
Niacin	0.18 mg
Vitamin C	30 mg
Vitamin A	750 retinol equivalent μg
Vitamin B_6	2.2 mg
Vitamin B_{12}	3.0 μg
Vitamin E	10 mg
Folate	200 μg
Sodium	40–100 mmol
Potassium	50–140 mmol
Calcium	600 mg
Iron	12 mg
Zinc	15 mg
Iodine	150 μg

Table 10.2 Criteria and management for starvation

	Weight ÷ height^2 (kg/m^2)	Management
Mild starvation	20–18	Feeding
Moderate starvation	18–16	Oral rehydration, feeding, and supplements
Severe starvation	< 16	Resuscitation in hospital

on children. In higher-income countries problems of malnutrition still occur, particularly in the elderly and the socially deprived, in association with alcohol abuse or food avoidance as in anorexia nervosa (see page 474). There is some risk also when diets are restricted to certain categories of food. For example, vegans who avoid all animal products are at considerable risk of vitamin B_{12} deficiency and may have inadequate intake of calcium, iron and zinc.

Many chronic diseases lead to inadequate nutrition. Disorders of the gastrointestinal tract may reduce appetite, cause discomfort on eating or interfere with absorption of food. Malignant diseases and some chronic diseases are associated with anorexia and weight loss.

Malnutrition in the Third World

The majority of the world's population lives in economically poor countries. These countries tend to have a relatively young population and an increasing population because of high birth rates. The problems related to an inadequate food supply are compounded by poor medical and public health resources, with increased risks of infection without facilities to cope with these. Malnutrition is a constant problem in such areas, with around 100 million children suffering moderate to severe starvation at any time. Major local disasters on top of this background problem are often related to drought or war.

Grades of starvation related to height and weight are shown in Table 10.2.

Clinical features

Malnutrition in children is separated into *marasmus* and *kwashiorkor*, although the two overlap often. Marasmus is equivalent to childhood starvation leading to severe weight loss with muscle wasting. In kwashiorkor the diet is particularly inadequate in protein compared with carbohydrate. Muscles tend to be spared but the liver is affected, leading to hypoalbuminaemia and oedema. The skin may show areas of depigmentation and hair loss.

Early features of malnutrition are weight loss in adults and a failure of normal growth in children. Thirst and hunger dvelop together with weakness and apathy. Nocturia may occur and there is intolerance to cold. The risk of infection is increased and compounds the problem.

As weight loss occurs the muscles become weak and wasted, hair thins and the skin becomes dry, pale and inelastic. There may be bradycardia, hypotension and hypothermia. The abdomen becomes distended and diarrhoea occurs. The associated apathy, weakness and depression increase the difficulties in obtaining food.

All organs and tissues other than the brain are reduced in size.

Investigations

There may be anaemia, leucopenia and thrombocytopenia. Albumin levels are often maintained, but blood sugar falls and ketones rise. The electrocardiogram shows a slow rate and small complexes. The basal metabolic rate slows, with a consequent reduction in oxygen consumption.

Treatment

The management depends upon the severity of the malnutrition (Table 10.2). The first essential in severe malnutrition is resuscitation with replacement of fluids, electrolytes and glucose. At the same time any associated infections must be dealt with. This phase should be followed by a gradual increase in the intake of calories and protein together with vitamin supplements.

Initial supplementation must be followed by plans for the future care and prevention. This involves questions of economics, public health and planning, including education on family planning, breast-feeding, oral re-hydration and growth monitoring.

Vitamins

Vitamins are organic substances or groups of substances that are required in the diet in very small quantities. They act as cofactors for metabolic processes. The necessary vitamins are shown in Table 10.3.

Vitamin A

Vitamin A (retinol) is available performed in some animal foods, particularly in liver, fish-liver oils and dairy products. Polar bear and seal liver have been a source of vitamin A toxicity in Arctic explorers. Coretenes are yellow or orange pigments found in vegetables and fruits and β carotene produces two molecules of vitamin A. This is then stored in the liver, where most adults hold a one to two year store of vitamin A.

Clinical features

Vitamin A is important in maintaining mucus-secreting epithelia, particularly the cornea and conjunctiva. Xeroph-thalmia and keratomalacia resulting from vitamin A deficiency are important causes of blindness in developing countries, particularly in Asia. There may be

Table 10.3 The essential vitamins

Vitamin	Alternative names
Vitamin A	Retinol
Thiamine	Vitamin B_1
Riboflavin	Vitamin B_2
Niacin	Nicotinic acid, nicotinamide
Vitamin B_6	Pyridoxine
Folate	
Pantothenic acid	
Biotin	
Vitamin B_{12}	Cobalamin
Vitamin C	Ascorbic acid
Vitamin D	Calciferol
Vitamin E	Tocoferols
Vitamin K	

an association also with skin tumours. Mild deficiency causes night blindness which responds rapidly to therapy, but more severe, destructive lesions are irreversible.

The toxic effects of excess vitamin A are desquamation of the skin, and raised intracranial pressure in acute toxicity and weakness, dry skin, liver damage and exostoses in chronic toxicity. Large intakes of carotene-containing vegetables produce carotenaemia, in which the skin and plasma are coloured yellow; but this is otherwise harmless. Carotenaemia also occurs in myxoedema, diabetes mellitus and anorexia nervosa.

Treatment

Treatment of vitamin A deficiency consists of retinol acetate orally (60 mg; 200 0000 units) or retinol palmitate intramuscularly. A retinoic acid derivative, etretinate, is used in the treatment of skin conditions such as psoriasis and acne.

Thiamine

Thiamine (vitamin B_1) is found in cereals and some meats. It is important in carbohydrate and amino acid metabolism. Deficiency occurs in the presence of poor nutrition with a diet mainly of polished rice and, par-ticularly in Western countries, in alcoholics.

Clinical features

In alcoholism and starvation for around one month, Wernicke-Korsakoff syndrome may occur. Wernicke's encephalopathy (see page 234) is made up of ataxia, external opthalmoplegia, nystagmus and suppression of consciousness; while Korsakoff's psychosis (see page 233) involves mainly memory problems, often with confabula-tion. Peripheral neuropathy or dry beriberi occurs with marked muscle tenderness. Cardiovascular beriberi involves high-output cardiac failure and is seen in areas of severe deficiency and when prolonged parenteral nutrition is given without supplementation.

Diagnosis

This is based on the clinical picture and the red cell transketolase level.

Treatment

The body's thiamine stores contain enough thiamine to last approximately one month. Cardiac failure and Wernicke-Korsakoff syndrome are treated with parenteral thiamine hydrochloride (50 mg daily). Peripheral neuropathy responds to oral therapy (30–50 mg daily). Other nutrition deficiencies will need to be dealt with at the same time, often using the parenteral combined vitamin B and C preparations.

Riboflavin

Riboflavin (vitamin B_2) comes from dairy products, liver, kidney and cereals and is an essential coenzyme in cellular oxidation.

Clinical features

Deficiency of riboflavin causes anaemia, angular cheilitis, a sore, atrophic oral mucosa and tongue, corneal vascularization and seborrhoeic dermatitis. The diagnosis can be confirmed by measuring the 24-hour urinary output of riboflavin.

Treatment

Treatment is by oral replacement (5–10 mg daily) and ensuring a suitable change in the diet to prevent future problems.

Niacin

Niacin (nicotinamide) acts as a coenzyme in a number of metabolic processes. It occurs in meat, fish and some cereals. Deficiencies of niacin occur in alcoholism, chronic renal failure, Hartnup disease and carcinoid tumours where tryptophan is converted to 5-hydroxytryptamine rather than niacin (see page 192). In Africa those on a predominantly maize diet are at particular risk.

Clinical features

The classic picture of niacin deficiency is *pellagra* consisting of dermatitis of exposed skin, dementia, diarrhoea, and a raw, red and painful tongue.

Diagnosis

This can be confirmed by the low urinary excretion of N-methyl nicotinamide and metabolites.

Treatment

Nicotinamide is used orally (50 mg in mild deficiency and up to 500 mg daily for severe cases).

Pyridoxine

Pyridoxine (vitamin B_6) is found in meat, fish, cereals and some fruits and nuts. Deficiencies occur in malabsorption and with certain drugs which antagonize pyridoxine, particularly isoniazid, hydralazine, penicillamine and, possibly, oestrogens.

Clinical features

Anaemia may develop in children deprived of pyridoxine. In adults cheilosis, glossitis, seborrhoeic dermatitis and peripheral neuropathy may occur.

Diagnosis

Plasma and urinary pyridoxine levels are low.

Treatment

This consists of pyridoxine replacement (10–50 mg daily) and attention to the underlying cause. Pyridoxine should be given prophylactically to patients on isoniazid therapy when high doses are used or nutrition is poor. Excess pyridoxine can itself produce a peripheral neuropathy.

Biotin

Biotin deficiency is rare. It produces a skin rash and painful tongue.

Folate

Folate is found in many vegetables and fruits and in bread and flour products. Deficiency occurs with a poor dietary intake, malabsorption, pregnancy, increased cell turnover in haematological malignancies and with antagonism by drugs such as methotrexate and alcohol. Body stores are small and folate deficiency can develop quickly.

Clinical features

Folate deficiency results in a megaloblastic anaemia similar to vitamin B_{12} deficiency. This is discussed further on page 360.

Vitamin B_{12}

Vitamin B_{12} is ingested preformed in animal foods, particularly liver, but including fish and milk. After combination with intrinsic factor in the stomach it is absorbed in the ileum. Considerable stores exist in the liver. Deficiency of vitamin B_{12} from dietary deficiency, lack of intrinsic factor, or small bowel disease can result in megaloblastic anaemia (see page 360), subacute combined degeneration of the cord (page 234), peripheral neuropathy, optic atrophy and dementia.

Vitamin C

Most of the vitamin C (as ascorbic acid) in the diet comes from fruits, green vegetables and potatoes. It is easily destroyed by heat and alkalis and dissolves in water, so cooking methods for vegetables should take account of this. The body has stores to last 2–3 months.

The recommended intake of vitamin C is 30 mg/day in the UK (60 mg in the USA). Ill patients require a large intake as needs increase with stress, surgery and various drugs. Lack of vitamin C affects collagen formation, capillary and platelet function and is responsible for the syndrome of scurvy.

Clinical features

In infants the features are anaemia, bone pains from subperiosteal bleeding and enlarged painful costochondral junctions (scorbutic rosary). Amongst adults the elderly are at greatest risk of *scurvy*. Bones, joints and muscles become painful and two characteristic features develop. The first is keratosis and haemorrhage at the hair follicles, and the second is swelling, infection and bleeding in the gums. The latter changes only occur in the presence of teeth or underlying roots and not in edentulous patients. Large spontaneous haemorrhages appear together with anaemia and delayed wound healing.

Diagnosis

Vitamin C can be measured in the plasma but is only unequivocally low in advanced disease. Better assessments come from measurement of vitamin C in the blood buffy coat or urinary excretion after a loading dose.

Treatment

In adult scurvy, 1 g of vitamin C should be given daily in divided doses. Larger doses have been recommended for prophylaxis of viral infections and tumours with very little supporting evidence. Large doses can produce diarrhoea and oxalate or urate stones in the urinary tract.

Vitamin D

Vitamin D3 (cholecalciferol) comes from fish oils and fortified margarine in the diet and from the action of ultraviolet light on dehydrocholesterol in the skin. Cholecalciferol is converted to 25-hydroxycholecalciferol in the liver and to 1, 25-dihydroxycholecalciferol in the kidney. Deficiency of vitamin D results in rickets in children and osteomalacia in adults, and the clinical features and treatment of these conditions are described in Chapter 9.

Vitamin E

Vitamin E in the diet comes from vegetable oils, wholegrain cereals, eggs and butter.

Clinical features

The vitamin prevents the oxidation of polyunsaturated fatty acids in cell membranes, and deficiency results in red cell fragility. A mild haemolytic anaemia occurs, and prolonged severe deficiency can produce ataxia, areflexia and retinal pigmentation.

Treatment

Treatment is with oral supplementation or by the intramuscular route in the presence of malabsorption. There is no evidence to support the popular belief that vitamin E supplements increase athletic or sexual performance.

Vitamin K

Dietary sources of vitamin K are mainly vegetables containing vitamin K_1 (phytomenadione). Bacteria produce vitamin K_2 (menaquinones) but this is not an important dietary source.

Clinical features

Vitamin K deficiency occurs in newborn infants and in adults in the presence of obstructive jaundice and malabsorption. Common oral anticoagulants act by antagonism of the formation of vitamin K dependent coagulation factors in the liver. Clinical features of vitamin K deficiency are hypoprothrombinaemia and haemorrhage. Vitamin K dependent factors, including prothrombin, will be low.

Treatment

Vitamin K_1 (10 mg) intramuscularly or, in emergency, slowly intravenously replaces the deficiency. In severe liver disease the lack of clotting factors is not helped by vitamin K.

Trace elements

Fifteen trace elements (by definition less than 0.005 per cent of body weight) are accepted as essential (Table 10.1). Iron and iodine are considered separately.

Copper

Children with malnutrition may develop anaemia, neutropenia and bone changes from copper deficiency. In adults the main problem is copper toxicity in Wilson's disease (hepatolenticular degeneration, page 186).

Fluorine

Dental caries is more common where the level in drinking water is below 1 ppm, and fluoridation of the supply or topical use reduces such caries.

Where the supply of fluoride is excessive, fluorosis develops with white patches on the teeth, pitting and discolouration of the enamel, and bone exostoses.

Zinc

Deficiency in children leads to impaired growth. An inherited disease, *acrodermatitis enteropathica*, is related to zinc malabsorption and produces diarrhoea, dermatitis and delayed growth. Zinc deficiency in adults occurs in liver disease and malabsorption and may produce night blindness and interfere with wound healing. Acute zinc deficiency during parenteral feeding can result in diarrhoea and dermatitis.

Adverse effects of food

Obesity (see page 330)

The body mass index (or Quetelet index) of weight in kilograms divided by the square of the height in meters (kg/m^2) is a suitable index of relative weight independent of height. Around 7 per cent of the population have a body mass index above 30, the threshold for obesity. Gross obesity occurs when the index exceeds 40. Mortality increases with body mass index over the desirable range of 20–25 but also at low weights (perhaps because of associated diseases causing the weight loss).

Obesity usually results primarily from taking in more calories than are consumed. Only rarely is it secondary to thyroid or hypothalamic disorders, although these must be considered.

There are many complications of obesity, particularly glucose intolerance, hypertension and cardiovascular disease, respiratory insufficiency and psychiatric problems.

The treatment of obesity is dealt with on page 331. Most patients require intensive support and encouragement to be successful.

Food intolerance

This may occur with a specific intolerance, such as the gluten sensitivity of coeliac disease (see page 158) or enzyme deficiencies such as lactose (page 146), or with various less-well-defined responses. Allergy to food has received a great deal of media attention and suggests a demonstrable immune response.

Clinical features

Symptoms of food intolerance vary. Early symptoms such as swelling of the lips and urticaria are easiest to pin down because of their close temporal relation to the food. It is much more difficult to be certain with responses like eczema or arthralgia. Most symptoms have been related to food intolerance at some time, but perhaps the best documentation is for urticaria, asthma, eczema, migraine and irritable bowel syndrome.

Diagnosis

When the patient is not certain about a relation to food, a food diary of everything eaten or drunk may help. The next step is to try eliminating foods: either selectively those suspected of giving trouble, or a general elimination of all but a few basic foods, with gradual reintroduction with assessment of individual items. Skin tests are often negative even in the face of documented food sensitivity, particularly if this is not immediate. Skin tests and the radio-allergosorbant test (RAST) look for specific IgE, but false positives and negatives are quite common.

The best way of diagnosing food sensitivity is by double-blind challenge. Usually this should be performed in hospital to deal with any late reactions.

Reactions to food vary. They include IgG and IgE antibodies, but may also occur as a direct response to chemicals in the food (such as histamine).

Treatment

This generally consists of identifying the particular problem or problems and then avoiding that substance. Patients often get on to their own complicated diets. It is important to check that these are nutritonally adequate. Introduction of a relevant allergen after a period of avoidance may result in an augmented reaction.

Therapeutic diets

Arterial disease (see also page 327)

Premature atherosclerosis is related to lipid abnormalities, which result in increased low-density lipoprotein (LDL) and cholesterol in the blood. This may be an inherited metabolic defect or may be related to diet. There seems little doubt that subjects with substantially abnormal levels of these substances should be encouraged to reduce them, and the earlier in life this treatment starts the better.

Although coronary artery disease is correlated with a country's median cholesterol intake, there is less-convincing evidence that changing the eating patterns of a nation can be successful and worth while. However, it seems likely to be helpful and should be encouraged, while greatest help is concentrated on those known to have very high levels.

Relevant foods are shown in Table 10.4.

Hypertension (see page 65)

Much attention has been devoted to sodium and potassium levels in hypertension. Each day the body requires approximately 20 mmol of sodium, although the average intake is much more than this. Reduction in sodium intake will produce a small drop in blood pressure; but the restriction needs to be quite severe to around 50–60 mmol/day, and some patients are not able to tolerate the diet. Substituting potassium and magnesium may help the palatability of the diet and, possibly, further reduce blood pressure.

Table 10.4 Reducing saturated fat and cholesterol

Avoid or reduce	Use
Butter, lard, suet	Polyunsaturated margarine
Cream	Skimmed or semi-skimmed milk
Meat, sausages	Poultry, fish
Cheese	Cottage cheese
Cakes	Vegetables, fruit
Pastries, biscuits	Cereals

Other conditions

Dietary manipulation in diabetes, renal disease and coeliac disease is described in the appropriate chapters of this book. Diet has been associated with malignancies of the oesophagus, stomach and large bowel, but not to a degree convincing enough to modify routine diets.

Enteral and parenteral feeding

Many patients who enter hospital for medical or surgical conditions suffer from poor nutrition related primarily to their underlying disease or to a secondary diminution in appetite. Substantial nutritional deficits interfere with recovery from operations and medical conditions. Guides to malnutrition are shown in Table 10.5.

The options for supplementing nutrition are to encourage suitable high-calorie high-protein feeds; to introduce feeds into the gastrointestinal tract by way of a tube, or to feed intravenously. They should be regarded in this same order of desirability.

Enteral feeding

Enteral feeding is used in patients who cannot or will not swallow appropriate nutrition readily, but in whom gastrointestinal absorption is adequate (Table 10.6). It is much safer and cheaper than parenteral feeding. Enteral feeding tubes are of fine bore and are able to take commercially designed feeds but not liquidized food.

Various commercial feeds are available for enteral feeding, providing approximately 2000 kcal in 2 litres of fluid with around 60–70 g of protein. Fat provides around one-third of the energy requirements. A higher calorie input is needed in the presence of severe sepsis or burns. Trace elements and vitamins need to be added when feeding is necessary for more than four weeks. A low-sodium feed may be necessary in patients with cardiac failure or renal failure.

Elemental feeds in which the protein is predigested to amino acids and oligopeptides may be necessary in the presence of severe intestinal or pancreatic disease.

Table 10.5 Criteria of malnutrition

Ten per cent recent weight loss
Bodyweight < 80 per cent ideal
Albumin < 30 g/l
Lymphocyte count < 1.2 × 10^9/l

Table 10.6 Indications for enteral feeding

Inadequate airway protection (unconsciousness, neurological
  defect)
Severe catabolic states (burns)
Chemotherapy
Short bowel syndrome
Inflammatory bowel disease
Intestinal fistulae

Table 10.7 Complications of parenteral nutrition

Pneumothorax
Air embolus
Catheter fracture
Catheter infection
Venous thrombosis
Fluid overload
Lack of essential nutrient
Increased CO_2 production
Hyperglycaemia

The complications of enteral feeding include
aspiration, vomiting, diarrhoea, hyperglycaemia, oesophageal erosions, and misplaced tubes. Patients who need
prolonged enteral feeding can learn to pass their own
nasogastric tubes so that they can continue treatment at
home.

Parenteral feeding

This is necessary where the gastrointestinal tract is no
longer able to cope with oral or enteral feeding. This may
occur in the short term after surgery, or in the longer term
with inadequate absorptive surface of the bowel. In the
latter situation it can be used for long-term outpatient
care. Access to the circulation is best into a large vein
such as the superior vena cava. The cannula should be
inserted by a strictly aseptic procedure and tunnelled
under the skin to reduce further risk of infection.

The constituents of the nutrition are nitrogen as amino
acids, carbohydrate and fat for calories, together with
electrolytes, vitamins and trace elements. Various
commercial preparations are available. The most suitable
arrangement is to have the hospital pharmacy produce
under sterile conditions a 2.5–3 litre bag containing each
day's supply. This will provide around 2500 kcal (30 per
cent as lipid) and 12 g of nitrogen. The details of feeds
needed in particular situations are best decided by a
designated parenteral feeding team in the hospital.

The complications of parenteral nutrition are shown in
Table 10.7.

Further reading

Davidson, S., Passmore, R., Brock, J.F. and Truswell, A.S. (1979)
  Human Nutrition and Dietetics, 7th edn. Churchill Livingstone,
  Edinburgh.
Silk, D.B.A. (1983) *Nutritional Support in Hospital Practice.*
  Blackwell Scientific, Oxford.

11
Disorders of the Blood

As it perfuses every organ, the blood reflects in both general and specific ways disease elsewhere in the body. In the United Kingdom, among the Caucasian population, intrinsic disease of the blood cells is rare, but changes in their number, shape, size and function can be detected in almost every illness. Among the black, Asian and oriental populations congenital disorders of blood cells are much commoner.

Because it is readily accessible, the function of the blood is better understood than that of any other tissue, and the understanding gained has led to advances in the management of blood diseases which have been both exciting and rewarding. From this understanding we have gained insight into a broad range of disorders of other tissues.

The blood cells

All blood cells are derived from a common, pluripotential stem cell. By a process of division and differentiation, distinct types of blood cells are formed. In the fetus this takes place in both liver and spleen, but from the fifth month of fetal life the medullary cavity of the bones

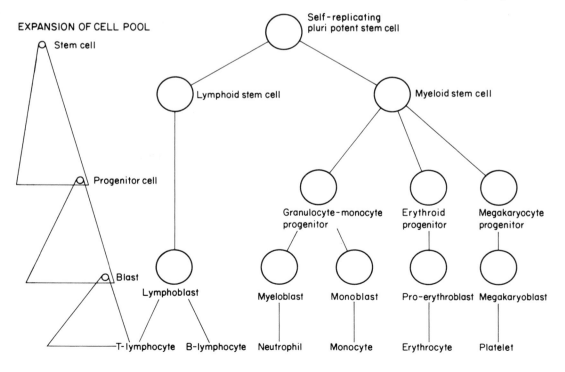

Figure 11.1 *Haemopoiesis.*

becomes increasingly responsible. In adults, the haemo-poietic bone marrow is mainly confined to the flat bones of the axial skeleton. Haemopoiesis is shown diagrammatically in Fig. 11.1.

All stem cells look like small lymphocytes and can only be distinguished from each other in functional assays. The pluripotential stem cell is self-perpetuating but is also capable of giving rise to a series of progenitor cells which are committed to a particular type of differentiation. This process responds to changes in demand and is under humoral control. A series of growth factors has recently been identified.

Red blood cells (Erythrocytes)

The earliest cell recognizably committed to red cell differentiation is the proerythroblast. This large cell will divide three to four times at roughly 24-hour intervals, becoming progressively smaller and acquiring increasing quantities of haemoglobin in the cytoplasm, while its nucleus condenses and is finally extruded. The newly formed erythrocyte when released from the bone marrow contains RNA which appears faintly bluish with Romanowsky stains. Supravital staining with cresyl blue reveals a reticular formation of condensed ribosomes, and such cells are therefore known as reticulocytes.

The mature red cell, a biconcave disc 7 μm in diameter, is extremely pliable and able to pass through spaces one-third of its size. It is a very simple cell comprising a membrane, haemoglobin, and a non-renewable enzyme system to maintain the integrity of the membrane and the respiratory pigment. The function of the cell is to transport oxygen from lungs to tissue by means of haemoglobin. This molecule consists of a protein (globin) which is made up of four folded polypeptide chains. In each chain, in a pocket between the folds, sits the red pigment, haem, which consists of four porphyrin rings surrounding a molecule of ferrous iron. Red cell production depends on the availability of iron salts, needed for haemoglobin; vitamin B_{12} and folic acid, required for DNA metabolism; and erythropoietin, a hormone produced by the kidney in response to hypoxia, which provides the erythroid 'drive' for the marrow.

Red cells survive in the circulation for about 120 days during which time their enzyme systems gradually decay. Effete cells are destroyed by macrophages in the bone marrow, liver and spleen. The iron from the haemoglobin is reutilized by the marrow, the porphyrin structures are broken down to bilirubin which is excreted by the liver, and the protein is recycled.

White blood cells (Leucocytes)

Whereas red cells spend their entire life span within the circulation, the white cells spend relatively short periods there en route to the tissues. There are three types of white cell: lymphocytes, monocytes and granulocytes.

Lymphocytes

The committed lymphoid progenitor cell is believed to arise from the pluripotent stem cell earlier than other committed cells. T lymphocytes migrate to the thymus where they are processed before circulating to the peripheral lymphoid organs. They are responsible for cellular immune responses and control of the immune system. B lymphocytes mature in the bone marrow before migrating to lymph nodes, spleen and other lymphoid tissue. They are programmed to produce specific antibody in response to antigenic stimuli, by differentiating into plasma cells. Lymphocytes are discussed more fully in Chapter 12.

Monocytes

Monocytes are large cells with irregular oval or horse-shoe-shaped nuclei and abundant cytoplasm with small numbers of granules. They derive from the same committed progenitor cell as granulocytes, and recognizable intermediate cells are monoblasts and promonocytes. Maturation takes 2–5 days within the bone marrow. Monocytes circulate in the blood for three days, before passing to the tissues where they become long-lived macrophages with a variety of names depending on the particular tissue: alveolar macrophages (lung), Langerhans cells (skin), microglial cells (brain), Kupfer cells (liver), littoral cells (spleen), osteoclasts (bone), and histiocytes (many tissues).

Granulocytes

Between the committed progenitor cell and the myeloblast, the earliest recognizable granulocyte precursor, at least five doubling divisions occur. Maturation of the myeloblast involves between four and six divisions over five or six days. The nucleus becomes eccentric, kidney-shaped and then lobulated. The cytoplasm becomes increasingly granular; the granules containing peroxidase, acid hydrolases, lysozyme and other enzymes hostile to bacteria.

Neutrophil polymorphonuclear phagocytes (often called 'polys') are held in the bone marrow as a 'reserve' pool for 5–10 days, but they eventually migrate into the blood where they circulate for six or seven hours before passing towards the margins of the blood vessels (the 'marginated' pool) and thence into the tissues, either to die, or when attracted by chemotactic factors, such as complement breakdown products, to act as effector cells in an immune response.

The number of circulating neutrophils increases in response to 'stress' factors: exercise, emotion, infection; and this increase comes from the mobilization of the reserve and marginated pools. Infection leads to the early release of neutrophils before nuclear lobulation has occurred (a shift to the left).

Eosinophil granulocytes have bilobed nuclei and large red granules in Romanowsky stained films. They are phagocytic for IgE-antigen complexes and parasites.

Basophil granulocytes are the blood phase of mast cells. They are involved in immediate hypersensitivity reactions. The Fc portion of IgE is bound to the basophil surface. Reaction of the IgE molecule with specific antigen causes the release of histamine and heparin from the basophilic granules.

Platelets

Platelets are small granular bodies 2–4 μm in diameter derived from cytoplasmic budding of megakaryocytes. The megakaryocyte is a very large cell with a multi-lobulated nucleus and abundant cytoplasm.

If they are not consumed in thrombosis, platelets survive in the circulation for ten days. Their function is to adhere to any break in the blood vessel wall, to aggregate to one another and to release factors which enhance the formation of the haemostatic plug.

Symptoms of blood disease

Although symptoms of blood diseases may be referred to almost any system of the body, a surprising number of disorders are asymptomatic.

Anaemia is frequently symptom-free, especially when it is of slow onset. Even when it does draw attention to itself many of its symptoms are non-specific (tiredness, lassitude, malaise and headache), while others are more clearly related to cardiac decompensation (angina, dyspnoea, orthopnoea and ankle oedema).

Infections are common in blood diseases because of lymphopenia, neutropenia and hypogammaglobulinaemia. Although there may be features which localize the infection to mouth, infusion sites or lung, such features are often absent and fever may be the only symptom of

infection in such patients. This causes diagnostic difficulties since it may also be caused by allergic reactions to drugs or blood products and sometimes as a direct consequence of the disease itself. Night sweats are often a symptom of low-grade fever and may occur in lymphoma and leukaemia.

External bleeding and bruising are features of platelet disorders, whereas clotting factor deficiencies are more likely to cause spontaneous bleeding into muscles and joints.

Pain in the left hypochondrium or left shoulder tip is a feature of splenic infarction, but patients otherwise seldom notice an enlarged spleen. On the other hand enlarged lymph nodes are often discovered by patients, although many such nodes have no serious pathological significance.

Signs of disease

Pallor

This is notoriously easy to misdiagnose since the colour of skin is the product of the pigment contained within it and the blood flowing through it. Facial colour is particularly difficult to assess since it varies with emotion, exposure to sunlight and covering with cosmetics. The mucous membranes give a better guide, although the conjunctivae and gums may be red because of inflammation and the tongue pale because of a coating. Nail beds and palmar creases have the advantage of being comparable with the examiner's own hands. Palmar creases remain pink in a fully opened hand unless the haemoglobin level is less than 70 g/l.

Purpura

The term refers to a haemorrhagic rash which may be due to platelet deficiency or damage to the vascular endothelium (vasculitis). It may consist of *Petechiae*, small (1–3 mm) round, red or brown lesions or *ecchymoses*, which are larger confluent areas of skin haemorrhage ranging from red or purple to blue or green in colour.

Lymphadenopathy

Lymph nodes are distributed widely throughout the body but are normally palpable only in the groins of adults, whereas in children they may also be felt in the cervical region. In the lymphomas and other blood disorders they may be enlarged and readily palpable in cervical, axillary, epitrochlear, inguinal and femoral regions. Very large para-aortic glands may sometimes be detected by deep palpation of the abdomen.

Splenomegaly

The normal adult spleen, which weighs about 150 g, is not palpable on physical examination. As it enlarges in disease states it appears from under the left costal margin advancing towards the right iliac fossa. It is dull to percussion and moves on respiration. The examining hand cannot get above it. The splenic notch may be felt along the medial border. Masses in stomach, colon, kidney, or pancreas, and the left lobe of the liver, are often mistaken for splenic enlargement.

Hepatomegaly

The normal liver may be palpable as much as 5 cm below the costal margin in certain normal individuals but is seldom normally palpable in the epigastrium. Hepatic enlargement below the costal margin should be measured in the mid-clavicular line. Hepatic size is best measured by determining both the upper and lower borders by percussion. The normal vertical span is up to about 11 cm.

Table 11.1 Red cell indices

Haemoglobin (Hb)	Measured by conversion to cyanmethaemoglobin and calculating absorbance at 540 nm Expressed in either g/l or g/dl
Red blood count (RBC)	Measured directly by light scattering or changes in potential difference Expressed as number $\times 10^{12}$ l
Packed cell volume (PCV)	May be measured by centrifuging blood in a capillary tube in a microhaematocrit or by calculation PCV (in %) = MCV × RBC
Mean cell volume (MCV)	Measured directly by electronic counters or derived from PCV and RBC Expressed in femtolitres (fl) = 10^{-15} l
Mean corpuscular haemoglobin (MCH)	Calculated from Hb ÷ RBC Expressed in pg
Mean corpuscular haemoglobin concentration (MCHC)	Calculated from Hb ÷ PCV Expressed in g/dl
Red cell distribution width (RDW)	Electronically derived estimate of degree of anisocytosis

Special investigations

Full blood count

This is normally performed on a blood sample anticoagulated with sodium EDTA. Nowadays, most laboratories are equipped with electronic blood cell counters which rapidly and reproducibly provide precise measurements of haemoglobin concentration, red cell, white cell and platelet number and mean red cell volume. They also calculate from these measurements a number of red cell indices (Table 11.1). More sophisticated machines are able to determine white cell differential counts. Normal ranges are given in the Appendix.

Blood film

Any examination of a blood film stained with one of the Romanowsky stains is the essence of diagnostic haematology. The sizes and shapes of red cells are noted and a differential white count performed. Abnormal cellular inclusions and the presence of certain parasites may be recognized. Terms used to describe abnormalities seen in the blood film are given in Table 11.2. Supravital staining with brilliant cresyl blue allows the detection of reticulocytes, Heinz bodies (denatured haemoglobin seen in certain haemolytic anaemias), and haemoglobin H inclusions (the golf-ball appearance seen in alpha thalassaemia).

Bone marrow examination

Examination of the bone marrow yields far more diagnostic information than the blood film, and it is usually done when investigating blood diseases.

Bone marrow aspirates may be obtained, using a hollow steel 'Salah' needle, from sternum or iliac crest. When adequate local anaesthetic is used together with a gentle technique patients are not deterred from having subsequent investigations should they be necessary. The aspirated bone marrow is spread, like blood, on glass slides and may be examined with Romanowsky stains. Cytochemical and immunochemical staining are useful to identify particular cells. Dispersed bone marrow cells may be examined by immunofluorescence to detect surface markers. They may also be examined cytogenetically to detect abnormal karyotypes (see Chapter 17).

Bone marrow trephine biopsies are usually obtained with the Jamshidi needle, a wide-bore hollow needle with a tapered tip which obtains a core of bone marrow from anterior or posterior iliac crest. The specimen is examined

Table 11.2 Terms used when reporting blood films

Term	Meaning	Significance
Hypochromia	Pale staining cells	Iron deficiency; thalassaemia trait; anaemia of chronic disorders
Microcytosis	Small red cells	
Macrocytosis	Large red cells	See Table 11.10
Anisocytosis	Variation in red cell size	Non-specific, but marked anisocytosis is seen in megaloblastic anaemia
Poikilocytosis	Variation in red cell shape	Seen in megaloblastic anaemia, severe iron deficiency, myelofibrosis, etc.
Spherocytes	Red cells are spherical instead of biconcave discs	Hereditary spherocytosis or autoimmune haemolytic anaemia
Elliptocytes	Red cells are elliptical	Hereditary elliptocytosis or myelofibrosis
Polychromasia	Some red cells appear bluish	Increased numbers of young red cells; haemolysis, haemorrhage or myelofibrosis
Target cells	Thin cells with dark central areas	Liver disease; thalassaemia; post-splenectomy; HbC disease
Tear drop cells	Red cells shaped like teardrops	Myelofibrosis
Anisochromasia	Two populations of palely and normally staining cells	Iron deficiency with treatment or sideroblastic anaemia
Leucoerythroblastic picture	Nucleated red cells and myeloid precursors seen	Marrow infiltration
Acanthocytosis	Irregularly shaped cells	Uraemia, microangiopathy, liver disease
Rouleaux	Red cells appear stacked like piles of pennies	Raised fibrinogen or immunoglobulin, especially seen in myeloma
Basophilic stippling	Fine blue staining inclusions	Lead poisoning; thalassaemia
Howell-Jolly bodies	Dark blue regular inclusions; remnants of nuclei	Splenectomy or splenic atrophy

histologically. Trephine biopsies are performed when aplastic anaemia, lymphoma, secondary cancer and myeloproliferative diseases are suspected or when aspiration have yielded a 'dry tap'.

Erythrocyte sedimentation rate

The ESR is a measure of the rate of settling of red cells in the patient's own plasma. The test must be performed in a standardized way. The rate is mainly determined by the fibrinogen level, but very high immunoglobulin levels will also accelerate settling. In patients over 60 the upper limit of normal increases and in pregnancy the test has no value. The test is mainly used as an index of inflammation and as a screening test for myeloma. In some laboratories plasma viscosity is measured as an alternative to the ESR.

Paul Bunnel test

This test is used to confirm the diagnosis of infectious mononucleosis and detects heterophile antibody which agglutinates sheep red blood cells. Most laboratories use the Monospot or similar test which relies on the agglutination of formalin-treated horse red cells, as a screening test.

Tests of iron metabolism

Serum iron is measured by a variety of colorimetric methods. Iron-containing medicines should be avoided for 72 hours before estimation. There is a diurnal variation with lower levels in the evening. Total iron-binding capacity (TIBC) is an indirect measurement of the serum transferrin content. Iron is stored as haemosiderin and ferritin. Haemosiderin may be visualized in bone marrow macrophages with Perl's stain and is the best indication of the presence of storage iron. A small fraction of the water-soluble iron-protein complex, ferritin, is present in the serum. Serum ferritin may be measured by a radio-immunoassay; in health it correlates with total body iron stores, but it also operates as an acute inflammatory protein and may be raised in connective tissue disorders and cancer.

Tests of megaloblastic anaemia

In some laboratories vitamin B$_{12}$ and folic acid are still measured by microbiological assays in which the vitamin in the patient's serum provides a critical growth factor for a particular micro-organism. However, these assays have largely been supplanted by methods making use of radio-

Table 11.3 Interpretation of B_{12} and folate measurements

	Serum B_{12}	Serum folate	Red cell folate
Vitamin B_{12} deficiency	Low	High or normal	Low
Folic acid deficiency	Normal	Low	Low
Poor diet recently	Normal	Low	Normal

isotope dilution. For a full assessment of megaloblastic anaemia it is necessary to assay serum B_{12} and both serum and red cell folate (Table 11.3).

The Schilling test is a measure of the absorption of vitamin B_{12}. Radio-actively labelled B_{12} is given orally and this is followed by an intramuscular injection of the unlabelled vitamin to flood the tissue stores. If the labelled B_{12} is absorbed it will be rapidly excreted in the urine (normals excrete more than 12 per cent in 24 hours). Those who malabsorb the B_{12} should be tested again with the addition of oral hog intrinsic factor. If this corrects the malabsorption it suggests that the absence of intrinsic factor is the problem and the diagnosis of pernicious anaemia is likely.

Tests of haemolysis

Tests of haemolysis are directed first to establishing that haemolysis is occurring, and then to finding out why. Evidence that haemolysis is occurring is gained from the following.

1 Increased red cell production
Signs of this are reticulocytosis and bone marrow erythroid hyperplasia.

2 Increased red cell breakdown
Signs of these are raised serum bilirubin, increased urinary urobilinogen, absent serum haptoglobins (the haemoglobin-binding proteins of serum) and decreased red cell survival. In the measurement of red cell survival the patient's red cells are labelled by incubating with radio-active chromium (^{51}Cr) and then reinjected. The radio-activity of samples taken on successive days is graphed to determine the rate of decay. The normal half chromium time is around 30 days: in significant haemolysis it is usually less than 15 days.

Variations on this test will yield further information. Surface counting over the liver, spleen and sacrum indicates where red cell destruction is taking place.

The measurement of radio-activity 30 minutes after reinfusion of the chromium-labelled red cells gives an indication of the total red cell content of the body (known as the red cell mass), and this usefully distinguishes between true and spontaneous polycythaemia. The total

body plasma volume may be estimated in a similar way using albumin labelled with radio-active iodine.

Tests for the cause of haemolysis

Clues to the causes of haemloysis may be found on the blood film, otherwise the following tests may be helpful.
1 Osmotic fragility
This tests for lysis of red cells in a series of salt solutions of decreasing concentration. Spherical cells are less able to swell under osmotic stress than are biconcave discs, and therefore lyse at a higher concentration of salt.
2 Coombs' test
The direct Coombs test is used to detect antibody or complement on the surface of cells. IgG antibodies are too small to bridge the gap between adjacent red cells and are unable to cause agglutination in the way that IgM antibodies do (Fig. 11.2). Washed red cells coated with immunoglobulin or complement may be agglutinated by

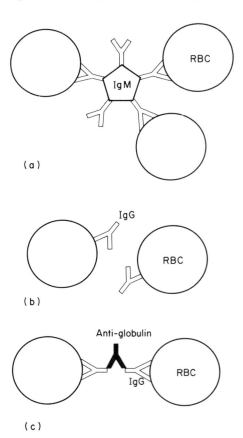

Figure 11.2 *The direct Coombs test. (a) IgM is large enough to agglutinate adjacent red cells. (b) Surface charge keeps red cells so far apart that the IgG molecule cannot react with adjacent cells. (c) Anti-globulin reagent bridges the gap.*

a second layer of antibody directed against the bound immunoglobulin.

An indirect Coombs test is employed in cross-matching blood as a means of detecting a putative anti-red cell antibody in the recipient's serum.

Tests of coagulation and bleeding

1 Bleeding time

This test is best performed in a standard way. The modified Ivy test uses a template to make a standard incision on the volar surface of the forearm while a sphygmomanometer cuff is pumped to a constant 40 mm Hg. The blood is absorbed every 30 seconds on to a piece of blotting paper which is not allowed to touch the incision. The result is mainly influenced by platelet number and platelet function.

Table 11.4 Classification of anaemia

Decreased production of red cells
Disturbed Hb synthesis
   iron deficiency
   anaemia of chronic disorders
   thalassaemias
Disturbed DNA synthesis
   vitamin B_{12} deficiency
   folic acid deficiency
Disturbed proliferation of stem cells
   aplastic anaemia
   dyserythropoietic anaemias
Insufficient humoral stimulus
   chronic renal failure
   thyroid deficiency
Bone marrow infiltration
   malignancy
   myelofibrosis

Increased loss or destruction of red cells
Red cell loss
   Acute bleeds
Intrinsic disorders of red cells
   membrane (hereditary spherocytosis)
   enzymes (G6PD deficiency)
   haemoglobin (sickle cell disease)
Extrinsic disorders affecting red cells
   Antibodies
   physical (heart valves)
   chemical (drugs)
   infections (malaria)
   hypersplenism

Spurious anaemia due to expanded plasma volume
   pregnancy
   splenomegaly
   macroglobulinaemia

2 Prothrombin time

The time taken for citrated plasma to clot after the addition of tissue thromboplastin (extracted from rabbit brain) and calcium is usually expressed as a ratio to a normal control, corrected by a reference value (the International Normalised Ratio, INR). It is prolonged by deficiencies of factors II, V, VII and X and fibrinogen.

3 The Kaolin Cephalin clotting time (KCCT)

This measures the activity of the intrinsic clotting system (see page 384). The steps in this pathway that are variable are the activation of contact factors and the release of phospholipid (platelet factor 3) from platelets. The test avoids these variables by fully activating contact factors with kaolin and providing a platelet substitute (cephalin). The test is sensitive to deficiencies of factors II, V, X, VIII, IX, XI and XII and fibrinogen.

Specialized imaging techniques

Visualization of retroperitoneal lymph nodes is obtained by *lymphography*. In this technique a radio-opaque lipid dye is injected into the lymphatics on the dorsum of each foot and accumulates in the abdominal lymph nodes. The dye remains in the nodes for up to three years so that successive abdominal X-rays allow comparison of the size of lymph nodes and the presence of filling defects. Coeliac axis nodes and mesenteric nodes are not well visualized by this technique, and so for these CT scanning or abdominal ultrasound is preferred.

The anaemias

Anaemia is defined as a level of haemoglobin lower than expected for the age and sex of the patient. Since the concept of a normal range is a statistical one the figures chosen are to a degree arbitrary. The newborn baby has an Hb as high as 200 g/l because the fetus has lived in a relatively hypoxic condition. By three months of age the Hb falls to just over 100 g/l. Because of the stimulating effect of androgens, after puberty males have Hbs on average 20 g/l higher than females. The anaemias are classified in Table 11.4, although this should be regarded as a tentative classification. Most anaemias are multifactorial. Even iron deficiency has a haemolytic element when it is severe.

Iron deficiency anaemia

Aetiology

Iron deficiency is the commonest cause of anaemia in every country in the world but myths about it abound

Table 11.5 Eight myths about iron

Myth	Truth
1 The MCHC is the best index of iron deficiency	A low MCHC was a methodological artefact; the MCV is the most useful index
2 Iron deficiency is a diagnosis	It is only an indication of an underlying abnormality
3 Poor diet is a common cause of iron deficiency	It is very rare in the UK; blood loss is the commonest cause
4 Spinach is a good source of iron	A nineteenth century chemist misplaced the decimal point; it is no better than lettuce leaves
5 Hiatus hernia is sufficient diagnosis for cause of blood loss	Significant numbers also have large bowel pathology
6 Malabsorption is an important cause of iron deficiency	Even in coeliac disease increased iron loss is more important
7 Sideroblastic anaemia is an important differential diagnosis of a low MCV	Most cases of sideroblastic anaemia are macrocytic
8 Parenteral iron raises the Hb faster than oral iron	Oral iron is just as quick and far safer

Table 11.7 Causes of iron deficiency

Inadequate intake	
Poor diet	Seldom the sole factor in the UK but may contribute when there is increased demand
Malabsorption	Contributes to anaemia of atrophic gastritis; post-gastrectomy syndrome; coeliac disease
Increased demand	
Growth	Growth spurts of childhood and puberty
Pregnancy	For uterus, fetus and increased blood volume
Blood loss	
Uterine	Fibroids; carcinoma; 10% normals
Gastrointestinal	Hiatus hernia; oesophageal varices; aspirin; hereditary telangiectasia; peptic ulcer; carcinoma of stomach; Meckel's diverticulum; angiodysplasia of colon; carcinoma of colon and rectum; hookworm; colitis; piles
Urological ·	Haematuria
Increased iron loss	
Gastrointestinal	Coeliac disease 3.5 mg/day post-gastrectomy syndrome 2 mg/day
Renal	Intravascular haemolysis leads to haemoglobinuria or haemosiderinuria

(Table 11.5). Although iron is one of the most plentiful elements on earth its absorption is carefully regulated according to what is needed (Table 11.6). This careful balance is disturbed in thalassaemia and haemochromatosis, and in these conditions excessive iron is absorbed and laid down in tissues.

Table 11.7 summarizes the main causes of iron deficiency. A normal diet which includes meat or fish every day provides most people with their requirements, and in the UK poor diet is seldom a cause of iron deficiency. Fresh vegetables are not a good source of iron (not even spinach). Most iron deficiency is caused by chronic blood loss and the commonest source is the uterus. More than 80 ml loss per month usually leads to anaemia, but most women find it difficult to know whether or not their periods are heavy. Passing clots or having to use both sanitary towels and tampons together are signs that they are. Heavy periods do not necessarily mean disease. Ten per cent of women without gynaecological pathology lose more than 80 ml of blood per month.

Gastrointestinal blood loss is the next most important cause of iron deficiency. Aspirin is a major cause of occult bleeding from the stomach. In the elderly, colonic cancer is common, clinically silent and often operable. Worldwide, hookworm is very common and the main cause of iron deficiency.

The iron deficiency associated with coeliac disease and the postgastrectomy syndrome is mainly caused by the

Table 11.6 Daily iron requirements

	Loss in faeces sweat and urine (mg)	Menstrual loss (mg)	Growth (mg)	Growth of fetus and uterus (mg)	Total (mg)
Men and post-menopausal women	0.5				0.5
Menstruating women	0.5	0.5–1.0			1.0–1.5
Children	0.5		0.5		1.0
Adolescent girls	0.5	0–1.0	0.5		1.5–2.0
Pregnant women	0.5			1.0–2.0	1.5–2.5

Table 11.8 Differential diagnosis of hypochromic anaemia

	Iron deficiency	Anaemia of chronic disorders	Thalassaemia trait	Sideroblastic anaemia
MCV	Reduced	Reduced	Reduced	Usually raised, reduced in rare congenital type
Serum iron	Reduced	Reduced	Normal	Raised
TIBC	Raised	Reduced	Normal	Normal
Serum ferritin	Reduced	Normal or raised	Normal or raised	Raised
Bone marrow: macrophage iron	Absent	Present	Present	Present
Erythroblast iron	Absent	Absent	Present	Ring forms

greatly increased iron loss from desquamating intestinal cells: 3.5 mg/day in coeliac disease and 2 mg/day in postgastrectomy syndrome.

Pathology

Iron absorption occurs mainly through the duodenum and is favoured by acid and reducing agents (like vitamin C). Phytates and phosphates (present in bread and rice) inhibit absorption. The iron content of the gut mucosal cells controls the amount of iron absorbed, which is therefore greater in iron deficiency. Iron passes from gut to bone marrow bound to transferrin. It is stored mainly in macrophages, first as ferritin, from which it is readily exchangeable, and then in its condensed form, haemosiderin. Most iron is delivered to developing erythroblasts for the manufacture of haemoglobin. In the absence of iron, erythroblasts are small with ragged cytoplasm and the red cells they produce are small, thin and irregularly shaped. In severe cases their survival is shortened. Iron is also required by other tissues, particularly for myoglobin and cytochrome C.

Clinical features

Mild cases are often asymptomatic, but as the Hb falls the symptoms of anaemia (see above) appear. In severe cases glossitis (smooth, sore, red tongue) and koilonychia (ridged, brittle, spoon-shaped nails) appear. Dysphagia due to postcricoid webs (Plummer-Vinson or Paterson-Kelly syndrome) is rare, as is pica (craving to eat unusual substances). Mild splenomegaly is sometimes present. Itching may be a feature even in the absence of anaemia.

Diagnosis

The blood count shows a low Hb, MCV and MCH. The low MCHC previously thought to be typical of iron deficiency was an artefact. The blood film shows hypochromia, microctosis with pencil-shaped poikilocytosis and some target cells. The main differential diagnoses are the anaemia of chronic disorders and thalassaemia traits. These can be distinguished by measurement of serum iron and TIBC. Serum ferritin may be helpful in sorting out difficult cases, but sometimes it is necessary to stain a bone marrow with Perl's stain in order to estimate iron stores (Table 11.8). The diagnosis of iron deficiency is not complete until the cause of the iron loss is determined. This may involve a complete investigation of the gastrointestinal tract.

Treatment

Treatment should be directed at the underlying condition. Heavy periods, in the absence of gynaecological pathology, may be reduced by the contraceptive pill or treatment with an anti-fibrinolytic agent such as tranexamic acid (500 mg t.d.s.) on the days of the period.

For replenishment of iron, oral ferrous sulphate (200 mg three times daily) is usually satisfactory. Its main side-effects are dyspepsia, constipation or diarrhoea. These are similar for all oral iron preparations. Those with less severe side-effects contain less iron (ferrous sulphate 200 mg = 62.5 mg elemental iron; ferrous gluconate 300 mg = 35 mg elemental iron). Slow-release tablets are often not absorbed at all. Parenteral iron has no real advantages except that the physician can be sure that it has been taken. (There is a small group of patients so intolerant of oral iron that they refuse it). The haemo-globin rises no more quickly than with oral iron. Intravenous iron may cause anaphylactic reactions, and some of it reaching macrophages is permanently locked within them, making it difficult to assess storage iron in the future. Intramuscular iron stains the skin and a small number of fibrosarcomas at injection sites has been reported.

Anaemias of chronic disorders

Chronic inflammatory diseases (particularly rheumatoid arthritis) and neoplastic diseases produce a blood picture that mimics iron deficiency anaemia, although the MCV seldom falls as low as it may in iron deficiency. The syndrome is produced by macrophage iron being unavailable for haemoglobin production. Measurement of serum iron and TIBC usually distinguishes between the two (Table 11.8), but in complicated cases (such as rheumatoid arthritis with chronic blood loss due to consumption of anti-inflammatory drugs) bone marrow iron stores should be estimated.

Not all anaemia in chronic disease is of this type. In uraemia, the anaemia is a product of shortened red cell survival and lack of erythroid drive from low erythropoietin production. The anaemia of myxoedema is often macrocytic and its origin complex. Thyroxine acts directly on the bone marrow but there is also a haemolytic element and frequently an associated iron deficiency due to menorrhagia or megaloblastic anaemia due to the coexistence of pernicious anaemia.

Treatment

This is of the underlying condition. Parenteral iron is inappropriate and may provoke a severe reaction with arthralgia, myalgia and fever.

Sideroblastic anaemias

The condition is characterized by the presence of rings of iron within mitochondria around the nucleus of developing erythroblasts in the bone marrow. Such rings may be seen in a minority of cells in some patients with haemolytic anaemia, lead poisoning, or rheumatoid arthritis or those on isoniazid treatment, but the commonest form of sideroblastic anaemia occurs in the elderly and is associated with a raised MCV. It is one of the myelodysplastic syndromes (see below). It is only the rare X-linked congenital type of sideroblastic anaemia that has microcytic red blood cells.

Treatment

Some of the congenital sideroblastic anaemias and some of those secondary to other conditions respond to treatment with pyridoxine 100–200 mg/day. Others may require regular blood transfusion but there is a danger of iron overload.

Megaloblastic anaemias

The megaloblastic anaemias are a group of disorders which display a characteristic abnormality in the erythroblasts of the bone marrow; the maturation of the nucleus being retarded compared with that of the cytoplasm. The underlying abnormality is a defect in DNA synthesis. In practice this is almost always due to a shortage of vitamin B_{12} or folic acid, although there are rare enzyme deficiencies and some cytotoxic drugs that produce the same effect. By far the commonest cause of megaloblastic anaemia in the UK is pernicious anaemia (PA), which was described first by Thomas Addison of Guy's Hospital in 1855 and has an incidence of 1:10000. It occurs predominantly in women over the age of 50, especially in those of blood group A and purportedly in those whose hair turns grey at an early age. There is frequently a family history of PA, and both patients and relatives have a high incidence of autoimmune thyroid disease and vitiligo.

Pathology

Vitamin B_{12} consists of a group of cobalt-containing compounds that are produced by micro-organisms. It is found in food of animal origin, especially in liver, but not in vegetables unless they are contaminated by bacteria. Vitamin B_{12} is released from food in the stomach where it binds to intrinsic factor (IF), a glycoprotein secreted by parietal cells. This B_{12}/IF complex binds to receptors in the terminal ileum from where the B_{12} is absorbed into portal blood. It is carried in the blood bound to transcobalamin II and thence transferred to the bone marrow. Storage of B_{12} is mainly in the liver but also in the blood bound to transcobalamin I which is produced mainly by granulocytes. Normally, enough B_{12} is stored in the body to sustain haemopoiesis for five years.

Folic acid (pteroylglutamic acid) is the parent compound of a large group of folates present in leafy vegetables and yeast products. Folates occur in food as polyglutamates and are absorbed as monoglutamates. They appear in the plasma as methyl tetrahydrofolate (methyl THF). In order to be taken-up from the plasma methyl, THF must be converted to 5, 10 methylene THF.

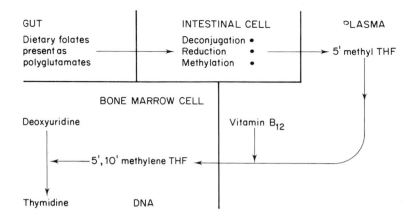

Figure 11.3 *Metabolism of folic acid.*

This reaction requires vitamin B_{12} as a co-enzyme. Once inside the cell 5, 10 methylene THF catalyses the conversion of deoxyuridine to thymidine, a step that is essential for DNA synthesis (Fig. 11.3).

Table 11.9 Causes of megaloblastic anaemia

Vitamin B_{12} deficiency

Decreased intake	Only in vegans whose food is uncontaminated by bacteria
Gastric causes	Pernicious anaemia
	Gastrectomy (total and partial)
	Congenital deficiency of IF
Intestinal causes	Consumption of B_{12} by bacteria in stagnant intestinal loops or by the fish tapeworm *Diphyllobothrium latum*
	Malabsorption due to coeliac disease or tropical sprue
	Disorders of the terminal ileum: resection, Crohn's disease, congenital malabsorption

Folate deficiency

Decreased intake	Old age; poverty; alcoholics; patients in intensive care units
Malabsorption	Coeliac disease; tropical sprue; bowel resection
Excessive utilization	Pregnancy; lactation
	Blood diseases: haemolytic anaemia; myelofibrosis
	Neoplasms: lymphoma; cancer
	Inflammation: rheumatoid arthritis; exfoliating skin disease; patients in intensive care units
Drugs	Anticonvulsants: phenytoin
	Antifolates: methotrexate

Unresponsive to B_{12} or folic acid

Rare congenital diseases	Orotic aciduria; Lesch-Nyhan syndrome
Metabolic inhibitors	6-mercaptopurine; 6-thioguanine; 5-fluorouracil; hydroxyurea; cytosine arabinoside

Pernicious anaemia is caused by a failure to secrete IF due to an immunological attack on the gastric parietal cells by autoantibodies and reactive lymphocytes. The gastric mucosa becomes atrophic and acid secretion is also reduced. Other mechanisms of B_{12} and folate deficiency together with a full list of causes are given in Table 11.9.

Clinical features

The onset of anaemia is usually insidious. Sometimes glossitis is present together with mild jaundice (a lemon-yellow tint). Purpura may be a presenting feature, and this is particularly likely in intensive care units where patients may become acutely and unexpectedly short of folate. Mild splenomegaly is sometimes present and the features of any underlying disease may be apparent. In B_{12} deficiency a neurological syndrome may dominate (see below).

Diagnosis

A macrocytic anaemia is usually apparent, although cases with a normal MCV undoubtedly occur. The blood film shows oval macrocytes, marked anisocytosis and poikilocytosis. Circulating megaloblasts may be seen. There is usually neutropenia and thrombocytopenia and occasionally this is severe. Hypersegmented neutrophils are usually seen. The differential diagnosis involves the other causes of macrocytosis (Table 11.10) and to establish the diagnosis of megaloblastic anaemia a bone marrow aspirate is necessary. This usually shows erythroid hyperplasia with the characteristic megaloblastic picture, the red cell precursors being large with lacey nuclear chromatin but normal haemoglobinisation and the white cell series showing giant metamyelocytes. Serum LDH

Table 11.10 Causes of macrocytosis

Megaloblastic anaemias
Reticulocytosis
    haemorrhage
    haemolysis
    response to treatment
Increased surface membrane
    liver disease
    myxoedema
    post-splenectomy
Dyshaemopoiesis
    myelodysplastic syndromes
    aplastic anaemia
    alcohol
    cytotoxic drugs (esp. hydroxyurea)

levels are high because of ineffective haemopoiesis. Both B_{12} and folate deficiency give the same blood and bone marrow picture, and to distinguish them serum B_{12} and folate and red cell folate measurements are necessary (see Table 11.3). A Schilling test will distinguish between malabsorption of B_{12} and lack of intrinsic factor. Antibodies to gastric parietal cells are present in the serum of 95 per cent of patients with pernicious anaemia (but are also present in large numbers of patients with thyroid disease, iron deficiency and Addison's disease and in 20 per cent of women over 40). Intrinsic factor antibodies are present in 50 per cent of patients with PA and are virtually confined to this condition.

Complications

B_{12} deficiency is associated with a number of neurological complications:

1 Subacute combined degeneration of the cord (see Page 234).
2 Glove and stocking peripheral neuropathy.
3 Dementia.
4 Optic atrophy (very rare).

Females with PA are usually infertile. Carcinoma of the stomach is commoner in PA than in the general populations, but it is still rare. There is an association with other organ-specific autoimmune conditions.

Treatment

In vitamin B_{12} deficiency, hydroxocobalamin (1 mg IM × 6) over two weeks should be given to replenish the stores. Thereafter 1 mg should be given every three months for life. In folate deficiency 5 mg of oral folic acid daily should be given at least for as long as the underlying condition persists. In either condition response is signified by a rise in the reticulocyte count, peaking at seven days, although there is often subjective improvement within 48 hours. B_{12} deficiency will also respond initially to folic acid treatment, but this is a hazardous enterprise since neurological complications are likely to be precipitated. If an urgent response is necessary before the full diagnosis is made, B_{12} and folic acid should be given together. In the elderly, potassium supplements may be necessary during the first ten days since hypokalaemia is common and may be fatal. Blood transfusion should be avoided unless absolutely essential, but if given, packed cells should be transfused slowly, perhaps isovolaemically. Prophylactic folic acid is often given during pregnancy, but physiological doses (0.5 mg/day) are all that are required.

Aplastic anaemia

This is a very rare but extremely serious disorder of bone marrow stem cells in which there is failure of production of erythrocytes, granulocytes and platelets. Each cell line may be affected individually, producing pure red cell aplasia, agranulocytosis or thrombocytopenia. The causes are given in Table 11.11.

Pathology

There is a destruction of stem cells and/or an inhibition of those remaining to divide and repopulate the bone marrow. In some cases this is immunologically mediated through antibodies or T suppressor cells. In others there is genetic damage.

Clinical features

The features are of anaemia, neutropenia and thrombocytopenia. The onset is insidious. Infections in the

Table 11.11 Causes of aplastic anaemia

Idiopathic
Radiation or cytotoxic drugs
Idiosyncratic reaction to drugs
    phenylbutazone and oxyphenbutazone
    chloramphenicol
    gold salts
    troxidone
    sulphonamides and derivatives including thiazides and sulphonylureas
Post-infection
    hepatitis; human parvovirus
Rare congenital conditions
    Fanconi syndrome, etc.

mouth with necrotic ulcers and thrush are very troublesome, and life-threatening haemorrhage—particularly intracranial—is a constant risk.

Diagnosis

Severe pancytopenia is characteristic. There is usually a normochromic, normocytic anaemia, although the MCV may be moderately raised. Reticulocytes are reduced. Granulocytes are fewer than 1.5×10^9 per litre and platelets reduced in severe cases to fewer than 10×10^9 per litre. A bone marrow trephine biopsy is essential to make the diagnosis. It shows patchy cellular areas on a fatty, hypocellular background.

Some cases are associated with paroxysmal nocturnal haemoglobinuria, and in these a positive Ham's test is found.

Treatment

Good supportive care as described for the treatment of acute leukaemia (see page 376) is the cornerstone of management. The milder cases sometimes respond to treatment with anabolic steroids in high doses (e.g. oxymethalone, up to 250 mg/day). Treatment for up to six months may be necessary before there is a response, and the side-effects are troublesome. All such drugs are androgenic to a degree and may cause cholestasis and fluid retention. Approximately 50 per cent of patients will respond to treatment with anti-T-cell antibodies (usually horse polyclonal antibodies, although mouse monoclonals are under evaluation). The best results are achieved by the centres that have the best supportive care.

Bone marrow transplantation (see page 377) should be considered in cases of severe aplasia where a suitable donor is available. The procedure differs from that used in acute leukaemia in that the recipient does not receive total body irradiation (TBI), since there is no leukaemic clone to obliterate, but only cyclophosphamide 50 mg/kg for four days for immunosuppression. Since the degree of immunosuppression obtained is less, rejection is more likely. However, this degree of immunosuppression may be sufficient to switch off the autoimmune process if this is the cause of the disease, and some patients regrow their own marrow rather than that of the donor.

Prognosis

More than 50 per cent of patients die in the first year. If the patient can be kept alive by good supportive care for more than a year, then improvement is likely. Bone marrow transplantation in the young is effective, with more than 70 per cent survival.

Haemolytic anaemias

Haemolytic anaemias are those anaemias caused primarily by increased red cell destruction. They may be caused by intrinsic disorders of the red cell or by external agents acting upon them. Many anaemias have a haemolytic element, but those with another major cause are not usually included within the classification (Table 11.12).

Clinical features

Pallor, mild jaundice and splenomegaly are the usual findings in 'haemolytic anaemia. Acute intravascular

Table 11.12 Types of haemolytic anaemia

Intrinsic red cell defects	
Disorders of haemoglobin	Sickle cell syndromes
	HbC disease
	Rare amino-acid substitutions (Thalassaemias)
Disorders of red cell membrane	Hereditary spherocytosis
	Hereditary elliptocytosis
	Other rare disorders
Disorders of red cell enzymes	G6PD deficiency
	PK deficiency
	Other very rare disorders
Extrinsic disorders	
Immune	
autoimmune	Warm antibodies
	Cold agglutinins
	Paroxysmal cold haemoglobinuria
isoimmune	Rhesus haemolytic disease of the newborn
	Incompatible transfusion
Non-immune	
Physical	March haemoglobinuria
	Heart valve damage
	Microangiopathic haemolytic anaemia (TTP, haemolytic uraemic syndrome, carcinomatosis, haemangiomas)
Chemical	Drugs
	Toxins
Infections	Malaria
	Clostridium welchii
Hyperactivity of monocyte-/macrophage system	Hypersplenism

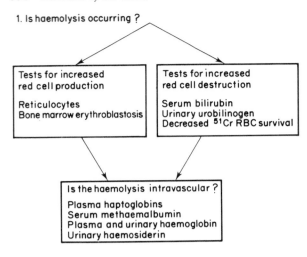

1. Is haemolysis occurring ?

Tests for increased
red cell production

Reticulocytes
Bone marrow erythroblastosis

Tests for increased
red cell destruction

Serum bilirubin
Urinary urobilinogen
Decreased ^{51}Cr RBC survival

Is the haemolysis intravascular ?

Plasma haptoglobins
Serum methaemalbumin
Plasma and urinary haemoglobin
Urinary haemosiderin

2. What is the cause of the haemolysis ?

Blood film
Special tests

Figure 11.4 *Investigation of haemolytic anaemia.*

haemolysis is often associated with back pain and dark urine.

Pathology

After a life-span of some 120 days red cells are destroyed, mainly in the bone marrow and spleen. Increased destruction leads to a compensatory increased production in the marrow which is capable of expanding up to eight times before anaemia results. When blood cells are destroyed within the circulation (intravascular haemolysis) the haemoglobin released is bound to haptoglobin and the complex cleared by the macrophages. Excess haemoglobin is filtered by the kidney; some will be processed by renal tubular cells and appear in the urine as haemosiderin. Some of the plasma haemoglobin is processed to methaemalbumin which circulates in the blood and may be detected spectroscopically. Extravascular haemolysis takes place mainly in the spleen, which is an environment especially hostile to damaged red cells.

Diagnosis

A scheme for the diagnosis of haemolytic anaemia is shown in Fig. 11.4.

Disorders of haemoglobin

The thalassaemias

The Thalassaemias are common in a broad band stretching from the Mediterranean to South East Asia. Generally speaking, alpha-thalassaemia is commoner in the east and beta-thalassaemia in the west. They are caused by inherited defects of globin chain synthesis. The heterozygous conditions (*thalassaemia minor*) manifest as abnormalities of the blood count which mimic iron deficiency, although anaemia is seldom present. The homozygous form (*thalassaemia major*) produce a severe anaemia which may be incompatible with life. *Thalassaemia intermedia* is a clinical term used to describe the condition of a number of patients with the blood features of thalassaemia minor who have a moderate to severe anaemia. It may be caused by the interaction of several congenital abnormalities of haemoglobin synthesis.

Pathology

Each molecule of haemoglobin A consists of two α chains and two non-α chains, either β, γ or δ. The major haemoglobin in the fetus is HbF (α_2, γ_2) which has a relatively high oxygen affinity. After three months of age, although small amounts of HbF continue to be made, the major haemoglobin is HbA (α_2, β_2). HbA$_2$ (α_2, δ_2) is also produced at low levels. Beta-thalassaemia trait is caused by the inheritance of an abnormal β-chain gene from one parent which results in a reduced synthesis of β chains, but their lack is compensated for to a degree by increased synthesis of γ and δ chains. Homozygous β thalassaemia is a much more severe condition characterized by the production of small dysplastic red cells with a short life-span.

Alpha-chain production is controlled by four α-chain genes, two from each parent. Therefore it is possible to have deficiencies of one, two, three or four α chains in alpha-thalassaemia. Four-gene deletion leads to death *in utero* from hydrops fetalis with the formation of Hb Barts (γ_4), and three-gene deletion produces HbH disease (β_4). One- and two-gene deletions produce alpha-thalassaemia minor.

Clinical features

Thalassaemia minor is a clinically silent condition which gives rise to an abnormal blood count, although the Hb remains near normal. Beta-thalassaemia major is not clinically apparent until the production of HbF decays at

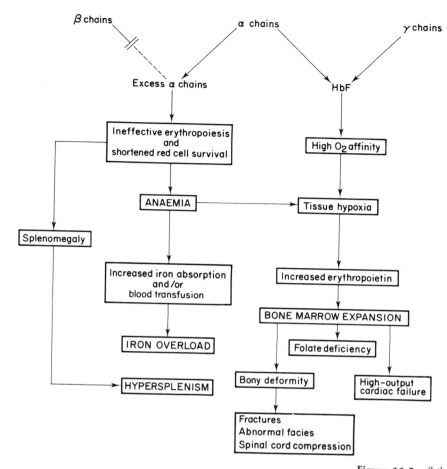

Figure 11.5 *β-thalassaemia major: mechanism of disease.*

about three months of age. The clinical features of the untreated disease are those of severe anaemia, hypersplenism, iron overload and marrow expansion (Fig. 11.5). The characteristic facial appearance is of bossing of the skull, prominent frontal and parietal bones and enlarged maxillae.

HbH disease is a chronic haemolytic anaemia with Hb levels between 80 and 100 g/l and splenomegaly.

Interaction between different types of thalassaemia and the haemoglobinopathies is common so that the phenotypic expression of any particular genotype is difficult to predict.

Diagnosis

The disease may be suspected from the blood count and film appearance which shows microcytosis, hypochromia, target cells, basophilic stippling and normoblasts. In beta-thalassaemia both HbA2 and HbF levels are raised, and in alpha-thalassaemia HbH inclusions may be seen by supravital staining with cresyl blue. In thalassaemia

major, X-rays show expansion of bones, the skull showing a typical 'hair-on-end' appearance. Precise genetic diagnoses are now possible with the use of cDNA probes, and these may be used on chorionic villus samples taken at the tenth week of pregnancy.

Treatment

Thalassaemia minor requires genetic counselling, especially in countries where the disease is common.

Beta-thalassaemia major should be treated with regular blood transfusions. The aim is to keep the Hb near normal so that the marrow may be sufficiently suppressed to prevent the bony changes. This policy leads to iron overload syndrome with diabetes, delayed puberty, liver damage and congestive cardiac failure, but the increased iron absorption found in the inadequately treated patient has a similar consequence. To prevent this iron chelation therapy is given: 2 g of desferrioxamine in each unit of blood transfused, together with pump-driven subcutaneous infusion of desferrioxamine (up to 4 g over 12 hours). Vitamin C (200 mg/day) enhances the urinary iron excretion produced by desferrioxamine. Folic acid supplements are also necessary. Splenectomy may be necessary for hypersplenism.

Prognosis

Thalassaemia minor and HbH disease are compatible with a normal life-span. Untreated thalassaemia major is fatal in childhood or adolescence. Transfusion and chelation therapy are expensive and beyond the reach of many of the countries where the disease is commonest, but they hold out hope for a prolongation of life to near normal.

Haemoglobinopathies

Aetiology

Point mutations of the genes coding for the α and β chains of globin lead to amino acid substitutions which may alter the structure and function of haemoglobin. Some of these have had a survival advantage (particularly in the heterozygous state) in malarious areas. The haemoglobinopathies are relatively common in patients whose origins are in Africa or Asia. In the third world they are a major health problem.

Sickle cell syndromes

These diseases are caused by an amino acid substitution at position 6 of the β chain (valine for glutamic acid). This gives rise to a haemoglobin molecule HbS that is insoluble in the reduced state and which when exposed to low oxygen tension forms crystals; the red cells adopt a sickle shape which prevents their normal circulation through small blood vessels and leads to microinfarcts in various organs.

Homozygous HbS disease is generally a severe disease, although it may be modified by conditions which increase the amount of HbF in the cell. The heterozygous condition, sickle cell trait, is a benign condition except in extreme anoxia. Combination of HbS with HbC or thalassaemia produces syndromes of varying severity.

Clinical features

There is a moderate haemolytic anaemia with an Hb of between 80 and 100 g/l in homozygous HbS disease. This steady state is punctuated by crises. Infarctive crises, which are characteristically severely painful, may occur in any organ but most frequently in the bones of the hand

and feet, the head of the femur, the lungs, and the spleen. They are precipitated by hypoxia, dehydration and infection. Aplastic crises occur either in association with human parvovirus infections or because of folate deficiency.

Diagnosis

The diagnosis may be suspected on the blood film, but this shows characteristic sickled red cells only in the homozygous condition. A solubility test rapidly screens for sickle cell disease and sickle cell trait, and this is valuable pre-operatively. The definitive test is haemoglobin electropheresis on cellulose acetate at pH 8.9, when HbA will migrate further towards the anode than HbS.

Complications

Pregnancy is hazardous in sickle cell disease but careful antenatal care has brought maternal mortality down from about 1 in 3 to 1 per cent. Leg ulcers are a feature of many haemolytic anaemias but are particularly common in adults with sickle cell disease. Most adults show features of hyposplenism. Painful priapism which usually results in impotence is one of the most unpleasant of the results of occlusion in the microvasculature.

Treatment

There is no specific treatment. Avoidance of the factors that precipitate crises is important together with the cultivation of a good standard of health and hygiene. Raising of living standards in the Third World helps to prevent crises. Infections should be treated promptly and acidosis and dehydration avoided. Pregnancy and anaesthesia carry special risks and for these prophylactic transfusions are often helpful. Patients should receive oral folic acid at a dose of 5 mg/day. Immunization against pneumococci and prophylactic oral penicillin reduce the sequelae of splenic infarction. Painful crises are treated with rest and adequate analgesia together with treatment of the precipitating cause. Genetic counselling may be necessary for patients with sickle cell trait.

Prognosis

In areas with a high standard of living sickle cell disease is compatible with an almost normal life-span, but in underdeveloped countries it is often a cause of early death.

Other haemoglobinopathies

Other amino acid substitutions lead to HbC, HbE and HbD. They are quite common in Africa and Asia but produce only mild haemolytic anaemias. There are over 100 different types of haemoglobinopathy that occur sporadically, most of which produce no clinical effect, although a minority cause a chronic haemolytic anaemia. The commonest of the latter is Hb Koln.

Red cell membrane abnormalities
Hereditary spherocytosis

This is the commonest hereditary haemolytic anaemia in Europe and is due to an abnormal structural protein in the red cell membrane. As a consequence the red cell loses its typical biconcave shape and becomes spherical. It is consequently less able to pass through small apertures and prone to destruction in the spleen. It is inherited as an autosomal dominant characteristic.

Clinical features

Hereditary spherocytosis may present at any age. The typical features of haemolytic anaemia are present and a family history is usual. The anaemia is sometimes revealed following a virus infection such as infectious mononucleosis. The severity varies from family to family. Pigment gallstones are common.

Diagnosis

The diagnosis is made by the finding of spherocytes on the blood film and confirmed if this finding is seen in the film of family members. The other common cause of spherocytosis is autoimmune haemolytic anaemia, and therefore in hereditary spherocytosis the direct Coombs test (see page 356) should be demonstrated to be negative. The presence of spherocytes is confirmed by the osmotic fragility test (page 356).

Treatment

Splenectomy results in complete · resolution of the anaemia and all other symptoms. It should certainly be offered to all patients who have suffered from the effects of anaemia or haemolysis, including those with pigment gallstones. Since splenectomy leads to an increased susceptibility to some infections (particularly those due to pneumococci and meningococci), it should be avoided in those with asymptomatic abnormalities and delayed in young children. Prophylaxis against such infection is indicated in young people by immunization with pneumococcal vaccine before splenectomy and long-term oral penicillin following it.

Hereditary elliptocytosis

Elliptical red cells are normal in camels but a rare finding in humans. This characteristic is inherited as an autosomal dominant trait but it seldom causes anaemia. Occasionally haemolysis is severe; when it is, splenectomy is indicated.

Disorders of red cell enzymes

The functions of the red cell enzyme systems are (a) the generation of hydrogen ions to prevent oxidation of the membrane and the haemoglobin molecule, and (b) the production of ATP to fuel the metabolic processes of the cell (Fig. 11.6).

Although congenital deficiency of many enzymes may occur, only two are likely to be encountered.

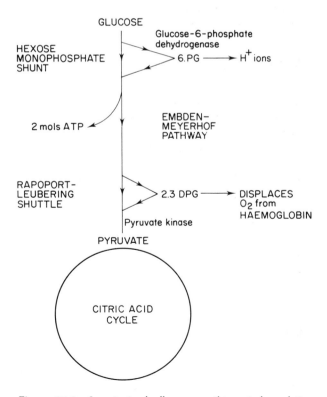

Figure 11.6 *Important red cell enzyme pathways in haemolytic anaemia.*

Glucose-6-phosphate dehydrogenase (G6PD) deficiency

G6PD deficiency is present in over 100 million people in the world. It is inherited as an X-linked recessive characteristic and there are three common abnormalities, the Negro, Mediterranean and Chinese variants, but over 160 sporadically occurring ones.

Pathology

Failure to generate hydrogen ions makes the red cell susceptible to oxidative stress causing denaturation of haemoglobin and the formation of Heinz bodies. Cells containing Heinz bodies cannot traverse the splenic pulp. In severe cases intravascular haemolysis occurs.

Clinical features

Three clinical syndromes are recognizable.
1 Chronic haemolytic anaemia.
This is mainly seen in the sporadic variants.
2 Episodes of acute intravascular haemolysis.
These are mainly in response to exposure to oxidative drugs or fava beans. The Mediterranean type is more susceptible than the Negro type to such stress. Most of the drugs quoted in large textbooks produce haemolysis that is only detectable in the test-tube. Those still in the British National Formulary that produce clinical haemolysis are given in Table 11.13.

Favism is confined to the Mediterranean type. The mechanism is unknown but is presumed to be in part allergic. Ingestion of beans or even inhalation of pollen leads to the most severe attack of intravascular haemolysis. Fava beans (Vicia Fava) are the common broad beans.
3 Haemolytic disease of the newborn.
This occurs particularly in the Chinese variant.

Diagnosis

Apart from the typical features of haemolytic anaemia, the changes on the blood film are minimal. A screening test for the integrity of the hexose monophosphate shunt may be performed and the level of the red cell G6PD may be estimated.

Treatment

Removal of the toxic agent is required together with blood transfusion as indicated.

Pyruvate kinase deficiency

This is the second commonest red cell enzyme defect; 250 cases have been described. It is inherited as an abnormal autosomal recessive characteristic and its chief unusual feature is the mildness of the symptoms for the degree of anaemia. This is because the block in the Embden Meyerhof pathway causes a build-up of 2,3 diphosphoglycerate. This displaces oxygen from the haem pocket making it more available to tissues. Diagnosis is by measurement of the specific enzyme.

Autoimmune haemolytic anaemia (AIHA)

Warm reacting antibodies

Pathology

Self-tolerance to red cell antigens may be bypassed in a variety of ways (Table 11.14), but in 50 per cent of cases the cause is unknown. Some drugs induce autoantibodies, and in most cases the presence of the drug is necessary to detect the antibody; but methyldopa produces a change in the immune system so that the patient's own red cells appear foreign. Thus about 20 per cent of patients taking methyldopa develop red cell autoantibodies although overt haemolysis is seen in fewer than 1 per cent.

Warm antibodies are most active at 37°C and are usually IgG in type. They are usually directed against rhesus antigens and a minority of them fix complement, although intravascular haemolysis is rare. Antibody-coated cells attach to macrophages in the spleen, whereas those coated with complement can also be destroyed by macrophages elsewhere.

Clinical features

The features are those of a haemolytic anaemia of variable severity with splenomegaly.

Table 11.13 Drugs inducing haemolysis in G6PD deficiency

Primaquine
Quinine*
Sulphamethoxazole
Nitrofurantoin
Nalidixic acid
Chloramphenicol*
Dapsone

*In Mediterranean type only.

Table 11.14 Causes of autoimmune haemolytic anaemias

Warm antibodies
Idiopathic (50% of cases)
Secondary to drugs
   methyldopa type
   hapten type
   immune complex type
Secondary to autoimmune disease
   SLE
   RA
   ulcerative colitis
Secondary to lymphoid malignancy
   CLL
   non-Hodgkin's lymphoma

Cold antibodies
Idiopathic (cold haemagglutination syndrome)
Secondary to infection
   mycoplasma pneumoniae
   infectious mononucleosus
Secondary to lymphoid malignancy
   non-Hodgkin's lymphoma

Paroxysmal cold haemoglobinuria
Secondary to
   syphilis
   measles
   varicella

Diagnosis

The blood film shows spherocytes and the direct Coombs test is positive. Features of any underlying disease should be sought.

Treatment

Most cases respond to treatment with oral prednisolone (60 mg/day). The dose is subsequently reduced to the lowest compatible with a normal Hb. If an acceptably low dose cannot be reached, then splenectomy may be indicated depending on results of the ^{51}Cr-labelled red cell splenic-uptake test. In some patients there is a place for immunosuppressive treatment with cyclophosphamide or azathioprine.

Cold reacting antibodies

Aetiology

Cold antibodies are most active at 4°C and are IgM in type. They may appear as part of the immune response to infections with EB virus of *Mycoplasma pneumoniae*, in which case they are polyclonal; or they may be a version of benign monoclonal gammopathy (see page 383) in which the antibody specificity of the monoclonal immunoglobulin happens to be directed against autologous red cells. Occasionally a monoclonal cold agglutinin is produced by malignant lymphoma. The specificity of the antibody is usually within the Ii blood group system. Antibody attaches to red cells in the cold (for example, when passing through skin blood vessels) and fixes the C3 component of complement. At body core temperatures the IgM antibody disassociates from the cell but the C3 remains. C3-coated cells may be cleared from the circulation by macrophages. Low-titre cold agglutinins are frequently present in normal people and complicate blood cross-matching done at room temperature. The only clinically significant antibodies are those of high titres which are active at temperatures greater than 30°C.

Clinical features

In most patients the haemolysis is minor, although after chilling severe intravascular haemolysis sometimes occurs. In many patients the major symptoms relate to sludging of red cells within the peripheral circulation, leading to acrocyanosis and Raynaud's phenomenon.

Diagnosis

The first clue to the presence of cold agglutinins is often a very high MCV caused by the electronic cell counter erroneously counting two cells for one. Red cell agglutination may be seen on the blood film. The direct Coombs test shows the presence complement (C3) on the red cells.

Treatment

The patient should be kept warm and is sometimes best advised to emigrate to a warm climate. Failing that, electrically heated gloves and socks may be a help. Corticosteroids, immunosuppressives, splenectomy and plasmapheresis all have their advocates for the chronic syndrome, but the treatment is generally unsatisfactory. Cases associated with acute infection resolve spontaneously within a few weeks.

Paroxysmal cold haemoglobinuria

This rare condition used to be seen in association with congenital syphilis but is now more frequently a transient complication of childhood virus infections. It is caused by the Donath-Landsteiner antibody (IgG with anti-P specificity) which reacts with red cells in the cold and fixes complement. When the temperature is raised, intravascular haemolysis occurs.

Isoimmune haemolytic anaemia

Haemolytic disease of the newborn (HDN)

Although only 20 years ago this was a major cause of infant mortality and morbidity, the widespread use of anti-D immunoglobulin has greatly reduced the prevalence, so that fewer than 70 infants per year die of this condition in the UK.

Incompatible blood transfusion

Transfusion of incompatible blood produces a haemolytic reaction which varies in severity from severe life-threatening intravascular haemolysis to a clinically inapparent shortened survival of transfused red cells.

Aetiology

Most incompatible transfusions arise from clerical errors. It is extremely important that request forms are filled in completely and accurately and that blood sample tubes are properly labelled. Tests of compatibility involve determination of the blood group of donor and recipient and screening of the recipient's serum for antibodies to red cells. This is supplemented by the cross-matching of donor cells with the recipient's serum. Agglutination is enhanced by the presence of a low-ionic-strength medium. In addition, reaction of the cells with IgG in the serum is tested for using an indirect Coombs test. However, even in the laboratory the commonest errors are clerical ones.

Clinical features

When there is a major incompatibility, symptoms begin after the transfusion of a few millilitres of blood. The patient complains of restlessness, nausea and back pain, and begins shivering and vomiting. The skin is cold and clammy and may be cyanosed. There is tachycardia, tachypnoea and pyrexia leading to prostration and shock. The features of acute intravascular haemolysis are present and this may give rise to acute renal failure due to acute tubular necrosis.

Diagnosis

The identification of all samples and of the patient should be checked. The cross-match should be repeated on pre- and post-transfusion samples. The plasma and urine are checked for free haemoglobin. A direct Coombs test is performed on the post-transfusion sample. Tests for disseminated intravascular coagulation are performed.

Management

The object is to maintain blood pressure and perfusion of the kidney. Intravenous hydrocortisone, saline and frusemide are usually required. Dialysis may be necessary until recovery occurs.

Prevention

The transfusion of blood must not be taken lightly. Check and recheck the identification of patient, sample and blood for transfusion. If in doubt start again. Legal action arising from mistakes cannot be successfully defended.

Red cell fragmentation syndromes

Red cells may be damaged by a variety of physical means within the circulation (see Table 11.12). The most important are prosthetic heart valves and intravascular fibrous strands laid down during disseminated intravascular coagulation. The blood film characteristically shows fragmented cells and microspherocytes. The features of acute or chronic intravascular haemolysis may be present. In infants a similar blood picture without anaemia is seen with vitamin E deficiency.

Polycythaemia

Polycythaemia is defined as the presence of a red cell count greater than normal for the age and sex of the patient. It is usually associated with a high haemoglobin and high haematocrit, but to rely on these can be misleading. Some alcoholics have a high haematocrit with a normal red cell count because they have larger than normal red cells, and some patients with polycythaemia who develop an associated iron deficiency are actually anaemic because their red cells are small (Fig. 11.7).

Polycythaemia may be *spurious*, with a normal red cell mass but a decreased plasma volume, or *true* due to an increased red cell mass. The causes of polycythaemia are given in Fig. 11.8.

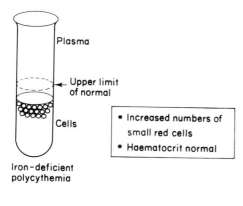

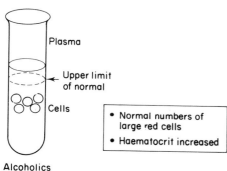

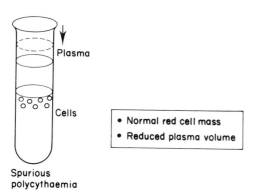

Figure 11.7   *Pitfalls in polycythaemia.*

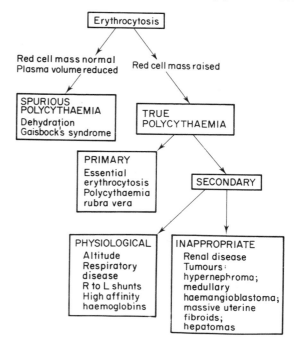

Figure 11.8   *Causes of polycythaemia.*

Primary proliferative polycythaemia (PPP)

This is one of the myeloproliferative disorders and is due to a clonal proliferation of erythroid progenitor cells. Megakaryocytes and granulocyte precursors are frequently involved in the proliferation.

Clinical features

The symptoms of polycythaemia are a feeling of fullness in the head or headache, shortness of breath, blurred vision, cold hands and feet together with those of any complication of polycythaemia present. Aquagenic pruritis—itching after a hot bath—is specific for PPP. Facial plethora frequently occurs but its appearance can be mimicked by exposure to the weather. Cyanosis, both central and peripheral, may be present. Splenomegaly is present in 75 per cent of patients and hepatomegaly in a third. Hypertension occurs in one-third of patients and small numbers have gout or peptic ulceration.

Diagnosis

Apart from the rise in Hb, RBC and PCV there may be a low MCV, since accompanying iron deficiency is common. There is frequently a neutrophil leucocytosis, a raised basophil count and a raised platelet count. The ESR is usually very low (1 mm in the first hour). The leucocyte alkaline phosphatase score is usually high and the serum B_{12} is high in a third of patients. Serum uric acid is often raised. Platelet function may be abnormal. The bone marrow aspirate is less helpful than the trephine biopsy, which shows hypercellularity with hyperplasia of erythropoiesis, granulopoiesis and thrombopoiesis.

Differential diagnosis

The patient with all of the features of the disease presents little diagnostic problem, but all of the features are seldom present. It is important to estimate the red cell mass and plasma volume (see page 356) to exclude spurious polycythaemia. The history and examination should point to underlying diseases of respiratory or cardiovascular systems and may reveal a tumor. Intravenous pyelography may be necessary to exclude a renal lesion, and arterial oxygen saturation measurements to exclude arteriovenous shunting.

Complications

The most frequent complications are cerebrovascular or peripheral ischaemia caused by the hyperviscosity of the blood. Some patients suffer bleeding manifestations owing to disorders of platelet function. Epistaxis, bruising and gastrointestinal haemorrhages may be seen. Myelofibrosis supervenes in 30 per cent of cases, and transformation to acute leukaemia occurs in 15 per cent.

Treatment

The most important aim of treatment is to lower the viscosity of the blood. This is best done by venesections, at least in the first instance. The aim should be to keep the PCV below 45 per cent (as measured by a centrifugal method). Some authorities prefer to manage the patient in the long-term by venesection, relying on the iron deficiency induced to keep the Hb low. Unfortunately, this policy may actually intensify the itching and the platelet count may rise and put the patient at risk from haemorrhage or thrombosis. Long-term low-dose aspirin (300 mg/day) has been recommended to reduce this risk.

Radioactive phosphorus (^{32}P) has been in use for many years. It is a beta-emitter which is concentrated in bone and from there irradiates the bone marrow. A single dose produces a remission lasting about two years and it may be repeated. There seems little doubt that ^{32}P increases the risk of leukaemic transformation, although others believe that this feature needs to be weighed against the longer survival in this group of patients compared with those treated by venesecton.

Cytotoxic drugs also have their advocates. Most carry a similar risk of leukaemic transformation as ^{32}P, although this may not be true for hydroxyurea (500–1000 mg/day) which is well-tolerated, easily reversible and has few side-effects.

Secondary polycythaemia

The control of haemoglobin level depends on oxygen receptors in the juxtaglomerular apparatus of the kidney.

Hypoxia leads to an increased secretion of erythropoietin, which is entirely appropriate if the hypoxia is caused by anaemia, but of less value in cardiac or respiratory disease and inappropriate when caused by distortion of the renal vasculature as in renal artery stenosis or polycystic kidneys. Inappropriate secretion of erythropoietin may also rarely arise from certain tumors (Fig. 11.8).

Treatment

Venesection is often indicated to give symtomatic relief and to reduce the risk of thrombosis, but a balance must be struck between oxygen carriage and viscosity. In patients with right-to-left cardiac shunts haematocrits of 70 per cent or more may occur. However, attempts to reduce viscosity by venesection are limited by symptoms of tissue hypoxia, particularly angina.

Spurious polycythaemia

Acute dehydration due to burns, vomiting or polyuria will raise the haematocrit. In stress polycythaemia (*Gaisbock's syndrome*), the plasma volume is chronically reduced for ill-understood reasons. Patients are usually middle-aged men, somewhat overweight, often with hypertension and are usually cigarette smokers. The condition is just as common in manual workers as in business executives. The disease mechanism is obscure but is almost certainly related to cigarette smoking. Untreated, about half of patients suffer a cardiac or cerebrovascular 'event' within 18 months of diagnosis.

Treatment

It is most important to stop smoking. In most patients who are able to stop the plasma volume rapidly returns to normal. The place of regular small-volume venesections is currently being investigated.

Primary proliferative thrombocythaemia

This condition is closely related to primary proliferative polycythaemia, being a clonal proliferation of stem cells mainly committed to the production of megakaryocytes.

Clinical features

Many patients are asymptomatic, but both haemorrhagic and thrombotic manifestations occur in cerebral and peripheral circulations. Splenomegaly is rare, possibly because of repeated small splenic infarctions.

Table 11.15 Causes of a raised platelet count

Proliferative
Primary proliferative thrombocythaemia
In association with other myeloproliferative disorders

Reactive
Haemorrhage
Chronic iron deficiency
Chronic infections
Chronic inflammatory conditions (esp. rheumatoid arthritis and Crohn's disease)
Malignancy
Post-splenectomy
Recovery from:
   megaloblsatic anaemia
   cytotoxic drugs
   alcohol
Treatment with vinca alkyloids

Investigations

The platelet count is usually greater than 1000×10^9 per litre. Since platelet function is abnormal, tests for chronic gastrointestinal haemorrhage may be positive and iron deficiency anaemia may be present. Bone marrow shows hypercellularity with increased numbers of megakaryocytes.

Differential diagnosis

The causes of a raised platelet count are given in Table 11.15. It may be difficult to distinguish reactive thrombocytosis from essential thrombocythaemia, but giant platelets and abnormal platelet function are more characteristic of the latter.

Treatment

There is no indication to treat asymptomatic patients. Haemorrhagic or thrombotic complications may be controlled or prevented by low-dose aspirin (300 mg/day). Radioactive phosphorus or hydroxyurea are both effective treatments of the myeloproliferation. Transformation to acute leukaemia is very rare.

Myelofibrosis

This condition masquerades under several names, including myelosclerosis, agnogenic myeloid metaplasia and myelofibrosis with myeloid metaplasia (MMM).

Pathology

Bone marrow fibrosis may occur in reaction to a number of stimuli, including infiltration with lymphoma, leukaemia or cancer. In the idiopathic type it seems to be in response to a proliferation of haemopoietic stem cells (possibly megakaryocyte precursors). The fibroblasts are not part of the clonal proliferation. Apparently in response to the marrow fibrosis, haemopoietic proliferation occurs in spleen, liver and sometimes lymph nodes.

Clinical features

Myelofibrosis is a disease of the elderly presenting with the symptoms of anaemia, weight loss, anorexia, night sweats and splenic pain. Bone pain, bruises, bleeding and infections may occur less frequently. There is almost invariably massive splenomegaly.

Diagnosis

Anaemia is usually present, often with a neutrophil leucocytosis, although neutropenia and thrombocytopenia occur late in the disease. The blood film shows a leuco-erythroblastic picture with a characteristic 'teardrop' poikilocytosis. Bone marrow aspirate often yields a 'dry tap', and trephine biopsy shows a hypercellular marrow with increased 'reticulin' demonstrated by silver stains. There is usually increased collagen and often increased bone formation. Megakaryocytes may be prominent.

Treatment

Blood transfusion and folic acid supplements may be all that is required, but the more proliferative cases often benefit from hydroxyurea treatment. Splenectomy is sometimes effective, but choosing when to offer it is difficult. Indications for splenectomy are increasing transfusion requirement, massive splenomegaly causing discomfort, and severe thrombocytopenia. Removing a massive spleen may be difficult (particularly if it has previously been irradiated). Early splenectomy is controversial. After splenectomy the liver often markedly enlarges because of extramedullary haemopoiesis, and this sometimes also causes lymphadenopathy.

Prognosis

Median survival is three years. Fewer than 10 per cent transform to acute leukaemia.

Infectious mononucleosis

In Western Europe and North America infection with the Epstein-Barr virus is either subclinical or produces infectious mononucleosis (sometimes known as glandular fever). In Africa the same virus is involved in the aetiology of Burkitt's lymphoma and in the Far East it plays a part in the development of nasopharyngeal carcinoma. The incidence of infectious mononucleosis is difficult to calculate, but most adults, when tested, show evidence of previous exposure to the virus.

The condition is discussed further on page 421.

Neutropenia

Mild neutropenia is one of the commonest findings in the routine blood count. Severe neutropenia (sometimes called agranulocytosis) is very rare and usually of grave significance. The causes of neutropenia are given in Table 11.16.

Pathology

The mechanisms of neutropenia are either decreased production or increased destruction. Drugs interact with antibodies and granulocytes in the same way that they react with antibodies and red cells to cause haemolytic anaemias.

Table 11.16 Causes of neutropenia

Infections	Most viruses can cause mild neutropenia which may persist for 6 weeks or longer
	Severe overwhelming infections with gram-negative bacteria
	Typhoid and tuberculosis
Drugs	Cytotoxic drugs
	Idiosyncratic reactions to many drugs; most important are phenothiazines, phenyl-butazone, chloramphenicol, sulphonamides, antithyroid drugs, indomethacin
Autoimmunity	SLE
	Felty's syndrome
	Autoimmune neutropenia
Blood diseases	Megaloblastic anaemia
	Aplastic anaemia
	Myelodysplastic syndrome
	Leukaemia
	Lymphoma
Splenomegaly	Any cause of a large spleen

Clinical features

Although the lower limit of normal for neutrophils is 2×10^9 per litre, infections are unlikely to be more common unless the neutrophil count falls below 10^9 per litre, and unlikely to be life-threatening unless it falls below 0.5×10^9 per litre. Most of the infections that occur are caused by endogenous organisms, typically Gram-negative coliforms and *Staphylococcus aureus*. Organisms not normally considered pathogenic, such as *Staphylococcus epidermidis* and *Candida albicans*, cause septicaemias, especially in patients who have already received antibiotics.

Diagnosis

For mild neutropenia (neutrophils more than 10^9 per litre), a drug history will often reveal the cause. White blood counts performed at weekly intervals will reveal cyclical neutropenia. Tests for neutrophil antibodies and anti-nuclear antibody should be performed. If neutropenia persists more than six weeks, then a bone marrow investigation is merited and this should be done at once in severe neutropenia of unknown cause. However, isolated neutropenia is rarely a presenting feature of leukaemia.

Treatment

Definitive treatment is directed at the cause. Mild neutropenia requires no special management. The management of severe neutropenia requires special skills and is dealt with under the management of acute leukaemia.

The myelodysplastic syndromes (MDS)

In the past these syndromes have been much neglected, mainly because they have gone under so many aliases: refractory anaemia, preleukaemia, sideroblastic anaemia, achrestic anaemia, oligoblastic leukaemia etc. They have now been recognized as belonging to a single group of conditions, diagnosable on morphological grounds and surprisingly common in the elderly (a prevalence of 1:1000 in the over-60s).

Pathology

MDS is now recognized as a clonal disorder of haemopoietic stem cells which retain the ability to differentiate into end cells, but do so in a disordered manner. All cells

Table 11.17 FAB classification of the myelodysplastic syndromes

Refractory sideroblastic anaemia (RAS)
Refractory anaemia (RA)
Chronic myelomonocytic leukaemia (CMML)
Refractory anaemia with excess of blasts (RAEB)
Refractory anaemia with excess of blasts
   in transformation (RAEBt)

deriving from the myeloid stem cell (see Fig. 11.1) are involved in the process. The French American British (FAB) group have classified the syndrome into five types, which are shown in ascending order of severity in Table 11.17.

The majority of cases of MDS are idiopathic; but with increasing use of cytotoxic drugs and radiotherapy more cases are being seen that are secondary to the use of these agents. Secondary MDS tends to occur in younger people.

Clinical features

The clinical features are related to anaemia, neutropenia and thrombocytopenia. Since granulocytes and platelets function poorly, infections and bleeding may occur even with relatively normal blood counts.

Diagnosis

The diagnosis is made on the characteristic appearances of blood and bone marrow, which include dyserythropoiesis, disorders of granulation and nuclear segmentation in white cells and abnormalities of megakaryocytes. Peripheral pancytopenia associated with bone marrow hypercellularity is the rule. Many patients have an abnormal karyotype in bone marrow metaphases.

Differential diagnosis

In the past many cases have been misdiagnosed as aplastic anaemia or megaloblastic anaemia. The characteristic features of MDS are now well known to haematologists.

Treatment

Supportive care with blood transfusions, antibiotics and platelet transfusions may be required. Aggressive chemotherapy may be offered for RAEB or RAEBt in young patients, but this is inappropriate for the majority. Low-dose chemotherapy with cytosine arabinoside has been recommended for the treatment of elderly patients.

The leukaemias

The leukaemias are a group of malignant neoplasms of the bone marrow in which the neoplastic clone replaces the normal tissue, frequently leading to anaemia, neutropenia and thrombocytopenia. Untreated, acute leukaemia is rapidly fatal, but chronic lymphocytic leukaemia is often compatible with a normal life of long duration.

For most leukaemias the cause is unknown, but in a few cases a cause has been determined.

1 Radiation.
Survivors of the Hiroshima explosion have a twenty-fold increase in most types of leukaemia (but not chronic lymphocytic). Patients with ankylosing spondylitis treated by irradiation of the spine have a sixfold increase in acute myeloid leukaemia. Children whose mothers received diagnostic X-rays in pregnancy have a slight increase in incidence of acute lymphoblastic leukaemia. The evidence does not support background radiation as a major cause for leukaemia.

2 Chemicals.
Benzene, toluene and related chemicals are leukaemogenic and an environmental hazard in some occupations. Cytotoxic drugs produce leukaemia in a small proportion of patients receiving them.

3 Viruses.
In cats, mice, cows and sheep leukaemogenic viruses have been identified. In humans, a T-cell leukaemia common in Japan is caused by a retrovirus.

4 Congenital factors.
There is a high coincidence rate in identical twins. Patients with Downs' syndrome have a twentyfold increase in incidence of acute myeloid leukaemia.

Leukaemia is classified according to the type of white cell affected and according to the rate of the clinical progression.

Acute myeloid leukaemia (AML)

This type of leukaemia occurs at any age. It is the commonest type of acute leukaemia in adults and in the first year of life.

Pathology

There is a proliferation of the myeloid stem cell, which shows greater or lesser degrees of differentiation that are recognized in the FAB classification (Table 11.18).

Table 11.18 FAB classification of the acute myeloid leukaemias

M1	Poorly differentiated myeloblastic leukaemia
M2	Well-differentiated myeloblastic leukaemia
M3	Promyelocytic leukaemia
M4	Myelomonocytic leukaemia
M5	Monocytic leukaemia
M6	Erythroleukaemia
M7	Megakaryoblastic leukaemia

The accumulation of leukaemic cells suppresses the growth of normal cells, leading to pancytopenia which usually occurs before the appearance of a leucocytosis. In the elderly and in patients with secondary acute leukaemia there is often a preceding myelodysplastic phase.

Clinical features

The clinical manifestations are those of pancytopenia. In M5 particularly there may be infiltrates of the skin and gums. Tender bones are sometimes noted. Splenomegaly and hepatomegaly are rare except in advanced disease.

Diagnosis

The diagnosis depends on the observation of more than 30 per cent blasts in the bone marrow. Auer rods (long, thin azurophil cytoplasmic inclusions) are characteristic of leukaemic myeloblasts, but cytochemical or immunocytochemical identification of the blasts may be necessary. Some subtypes of AML have a characteristically abnormal karyotype; for example, in M3 a translocation between chromosomes 15 and 17 is almost always seen.

Complications

In M3 the granules of the promyelocytes contain a procoagulant which is capable of inducing disseminated intravascular coagulation (see page 389).

Treatment

There are three elements to treatment: remission induction; supportive care; and consolidation and maintenance.

1 Remission induction.

In patients below the age of 60, complete remission, defined as the return of blood and bone marrow to normal, is achievable in upwards of 70 per cent of patients. However, even in complete remission up to 10^8 leukaemic cells may remain in the body compared with between 10^{10} and 10^{12} in the patient with frank leukaemia and marrow failure.

A number of induction regimens are in current use, most involving a combination of daunorubicin, cytosine arabinoside and 6-thioguanine.

2 Supportive care.

The induction regimen induces severe pancytopenia which may last for several weeks. Effective supportive care is the cornerstone of successful treatment. Of prime importance is good vascular access. It is usual to introduce a right atrial cannula via one of the subclavian veins. This is left *in situ* for the duration of the induction and consolidation regimen. In order to diminish the risk of cannula-associated infections, the cannula is taken through a subcutaneous tunnel before exiting from the skin.

The treatment of anaemia is by red cell transfusion. Prevention of haemorrhage requires platelet transfusions. Most units use platelets prophylactically when the count drops below 20×10^9 per litre. Some patients become refractory to platelet transfusions owing to the development of isoantibodies. In these, single-donor HL-A matched platelets collected on a cell separator are indicated.

Infection is very likely in patients with fewer than 0.5×10^9 neutrophils per litre. Most infections are with endogenous organisms so that the value of reversed barrier nursing in rooms with laminar flow ventilation is questionable. However, single rooms are preferable to the open ward and reasonable care (such as nurses washing hands between patients) to prevent the spread of infection is essential. Reduction of gut flora by prophylactic oral non-absorbable antibiotics, or by co-trimoxazole, is practised in many units. Regular cultures of urine, faeces, sputum, and of swabs from vagina, throat, nose and other sites document the patient's commensal bacteria and their sensitivity to antibiotics.

Fever is the best indication that infection is present and thorough attempts to identify the cause of any organism causing a temperature of 38°C presenting for two hours should be made, at the same time beginning treatment with empirical antibiotics such as a broad-spectrum penicillin and an aminoglycoside which will cover likely organisms. If no response occurs the possibility of viral or fungal organisms or *Staphylococcus epidermidis* should be considered. Granulocyte transfusions have a limited place in the treatment of infections refractory to antibiotics.

3 Maintenance.

Remissions are prolonged by two consolidation courses

of the induction regimen, but probably not by prolonged treatment with low doses of cytotoxics. Allogeneic bone marrow transplantation should be considered in patients aged 45 and under who are in remission and have an HL-A compatible sibling. The patient is prepared with total body irradiation and cyclophosphamide which it is hoped will remove any residual leukaemia. Donor bone marrow drawn from the pelvic bones is filtered and then infused intravenously into the recipient. Recovery of bone marrow function occurs in 2–3 weeks. Bone marrow transplantation remains a hazardous procedure. About 25 per cent of patients die from complications of the treatment, and in a further 25 per cent the leukaemia relapses despite the treatment. The major risks are:

(a) infection, particularly with cytomegalovirus (CMV);
(b) graft versus host disease (GVHD), an immune attack by the graft on the host causing rash, diarrhoea and hepatitis as well as increased susceptibility to infection;
(c) interstitial pneumonitis, a usually fatal lung condition possibly related to GVHD, CMV or lung irradiation;
(d) failure of engraftment or rejection of the graft.

The incidence of GVHD may be reduced by depletion of T cells from the graft or by the immunosuppressive drug cyclosporin A. Bone marrow allografts from HL-A compatible unrelated donors or partially mismatched related donors are experimental procedures.

Bone marrow autografts using bone marrow collected in first remission may have a role in increasing the number of long-term survivors.

Prognosis

In patients not receiving bone marrow transplants the survival rates for patients under 25 are between 10 and 30 per cent alive at five years. For patients receiving bone marrow transplants, survivals of between 30 and 50 per cent have been achieved.

In older patients the prognosis is much worse. In patients over 60 years, fewer than 50 per cent achieve complete remissions, and these are not usually sustained for much more than twelve months.

Acute lymphoblastic leukaemia (ALL)

ALL is the commonest leukaemia of childhood but it may occur at any age. The most useful classification is according to the cell of origin.

1 Common ALL.

This has a peak incidence between the ages of 2 and 5. It comprises 70 per cent of ALL and has the best prognosis. The cell of origin has recently been identified as a pre-B cell. Most cases bear the cALLa surface marker (CD10).

2 T-cell ALL.

This is five times commoner in boys than girls and has a peak age of incidence between 10 and 15. It is frequently associated with a mediastinal mass (Sternberg sarcoma).

3 B-cell ALL.

This is very rare (less than 2 per cent of total) and may be regarded as the blood phase of Burkitt's lymphoma.

Clinical features

These are similar to AML except that tender bones are more common, meningeal involvement (headache, vomiting, diplopia) is much more common, and testicular involvement is a feature. Hepatomegaly and splenomegaly are also more likely to be seen.

Diagnosis

This is made on bone marrow appearances with the help of immunochemical markers.

Treatment

Treatment of ALL, especially in children, is more effective than of AML. Complete remission is achieved in 95 per cent of patients. A combination of drugs is used that always includes vincristine and prednisolone, which are minimally toxic to normal marrow, together with a permutation from asparaginase, daunorubicin, cytosine arabinoside and cyclophosphamide.

Once remission is achieved prophylaxis against meningeal leukaemia is necessary and skull irradiation and intrathecal methotrexate are important adjuncts to treatment. Maintenance chemotherapy with methotrexate and 6-mercaptopurine together is continued for two to two-and-a-half years with three-monthly vincristine and prednisolone. Bone marrow transplants are offered to patients in second remission or those in first remission with a poor prognosis.

Prognosis

Among children the five-year survival rate is greater than 50 per cent, and many of these may be regarded as cured. Poor prognostic features include a high white count, age greater than 16 and T or B cell surface markers.

Chronic myeloid leukaemia

Pathology

The disease, which may be seen at any age, has two phases. In the chronic phase there is uncontrolled proliferation of a stem cell which retains the ability to differentiate. Red cells, granulocytes and platelets all derive from the malignant clone which is characterized by an abnormal karyotype. There is a reciprocal translocation between the long arms of chromosome 9 and 22. The small chromosome 22 resulting is known as the Philadelphia chromosome. The translocation produces a hybrid gene, *c-abl-bcr*, the product of which functions as a protein kinase. In most patients, the disorder eventually transforms into an acute leukaemia, on average three years after diagnosis. In 70 per cent of cases this is acute myeloblastic leukaemia and is generally refractory to treatment. In 25 per cent of cases, ALL ensues with a response to treatment typical of other cases of ALL (see above), although remission seldom exceeds one year.

Clinical features

The features of anaemia are usually present together with those of hypermetabolism, weight loss, night sweats and lassitude. In patients with white cell counts greater than 80×10^9 per litre, splenomegaly is almost always present and it may be massive and associated with pain and discomfort. Bruising and haemorrhage may occur even in the presence of a normal platelet count. A significant number present with gout, neurological symptoms caused by hyperviscosity and priapism.

Diagnosis

There is usually a leucocytosis with a WBC above 100×10^9 per litre. A complete range of granulocyte precursors from myeloblasts to metamyelocytes is seen together with increased numbers of neutrophils, eosinophils and basophils. The bone marrow is hypercellular with a predominance of myeloid precursors. The neutrophil alkaline phosphatase score is zero, serum B_{12} is high and the Ph′ chromosome is present in over 95 per cent of cases.

Differential diagnosis

A similar blood picture may be seen in leukaemoid reactions due to marrow infiltration and cancer, in some cases of myelofibrosis, and in atypical chronic myeloid leukaemia. In all of these the Ph′ chromosome is absent.

Treatment

Busulphan is the drug which has been used most commonly for the chronic phase. It controls the white count, the anaemia and the splenomegaly, but does not delay the onset of the acute phase. Among the side-effects are aplastic anaemia, skin pigmentation, lung fibrosis and cataract. Hydroxyurea is equally effective and is easier to control with fewer side-effects. Splenic irradiation may be useful in controlling the disease when it becomes refractory to chemotherapy. Bone marrow transplantation may be curative if the criteria of age and availability of an HL-A compatible sibling can be fulfilled. Treatment of the acute phase is disappointing.

Prognosis

The median survival is 3–5 years. Ten per cent of patients survive ten years.

Chronic lymphocytic leukaemia

This is the commonest of the leukaemias. It mainly occurs after the age of 55 and becomes more common in each succeeding decade. The incidence in men at any particular age is twice that of women.

Pathology

There is a monoclonal proliferation of early B lymphocytes which characteristically bear small amounts of surface IgM and IgD, a receptor for mouse red blood cells and the CD5 antigen. The disease apparently starts in the bone marrow and may be non-progressive. If it does progress it involves lymph nodes in cervical, axillary and inguinal regions, the spleen and the liver. Eventually marrow failure may ensue.

Clinical features

In one large series from a single centre, over 70 per cent of patients were detected incidentally on routine blood counts. In the remainder the main features were of anaemia, lymphadenopathy and splenomegaly.

Complications

Autoimmune haemolytic anaemia occurs in about 8 per cent of patients. Autoimmune thrombocytopenia is found in 2 per cent. In patients with low serum immunoglobulins infections are common, particularly chest infections and herpes zoster, which occurs in about 20 per cent of patients. It is often severe, sometimes affecting motor nerve roots and frequently being followed by postherpetic neuralgia.

Diagnosis

A lymphocytosis is seen on the blood film together with smear cells. Bone marrow trephine may show interstitial, nodular or diffuse infiltration. Cell markers confirm the diagnosis. Serum immunoglobulins are reduced in over 60 per cent of patients.

Treatment

Most patients do not require treatment. Patients with signs of marrow failure and those who have unacceptable organomegaly may be successfully treated by chlorambucil (up to 10 mg/day for two weeks every four weeks). Prednisolone (10 mg/day) is often added to this regimen.

Herpes zoster infections should be treated promptly with acyclovir infusions.

T-cell CLL

About 2 per cent of CLL has T cell markers. Not all T cell proliferations are neoplastic and clonality can only be determined by the finding of an abnormal karyotype or rearrangement of T receptor gene. There is a clinical association with rheumatoid arthritis and coeliac disease. Some patients develop pure red cell aplasia which improves with treatment of the leukaemia.

Prolymphocytic leukaemia

This is a more aggressive varient of CLL almost invariably associated with splenomegaly. Most cases are B cell in type.

Hairy cell leukaemia

This variant of CLL is characterized by small numbers of B cells with filamentous pili protruding from the cytoplasm. There is usually neutropenia and splenomegaly, the bone marrow aspirate showing a 'dry tap' and the trephine a characteristic regular infiltrate. Treatment by splenectomy is often helpful, but more recently very satisfactory remissions in almost all patients have been achieved with either interferon-α or deoxycoformycin therapy.

Adult T leukaemia-lymphoma

This unusual tumour of Japanese and of blacks from the Carribean is caused by infection with the retrovirus HTLVI. It is generally associated with hypercalcaemia and is refractory to treatment.

The lymphomas

Hodgkin's disease

First described by Thomas Hodgkin of Guys Hospital, in 1832, this has been one of the greatest successes of modern cancer treatment. There are two peak ages of incidence: between the ages of 20 and 40 and in the over 60s. Although the pathological picture in both is similar the outlook in each is so very different that a different aetiology has been postulated. However, the cause is unknown.

Pathology

The characteristic histological abnormality is the *Reed-Sternberg cell*, a large binucleate cell with acidophilic nucleoli. Just what the normal counterpart for this cell is, is vigorously disputed. Reed-Sternberg cells are surrounded by large numbers of T lymphocytes, plasma cells, neutrophils, monocytes and eosinophils which are not part of the tumor clone, but appear to be the host's defence against the tumour. Histological grading (Table 11.19) is according to the relative numbers of Reed-Sternberg cells and host defence cells. In some cases the lymph node is broken into nodules by fibrous tissue.

The disease progresses in a regular fashion from lymph node to contiguous lymph node, usually beginning above the diaphragm. The spleen is always involved before the liver and the bone marrow.

Clinical features

Most patients present with discrete asymmetrical enlargement of superficial lymph nodes. The nodes are firm and painless. Splenomegaly is present in up to 50 per cent and the liver may be enlarged in more advanced cases.

Table 11.19 Histological grading of Hodgkin's disease

Lymphocyte predominant	Increasing
Nodular sclerosing	malignancy
Mixed cellularity	
Lymphocyte depleted	↓

Table 11.20 Staging of Hodgkin's disease

Stage 1	Disease confined to one lymph node site
Stage 2	Disease in more than one lymph node site but confined to one side of the diaphragm
Stage 3	Involvement of lymph nodes and/or spleen on both sides of the diaphragm
Stage 4	Involvement of sites outside the lymphatic system

Suffixes
A = Symptom free
B = symptoms present
     loss of more than 10% body
     weight in six months
     unexplained fever above 38°C
     night sweats
E = local extranodal spread within the range of radiotherapy

Fever is present in a third of patients. The Pel Ebstein fever (pyrexia alternating with days with a normal temperature) is said to be typical but is rather uncommon. Pruritis and alcohol-induced pain occur in some patients but have no prognostic significance. Weight loss and night sweats are typical in more advanced cases.

Diagnosis

The diagnosis is made on lymph node biopsy. The blood count may show a neutrophil leucocytosis, sometimes with eosinophilia. Anaemia, lymphopenia and bone marrow failure are evidence of advanced disease. It is important to stage the disease carefully since the success of particular forms of treatment depends on knowing accurately the extent of the disease (Table 11.20). The presence of retroperitoneal lymph nodes is best assessed by lymphography, perhaps supplemented by a CT scan. Patients for whom radiotherapy is planned (stages I–IIA) will probably need to have staging confirmed by laparotomy with splenectomy and lymph node and liver biopsy. Bone marrow trephine shows marrow involvement in 4 per cent of cases.

Complications

Patients with Hodgkin's disease have deficiencies in cell-mediated immunity. Infections with herpes zoster, cytomegalovirus, candida and mycobacteria are common.

Treatment

Patients with stage I or IIA may be cured by radiotherapy alone (4000 rad). A single upper mantle field treats disease above the diaphragm, and below the diaphragm an inverted Y is used. Stages IIB, III or IV should be treated by chemotherapy. The benchmark regimen is MOPP, consisting of mustine, vincristine (oncovin), prednisolone and procarbazine. The good results obtained with this regimen depend on the recommended dosage being given, but it may be very toxic and regimens with fewer side-effects such as ChIVPP (chlorambucil, vinblastine, prednisolone and procarbazine) have been substituted in some centres. Chemotherapy virtually always leads to sterility in males.

Prognosis

Five-year survival rates for stages I and II are 85 per cent, for stage IIIA 70 per cent, for stage IIIb 50 per cent and for stage IV 40 per cent. However, these rates are very age-dependent. Young people usually do well; old people less often.

Non-Hodgkin's lymphoma

The variety of non-Hodgkin's lymphomas is extremely wide and made confusing by the fact that at least six different histological classifications are currently in use.

Pathology

The distinction between leukaemias and lymphomas is to some extent arbitrary since many lymphomas involve the blood and many leukaemias involve the lymph nodes and spleen. The differentiation pathways of lymphocytes are complex, and lymphomas may theoretically arise from lymphocytes frozen at any stage of differentiation.

In general, lymphomas with large cells are more malignant than those with small cells, and those with diffuse histology more malignant than those with nodular histology. A recent working formulation recognizes *low-grade lymphomas*, which have an indolent clinical course, relatively long survival, a non-destructive growth pattern and a tendency to respect privileged sites such as the brain and testes, but which are not curable with chemotherapy; and *high-grade lymphomas* which have an aggressive clinical course, a short survival without therapy, a destructive growth pattern and a tendency to invade privileged sites but which may be cured by chemotherapy. Low-grade and high-grade lymphomas each comprise about 35 per cent of all lymphomas. Unfortunately a large minority of lymphomas fall into an intermediate group (Table 11.21). In the UK about 20 per cent of lymphomas are of T cell origin but their classification is unsatisfactory.

Table 11.21 Classification of non-Hodgkin's lymphomas

Low-grade (35%)
Lymphocytic diffuse (CLL)
Lymphoplasmacytic diffuse
Centroblastic/centrocytic nodular

Intermediate-grade (20%)
Centroblastic/centrocytic diffuse
Centrocytic diffuse

High-grade (35%)
Centroblastic diffuse
Immunoblastic diffuse
Lymphoblastic diffuse
Burkitt's lymphoma

Miscellaneous (10%)
Mycoses fungoides
Histiocytic
Unclassifiable

Clinical features

Two-thirds of patients present over the age of 50. Most patients have asymmetric, painless, superficial lymphadenopathy. Between 5 and 10 per cent have involvement of oropharyngeal lymphoid structures (Waldeyer's ring). Hepatosplenomegaly is more common than in Hodgkin's disease, and massive enlargement of retroperitoneal lymph nodes can sometimes be felt in the abdomen. Extranodal involvement is more common than in Hodgkin's disease, and characteristic lymphomas of skin, stomach, lung and thyroid are recognized.

Diagnosis

Diagnosis is made by lymph node biopsy. Eighty-five per cent of patients have disseminated disease. In 50 per cent, tumour cells are detectable immunologically in blood and bone marrow. In the UK most patients have B cell lymphomas and in these serum immunoglobulins may be low. In about 15 per cent a monoclonal immunoglobulin is detectable in the serum.

Treatment

Radiotherapy is only recommended in the minority of patients (5 per cent) with stage I disease. Low-grade lymphomas should be managed by observation until systemic symptoms, bone marrow failure or uncomfortable or compressive organomegaly ensue. They usually respond to single-agent chemotherapy (e.g. chlorambucil 10 mg daily for two weeks of every four).

High-grade lymphomas should be treated with aggressive chemotherapeutic regimens. Experimental treatment includes supralethal chemotherapy with bone marrow allograft or autograft.

Prognosis

Median survival in low-grade lymphomas is seven years. In many of these, transformation to high-grade lymphoma occurs. High-grade lymphomas have 'cure' rates of 30 per cent but the majority fail to survive two years.

Burkitt's lymphoma

This is a B cell lymphoblastic lymphoma, endemic in malarious areas of tropical Africa and New Guinea. Sporadic cases occur elsewhere. It is a disease of children and young people with a peak age of incidence between 4 and 8 years.

Epstein-Barr virus infections are involved in the genesis of the lymphoma, which is almost always associated with a chromosomal translocation between a site on the long arm of chromosome 8 near to the locus coding for the c-myc oncogene and a site on the long arm of chromosome 14 near to the locus coding for the heavy chains of immunoglobulin.

The lymphoma involves extranodal sites, particularly the jaws, kidney, adrenals and ovaries. In young women the lactating breast is frequently a site of involvement. Histologically, there is a characteristic 'starry sky' appearance formed by pale histiocytes in sheets of darkly staining lymphoblasts. Localized tumours respond well to aggressive chemotherapy, but disseminated disease, particularly when it takes the form of a B cell lymphoblastic leukaemia, has a grave prognosis.

Multiple myeloma

Multiple myeloma is a malignant disease of bone marrow plasma cells. It gives insight into the concept of clonality. Its incidence of 2.6 per 100000 in the UK.

Pathology

The serum immunoglobulins are a mixture of antibody molecules each committed to a different antigen. This commitment occurs as a genetic event in the early B cell precursors of the plasma cells that secrete immunoglobulin. Neoplastic proliferation begins in one cell and all its progeny secrete one type of immunoglobulin molecule, which is therefore monoclonal. Normal serum electrophoresis demonstrates the immunoglobulins as a broad band towards the cathode, reflecting the molecular heterogeneity. In myeloma the immunoglobulin has a single molecular structure, and serum electrophoresis therefore demonstrates it as a narrow band (which is sometimes called a paraprotein). In myeloma the majority of tumours produces IgG or IgA. IgD, IgE and IgM producing myelomas are rare. There is usually an excessive production of immunoglobulin light chains and 25 per cent secrete light chains only. About 5 per cent of myelomas are non-secretory. The malignant plasma cells also secrete an osteoclast activating factor (now known to be 'tumour necrosis factor B') which is responsible for bony destruction around nests of plasma cells and the mobilization of bony calcium.

Clinical features

Myeloma has a peak incidence between the ages of 60 and 70. The clinical features are wide-ranging, although perhaps 20 per cent are discovered by an incidental blood test. Bone pain is frequently present. Pathological fractures and collapsed vertebrae are not common. Since the axial skeleton is involved, neurological symptoms are common, with severe root pain and paraplegia occurring. Hypercalcaemia causes constipation, vomiting, thirst, polyuria, drowsiness and coma together with renal failure which is usually the result of a combination of causes (Table 11.22).

Bone marrow failure is present in the most advanced cases. Recurrent infections are the consequence of both neutropenia and low levels of normal immunoglobulins. High levels of paraprotein may be associated with the hyperviscosity syndrome, characterized by purpura, haemorrhages, visual defects and heart failure.

Fundoscopy reveals dilated veins with a 'string of sausages' appearance. Amyloidosis may occur leading to macroglossia, carpal tunnel syndrome, purpura (skin pinch syndrome and postproctoscopic periorbital purpura which is self-explanatory), renal failure and cardiomyopathy.

Table 11.22 Causes of renal failure in myeloma (renal failure is usually precipitated by infection and dehydration)

Precipitation of immunoglobulin light chains in renal tubules
Hypercalcaemia
Hyperuricaemia
Recurrent urinary tract infections
Amyloidosis

Diagnosis

The blood count may be normal but frequently shows a degree of anaemia with pancytopenia in the more advanced cases. There is usually rouleaux formation, and the high level of immunoglobulin can often be predicted by a blue background staining. The ESR is frequently greater than 140 mm in the first hour but may be normal in light-chain myeloma. Bone marrow shows increased numbers of plasma cells which may be binucleate or otherwise abnormal, and which on immunostaining show a single heavy- and light-chain type of immunoglobulin.

Serum electrophoresis shows a monoclonal band in 70 per cent of cases, and measurement of specific immunoglobulins shows a rise in one class while the others are depressed. Rarely, all classes are depressed. Urinary electrophoresis may demonstrate a monoclonal band representing free light chains (*Bence Jones proteinuria*). The heat test for Bence Jones protein is now only used to entertain students.

Serum calcium is raised in 45 per cent, but alkaline phosphatase levels are usually normal. Serum uric acid may be raised. Skeletal X-rays show osteolytic areas in 60 per cent of patients or generalized osteoporosis in 20 per cent.

Differential diagnosis

Monoclonal proteins may be found in a number of conditions (Table 11.23). It is important to distinguish myeloma from non-progressive conditions. Two of the following should be present in order to confirm the diagnosis: osteolytic bone disease, paraprotein, and/or more than 10 per cent plasma cells in the bone marrow.

Treatment

1 Acute.
Myeloma may be a medical emergency. Renal failure should be treated by rehydration, the correction of hyper-

Table 11.23 Conditions associated with monoclonal immunoglobulins

Myeloma
Waldenstrom's macroglobulinaemia
Smouldering myeloma
Benign monoclonal gammopathy
Cold haemagglutination syndrome
Cryoglobulinaemia
B-cell non-Hodgkin's lymphoma
Chronic lymphocytic leukaemia
Prolymphocytic leukaemia

calcaemia or hyperuricaemia and the treatment of any infection. Plasmapheresis may be effective in reducing the excretion of immunoglobulin light chains, but early treatment of the myeloma is the ideal way of reducing their production.

Hypercalcaemia should be treated by rehydration, corticosteroids and, if required, calcitonin or mithramycin. Compression paraplegia should be treated by either laminectomy or radiotherapy; whichever can be done the soonest.

Locally painful skeletal lesions require radiotherapy.

2 Chronic.

For many years the standard treatment has been melphalan (0.25 mg/kg for four days) together with prednisolone (100 mg/day for four days), repeated every six weeks, together with allopurinol. More intensive regimens produce very little better results with greater side-effects. Recently treatment with high-dose melphalan (140 mg/m^2) with or without autologous bone marrow graft has been recommended for younger patients.

Prognosis

The median survival is two years. Although there are long-term survivors nobody is cured. Uraemia and anaemia are bad prognostic features.

Waldenstrom's macroglobulinaemia

This is a malignant tumour of bone marrow composed of lymphoplasmacytoid cells which secrete IgM.

Clinical features

In many patients it is an incidental finding. When they are present clinical features are related to marrow failure or hyperviscosity, which results in visual disturbances, muscle weakness, confusion, congestive cardiac failure and coma. The retinal changes are characteristic with engorged veins, haemorrhages and exudates and blurred discs.

Diagnosis

There may be a spurious anaemia owing to increased plasma volume. Rouleaux and a blue background may be seen on the blood film. The features of marrow failure may be present. Bone marrow shows a diffuse infiltrate of small lymphocytes and plasma cells or of lymphoplasmacytoid cells which on immunostaining contain IgM

and either κ or λ light chains. The ESR is very high. Serum electrophoresis shows a monoclonal protein which may be identified as IgM. Hypercalcaemia and bony disease are not seen.

Treatment

The treatment of hyperviscosity is plasmapheresis supplemented as required by cytotoxic drugs. Chlorambucil and cyclophosphamide are the most widely used drugs.

Benign monoclonal gammopathy

This name is applied to a paraprotein discovered in the serum in the absence of other features of myeloma or Waldenstrom's macroglobulinaemia (see above). The level of paraprotein is less than 30 g/l and normal immunoglobulins are not suppressed. When followed for 15 years, 30 per cent show signs of myeloma.

Smouldering myeloma

Cases intermediate between multiple myeloma and benign monoclonal gammopathy are sometimes seen. The level of the paraprotein may be greater than 30 g/l, there may be a degree of Bence Jones proteinuria or suppression of normal immunoglobulins. There may be increased numbers of plasma cells in the marrow. However, there is no evidence of bony destruction, renal damage or bone marrow failure, nor of progression. In such cases the term 'smouldering myeloma' is sometimes used and the correct management is observation.

The haemorrhagic disorders

As it circulates the blood must remain in a fluid state, yet when the circulation is breached the blood that leaks out must rapidly solidify to staunch the flow. The system of checks and balances that achieves this (Fig. 11.9) is a complex one which is prone to failure. A series of amplification cascades, designed to ensure that a small stimulus has a large effect, is held in check by a range of inhibitors. A bleeding diathesis may result from disorders of blood vessels, platelets or the coagulation system.

1 Disorders of blood vessels.

Clinically important disorders of blood vessels are rare and common ones are clinically insignificant. They are classified in Table 11.24.

2 Disorders of platelets (Table 11.25).

Mild thrombocytopenia is a relatively common finding

Table 11.24 Disorders of blood vessels

Structural malformations
Hereditary haemorrhagic telangiectasia
Hereditary disorders of connective tissue (Ehlers Danlos syndrome, pseudoxanthoma elasticum)
Acquired disorder of connective tissue (scurvy, steroids, senile purpura, rheumatoid arthritis, scleroderma, amyloidosis)

Immune vasculitis
Henoch Schönlein purpura
Drug-induced vasculitis (iodides, quinine, aspirin)
Autoimmune disorders (polyarteritis nodosa, systemic lupus erythematosus, rheumatoid arthritis, cryoglobulinaemia)
Infections (subacute bacterial endocarditis, meningococcal septicaemia, Rocky mountain spotted fever)
Autoerythrocyte sensitization

on blood counts and it is usually insignificant. Severe thrombocytopenia may be caused by a failure of production or increased destruction of platelets.

Hereditary haemorrhagic telangiectasia

This rare syndrome is inherited as an autosomal dominant characteristic, the number of lesions increasing with age. Thin-walled dilated capillaries and arterioles may be recognized on skin and mucous membranes, and may characteristically be seen on the lips and tongue. They blanch on compression. Spontaneous epistaxis and gastrointestinal bleeding frequently cause chronic iron-deficiency anaemia. Treatment is difficult, although nasal

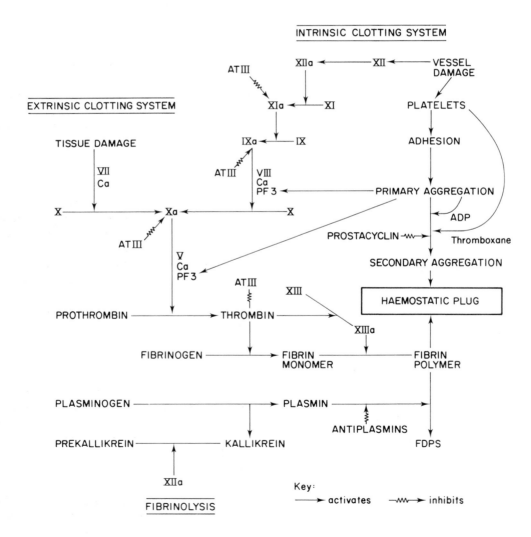

Figure 11.9 *Mechanisms of coagulation and fibrinolysis. Ca, calcium; PF3, platelet factor 3; ATIII, anti-thrombin III; ADP, adenosine diphosphate; FDPs, fibrin degradation products.*

Table 11.25 Disorders of platelets

Reduced platelet production
Selective megakaryocytic suppression
   congenital (Fanconi's syndrome)
   drugs (thiazides, sulphonamides)
Part of generalized bone marrow failure
   see Table 11.11

Increased platelet destruction
Immunological causes
   autoimmune
      idiopathic
      drugs
      systemic lupus erythematosus
      lymphoid tumours
   isoimmune
      fetomaternal incompatibility
      post-transfusion purpura
Non-immunological causes
   disseminated intravascular coagulation
   thrombotic thrombocytopenic purpura
   splenomegaly
   dilution by massive transfusion

Abnormal platelet function
Congenital
   Von Willebrand's disease
   Glanzman's thrombasthenia
   Bernard Soulier syndrome
Acquired
   aspirin therapy
   mycloproliferative disorders
   paraproteinaemia
   uraemia

cautery may be helpful. Blood loss may be so great that parenteral iron replacement may be necessary to keep up with it.

Henoch Schönlein purpura (see page 274)

This is an immune complex vasculitis occurring as an acute disorder, often after an infection, and most commonly in children. Large, often confluent, areas of palpable purpura, accompanied by urticaria, appear on the buttocks and extensor surfaces of the legs. Itching is common. Gastrointestinal involvement may lead to haemorrhage or intussusception; arthritis is common and glomerulonephritis less so. Most cases resolve spontaneously within a few weeks.

Immune thrombocytopenic purpura (ITP)

Acute ITP is a self-limiting condition seen mainly in children. There may be a history of a recent upper res-
piratory infection. Chronic ITP is seen more commonly in women than men, particularly between the ages of 20 and 50. In about 40 per cent of cases an underlying cause (systemic lupus erythematosus, CLL or drugs) is found.

Pathology

Autoantibodies to platelet antigens are produced by the patient, usually for unknown reasons. Sometimes an underlying lymphoid tumour is found or antiplatelet antibodies, as in systemic lupus erythematosus or infectious mononucleosis. Drugs may be implicated in three ways as indicated for autoimmune haemolytic anaemia (Table 11.14). Antibody-coated platelets are cleared rapidly by the spleen.

Clinical features

Petechiae and echymoses are seen on skin and mucous membranes. In children with acute ITP serious bleeding is very rare. Chronic ITP is more troublesome with epistaxis, menorrhagia, gastrointestinal haemorrhage and even intracranial haemorrhages occurring. The spleen is not enlarged in primary ITP.

Diagnosis

The platelets count is usually less than 10×10^9 per litre. On the blood film, platelets frequently appear larger than normal. Bone marrow shows increased numbers of megakaryocytes which are frequently small with few nuclear lobulations. IgG may be detected on the surface of platelets using a variety of tests which are only available in specialized laboratories. In about 5 per cent of patients an autoimmune haemolytic anaemia is also present (*Evans' syndrome*).

Treatment

Acute ITP in children usually recovers spontaneously within six weeks to six months. Although opinions differ, many authorities prefer to offer no specific treatment but simply to restrict the activities of the children so as to avoid the risk of injury.

In chronic ITP spontaneous remission is rare. Most patients respond to oral prednisolone (60 mg/day). Gradual reduction of steroid dosage is often possible, but in a large minority relapse occurs while still on an unacceptably high dose. In these patients splenectomy is usually indicated and is successful in restoring a normal platelet count in 75 per cent. Those patients with dangerously low platelet counts despite steroids and splenectomy should be treated with immunosuppressive drugs. Cyclophosphamide and azathioprine have been successfully used, while vincristine is an experimental agent of promise.

High doses of intravenous immunoglobulin (0.4 g/kg daily for four days) has been successfully used in childhood ITP, but it is difficult to justify its use here. In chronic ITP it may be used to restore the platelet count temporarily prior to splenectomy in patients refractory to steroids.

In post-transfusion purpura in which the patient's own platelets are caught up in an isoimmune reaction against transfusion platelets, there is no response to either steroids or splenectomy and high-dose intravenous immunoglobulin is the treatment of choice.

Platelet transfusions are usually ineffective in immune thrombocytopenia since they are themselves destroyed by the immune reaction.

Thrombotic thrombocytopenic purpura

This rare, frequently lethal, condition is characterized by a microangiopathic haemolytic anaemia, severe thrombocytopenia, fever, renal failure and fluctuating neurological features. In children a similar syndrome is known as the haemolytic uraemic syndrome. The cause of both these disorders is unknown, but abnormalities of prostacyclin metabolism have been found. Treatment is unsatisfactory, but roughly 50 per cent of cases respond to plasma exchange using fresh frozen plasma as the exchange fluid.

Massive transfusion syndrome

Platelets do not survive in blood stored at 4°C for more than 24 hours. Following transfusion with more than ten units of stored blood in a 24-hour period, a bleeding diathesis is likely. The clotting factors V and VIII also store poorly and bleeding is caused by a combination of deficiencies of these factors and thrombocytopenia. Treatment is by including two units of fresh frozen plasma for every ten units of blood transfused, and platelet transfusion as required.

Hypersplenism

The normal spleen weighs between 150 and 250 g. The pathological spleen may be up to twenty times larger. In very large spleens 90 per cent of the body's platelets may

Table 11.26 Causes of massive splenomegaly

Chronic myeloid leukaemia
Myelofibrosis
Primary proliferative polycythaemia
Chronic lymphocytic leukaemia
Prolymphocytic leukaemia
Hairy cell leukaemia
Non-Hodgkin's lymphoma
Hodgkin's disease (rarely)
Thalassaemia major
Gaucher's disease
Kala azar
Malaria
Sarcoidosis (rarely)
Felty's syndrome (rarely)

be pooled in the spleen. This contrasts with red cell pooling which usually accounts for no more than 20 per cent of the red cell mass. On the other hand, normal platelets are not injured by their sojourn in the spleen, whereas red cell life-span is noticably shortened. The causes of massive splenomegaly are shown in Table 11.26.

Treatment

Thrombocytopenia due to hypersplenism is seldom the cause of bleeding unless platelet function is also abnormal. Splenectomy may be indicated if the hypersplenism is symptomatic.

Coagulation disorders

Hereditary disorders of each of the coagulation factors have been described. Most are rare, but haemophilia A or B and Von Willebrand's disease are merely uncommon.

Haemophilia A and B

Both types of haemophilia are inherited as X-linked recessive disorders. The diseases are therefore virtually confined to boys. Haemophilia A (factor VIII deficiency) has an incidence of 1 in 10000 and is five times as common as haemophilia B (factor IX deficiency or *Christmas disease*).

Pathology

Both factor VIII and factor IX are essential elements of the intrinsic clotting pathway (Fig. 11.9). Reduced levels of

Table 11.27 Severity of haemophilia related to levels of clotting factors

Level of factor VIII or factor IX (% of normal)	Clinical features
< 1	Severe disease; spontaneous bleeding into muscles and joints every few days from an early age; crippling joint deformities
1–5	Moderate disease; serious bleeding from trivial operation or injury; occasional spontaneous bleeding
5–20	Mild disease; serious bleeding after trauma or surgery
25–50	Subclinical disease; moderate bleeding after surgery; some female carriers fall within this group

either factor prolongs the time taken for coagulation to occur. Factor VIII is extremely labile with a short half-life. Factor IX is more stable.

Clinical features

Clinical features are identical in both types of haemophilia. The severity of the disease depends on the levels of the factor concerned (Table 11.27). The most common feature is spontaneous haemarthrosis of knee, ankle, elbow and shoulder. Acutely inflamed joints are immobile, which leads to disuse atrophy of the surrounding muscles. This in turn makes the joints more unstable and increases the risk of further haemarthroses. A succession of joint bleeds often leads to permanent damage. Bleeding also occurs into muscles; ileopsoas and retroperitoneal bleeds may mimic acute abdominal emergencies. Gastrointestinal haemorrhage is usually consequent on a local lesion. Intracranial bleeds occur mainly in younger haemophiliacs and are usually secondary to trauma. In milder haemophiliacs bleeding is most often related to accidental or surgical trauma. Bleeding is often delayed since the vascular and platelet responses to haemorrhage are normal.

Diagnosis

The bleeding time is normal in haemophilia. The prothrombin time is normal but the kaolin cephalin time (see page 357) is prolonged. Measurement of specific clotting factors VIII and IX will distinguish haemophilia A and B. About 7 per cent of patients with haemophilia A develop antibodies to isologous factor VIII (known as inhibitors). These are detected by the failure of an admixture of normal plasma to correct the KCCT and make management much more difficult.

Differential diagnosis

The major differential diagnosis is between haemophilia A and Von Willebrand's disease in which factor VIIIc levels are also low.

Treatment

The basis of treatment is the adequate replacement of the missing coagulation factor. The short half-life and limited availability of factor VIII means that prophylactic treatment is not feasible for any but a selected minority of patients with a history of recurrent severe bleeds. For the rest it is important to treat as early as possible after each bleed.

The haemophiliac himself is usually the best judge of when a bleed is occurring and for this reason most severe haemophiliacs are on home treatment.

For haemophilia A concentrates of factor VIII extracted from screened donor blood are available. Those in current use have been heat-treated so as to eliminate as far as possible the risk of virus transmission. For spontaneous joint haemorrhage the aim is to raise the factor VIII level above 20 per cent of normal. For major surgery and post-traumatic bleeding the level should be raised to 100 per cent until the haemorrhage has stopped and then maintained above 60 percent until the risk of haemorrhage has passed. The half-life of factor VIII is only ten hours so that twice daily treatment is required. Minor surgery such as tooth extraction is usually undertaken under the cover of tranexamic acid which inhibits fibrinolysis and greatly reduces the need for factor VIII. The vasopressin analogue desmopressin (DDAVP) produces an approximately threefold rise in factor VIII activity, and this may be sufficient to permit surgery in mild haemophiliacs.

Factor VIII concentrate is expensive, and although the risk of HIV transmission is now much less than previously, transmission of non-A non-B hepatitis may still be a hazard. For this reason some centres prefer to use cryoprecipitate, a crude extract of factor VIII and fibrinogen prepared from a small number of donors for the treatment of mild and moderate haemophilia.

Patients with inhibitors require huge amounts of factor VIII to overcome the antibody and this has only a temporary effect since the immune response is boosted by the infused material. Plasmapheresis to remove the inhibitor may be helpful.

Haemophilia B is treated with factor IX concentrate. This has a longer half-life than factor VIII and may therefore be given less frequently. Cryoprecipitate does not contain factor IX.

Prevention of crippling joint disease is only achieved by careful attention to detail and prompt treatment. Muscle and joint bleeds are managed by rest for the first 36 hours, splinting sometimes being necessary. Thereafter mobilization under the guidance of a physiotherapist is ideal. Pain relief is usually achievable with paracetamol-based products. Aspirin should be avoided because of its effect on platelets, and strong analgesics carry the real risk of addiction.

Complications

Owing to virus contamination of clotting concentrates in the past many severely affected haemophiliacs have been exposed to hepatitis B, non-A non-B hepatitis and human immunodeficiency virus. Disordered liver function tests are common as are imbalances of T cell subsets. About 40 per cent have antibodies to HIV; some have already developed AIDS and others are bound to do so.

Even without the spectre of AIDS many haemophiliacs suffer from psychological problems. The Haemophilia Society provides valuable social and psychological support.

Screening

Daughters of haemophiliac fathers and mothers of two haemophiliac sons are obligate carriers of the abnormal gene. However, about 30 per cent of cases of haemophilia are thought to arise from new mutations which makes genetic counselling difficult. The detection of haemophilia carriers may be aided by the finding of a disparity between factor VIII:C and factor VIII:Ag levels in female relatives. Measurement of factor VIII:C in fetal blood and cDNA probes on chorionic villi permit the diagnosis of affected fetuses.

Von Willebrand's disease (VWD)

Von Willebrand's disease is an autosomally transmitted deficiency of Von Willebrand's factor (VWF). In most cases the inheritance is dominant, although recessive forms exist. The incidence is 1:25000, although many of these cases are not clinically important. A number of VWD variants exist.

Pathology

Von Willebrand's factor is a high-molecular-weight protein which binds avidly to factor VIII and prolongs its half-life in the circulation. It also binds to platelet membranes and vessel wall collagen and here helps to stabilize the platelet plug. Deficiency of VWF shortens the factor VIII half-life so that its plasma level falls. In addition platelet function is impaired.

Clinical features

The main features are menorrhagia, epistaxis and easy bruising, together with haemorrhage after trauma or surgery. In severe cases, particularly in rare homozygous patients, the factor VIII level may be low enough to lead to muscle and joint bleeds.

Diagnosis

The bleeding time is prolonged. Clotting tests are also abnormal: the KCCT is prolonged and the factor VIIIc level reduced. VWF is measured immunologically as factor VIII related antigen (F.VIIIRag). It is reduced in Von Willebrand's disease, whereas in Haemophilia A it is present in close to normal levels. Platelets will normally aggregate in the presence of the antibiotic ristocetin; in VWD they fail to do so.

Treatment

Cryoprecipitate is the treatment of choice since it contains much higher levels of VWF than factor VIII concentrates. Single infusions raise the factor VIII level for 48 hours.

Acquired defects of coagulation

Vitamin K deficiency

Vitamin K, a fat-soluble substance obtained from green vegetables, is required by the liver for the formation of factors II, VII, IX and X. Levels are low in the first days of life, especially in premature infants. In adults dietary deficiency is rare, but malabsorption may occur in obstructive jaundice and pancreatic or small bowel disease. In severely affected cases a haemophilia-like syndrome occurs which is on rare occasions fatal. Both the prothrombin time and the KCCT are prolonged. Vitamin K (1 mg IM) is administered prophylactically to all newborn babies (the synthetic vitamin should not be used as it may cause haemolysis and kernicterus). In adults either form given orally or intravenously is satisfactory.

Liver disease

The bleeding diathesis of liver disease is complex. The component parts are:

1 malabsorption of vitamin K because of obstructive jaundice;
2 reduced synthesis of all clotting factors except factor VIII;
3 production of a functionally abnormal fibrinogen (dysfibrinogenaemia);
4 hypersplenism due to portal hypertension leading to thrombocytopenia;
5 low-level disseminated intravascular coagulation.

In addition there is a thrombotic element due to reduced synthesis of antithrombin III.

Disseminated intravascular coagulation (DIC)

The conversion of fibrinogen to fibrin within the circulation leads to the consumption of coagulation factors and platelets and an acute or chronic haemorrhagic state. There are many causes (Table 11.28).

Table 11.28 Causes of disseminated intravascular coagulation

Obstetric
Amniotic fluid embolus
Premature separation of placenta
Septic abortion
Intrauterine death
Eclampsia

Infection
Gram-negative shock
Meningococcal septicaemia
Falciparum malaria
Rocky Mountain spotted fever
Subacute bacterial endocarditis

Malignancy
Carcinoma of prostate
Acute promyelocytic leukaemia (M3)
Mucin secreting adenocarcinoma

Miscellaneous
Haemolytic transfusion reaction
Burns
Liver failure
Snake venoms
Hypothermia
Anaphylaxis

Pathology

Intravascular coagulation is triggered by the liberation of a thrombogenic substance into the circulation. Platelets and coagulation factors are consumed. A secondary fibrinolysis is induced which further depletes clotting factors. Fibrin degradation products are themselves antithrombins.

Clinical features

In severe cases there is bleeding from nose, mouth and venepuncture sites. Petechiae and ecchymoses are found.

Diagnosis

The blood film shows anisocytosis, red cell fragments, polychromasia, nucleated red cells and microspherocytes. The platelet count is low and there is prolongation of the prothrombin time, KCCT and thrombin time. The concentration of fibrinogen is reduced. High levels of fibrin degradation products are found in serum and urine.

Treatment

It is important to treat the underlying cause. When DIC is severe, replacement therapy with clotting factors and platelet transfusion is necessary. In some cases heparin may be carefully administered to control the ongoing coagulation.

Inhibitors of coagulation

Inhibitors of coagulation factors are generally antibodies. In congenital clotting factor deficiencies such as haemophilia A and B, they arise in between 5 and 10 per cent of patients against the clotting factor used for treatment; and although they do not cross-react with the patient's own factor VIII or IX, they may be serious barriers to treatment and may need to be lowered by plasmapheresis before clotting factors are given. Factor VIII autoantibodies may occasionally be seen post-partum and as the antibody activity of the monoclonal protein in Waldenstrom's macroglobulinaemia.

In systemic lupus erythematosus, the 'lupus anticoagulant' is an antibody against phospholipid that causes prolongation of the KCCT. It is not associated with haemorrhage but paradoxically with an increased risk of venous thrombosis. There is also an association with recurrent mid-trimester abortions.

Anticoagulant drugs

Heparin

Heparin acts by potentiating the inhibitory effects of antithrombin III on activated factors XII, IX, X and thrombin. It is used as a treatment for venous thromboembolism. For preference it should be given as a continuous intravenous infusion. Doses of 30–40000 units over 24 hours are usually necessary to keep the KCCT in the desired range, 1.5–2.5 times normal. It is frequently used as the initial treatment of venous thrombosis until concurrently administered oral anticoagulants have their maximal effect.

Overdosage may be reversed by protamine sulphate in a dose of 1 mg for each 100 units of heparin. Heparin is ineffective in antithrombin III deficiency. Low-dose sub-

cutaneous heparin is used for the prophylaxis of venous thrombosis perioperatively and during periods of immobilization. The dose is 5000 units twice or three times daily. The calcium derivative should be used since the usual sodium derivative is as painful as a bee sting. Complications include rare cases of immune thrombocytopenia and osteoporosis with long-term use.

Oral anticoagulants

The oral anticoagulants are mainly coumarin derivatives and act as vitamin K antagonists. They inhibit the gamma carboxylation of the terminal glutamic acid residues of factors II, VII, IX and X. These abnormal proteins (known as PIVKAs) have a poor affinity for calcium and thus are poorly able to participate in coagulation. Anticoagulation is controlled using the prothombin time, results being expressed in a standardized way (the INR) which is comparable between laboratories. An INR of between 2 and 4 is considered to produce a therapeutic effect with little risk of haemorrhage. Almost all patients are treated with warfarin. It is usual to start with 10 mg daily for three days, followed by a dose between 1 mg and 10 mg according to the INR. Anticoagulation is not effective until the third day.

The major cause of lack of control is interaction with other drugs which may potentiate or inhibit the effect of oral anticoagulants (Table 11.29). Overdosage may be reduced by treatment with 10 mg of vitamin K, although this should be avoided if possible since the patient is then made refractory to further oral anticoagulants for several days.

A few patients develop skin necrosis on warfarin treatment. Warfarin should not be given during pregnancy as it causes fetal abnormalities. Heparin should be used instead.

Fibrinolytic agents

Streptokinase and urokinase are enzymes capable of activating the fibrinolytic system. They are used therapeutically for massive pulmonary embolus, for large vessel venous thrombosis, to limit the myocardial damage following coronary thrombosis, and to dissolve thrombus in arteriovenous shunts.

Table 11.29 Drugs causing serious interactions with oral anticoagulants

Potentiation of anticoagulants	Inhibition of anticoagulants
Analgesics	
Aspirin	
Phenylbutazone	
Azapropazone	
Indomethacin	
Co-proxamol	
Antibiotics	
Sulphonamides	Rifampicin
Erythromycin	Griseofulvin
Metronidazole	
Ketoconazole	
Miconazole	
Latamoxef sodium	
Cephamandole	
Hypnotics	
	Barbiturates
	Dichloralphenazone
Anticonvulsants	
	Primidone
	Carbamazepine
Lipid-lowering agents	
Clofibrate	Cholestyramine
Bezafibrate	
Dextrothyroxine sodium	
Gastrointestinal drugs	
Cimetidine	Sucralfate
Hormones	
Anabolic steroids	Oestrogens
Danazol	
Miscellaneous	
Sulphinpyrazone	
Amiodarone	

Further reading

Wintrobe, M.M. (1981) *Clinical haematology*, 8th edn. Kimpton, London.

12
Immunology in Clinical Medicine

Immunology has its roots in the observation that persons surviving certain infectious diseases seldom suffer from the same disease again. Apart from conferring specific resistance to various pathogens, it is now realized that the immune system plays a fundamental role in other biological reactions of great clinical importance.

Nature of the immune response

The immune response (Fig. 12.1) is initiated by a variety of substances referred to as antigens. These are classified according to their origin:

1 Heteroantigens originate in a foreign species (e.g. pathogenic organisms or their products).
2 Isoantigens originate in a genetically dissimilar member of the same species (e.g. blood group substances).
3 Autoantigens originate in the sensitized host (e.g. thyroglobulin).

Antigenic compounds may be complex proteins or carbohydrates of large molecular size. Many antigens which initiate a specific antibody response can be observed to undergo phagocytosis by tissue macrophages. These cells do not synthesize antibody but appear to participate in the immune response by concentrating antigen and presenting it to adjacent lymphocytes; they are therefore called antigen-presenting cells. The latter cells, which are derived from precursors in bone marrow, are widely distributed in lymph nodes, spleen, marrow, skin and lymphoid tissues of the lung and gastrointestinal tract.

Adaptive immune responses are initiated by interaction of antigen with specific receptors on the surfaces of lymphoid cells. Two major classes of lymphocytes are recognized and these behave differently after reaction with antigen. T-lymphocytes undergo transformation

and mitosis, generating a population of cells specifically reactive with the inducing antigen; B-lymphocytes differentiate into plasma cells which secrete humoral antibody, but this process usually requires cooperation with T_H (T-helper) cells. Another subpopulation designated T_S (T-suppressor) cells interact with T_H cells to inhibit antibody synthesis. The immune reactions generated by these cellular responses therefore fall into two major categories. One is mediated by specific humoral antibody and the other by specifically sensitized T-lymphocytes (cell-mediated immunity). Antibody action may, in certain circumstances, be independent of cells (e.g. neutralization of toxins) and certain specific cell-mediated reactions are independent of antibody (e.g. T_C (T-cytotoxic) killing of viral-infected or tumour cells).

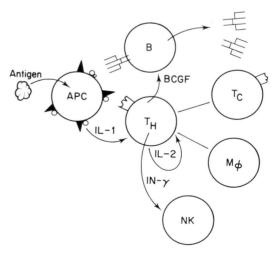

Figure 12.1 *Schematic representation of the immune response. APC, antigen presenting cell; B, B-lymphocyte; T_H, T-helper cell; T_C, T-cytotoxic cell; M_ϕ, macrophage; NK, natural killer cell; IL-1, interleukin-1; IL-2; interleukin-2; IF-γ, γ-interferon; BCGF, B-cell growth factor.*

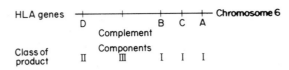

Figure 12.2   *The HLA system.*

Several other specific immune mechanisms require the interaction of humoral antibody with cells. Such antibody-dependent cell reactions include macrophage endocytosis, mast-cell degranulation and ADCC (antibody-dependent cell-mediated cytotoxicity). In addition, the immune response generated by the interaction of antigen with lymphocytes may locally affect other cells which do not carry the specific antigen (non-specific immunity).

The major histocompatibility (HLA) system

The HLA system includes a number of closely linked genetic loci which control the synthesis of cell surface antigens concerned with immune responses and certain complement components. Three loci, HLA-A, B and C, control class I antigens present on all nucleated cells and recognized during graft rejection; HLA-D codes for a structurally distinct set of class II antigens found only on lymphocytes and monocytes (Fig. 12.2). Class I and II HLA antigens have a structure analogous to immunoglobulin (see below).

Histocompatibility antigens have a fundamental physiological role in the control of the cell interactions mentioned above. Thus, T-helper (T_H) or T-suppressor (T_S) cells and antigen presenting cells (APC) can interact functionally only if compatible at the HLA-D locus. Similarly, T_C (cytotoxic) cells can kill only target cells with corresponding specificities at the B, C and A loci. Several diseases, such as ankylosing spondylitis, multiple sclerosis, juvenile diabetes, Reiter's syndrome and gluten-sensitive enteropathy, associate strongly with certain class II genes, suggesting that these enable T_H cells to react against self-antigens.

End products of the immune response

Serum immunoglobulins

Serum antibodies are confined to the gammaglobulin fraction of serum proteins and are referred to as immunoglobulins (Ig). They are large proteins containing two

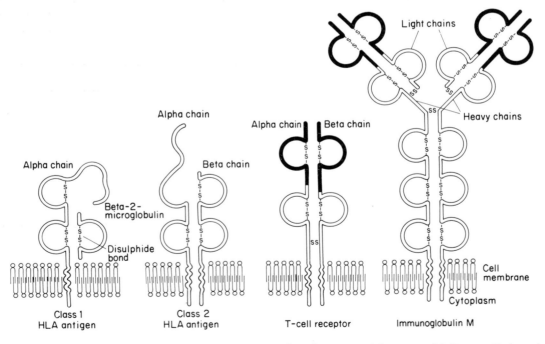

Figure 12.3   *Structures of the HLA class 1 and the class 2 proteins and T-cell receptor and the immunoglobulin, or antibody, molecule are similar. The molecules are characterized by loops made up of about 70 amino acids within each chain. Class 1 proteins are expressed on the surface of every nucleated cell in association with beta-2-microglobulin. Class 2 proteins are expressed only on the surface of selected cells, such as lymphocytes and macrophages. The variable regions of Ig and the T-cell receptor (shaded areas) generate individually specific antigen combining sites.*

heavy and two light polypeptide chains (Fig. 12.3). The different classes of immunoglobulin (IgG, IgA, IgM, IgD, IgE) are distinguished by the structure of their heavy chains. Each Ig chain is made up of repeating units of about 70 amino acids enclosed by a disulphide bond. This arrangement is of interest since antibodies have evolved to perform two distinct functions that are separately localized in the molecule.

First, each antibody combines with a specific antigen. Every individual can probably make at least 10^6 antibodies with different specificities. The portions of the molecule which interact with antigen are called combining sites, and there are two on each four-chain molecule. These sites are generated by the interaction of the N-terminal units (V_H and V_L) of heavy and light chains, which show great variability of structure and are different in antibodies of distinct specificities. The V regions are common to all classes of immunoglobulins so that antibodies of a given specificity may be distributed in all the major Ig classes.

Second, antibodies also carry out various effector functions which are consequent upon interaction with complement or with specific cells or membranes of the body. These effector sites are in C regions of the antibody molecule and given sites are present on some immunoglobulin classes but absent from others. Only IgG and IgM have sites for complement fixation, and only IgE has a site for attachment to mast cells, which is the basis for sensitization of autologous tissues. Both IgG and IgM attach to the surface of macrophages and mediate endocytosis, while IgG alone attaches to K (killer) cells to initiate antibody-dependent cell-mediated cytotoxicity (ADCC). These differences between the immunoglobulin classes account for the remarkable diversity of biological reactions mediated by serum antibody (Table 12.1).

Monocolonal antibodies produced by hybridomas

Antigens carry several different antigenic sites each of which stimulates antibody production by several clones of B cells. Antisera specific for a given antigen therefore contain a broad spectrum of polyclonal antibodies which have different combining specificities and may be of different classes. Individual B cells and their clonal progeny, by contrast, produce a single antibody species, but such cells cannot be readily cultured *in vitro*. However, if B cells are fused with myeloma cells the resulting hybridoma has the capacity to produce antibody and to proliferate *in vitro*. Such antibody comprises a single molecular species having defined specificity and class and can be produced in limitless amounts. The products of hybridomas therefore comprise standard immunological reagents previously unobtain-

Table 12.1 Properties of human immunoglobins

	IgG	IgA	IgM	IgD	IgE
Structural					
Molecular weight	150 000	160 000 (serum) 370 000 (secretory)	900 000	170 000	200 000
Heavy chain classes	γ	α	μ	δ	ε
Light chain types	κ, λ	κ, λ	κ, λ	κ, λ	κ, λ
Carbohydrate (%)	2.9	7.5	11.8	11.3	10.7
Biological					
Serum concentration (g/l)	8–17	1.5–4.5	0.5–1.5	0.003–0.40	0.10–1.3 μg/l
Antibody activity	+	+	+	+	+
C fixation	+	0	+	0	0
Placental transfer	+	0	0	0	0
Seromucous secretion	0	+	0		+
Tissue sensitization	0	0	0	0	+
Combination rheumatoid factor	+	0	0		
Attachment to macrophages	+	0	+		+
B-cell receptor	0	0	+ (monomer)	+	0
Attachment to K cells (ADCC)	+	0	0	0	0

Table 12.2 Clinical uses of monoclonal antibodies

Immunodiagnosis	Blood grouping; tissue typing; immunodiagnosis of infections and tumors
Experimental analysis	Cell products (e.g. interferon); cell constituents (e.g. for vaccine development); cell subsets (e.g. of lymphocytes and neurones)
Therapeutic agents	Drug targeting; immunotherapy

able by conventional immunization. Such antibodies have many increasingly important applications in clinical medicine (Table 12.2).

Specific cell-mediated immunity

In addition to the immunoglobulin response outlined above, antigenic stimulation leads to the proliferation of T cells. These T cells originate in bone marrow but are modified in some way by passage through the thymus gland. The antigen receptor of the T cell consists of alpha and beta chains and has a structure analogous to Ig (Fig. 12.3). The N-terminal variable regions of the chains generate the antigen combining site. This differs from the combining site of Ig in recognizing only cell-surface antigen which is associated with class I or class II HLA antigens.

T cells comprise 80 per cent of circulating lymphocytes. Functional subsets of T cells include T_H (helper) cells which cooperate with B cells in Ig synthesis, T_S (suppressor) cells which inhibit B cells, and T_C (cytotoxic) cells which can specifically kill virally infected target cells and some tumour cells. Sensitized lymphocytes after combination with antigen can also exert widespread effects by producing factors which are called lymphokines and act upon other cell types (Table 12.3). For example, macrophages are attracted to the site of T cell antigen interaction by chemotactic factor, immobilized there by MIF and activated by MAF which is identical to γ-interferon. Activated macrophages in turn secrete soluble factors which act upon other cell types—notably, interleukin-1 which influences proliferation of lymphocytes.

Cell-mediated immune responses are directed predominantly against intracellular pathogens and organized tissue targets, and are associated with delayed hypersensitivity responses to specific antigen.

Natural killer (NK) cells

There are a subpopulation of lymphoid cells comprising mainly large, granular lymphocytes. NK cells are able to kill some infected target cells and a range of tumour cells and do not require the presence of antibody. They are found in normal people and their activity does not depend on previous sensitization. NK cells possess an oxygen-dependent killing system which generates superoxide radicals and in this respect are akin to mononuclear phagocytes and granulocytes. NK cells are thought to be important in defence against tumour cells and their activity is augmented by interferons.

Immunological paralysis

Cells of the immunological system can respond in two alternative ways to the presence of antigen. On the one hand, antigenic stimulation, as outlined above, may induce the cycle of cell proliferation and differentiation which culminates in humoral or cell-mediated immunity. On the other hand, antigen may lead to specific immunological paralysis; this is not merely a failure to produce specific antibody, but is characterized by long-lasting loss of the capacity to synthesize antibodies specific for the paralysing antigen. Injection of antigens during fetal life tends to induce specific paralysis rather than antibody production, but specific paralysis can also be induced in adults by using the appropriate antigen dose or by modifying the physical character of the antigen.

The mechanisms that determine whether an antigen will induce specific paralysis rather than antibody production are not fully understood. In some instances, the removal from antigen preparations of aggregated material liable to phagocytosis converts an immunizing protein antigen into one inducing specific paralysis. This suggests that, at least in these instances, the immune response is initiated by antigen which has been modified by passage through macrophages while specific paralysis follows the direct interaction of antigen with lymphocytes.

Non-specific cell-mediated immunity

Sensitized T-lymphocytes reacting with antigen undergo blast transformation and may produce cytotoxic agents capable of damaging bystander cells. In addition, other lymphocyte products may activate macrophages which become cytotoxic for a wide range of pathogens and cells.

Disorders of the immune function

Clinical disorders may be associated with either diminished or increased production of antibody or lym-

Table 12.3 Lymphokines

Cells affected	Active lymphokine
Macrophages and monocytes	Migration inhibition factor (MIF)
	Macrophage activating factor (MAF)
	Chemotactic factor for macrophages
Lymphocytes	Enhancement of antibody formation (helper factors)
	Suppression of antibody formation (suppressor factors)
	T-cell growth factors (interleukin-2)
Polymorphouclear leucocytes	Chemotactic factors
Other cell types	Lymphotoxin
	γ-interferon
	Collagen producing factor
	Osteoclast activating factor (OAF)

phocytes (Table 12.6). The most severe forms of antibody deficiency affect both cell-mediated and humoral immunity, but in other syndromes only one of these immune responses may be affected while the other remains relatively intact. Ig deficiency is associated with unusual susceptibility to bacterial infections, whereas cell-mediated immune deficiency induces susceptibility to viral, protozoal and fungal infections. Patients with intact immune responses may rarely show increased susceptibility to infection associated with absence of complement components or defects of polymorph function.

Clinical immunodeficiency occurs in several rare congenital syndromes but more frequently is a complication of acquired disorders of the lymphoid system (e.g. Hodgkin's disease, myelomatosis, lymphatic leukaemia, and AIDS).

Human immunodeficiency virus (HIV) and acquired immunodeficiency syndrome (AIDS)

HIV is a retrovirus which has emerged since 1980 as an important cause of human disease. One of the consequences of such infection is the acquired immunodeficiency syndrome (AIDS). Early in 1988 well over 50,000 cases had been reported worldwide with nearly 800 deaths in the UK. In many countries these figures seem likely to increase for some years to come. In parts of Africa there are high rates of infection with HIV, although the number

of cases of AIDS is uncertain because of under-reporting. The HIV virus infects and destroys T_H cells and severely compromises cell-mediated immune responses.

Incidence and spread of infection

The infection is spread predominantly by sexual transmission during anal intercourse between male homosexuals. Such cases make up around 80 per cent of the current numbers in Europe and the USA (Table 12.4). Infection by blood or blood products occurs in haemophiliacs and intravenous drug abusers and occasionally after organ transplantation or blood transfusion. The incidence among female partners of infected men has been low in Europe and the USA, but HIV infection occurs equally in men and women in some parts of Africa. Infected mothers may transmit the disease perinatally to their infants. Infection of children born before the onset of infection is rare, confirming that spread among non-sexual contacts of infected subjects is very uncommon.

The incubation period from HIV infection to development of AIDS varies and is generally shorter after sexual transmission than blood product spread. However, experience of the disease is relatively short and the full natural history remains to be seen.

The HIV virus has been isolated from semen, blood, saliva, tears, breast milk and vaginal secretions. However, transmission has been attributable only to infected semen and blood or blood products. The virus is readily inactivated by heat and treatment with hypochlorite or alcohol, so that blood products such as factor VIII can now be suitably treated and safely administered.

The lack of effective treatment for AIDS and the mortality of the disease indicate that strenuous efforts must be made to prevent its spread. Spread should no longer occur with suitably screened and treated blood and blood products given for medical reasons. Intravenous drug users need to avoid sharing needles and syringes. It is hoped that the use of condoms and restriction in sexual partners will limit homosexual cases and prevent spread into the heterosexual community. This will require continued education programmes.

Clinical features

There are a number of clinical manifestations of HIV infection (Table 12.5). Infection is often followed within weeks by an acute, febrile, 'flu-like' illness with no distin-

Table 12.4 USA cases of AIDS by risk group February 1986 (Source: Center for Disease Control)

Group	Males		Females	
Homosexual/bisexual men	12 689	(79%)		
IV drug users	2 340	(15%)	600	(53%)
Haemophiliacs/coagulation disorder	135	(1%)	3	(0%)
Heterosexual contact	39	(0%)	185	(16%)
Blood transfusion	169	(1%)	108	(10%)
Other	765	(5%)	233	(21%)
Totals	16 137	(100%)	1 129	(100%)

guishing features. There follows an asymptomatic period of infectivity which usually lasts around three years when further problems develop. Asymptomatic infection may continue longer than this and it is still unclear how many carriers of the HIV virus eventually develop the clinical problems of AIDS.

Around 25 per cent develop signs and symptoms of persistent generalized lymphadenopathy (PGL). Present estimates are of more than 30 per cent developing AIDS, but these numbers may have to be revised upwards with further experience. AIDS consists of the development of specified opportunistic infections (Table 12.5) or tumours. Other conditions such as chronic ill health and weight loss and progressive dementia also occur. The eventual mortality rate of AIDS is probably 100 per cent.

The commonest infection is pneumonia caused by the protozoan *Pneumocystis carinii*. Other frequent infections are Cytomegalovirus, *Mycobacterium tuberculosis* or *Mycobacterium avium-intracellulare* and Cryptosporidium infection of the gastrointestinal tract. Infection with common pathogens is also increased. The characteristic tumour is Kaposi's sarcoma and lymphomas and oral carcinomas also occur. Median survival is around nine months from the first episode of pneumocystis

Table 12.5 Major clinical manifestations of HIV infection

Acute febrile illness
Asymptomatic infection
Persistent generalized lymphadenopathy (PGL): lethargy;
   weight loss; night sweats; fever; joint pains; skin rashes;
   diarrhoea; lymphadenopathy; splenomegaly; lymphopenia
AIDS
   Opportunist infection: *Pneumocystis carinii* pneumonia;
                          Mycobacterium avium-intracellulare;
                          Mycobacterium tuberculosis;
                          Cytomegalovirus; Cryptococcus
                          meningitis; Cryptosporidium
   Tumours: Kaposi's sarcoma; intracranial lymphoma; oral
            and anal carcinoma
   Neurological disease: progressive encephalopathy
   General progressive ill-health

pneumonia and about two years from the diagnosis of Kaposi's sarcoma. Chronic diarrhoea may be a problem and neurological manifestations are being recognized increasingly.

A test for specific antibodies to HIV in the form of an immunoassay based on viral antigen has, since October 1985, been carried out on all blood donations in the UK. Testing individuals suspected of HIV infection or AIDS requires careful consideration. Experienced counsellors should be available to discuss the consequences of the findings with patients before and after such testing.

Treatment

Several agents have been shown to inhibit replication of HIV, but viral multiplication resumes as soon as the therapy, often toxic, has been stopped. Therapy combining antiviral agents with immune-enhancing agents such as gamma-interferon and interleukin II is under investigation. Structural variation in the coat of the different isolates of the virus complicates the development of a vaccine which could protect against primary infection. Vaccines would be unlikely to prevent progress of the disease in those infected since the immune system would already be compromised.

Treatment of pneumocystis pneumonia consists of high-dose co-trimoxazole or pentamidine. Co-trimoxazole produces skin rashes and bone marrow suppression while pentamidine shows renal toxicity. Corticosteroids may help in severe disease. Nebulized pentamidine is much less toxic and may be useful in treatment and prophylaxis. Recovery from the first episode occurs in around 80 per cent of cases with this treatment, but few patients go on to survive for longer than one year because of the development of other infections or tumours. Pneumocystis pneumonia itself recurs in 20 per cent. Kaposi's sarcoma may respond to interferon treatment or chemotherapy. The universally fatal outcome of the disease with current therapy means that intensive care to the extent of ventilatory support is inappropriate in most cases.

Table 12.6 Disorders of antibody production

Deficient production
Reduced cell-mediated and Ig responses:
    Combined immunodeficiency
    Combined immunodeficiency (with thymoma)
    Wiskott–Aldrich syndrome (with thrombocytopenia and
       eczema)
Reduced Ig response only:
    Transient hypogammaglobulinaemia of infancy
    Congenital agammaglobulinaemia
    Secondary hypogammaglobulinaemia (e.g. in Hodgkin's
       disease, nephrosis)
Reduced cell-mediated response only:
    Thymic aplasia (di George's syndrome)
    AIDS (acquired immunodeficiency syndrome)

Excessive production
Diffuse hypergammaglobulinaemia:
    Chronic infections
    Granulomata
    Hepatic disease
    'Connective tissue' disease
'Monoclonal' Ig production:
    Multiple myelomatosis (IgG, IgA, IgD or IgE)
    Macroglobulinaemia (IgM)
    Lymphoma
    Idiopathic 'gammopathy'
Clonal lymphocyte proliferation:
    Acute lymphatic leukaemia
    Chronic lymphatic leukaemia
    Burkitt's lymphoma

Agents such as zidovudine (AZT) may slow the course of the disease.

Excessive production of Ig

A diffuse increase of gammaglobulin detected on electrophoresis of serum is seen in many clinical disorders and results from proliferation of many different clones of lymphoid cells. The proliferation of a single clone, on the other hand, leads to production of monoclonal Ig which is homogeneous on electrophoresis and belongs to a single Ig class. This occurs in multiple myelomatosis and macroglobulinaemia, in association with various lymphomata and unrelated neoplasms and also, quite commonly, as an 'idiopathic' condition without detectable underlying pathology. Clonal proliferation of lymphocytes also occurs in acute and chronic lymphatic leukaemia, but these cells rarely produce immunoglobulin.

Reactions mediated by immune responses

Humoral antibodies and cell-mediated immunity are of fundamental clinical importance, not only in regard to protective immunity, but also in a wide range of pathological states involving immediate hypersensitivity reactions, autoantibody formation or reactions to circulating immune complexes.

Protective immunity

The primary interaction of antibody with the pathogen or its toxic products is the basis of protective immunity only in rare instances (e.g. some forms of viral immunity and toxin neutralization). Immunity is usually dependent on subsequent reactions of the bound antibody either with complement which leads to cell lysis (e.g. of Gram-negative bacteria) or with the surface of macrophages which promotes phagocytosis of the pathogen (e.g. pneumococci or with K cells responsible for antibody-dependent cell-mediated cytotoxicity). It follows that protective immunity in systemic infections is mainly dependent upon IgG and IgM antibodies since only these can fix complement and attach to effector cells. IgA is the predominant antibody of seromucous secretions and fulfils an important protective role at the epithelial surface of pulmonary and gastrointestinal tracts. Although IgA does not fix complement, it can act synergistically with lysozyme, present in seromucous secretions, and activate complement by the alternative pathway to cause bacterial lysis. Cell-mediated immunity plays an important role in specific resistance to intracellular infections, including tuberculosis, leishmaniasis, leprosy and some viral infections, and may be responsible for many of the papular and vesicular rashes which accompany common infectious diseases. The presence of cell-mediated immunity is indicated by the delayed hypersensitivity response (an inflammatory lesion appearing 24 hours after intradermal challenge with the antigen) and characterized by local infiltration of the tissue with mononuclear cells.

Whether the immune response to infection is clinically effective or not depends mainly on the serological character of the pathogen and its distribution in the body (Table 12.7). Lasting immunity occurs with organisms of uniform antigenicity widely distributed in the circulation (e.g. pertussis infection). Recurrent infections may be caused by serological variants of the original infecting pathogen (e.g. pneumococcal infections), or may occur after localized infections which evoke a feeble immune response (e.g. diphtheria). Immunity may be totally ineffective where the organisms persist in modified form (e.g. the herpes virus as DNA) or where the lethal dose of a toxic product (e.g. tetanus toxin) is less than the immunizing dose.

Table 12.7 Immune response to various infections

Clinical immunity	Serology	Distribution of pathogen	Infections			
			Bacterial	Rickettsial	Viral	Protozoal
Lasting	Uniform	Systemic or localized	Pertussis	Q fever	Measles; mumps; rubella; smallpox; yellow fever; chickenpox	Cutaneous leishmaniasis
Strain-specific	Varied	Systemic or localized	Streptococcal Staphylococcal Pneumococcal	Typhus	Polio; common cold; Influenza	African trypanosomiasis
Poor	Uniform or varied	Localized (or intra-cellular)	Brucella		Common cold; influenza; trachoma; gonorrhoea	Malaria S. American trypanosomiasis
Ineffective			Tetanus		Herpes	Visceral leishmaniasis Schistosomiasis

The secretion of soluble cell surface antigens which combine with specific antibody or T cells may effectively block immunity and promote survival of the pathogen (e.g. in schistosomiasis). Some intracellular pathogens are able to survive within phagocytic cells. Such survival may occur when a pathogen escapes from the ingested phagosome and lies free in the cytoplasm of the phagocyte (e.g. *Trypanosoma cruzi*); or when phagosomes fail to fuse with lysosomes and ingested organisms are therefore shielded from the potentially lethal lysosomal enzymes (e.g. *Toxoplasma*); or when fusion of phagosomes with lysosomes occurs, but the organisms are resistant to enzyme action (e.g. tubercle bacilli and *Leishmania*).

Immunity to tumours leading to involution of their growth may occur with virally induced and chemically induced tumours which carry recognizable foreign surface antigens. Unfortunately, tumours which arise spontaneously are not usually recognized as foreign and produce no effective immune response. The incidence of cancer may be increased in immunosuppressed subjects (e.g. Kaposi sarcoma in AIDS), but the occurrence of

Table 12.8 Immunopathology—mechanisms and clinical associations

Mechanism	Antibody	Antigens	Clinical
Anaphylactic (Type I)	IgE	Allergens (e.g. drugs, pollen)	Systemic anaphylaxis; bronchial asthma; hay fever; urticaria
Cytotoxic (Type II)	IgG or IgM	Host tissue	Hyperthyroidism; Goodpasture's syndrome; myasthenia gravis; autoimmune haemolytic anaemia
		Viral	Post-measles encephalitis
		Drugs	Haemolytic anaemia; thrombocytopenia
Immune complex (Type III)	IgG or IgM	DNA	Lupus erythematosus nephritis
		Serum, drugs	Serum sickness, Arthus reaction
		Viral	Serum hepatitis (arthritis, nephritis)
		Bacterial	Glomerulonephritis; lepromatous leprosy
		Protozoal	Malarial nephrosis
		Fungal	Farmer's lung
Cell-mediated (Type IV)	Cell-mediated	Host	Hashimoto's disease
		Chemical	Nickel sensitivity
		Viral	Herpes simplex
		Bacterial	Tuberculosis; leprosy
		Protozoal	Cutaneous leishmaniasis
		Helminth	Schistosomiasis (cirrhosis)

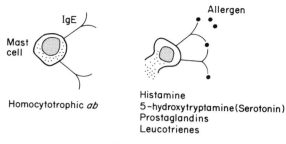

Figure 12.4 *Mechanism of local and generalized anaphylaxis. Antigenic stimulation of a susceptible subject leads to synthesis of IgE antibody which becomes attached to mast cells. A subsequent exposure to the same antigen leads to its combination with cell-bound IgE and consequent degranulation of mast cells and discharge of pharmacologically active compounds which cause anaphylaxis.*

lymphoid tumours in these patients could be related directly to the immunosuppressive agents used. NK cells (see page 394) are able to kill some tumour cell lines, and interferon enhances their activity, thus raising hopes for more effective tumour thepary.

Immunopathology

In addition to specific protection, immune response can cause tissue damage in several different ways (Table 12.8).

Anaphylactic (type I reactions)

These reactions, which include general and localized forms of anaphylaxis, depend on an immune response fundamentally similar to that responsible for protective immunity. There has long been speculation regarding the underlying mechanism producing such dramatically divergent reactions. It is now established that immediate hypersensitivity is mediated by one class of immunoglobulin, IgE (Table 12.1), and atopic individuals tend to produce this antibody in response to antigenic stimulation. The serum concentration of IgE is very low (see page 393) and most of this antibody is attached to tissue mast cells which are then said to be sensitized. On subsequent exposure, the antigen (allergen) reacts with tissue bound IgE and as a result the sensitized mast cells undergo degranulation, liberating various pharmacologically active compounds (Fig. 12.4) which cause the characteristic allergic symptoms (Table 12.8).

In addition to the release of histamine and 5-hydroxytryptamine, triggering of mast cells leads to the activation of membrane phospholipase A with release of arachidonic acid, which produces prostaglandins and thromboxanes via the cyclo-oxygenase pathway and leukotrienes via the lipoxygenase pathway. A mixture of leukotrienes C4 and D constitutes slow-reacting substance (SRS-A) which induces sustained contraction of some smooth muscles.

Desensitization of atopic individuals can sometimes be achieved by injecting very small doses of the allergen. This stimulates the production of IgG antibody and on subsequent, natural exposure the allergen combines mainly with the predominant IgG (blocking) antibody so that reactions due to combination with IgE are prevented (Fig. 12.5). It is apparent that the biological consequences of antibody reactions depend fundamentally on the relative proportions of the reacting Ig classes.

Autoantibodies (cytotoxic type II reactions)

The remarkable ability of the immunological system to distinguish 'self' and 'non-self' is thought to depend on the development during fetal life of specific paralysis to autoantigens. The appearance of autoantibodies could, therefore, result from changes in the structure of autoantigens (e.g. by drugs or infectious agents), entry into the circulation of antigens normally shielded from the immune system (e.g. spermatozoa, lens protein or thyroglobulin), the presence of cross-reacting heteroantigens (e.g. group A streptococci, which have antigens also present in human heart tissue) or loss of T_S (suppressor) activity (as in systemic lupus erythematosis). Viral infections which cause antigenic modification of cell surfaces may also induce antibody formation against the infected tissues (e.g. as probably occurs in post-measles encephalitis).

Autoantibodies are being found in association with an increasing number of pathological states. In many instances these antibodies (Table 12.9) are directly res-

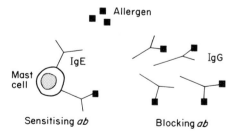

Figure 12.5 *Desensitization of an atopic subject by injecting small amounts of the allergen may induce the formation of IgG antibody. By combining with this allergen after natural exposure the IgG acts as a 'blocking' antibody and prevents combination with IgE on sensitized mast cells.*

Table 12.9 Properties of some common autoantibodies

Disease	Antibody	Antigen	Test	Positive in
Rheumatoid arthritis	Rheumatoid factor (IgM)	IgG	Rose-Waaler } Latex-particle } agglutination	Rheumatoid arthritis 70%; SLE 20%; normal 5%; Sjøgren's syndrome 75%
Systemic lupus erythematosus	L.E. factor (IgG, IgA or IgM)	Deoxyribonucleohistose (nuclear protein)	LE cell phenomenon or immunofluorescence	SLE 90%; rheumatoid arthritis 50%; Sjøgren's syndrome 75%
Thyroiditis	IgG or IgM	Thyroglobulin; thyroid microsomes	Precipitin reaction or agglutination C^1 fixation	Hashimoto's disease 100%; Thyrotoxicosis, Ca thyroid, non-toxic goitre 60%; normal females 15%; pernicious anaemia 40%
Thyrotoxicosis	LATS (IgG)		Release of labelled hormone from thyroid	Thyrotoxicosis 60%
Acquired haemolytic anaemia	IgG (non-agglutinating)	rH	Indirect haemagglutination (Coombs' test)	AHA 80%
Pernicious anaemia		Intrinsic factor; parietal cell	Binding of radioactive vitamin B_{12}; immunofluorescence	Pernicious anaemia 50%; thyroiditis 30%
Myasthenia gravis	IgG	Accetylcholine receptor of motor end plate	Immunofluorescence	Myasthenia gravis 85%
Goodpasture's syndrome	IgG	Glomerular and pulmonary basement membrane	Immunofluorescence	Goodpasture's syndrome 100%

ponsible for the pathological lesions (e.g. in hyperthyroidism, myasthenia gravis and Goodpasture's syndrome). In other instances their presence is of diagnostic value, but several facts throw doubt upon the role of most of these antibodies in the *initiation* of pathological lesions. Many autoantibodies occur in only a proportion of patients with the particular clinical syndrome and, conversely, specific autoantibodies are often found in the absence of the relevant disease (Table 12.9). In addition, their presence or level may show little correlation with the clinical state and autoimmune lesions are not usually induced by passive transfer of autoantibodies. Thyroid stimulating antibody is an exception to this statement since thyrotoxicosis may occur in newborn offspring of thyrotoxic mothers who have circulating antibody. Muscle weakness may occur in babies born to mothers with myasthenia gravis associated with antibodies to acetylcholine receptors. These observations strongly support the idea that some forms of thyrotoxicosis and myasthenia gravis are caused by autoimmune reactions involving serum IgG antibody.

Immune complex (type III reactions)

Antigen–antibody complexes present in the circulation may form microprecipitates in small blood vessels, fix complement and lead to accumulation of polymorphonuclear leucocytes, vascular occlusion and perivascular inflammation. Such lesions may occur in individuals injected with large doses of penicillin or horse serum (e.g. during passive immunization for diphtheria or tetanus) who form antibodies which combine with the circulating antigen. The resulting syndrome, which is known as *serum sickness*, is characterized by glomerulonephritis, myocarditis, joint effusions, urticaria and pyrexia. Certain forms of pulmonary alveolitis which follow inhalation of fungal antigens (e.g. farmer's lung) also represent a reaction to circulating immune complexes. There is at present considerable interest in the possibility that various forms of renal disease, arthritis and periarteritis of obscure aetiology are caused by a similar immune mechanism.

Cell-mediated immunity (type IV reactions)

Sensitized lymphocytes of thymic origin are involved especially in immunological reactions against organized tissues carrying foreign antigens. Such cell-mediated reactions are primarily responsible for rejection of foreign grafts, immunological responses to tumours and for certain forms of immunopathology (e.g. hepatic cirrhosis associated with schistosomiasis, granulomatous lesions in leprosy and sensitivity reactions to nickel, picryl chloride and poison ivy—see Table 12.8). The presence of cell-mediated immunity is indicated by the delayed hypersensitivity response (i.e. an inflammatory lesion appearing 24 hours after intradermal challenge with the antigen) and characterized by local infiltration of the tissue with round cells.

Summary

The immune system embodies an array of sensing cells which, through a wide repertoire of receptors, recognize antigens foreign to the host. This recognition event triggers a series of responses involving specific antibody formation and the production of a complex set of lymphokines which regulate the activities of many cell types. These reactions act individually and in concert to establish immunity to a variety of pathogens and to some tumours with recognizable antigenicity. Congenital and acquired disorders of the immune system may produce life-threatening susceptibility to microbial invaders. In addition, immune reactions can under circumstances outlined above cause damage to host tissue and generate a wide spectrum of pathological processes. Better understanding of factors which regulate immune responsiveness may permit more effective treatment of immunodeficiency and control of immunopathology.

Further reading

Holborrow, E.J. and Reeves, W.G. (1983) *Immunology in Medicine: a Comprehensive Guide to Clinical Immunology*. Grune & Stratton, London.
Roitt, I.M. (1984) *Essential Immunology*. Blackwell Scientific, Oxford.

13
Disorders of the Skin

Introduction

Skin diseases constitute a very significant proportion of the total of all diseases. Many are of minor importance, but some can give rise to significant illness or even death if untreated. Perhaps the commonest are the so-called tropical diseases, and many of these have a major dermatological component. It is likely that these diseases are the ones where the most significant advances in therapy will be made in the next 20 years. It is also probable that many diseases could be eliminated at present if it were possible to provide a uniform service throughout the world.

Two advantages that skin diseases have over other disorders is that the morphology can be examined in any one individual and the lesions are readily available for histological examination if this is appropriate. A wrong diagnosis is generally made because the patient is not examined carefully and completely. Well over 80 per cent of skin diseases could be easily diagnosed and treated by a general practitioner. Hospital referral is seldom necessary, but it is significant that, annually, 1 per cent of the population in the British Isles are seen by a hospital consultant as new referrals. This figure could be significantly reduced, in many instances, by a simple diagnosis and application of sensible treatment by the primary health care doctor.

As topical and systemic treatments have improved over the last 20 years, far fewer patients are sufficiently sick to need hospital admission. It is to be hoped that in the next two decades the need for hospital admission will be almost eliminated for dermatological disorders. Treatment in the patient's home is certainly cheaper and often more effective.

Most dermatologists would agree that it is best to keep treatment safe and simple. New remedies are not necessarily the most successful, and often result in a dermatitis medicamentosa — that is, a contact dermatitis to the topical application.

Moist, exudative lesions need a lotion to dry them, and chronic, scaly lesions are best treated with an ointment or cream. Some diseases require appropriate systemic therapy such as oral steroids.

Common symptoms

Pruritus

This is the single most significant dermatological symptom. It is totally subjective, and so there is no satisfactory way in which the patient's response to treatment can be measured. It can be of very great severity (as in scabies) or fairly mild (as in some individuals with pemphigoid). Pruritus may result in severe excoriation (scratching) and thence secondary bacterial infection (e.g. impetigo). Many legions will greatly improve if the pruritus can be controlled, so that they are removed from the itch–scratch cycle.

Pain

This is not a prominent feature of dermatological disorders, although it may be very marked in some conditions such as herpes zoster (shingles). Deep fissures (chapping) of the hands and feet may be a complication of some occupations, but often the patient complains of *soreness* rather than pain. For instance, two epithelial surfaces rubbing together (intertrigo) with some loss of the epidermis may be very sore. Similarly, bullae in the mouth or vulva quickly burst, leaving erosions that are very sore, and the former may make eating difficult.

Relevant signs

The morphological features of dermatological disorders are classically described by various terms. A *macule* is a localized discolouration of the skin with no change in texture or palpable thickening. A *nodule* is a circumscribed, palpable, usually solid lesion, larger than 1 cm in diameter affecting the epidermis, dermis and subcutis or only the dermis and subcutis. A *papule* is a small, solid lesion, up to 1 cm in diameter, which is raised and palpable. A *vesicle* is a small (up to 1 cm. diameter) fluid-filled superficial lesion. A *bulla* (or blister) is a larger (more than 1 cm diameter) fluid-filled and raised lesion. A *pustule* is a vesicle or bulla containing pus.

Erythema, or redness, of the skin results from an increase in blood within the small, superficial blood vessels, whereas a *wheal* is a raised, often transient, area of dermal and hypodermal oedema. Dried serum and other exudates result in a *crust*. With *hyperkeratosis* there is thickening of the horny layer of the epidermis, and in *lichenification* there is a thickening of all layers of the epidermis, shown clinically by an increase in normal skin markings. *Telangiectasia* results from permanently dilated small blood vessels. Haemorrhage into the skin, if from 2 to 5 mm in diameter, is called *purpura*.

Investigations

Many standard investigations, such as a chest X-ray, may be indicated for various dermatological disorders, such as erythema nodosum or sarcoid. A full blood picture and ESR may also be useful. However, a number of tests are carried out specifically in dermatological disorders.

Bacteriological disorders may be suspected and a *skin swab* taken in many disorders where infection is likely. Virological studies may be indicated in herpetic disorders.

Skin scrapings are useful for fungal infections. Scrapings taken from a lesion are immersed in potassium hydroxide and examined with a microscope if a tinea is suspected. This should be virtually a routine procedure in any scaly lesion. Nail clippings are examined in the same way. Skin and nail can also be cultured on an appropriate medium. If a fungal infection of hair is suspected the patient should be examined with a *Wood's light*.

Histological examination of a lesion is certainly helpful in most skin diseases where there is any doubt as to the diagnosis. This is so important that 'every dermatologist should be his own histopathologist'. *Immunofluorescent* studies on skin sections may also be indicated, for bullous diseases and vasculitides.

If scabies is suspected, an attempt should be made to confirm the diagnosis by seeing an acarus or an egg *under the microscope*. With a needle a suitable lesion (such as a burrow) should be scraped. Pediculosis pubis, and other pediculoses, can also be examined under a microscope.

Red and scaly eruptions

A very large proportion of skin diseases comes under the heading of an erythemato-squamous dermatopathy – that is, characterized by red, scaly lesions. There are seven important conditions in this group:

>   All the eczemas
>   Superficial fungal diseases
>   Psoriasis
>   Pityriasis rosea
>   Secondary syphilis
>   Discoid lupus erythematosus
>   Lichen planus.

Eczema and dermatitis

The words 'eczema' and 'dermatitis' have been a source of confusion for many years. It is now generally accepted that they are synonymous and clinically and histologically refer to the same condition. However, because of long usage, the two words are sometimes retained, and then eczema is used if the cause is endogenous (as in atopic eczema) and dermatitis if the cause is exogenous (such as in a contact dermatitis due to nickel).

Atopic eczema

This generally begins after the age of three months and before the age of two years. It is frequently associated with asthma and hay fever, and the predisposition to all these conditions is probably genetically determined. The eczematous lesions may develop first on the face in very young children, but subsequently the antecubital and popliteal fossae are the sites most commonly affected.

Contact dermatitis

Some substances provoke a dermatitic reaction when applied to the skin of normal people, others only when applied to the skin of a sensitized individual. The former is often referred to as a *primary irritant dermatitis* and the latter as a *contact dermatitis*, followed by the name of the causative agent. A very common cause of a primary irritant dermatitis is detergents, which are often too strong to be applied undiluted to the skin.

Contact dermatitis is extremely common, and the substances which provoke this reaction can be classified into the following groups:

1 Chemicals

Almost any therapeutic agent applied to the skin may induce a dermatitic response, particularly if it is applied repeatedly over a period of time. Drugs such as neomycin, penicillin and streptomycin are common causes. Doctors, nurses and students should be very careful when giving injections of the last two substances not to allow any of the solution to come into contact with their own hands. Nickel (on rings, necklaces and brassiere clips), lipstick, nail varnish and hair dyes are common causes of a contact dermatitis, and so are furs and some articles of clothing. Soaps, bleaching agents and detergents usually cause a primary irritant dermatitis rather than a true contact dermatitis.

2 Substances of plant origin

In the UK the plants that may give rise to a contact dermatitis are primula obconica and chrysanthemums.

3 Micro-organisms

Skin infections such as impetigo and ringworm (tinea) may be complicated by an eczematous reaction.

The diagnosis of contact dermatitis is usually suggested by a careful history, and by the site and distribution of the lesions. It may be confirmed by a patch test: appropriate dilutions of the suspected substance are applied to an area of normal skin (usually on the back), covered with a micropore dressing, left for 48 hours and then removed. The tested area should be reviewed another 48 hours later. A positive result is seen with the development of a dermatitic response in the area of skin covered by the testing substance.

The most important point in treatment is the removal of the cause if this is known. Contact with the offending agents must be prevented. If there are several possible causes (for example, if the patient is a hairdresser or dentist), patch tests must be done to determine the exact cause.

For local therapy, treatment with a 1% hydrocortisone ointment is the safest remedy. However, 2½% hydrocortisone, betamethasone valerate or triamcinolone acetonide are often more effective and may be needed; but these agents can induce striae formation, atrophy of the skin and telangiectasia if they are used for too long, and particularly if they are applied under polythene occlusion. The stronger steroid ointments should never be used in children.

If the dermatitic lesions are secondarily infected then the steroid should be combined with an antibiotic such as tetracycline. Neomycin should not be used on the skin because of the danger of sensitization. Some other antibiotics should be avoided in topical applications because they may need to be used systemically.

Seborrhoeic eczema

It is difficult to give an exact cause of this condition. It is often considered constitutional in origin, because some individuals seem to be more prone to be affected than others. However, a reasonable definition might be a low-grade infected eczema, with three main clinical components.

1 Severe pityriasis capitis

Scaling of the scalp (dandruff) is extremely common and in most cases is probably due to inadequate hygiene; that is, the individual does not shampoo often enough. However, an extremely crusted and infected scalp is undoubtedly pathological, the condition being called pityriasis capitis.

2 Flexural infected eczema

Lesions are situated behind the ears, on the cheeks next to the nose, in the axillae and groins.

3 Presternal petaloid dermatitis

Red, scaly lesions on the front of the chest are particularly common in older men.

Discoid (nummular) eczema

In older individuals disc-like lesions are seen predominantly on the legs, and occasionally the arms and trunk. They are notoriously unresponsive to treatment and cause a great deal of distress because of the pruritus. They are not associated with systemic disease.

Classical treatment was with tar applications; but the stronger steroids (e.g. betamethasone valerate and triamcinolone acetonide), if necessary under polythene occlusion at night, are usually helpful.

Stasis eczema

Most patients with chronic varicose veins develop stasis eczema, classically just above the medial malleolus. If untreated the eczema may progress to a varicose ulcer. Similarly, most chronic leg ulcers are surrounded by an area of eczema which may need treatment different from the ulcer itself. Ultimately, resolution of the eczema depends on appropriate treatment for the veins which are responsible for its development.

Chronic hand and foot eczema

Many patients present with this type of lesion, which is characterized by its non-responsiveness to ordinary therapy. Occasionally these individuals, infact, have psoriasis, but often the cause is unknown, because patch tests are negative and scrapings for a fungus infection are negative.

Syphilis and the skin (see page 432)

The skin can be affected in all three stages of syphilis. The first stage, the primary chancre, is at the point of infection and is a small button-like ulcer. Microscopic examination of scrapings confirms the diagnosis: the spirochete is observed with dark-ground illumination. The secondary stage may present with an extensive eruption over the trunk which is red and scaly and may have a slightly beefy or brown tint to the eruption. There may also be ulcers in the mouth, a lymphadenopathy, general malaise and pyrexia. Loss of scalp hair may be a diagnostic feature. The third stage is characterized by gummatous lesions over the trunk, limbs or face.

Psoriasis

The cause of this common chronic skin disorder is unknown, although heredity (multifactorial inheritance) undoubtedly plays some part in its aetiology. In some patients the onset appears to be precipitated by an acute infection, by pregnancy, or by minor trauma.

Clinical features

The typical lesion is a red spot or patch of varying size covered with a thick layer of scales, which can be scraped off with the finger nail or curette, and which exhibits a characteristic silvery sheen. Further gentle scraping of the exposed red, shiny surface causes bleeding, but there is no exudation of serum. The lesions are most often seen on the extensor aspect of the knees and elbows, but practically the whole surface of the body may be involved. The scalp is a common site and there may be hyperkeratotic patches on the palms and soles. Affection of the nails causes them to be thickened, pitted and striated. The condition may persist for life, with occasional remissions and exacerbations.

Arthropathic psoriasis is often seen in middle-aged or elderly patients. There is a characteristic seronegative polyarthritis of the hands and feet, associated with the skin lesions as described above; it may be similar to that seen in rheumatoid arthritis (see page 238). Other types are distal (where the distal interphalangeal joints are primarily affected), spondylitic, monoarthropathic, and arthritis mutilans.

Treatment

The appearance of the lesions on exposed parts and the profuse scaling may cause great social embarrassment. It is important to stress to the patient and his relatives that the disorder is neither contagious nor infectious. He should also be encouraged to live an active normal life with as much sunshine as possible, though a period of bed-rest may be very beneficial during acute exacerbations. At such times a 1% hydrocortisone, ung. emulsificans (BP) baths or even yellow vaseline (Paraff. molle flav.) should be used; but in the chronic stage preparations such as 0.1% dithranol in Lassar's Paste should be applied twice daily. If this causes inflammation of the skin, 3% crude coal tar in a zinc or starch paste may be more suitable.

Application of the newer absorbable corticosteroids under polythene occlusion at night may clear the lesions, but they should be used with caution because of the danger of secondary infection. It is wise to treat only one area at a time, to use the ointment sparingly, and to watch for the development of striae or atrophy of the skin. Topical steroids are helpful in the treatment of psoriasis, but the lesions are more liable to relapse than if they are treated with dithranol.

Pityriasis rosea

This is probably due to a virus infection and occasionally groups of three or four cases are seen in hostels and similar institutions. It produces one of the most characteristic rashes in dermatology. The first lesion (or herald patch) is an oval erythematous area about 25 mm across with a collarette of inward-facing scale. It is often situated on the front of the chest. A few days later other similar, but smaller, oval patches appear, mainly on the trunk with their long axes in line with the ribs, though there may be a few on the upper arms and thighs. There may be slight itching, but this is not a striking feature and the general health is unimpaired. Complete spontaneous recovery is the rule within about 6–8 weeks. No treatment is necessary, but if irritation is troublesome 1% hydrocortisone ointment may be used.

Exfoliative dermatitis
Clinical features

Exfoliative dermatitis is a syndrome in which there is a progressive desquamation involving the whole skin. It is characterized by the shedding of large amounts of the

Table 13.1 Causes of exfoliative dermatitis

Medicamentosa (e.g. from arsenic, gold, streptomycin, penicillin)
External applications (penicillin, sulphonamides, dithranol, streptomycin)
Generalized atopic eczema
Generalized psoriasis (often after therapy which is too strong has been applied)
Generalized erythroderma may complicate Hodgkin's disease, leukaemias and lymphomas
Two rare conditions, mycosis fungoides and pityriasis rubra pilaris
An idiopathic group, which is by far the largest group

superficial layers of the skin, and is complicated by excessive heat loss and almost always by secondary infection. There may be a generalized lymphadenopathy. If long-standing, the constant skin loss causes a negative nitrogen balance and hypoproteinaemia, which may result in oedema. Special skin structures (sweat and sebaceous glands and hair follicles) may be destroyed, sometimes permanently.

Many causes of exfoliative dermatitis are recognized, and the more common are listed in Table 13.1.

Treatment

Secondary infection should be treated appropriately, and the patient's body kept clean and warm. All other drugs should be withdrawn. If heavy-metal poisoning is suspected a course of dimercaprol (BAL) may be given (see page 509). Some cases have responded well to local and systemic application of steroids, but with the exception of the iatrogenic group treatment often has to be continued for months or even years.

Drug eruptions

In theory nearly every drug can produce any type of skin reaction, but in practice a particular drug often produces a particular response, such as purpura. Problems must arise when a patient is on several drugs and it is often not possible to say which is the cause of his reaction. All drug therapy may have to be stopped and reintroduced one by one, when the eruption has faded.

Drug eruptions are very common and may mimic the rashes of many other diseases, such as measles and scarlet fever. The barbiturates, sulphonamides, streptomycin, penicillin, gold and aspirin commonly do so, and para-aminosalicylic acid (PAS), isoniazid and phenylbutazone may also cause skin rashes.

Iodides are usually taken in the form of potassium iodide in a cough mixture, and if taken for a long time this can cause remarkable, large fungating lesions. The heavy metals such as gold and arsenic may cause a severe, generalized exfoliative dermatitis which can be fatal is untreated. Twenty-five per cent of the patients on gold therapy will develop a skin eruption in time. In a sensitized individual an injection of penicillin may cause an urticarial rash, angioneurotic oedema or even death within a few minutes from anaphylactic shock. The last complication may occur in people who are atopic — that is, they have asthma, eczema and hay fever. If a patient says he has a rash from penicillin on no account should any more be given.

Treatment

In mild cases withdrawal of the drug is all that is needed. For relief of irritation an antihistamine tablet should be given, such as promethazine hydrochloride (25 mg) two or three times a day. Most antihistamines cause drowsiness and motor-car drivers and others should be warned of this side-effect. Chlorpheniramine maleate (4 mg three times daily) is an alternative which is said to cause less drowsiness. Promethazine (50 mg) or chlorpheniramine (10 mg) may be given intramuscularly if the need is urgent. Very severe cases should be treated with cortisone or an analogue such as prednisolone (30–40 mg daily). The dosage is gradually tailed off over a period of two or three weeks. Dermatitis due to heavy metals such as gold can be treated with dimercaprol (BAL; 3 mg/kg 1 M every 6 hours for 3 days).

For anaphylactic shock following injection of a drug, an immediate injection of 1:1000 adrenaline (0.5 ml) should be given subcutaneously, after which it may be necessary for an intravenous infusion of saline containing noradrenaline or aminophylline to be set up. It is a very good rule never to give any drug by injection without having a solution of adrenaline ready for use if needed.

Urticaria

In susceptible subjects local urticaria may follow trauma, stings or insect bites. Generalized urticaria may be due to sensitivity to certain foods, particularly shellfish and strawberries, or due to drugs, notably penicillin and aspirin, or to parenteral serum or blood. In other patients the condition is associated with worm infestation; but in more than half of the cases seen with chronic urticaria the cause is never found.

Clinical features

The typical lesion is an extremely itchy wheal surrounded by a zone of erythema. The wheals, which may be of any size and shape, may cover the greater part of the body. There may be associated swelling (angioneurotic oedema) in the subcutaneous tissue and mucous membranes, particularly in the mouth and throat.

Treatment

Quick relief can usually be obtained by giving 0.5 ml of 1:1000 adrenaline hydrochloride subcutaneously. An intramuscular antihistamine, such as promethazine hydrochloride (50 mg), may also be given. If there is laryngeal obstruction which is not quickly relieved by these measures, emergency tracheotomy must be performed. Antihistamines are given by mouth for more sustained effect: promethazine hydrochloride (25 mg) is the most powerful of these but often causes troublesome drowsiness. Chlorpheniramine maleate (4 mg three times daily), or terfenadine (60 mg twice daily) are less sedative. The tablets are given two or three times daily. Cortisone suppresses the lesions, but its administration is rarely justified in this condition. The best local application is calamine lotion or 1% hydrocortisone ointment.

Erythema multiforme

This eruption consists of raised erythematous areas of irregular outline and varying size and shape; sometimes in addition there are vesicular, bullous, nodular or 'target' lesions. There may be associated ulcerative lesions on the buccal mucosa. Sometimes it appears as a cutaneous reaction to a focus of infection in the skin or elsewhere; sometimes it is a drug reaction; but usually the cause is never discovered. It may be preceded by *Herpes simplex*, which is often the precipitating factor.

Apart from slight fever there is little constitutional upset and spontaneous healing occurs within a couple of weeks, though recurrent attacks are common.

Stevens–Johnson syndrome

This is the severest variety of erythema multiforme, presenting acutely with fever, followed by the appearance of ulcers in the mouth and sometimes on the conjunctivae. The mucosa of the genitalia may also be affected. The patient may be gravely ill for a week or two, but rapidly recovers when the temperature settles.

Ophthalmic scarring, however, may lead to blindness. Prednisolone should be given, particularly if there is a rising pulse rate or falling blood pressure.

Erythema nodosum

Clinical features

In this condition there are painful, red, tender nodules usually affecting the front of the lower legs, and occasionally the thighs and forearms. These subside spontaneously in 3–6 weeks, with some scaling of the skin and colour changes like a bruise. The nodules do not leave permanent skin changes. Occasionally the patient is pyrexial.

Aetiology

Women are affected more commonly than men, with a peak incidence in the third decade of life.

The commonest cause is a streptococcal infection of the throat, but it is also often due to sarcoidosis or a drug such as a sulphonamide. Pulmonary tuberculosis is no longer a common cause, but it must be excluded. Less common causes are ulcerative colitis, Crohn's disease, deep fungus infections such as coccidioidomycosis and Hodgkin's disease. In Africa and Asia leprosy is a common cause, but often the aetiology is unknown.

Treatment

Erythema nodosum is an important condition to recognize because most patients need further investigations. The treatment is for the underlying condition.

Ichthyosis

Ichthyosis of the skin implies that there is scaling, often generalized, which can be removed. This is to be contrasted with dry skin (xeroderma). Most patients with ichthyosis have inherited the disorder; it is, therefore, apparent before the age of five years. Ichthyosis coming on later in life should suggest an internal malignancy (Hodgkin's disease) or occasionally may be due to a drug.

Clinical features

Ichthyosis vulgaris is the commonest type, which is inherited as an autosomal dominant trait. The scales are fine, white and branny and patients may show a shiny hyperkeratosis of the elbows and kness, together with increased palmar and plantar markings. It generally improves as the patients grow older. *X-linked ichthyosis* is more widespread and the scales are darker. It only affects males because the inheritance is that of an X-linked recessive trait. It is associated with a steroid sulphatase deficiency. The autosomal recessive type of ichthyosis is usually very severe, with very marked scaling, and does not improve as the patients age.

Treatment

This is usually by safe topical emollients (i.e. not steroids). They should be applied after the skin has been hydrated, that is after a bath or shower, for maximum effect. There are a number of emollients to choose from, such as emulsificans (best put in the bath) and ung. aquosum.

Infections of the skin

Infection with coagulase-positive staphylococci is responsible for furunculosis (boils), sycosis barbae (folliculitis of the beard area), carbuncles, axillary hidradenitis, pemphigus neonatorum, and impetigo contagiosa (which may also be due to streptococcal infection). Only the last of these will be described here.

Impetigo contagiosa

This very common condition is due to a bacterial infection of the superficial layers of the skin. If the condition does not respond to treatment, an underlying cause such as scabies or prediculosis should be suspected. As the name implies it is spread by direct contact or by the use of contaminated towels or clothes.

Clinical features

The first lesion is a pink macule up to half-an-inch in diameter, but within a few hours this becomes coverted into a superficial vesicle, then a pustule which ruptures with the formation of a typical bright yellow crust. Bullous lesions may occur in children. The face is a common site. There is rarely any fever or constitutional disturbance.

Treatment

Patients with severe infection should be given flucloxacillin (250 mg 6-hourly) by mouth. The essential local treatment is to remove the crusts with 1% cetrimide.

Topical antibiotic preparations should be avoided because of the risk of sensitization. In many cases it is essential to give a systemic antibiotic. It is important to search for and treat any associated condition, such as scabies or pediculosis capitis. The latter is particularly likely to be found in girls with long hair. The patient must, of course, be kept away from other children and must have his own towel and pillow-case, which should subsequently be sterilized by boiling.

Viral diseases

The commonest viral disease of the skin is the common wart or verruca vulgaris. *Warts* can occur on any part of the skin, but are particularly common on the hands and soles of the feet (plantar warts). Untreated most warts will spontaneously remit in about 18 months, presumably because the body develops some resistance to the wart virus. Warts on the genitalia are often known as venereal warts and may be due to a different virus. Perianal warts can be very difficult to treat.

Little is known for certain about the aetiology of warts. However, there is strong circumstantial evidence that plantar warts may be acquired at swimming pools and in changing rooms. Contact may be a factor, but their contagiousness is low.

Treatment of warts can be legion, which suggests that there is no really effective remedy. Magic-type treatments probably owe a great deal to the fact that they are given when the wart is spontaneously remitting. Hypnotism is of unproven value. Surgical removal is often apparently beneficial at first, but then many warts may develop around the site of the original lesion. Carbon dioxide snow and liquid nitrogen are probably as quick and effective as any other remedy. 40% salicylic acid plasters applied every night can be useful for their keratolytic action. Podophyllin application can be very helpful for penile, vulval and perianal warts, but the patients must be warned to wash off the application a few hours later or ulceration may result.

If the patient can be persuaded, no treatment is often the best treatment.

Herpes simplex (see page 418)

This very common, localized vesicular lesion must be known to everyone (the 'cold sore'). The lesions are generally on the face about the lips, and the virus may be activated by an upper respiratory tract infection or sunlight. However, lesions can occur anywhere (for example, on the ear, the point of the shoulder (type I) or the penis (type II). The last site may be particularly difficult to treat because they often occur after sexual intercourse. 3% acyclovir ointment may have some effect in cutting short an attack if applied immediately it is apparent the lesions are developing. For the developed lesion, some patients prefer a spirit lotion and others an antibiotic (aureomycin) cream to eradicate secondary bacterial infection.

Herpes zoster (shingles) (see page 418)

This is caused by the same virus as that responsible for chicken pox and occurs commonly, but not exclusively, in adults. The characteristic lesion of *herpes zoster* is preceded by pain, which may result in misdiagnosis of other disorders such as an acute appendicitis. However, once the vesicles have erupted in the distribution of a cutaneous dermatome the diagnosis is readily made.

Ringworm

This is a group of common superficial fungus infections of the skin which affect mainly the scalp, the groin and the feet.

Tinea capitis (ringworm of the scalp)

The infection is seen mainly in children under ten, particularly boys, and never persists beyond adolescence. The scalp shows a number of rounded or oval patches which are covered with fine greyish-white scales and from which most of the hairs have fallen out. The ringworm fungus fluoresces a bright green colour under Wood's light, and this examination is therefore helpful in diagnosis. The fungus can also be identified microscopically in stumps of hair removed from one of the patches.

Griseofulvin (125 mg four times daily) for a month or six weeks is now the treatment of choice. Very occasionally it may cause headache and urticaria, and should be used with caution in patients sensitive to penicillin.

Tinea cruris (ringworm of the groins)

This infection occurs mainly in young adults, particularly men, and may be acquired by direct contact, from infected clothing or spread from between the toes. It causes a red, slightly raised patch extending from the crutch for two or three inches down the inner aspect of each thigh. There is sometimes itching in the affected area. The infection is seen mainly in hot weather and is more common therefore in the tropics.

Half-strength Whitfield's ointment is usually a very effective treatment, but relapses in subsequent spells of hot weather are common. Griseofulvin may also prove effective.

Tinea pedis (athlete's foot)

This infection occurs with two characteristic distribution patterns; but both may occur together, the first showing vesicles and subsequent desquamation on the sole of the foot, and the second causing fissuring and maceration of the skin in the clefts between the toes. Like tinea cruris, with which it may be associated, this infection is often seen in young adults and is acquired from floors of swimming baths and changing rooms.

Whitfield's ointment, clotrimazole 1% cream, and undecylenic acid ointment are three among a number of effective remedies. Relapse is common, however, and to try to prevent it careful attention to the hygiene of the feet is important. They should be washed daily, carefully dried and powdered and the socks should be changed every day.

Scabies

The parasite causing scabies is a mite (Sarcoptes scabei hominis). It has four pairs of legs and the female, which causes the trouble, is about 0.3 mm long — therefore just being visible to the naked eye. The male is smaller. The female makes a burrow up to a centimetre in length in the epidermis and lays about 30–40 eggs in it. Each egg hatches out in 4–8 days into a larval form which leaves the burrow and eventually matures into the adult form.

Infection is usually acquired by contact (for example, by sleeping with an infected person). It may therefore be a venereal infection, or children may acquire it from their parents or from each other. Less often, infected blankets, bedding or clothes may transmit the infection.

Clinical features

The burrow is the characteristic lesion of scabies and appears as a fine, often zig-zag, hair-like line in the epidermis, greyish or whitish in colour and 0.5–1 cm in length. At the far end a tiny pinhead vesicle may be seen. These burrows occur mainly in the webs and sides of the fingers, the ulnar sides of the hands, the anterior axillary folds, the lower abdomen and penis and the lower part of the buttocks. They cause intense itching, particularly when the patient is warm in bed. As a result of scratching secondary infection is common and there may be an extensive papular and pustular eruption.

Diagnosis

This is usually easy from the history of intense itching and the discovery of topical burrows. It may be confirmed by identifying the female acarus or its eggs in a microscopical preparation of scrapings from a burrow.

Treatment

Malathion 0.5 per cent aqueous solution is the most effective and least toxic preparation available. It should be applied to the whole body from the neck downwards. It is very rare for the face and hair to be affected in adults, but if malathion is applied to the face great care must be taken to avoid the eyes. It is left on for 24 hours then the patient may take a bath. All clsoe contacts should be treated whether they have symptoms or not. Although the mite dies very quickly away from the body it is worth laundering sheets, clothes, etc. Itching often lasts for several weeks after treatment and may be relieved by calamine lotion or 1 per cent hydrocortisone ointment.

An alternative treatment is crotamiton which is applied to the body as above daily for 2 days and is less irritant but less effective.

Pediculosis

Lice are blood-sucking parasites which mainly infect hairy parts of the body. The female produces several hundred eggs, each of which is attached to a hair and is commonly known as a nit. A larva is hatched out from the egg in 6–9 days and develops into a mature louse in one or two weeks.

Head lice

In pediculosis capitis infestation, the louse concerned is *Pediculus humanus capitis*, which is about 3 mm long and 1 mm broad. It infests the scalp, the nits being attached mainly to hairs at the back and sides of the head. Since the louse deposits the eggs on hairs close to the scalp, and since they have hatched out by the time the hair has grown an inch or so, the search for nits should be concentrated on hair close to the head. The diagnosis depends usually on the discovery of nits, since the lice themselves are few in number and difficult to find. Nits are greyish-white, shiny, oval, opalescent structures firmly attached to the hairs.

Infection may be acquired by direct transmission from person to person or by wearing infected headgear; and since the lice flourish particularly in long hair which is seldom washed, it is now often seen in young men as well as in women living under poor hygienic conditions. However, school-children are particularly liable to be infested. Patients recently infected usually complain of irritation of the scalp, but those who have had head lice for a long time often seem to suffer no inconvenience at all. When there has been much scratching septic lesions of the scalp are a common complication.

Treatment

Resistant strains of lice can develop and to prevent this carbaryl alcoholic solution and malathion alcoholic solution should be used in rotation, changing the preparation every two to three years. If the skin is abraded use aqueous solution. Both preparations are applied to the affected areas and allowed to dry naturally. After 12 hours the hair is washed with soap and a Secker comb can be used to remove nits. It is much easier to treat short hair.

Body lice

Pediculus humanus corporis is similar to the head louse but slightly bigger. It normally lives in the clothes and deposits its eggs in the seams and folds of woollen undergarments.

Clinical features

Infestation causes a variable amount of itching; scratch marks are seen mainly around the shoulders, buttocks, and the fronts of the thighs and there may be a widespread eruption from secondary bacterial infection in these situations. Tramps and vagrants after life-long infestation may develop a generalized pigmentation of the skin like that seen in Addison's disease ('vagabond's disease'). The diagnosis is established by finding the louse or its ova in the seams of the patient's underclothes.

Treatment

Carbamyl or malathion are applied as above.

Underclothes must be washed and bedding and other clothing autoclaved.

In some countries, in addition to their direct effects, infestation with head and body lice is important in the spread of typhus and relapsing fever (see page 447).

Crab lice

This louse is not in fact of the species pediculus, its scientific name being *Phthirus pubis*. Its life history is similar to that of the pediculi, but it is smaller (about 2 mm by 1.5 mm) and does not spread typhus or any other disease.

Clinical features

The louse infests the pubic region, but in very hairy men the whole of the trunk, the thighs and the upper arms may be involved. On close inspection the adult lice can be seen, lying flat on the skin and holding on to a hair at each side; the nits are very similar to those of *Pediculus humanus* and are closely attached to the body hairs. Infection is acquired mainly by sexual intercourse and occurs usually therefore in young adults.

Treatment

This is as for pediculosis corporis. Crotamiton lotion or even benzyl benzoate are alternative applications.

Acne vulgaris

Acne is often associated with seborrhoea (that is excessive sebaceous secretion). The essential lesion is the comedo, which is a sebaceous follicle whose opening has been blocked with sebum mixed with epithelial debris. These comedones frequently become pustular from infection of the retained sebaceous material. They are found on the face, chest, shoulders, and back. Their formation appears to be favoured by androgens and they appear therefore in the years following puberty. Adolescent acne tends to disappear spontaneously in early adult life, though when it is very severe it may persist and healing of the lesions may leave permanent scarring.

Treatment

The treatment of acne falls under two headings: applications which degrease the skin, and those that treat the

secondary infection. Natural sunlight (or ultraviolet light therapy) combines the two actions and is the best single treatment for acne. A hair-style which keeps the hair from falling over the face is important. Daily washing with soap and water is a help in mild cases, and the patient should shampoo his scalp at least three times a week. Oral tetracycline (500 mg twice daily) for two months or longer may be of great benefit for patients with grossly infected lesions. All patients, particularly women, must be discouraged from picking and squeezing the lesions, and they should realize there is no magic cure, but patient, persistent therapy can achieve remarkable results.

Rosacea

This is a chronic hyperaemia of the face, particularly the cheeks and central part of the forehead, leading to permanent dilatation of capillaries and the formation of telangiectases. The patients are often middle-aged women, many of whom also have vague digestive symptoms for which no definite cause can be found. The cosmetic disability is aggravated by the flushing associated with the menopause and with the taking of alcohol or hot spicy food; that is, anything which tends to make the face flush. There may be associated papules and pustules and sometimes hyperplasia of the sebaceous glands.

Oral tetracycline (250 mg twice daily) for two months and application of 2% sulphur in aqueous cream may be of benefit.

Lichen planus

The cause of lichen planus is unknown. The eruption is seen only in adults. Although it usually clears up spontaneously in 6–18 months, relapses are common and in some patients the lesions may persist for years. A lichenoid eruption, indistinguishable from lichen planus, may be caused by some drugs.

Clinical features

The typical lesion is a small, flat-topped violaceous papule, often little bigger than a pin's head. The papules may be limited to certain situations, such as the anterior aspect of the wrists and forearms, the genitalia, or the legs, or they may be very profuse and widespread over most of the body, though the face and other exposed parts are rarely affected. Linear disposition of the lesions along scratch marks (*Koëbner phenomenon*) is common. In some of the patients bluish-white reticulate streaks or patches may be seen on the buccal mucosa. There is usually some irritation of the skin and sometimes this is severe.

Treatment

Confinement to bed and sedation may be necessary in very severe acute cases, but usually all that is necessary is an application such as calamine lotion to allay irritation. An antihistamine tablet such as promethazine hydrochloride (25 mg) may help in this respect. If itching continues, 1% hydrocortisone ointment may be tried. If the mouth, scalp or genitalia are affected, about a month's course of oral steroids may be given, but this is seldom necessary.

Pemphigus vulgaris

The cause of this very serious disease is unknown. Fortunately rare, it occurs equally in men and women and seldom appears before late middle age. Before cortisone therapy it was nearly always fatal within two years.

Clinical features

The essential lesion is a bulla which appears on normal skin with no surrounding erythema. Crops of these bullae appear on the skin and mucous membranes and soon rupture and become infected. Constitutional disturbance is severe.

Treatment

Cortisone or an equivalent must be given in high dosage; for example, prednisolone (80 mg daily). The dose is slowly reduced when fresh blisters cease to appear, but at least 15 mg daily should be continued until the patient has been free of symptoms for three months, when the drug may be further reduced in dosage. With this treatment a fatal outcome is not so common.

Dermatitis herpetiformis
Clinical features

This disease of unknown cause has a clinical similarity to pemphigus (see above), since the lesions are predominantly vesicular or bullous and it tends to run a chronic or relapsing course.

There are, however, important differences. First, the vesicles and bullae are set on an erythematous base and are often accompanied by urticarial and erythematous lesions. Second, the blisters tend to appear in clusters, particularly on the elbows, buttocks and posterior aspect of the thorax. Third, there are seldom lesions in the mouth. Fourth, constitutional upset is slight and, fifth, irritation of the skin is usually severe. This disease is associated in many patients with a gluten sensitive enteropathy.

Treatment

Dapsone (diamino-diphenyl sulphone) is the drug of choice and so often successful that it is sometimes used as a diagnostic test in this condition. The dose is 100–200 mg a day by mouth. Prednisolone is now less often used.

Further reading

Burton, J.L. (1985) *Essentials of Dermatology*, 2nd edn. Churchill Livingstone, Edinburgh.

MacKie, R.M. (1986) *Clinical Dermatology*, 2nd edn. Oxford University Press, London.

Sneddon, I.B. and Church, R.E. (1983) *Practical Dermatology*, 4th edn. Edward Arnold, London.

14
Infectious Diseases

Introduction

The term 'infectious disease' might be applied to any illness which results from invasion of the body by a micro-organism. The term is sometimes limited to diseases which spread from patient to patient. This chapter deals mainly with such diseases but includes some infections that do not fit easily into other chapters on specific systems. Other infections are best dealt with under the relevant system and are not covered in this chapter.

Infection and immunity

The results of any infection depend partly on the virulence and numbers of the invading organisms, and partly on the state of the patient's defences against them. The defences are a combination of natural immunity, which may vary with factors such as race, heredity and nutrition, and aquired immunity resulting from previous infection or prophylactic immunization against this particular organism. Various body surfaces are colonized by micro-organisms which cause no problems but can produce infections if they penetrate the surface barriers.

Natural defences are made up of a number of elements which prevent entry of micro-organisms or counteract their establishment. The surface barrier of the skin is very resistant to penetration, and so entry is more likely through the mucosae of the respiratory or alimentary tract. Tears, urine and mucus contain antibodies and substances such as lysozymes which destroy organisms. In the blood and tissue fluids, cells such as phagocytes and eosinophils can act non-specifically against invasion.

Resistance to specific micro-organisms is stimulated as antibody-mediated humoral immunity or as cell-mediated immunity. These aspects are dealt with in chapter 12.

Notification

Certain infectious diseases require notification in writing to the Medical Officers of Environmental Health

Table 14.1 Notifiable diseases in the United Kingdom

Anthrax
Cholera
Diphtheria
Dysentry
Encephalitis
Food poisoning
Infective jaundice
Lassa fever
Leptospirosis*
Malaria
Marburg disease
Measles
Meningitis
Opthalmia neonatorum
Pertussis
Plague
Poliomyelitis
Rabies
Relapsing fever*
Scarlet fever
Smallpox
Tetanus*
Tuberculosis
Typhoid and paratyphoid
Typhus fever
Viral haemorrhagic diseases
Yellow fever*

Additional diseases notifiable in Scotland only

Chickenpox
Continued fever
Encephalitis lethargica
Erysipelas
Pneumonia
Puerperal fever

*Not notifiable in Scotland.

(MOEH). This is a statutory requirement of the attending doctor. Regular records of numbers of notifiable diseases are produced by the Office of Population Censuses and Surveys. Appropriate forms for notification are provided by the MOEH.

Notifiable diseases are listed in Table 14.1.

Immunization

Two main forms of immunization are practised. In *passive immunization* serum containing specific antibodies is given. This provides a degree of immediate immunity but is only temporary, disappearing as the antibodies are broken down. The antiserum is obtained from humans who have recovered from the disease or from horses actively immunized for this purpose.

Active immunization applies to the induction of immunity by administration of antigen. This technique is widely used with (a) *live* vaccines using an avirulent form of the organism, or (b) *inactive* vaccines that consist of killed organisms or extracts or toxoids which are altered bacterial toxin.

Scheme of prophylactic inoculations in the UK

First year of life

Triple vaccine: diptheria toxoid, tetanus toxoid and pertussis vaccine together with oral polio vaccine. This is given in three consecutive doses, the first at three months, the second 6–8 weeks later, and the third 4–6 months after the second.

Pertussis vaccine is complicated rarely by encephalopathy. This is more likely to occur in infants with a history of convulsions.

Absolute contraindications to pertussis are a severe reaction (local, neurological or generalized) to a previous dose, or a history of cerebral irritation, neonatal neurological injury, fits or convulsions.

Relative contraindications are a parental or sibling history of epilepsy, developmental delay through neurological causes, or existing neurological disease.

Worries about encephalopathy in recent years have led to a decrease in the uptake of perussis vaccination. However, in the absence of these specific contraindications the risks of the disease outweigh those of the vaccine.

Second year of life

Measles vaccine: a live vaccine given at around 13 months. It may be inactivated by maternal antibodies if given in the first year.

Fifth year of life or School Entry

Triple vaccine; poliomyelitis.

Girls aged 10–14

Rubella: a live vaccine given to all girls. A history of previous rubella is not reliable.

Children aged 11–13

BCG: live bacilli (*bacillus Calmette–Guerin*). This is given intradermally to tuberculin-negative children, and to neonates in high-risk groups.

School leaving

Poliomyelitis; tetanus toxoid. This is usually given between the ages of 15 and 19.

Adults

Tetanus toxoid: a booster in 'at-risk' occupations.

Poliomyelitis: before travel abroad to endemic areas. Inactivated Salk vaccine is used when live vaccine is contraindicated (e.g. in pregnancy, immune deficiency).

Rabies: for exposed individuals.

Influenza: for individuals at risk of severe chest infection.

Hepatitis B: for high-risk groups (e.g. in renal transplant units).

Fever

This is a feature of many body reactions other than immunological responses to infections. For example, fever is a typical finding in the days after a myocardial infarction. The body temperature is kept in a stable range by the interaction of the hypothalamus and the autonomic nervous system. The oral temperature lies usually between 36 and 37 °C with a diurnal variation producing lowest levels at between 3 and 5 a.m. Rectal temperatures are around 0.6 °C higher than oral ones, while axillary temperatures are 0.2 °C or more lower.

Fever is produced by an endogenous pyrogen derived from macrophages which acts on the hypothalamus. Endogenous pyrogen is produced in response to exogenous pyrogens produced by micro-organisms or to a lymphokine produced by sensitized T cells. Specific patterns of fever in particular disorders are rarely helpful except, perhaps, in malaria. In epileptics and in children aged 1–6 years, a rising fever may produce convulsions.

Fever can be reduced by tepid sponging or by anti-pyretic drugs, aspirin or paracetamol.

Incubation period

This is the time which elapses between the access of organisms to the tissues of a susceptible individual and the onset of the first clinical symptoms. Its duration varies widely in the different infectious diseases but remains fairly constant in each of them. The approximate length of the incubation period of the common specific fevers is shown in Table 14.2.

Childhood viral infections

Measles

Measles is caused by a morbillivirus transmitted by droplets entering through conjunctiva or respiratory mucosa. Passive immunity from the mother prevents infection in the first three months of life, but thereafter the child becomes highly susceptible.

Clinical features

About 10–14 days after exposure to infection the prodromal illness develops. This is similar to a common cold, with fever, running nose and eyes, sneezing and cough. Examination of the mouth, however, reveals an eruption of tiny white spots like grains of salt set on a slightly reddened base, usually best seen on the mucous membrane inside the cheeks opposite the molar teeth. These are *Koplik's spots* and they are diagnostic of measles. If they are overlooked the erroneous impression that the child simply has a cold may appear to be confirmed on the third day, when the temperature may come down to normal, but on the fourth day the typical rash appears on the skin.

Transient prodromal rashes are sometimes seen during the first three days, but the true morbilliform eruption appears on the fourth day as pink macules, about 3–5 mm in diameter, which first appear behind the ears and spread over the face, trunk and limbs over the next two days. Within a day or two the lesions enlarge and become papular, many of them coalesce into large, irregular, blotchy areas, and their colour gradually changes to a darker red. The temperature rises again with the appearance of the rash and continues for several days before finally subsiding as the lesions fade. The Koplik's spots disappear as the rash is developing. The child is infectious from two days before the prodrome until 'staining', when the red rash changes to an orange-brown colour. Lymphadenopathy may occur. Encephalitis is sometimes seen in the prodromal period, and in 0.1 per cent of cases around the third day of the rash, when it may leave permanent neurological sequelae.

Complications

These are mainly due to secondary bacterial infection of the respiratory tract. A viral measles pneumonia is common but of minor importance and usually resolves completely. However, bacterial bronchopneumonia is a serious development, particularly in very young children. It should always be suspected in a severely ill child with a persistent cough and should be treated with antibiotics. Otitis media is fairly common. Corneal ulceration and potential blindness should be prevented by careful treatment of any conjunctival inflammation that occurs. Subacute sclerosing panencephalitis (SSPE) occurs months to years later in 1 in 100 000 cases (see page 222).

Treatment

The virus of measles is not susceptible to any form of specific treatment, but antibodies are of value as soon as any secondary bacterial complication is suspected. This may be penicillin, amoxycillin, erythromycin or co-trimoxazole.

Table 14.2 Incubation periods of common infections

Less than 7 days (usually 1–3)	Meningococcal meningitis Diphtheria (1–3) Scarlet fever (2–3)
10 to 14 days	Measles (10–14) Whooping cough (7–14) Enteric fever (10–14)
14 to 21 days	Chickenpox (14–17) German measles (17–18) Mumps (18–21)

Prevention

Effective measles vaccines are now available and have nearly eradicated the disease in the USA where they are given to children before school entry. A live attenuated vaccine is offered in the UK in the second year of life.

Rubella (german measles)

Rubella is caused by a ribivirus of the family Togaviridae. It is a less infectious disease than true measles and even in towns many people reach adult life without acquiring it. It causes little constitutional upset and is never fatal, but its importance lies in the effects on the fetus when acquired by women in the first four months of pregnancy. Cataract, glaucoma, disorders of retinal pigmentation, deaf mutism, and congential heart disease are the lesions commonly caused. There is also an increased incidence of abortion, miscarriage and stillbirth, but fetal injury is not inevitable and a proportion of women who have had rubella early in pregnancy do produce healthy live babies.

Girls should be given a single dose of live attenuated rubella virus between the ages of 11 and 14. No other vaccine should be given within 3–4 weeks. This vaccine must not be given to pregnant women because of the risk of fetal damage, or to patients with Hodgkin's disease or leukaemia, or to those on immunosuppressive therapy.

Clinical features

After an incubation period of 2–3 weeks (usually 17–18 days) the rash is usually the first indication of the disease, and takes the form of small pink macules and papules which remain distinct units and do not run together as in true measles. The rash begins on the forehead and face. There is a sore throat and mild conjunctivitis. There are no Koplik's spots in the mouth. Lymph node enlargement is common affecting particularly the occipital and cervical nodes. There are rarely any general symptoms of illness and the rash usually fades in two or three days. In adults a transient mild arthritis is common. Encephalitis is a rare complication.

Treatment

Clinical diagnosis may be uncertain and can be confirmed by finding rising antibody titres in the blood, or measurement of IgM antibodies. High-titre immunoglobulin may prevent infection in exposed women.

Mumps (epidermic parotitis)

Mumps is a relatively trivial illness in young children, but if contracted after puberty it may have serious complications. There may be advantages, therefore, in 'getting it over with' early in life, and only if a child is in a weak state of health from some other illness should any steps be taken to isolate him from this infection. Around 20 per cent of adults leave childhood without serological evidence of previous infection. A live attenuated vaccine is available for children over one year of age.

Clinical features

After an incubation period of three weeks or a little longer the patient develops fever, malaise and stiffness in the jaw, and examination reveals swelling of one or more of the salivary glands. Usually the parotid glands are affected and fill out the hollow between the angle of the jaw and the mastoid process. Sometimes the submandibular glands are affected too, or occasionally they are involved alone. There is no rash and usually the fever and glandular swellings subside within a few days.

Diagnosis

The diagnosis is usually easy, but if there is doubt it can be confirmed by isolation of the virus from saliva, or by demonstrating a rising antibody titre in two specimens of serum taken at the onset of illness and a fortnight later.

Complications

These are almost confined to adolescent and adult patients and usually arise a few days after the swelling of the salivary glands.

1 Orchitis

This is the commonest complication, being seen in about 25 per cent of patients. It may develop after initial improvement. It is usually unilateral and causes severe pain and swelling of the testicle. Rarely it may be bilateral and result in sterility.

2 Oophoritis

This is less common and causes severe lower abdominal pain and vomiting.

3 Prostatitis

This should be suspected in patients with unexplained fever and perhaps some frequency of micturition.

4 Mastitis

Pain and swelling of the breast may be seen in either sex.

5 Pancreatitis

This is characterized by severe upper abdominal pain, fever and vomiting. Milder forms often occur.

6 Meningitis

Routine lumbar puncture in patients with mumps usually reveals a pleocytosis in the CSF, so that invasion of the nervous system by the virus is common; but only in about 10 per cent of cases is there clinical evidence of meningitis (headache, fever, vomiting and neck rigidity). These symptoms usually subside within two or three days and the prognosis is excellent.

7 Encephalitis

Characterized by severe headache, fever, vomiting, perhaps cranial nerve palsies, drowsiness and coma, this is much more serious and carries a mortality of about 50 per cent. Cranial nerve palsies such as deafness may occasionally be permanent.

Treatment

There is no specific treatment. However, patients with orchitis gain relief from systemic steroids.

Hand, foot and mouth disease

Coxsackie A viruses produce acute oropharyngeal infections, and Coxsackie A16 causes a highly infectious disease in children – hand, foot and mouth disease. (This is quite distinct from foot and mouth disease of animals, which is caused by quite another picornavirus). It is seen mainly in young children, but adults in the family are often affected too. It occurs mainly in summer and autumn.

Clinical features

After an incubation period of 3–6 days there is a mild febrile illness lasting only a few days. On the second or third day a maculopapular rash, later becoming vesicular, appears on the fingers, toes and lateral borders of the feet, and painful ulcers develop in the mouth. These lesions heal within about a week.

Diagnosis

The clinical picture is quite characteristic but if necessary the diagnosis can be confirmed by virus studies. The virus may be present in the faeces for several weeks after infection. Other ECHO and Coxsackie viruses occasionally produce a generalized rash, usually maculopapular but rarely vesicular.

Varicella

Chickenpox is caused by the varicella-zoster virus, part of the herpes group spread by droplet transmission from pharyngeal secretions or vesicle fluid: susceptible children who come into contact with shingles may develop chickenpox. The virus lies dormant in dorsal root ganglia, from where it may be reactivated as herpes zoster (shingles).

Clinical features

After an incubation period of up to three weeks the illness may start with a day of vague malaise, headache, fever and a transient prodromal rash, before the specific eruption appears. The prodrome occurs in adults particularly, and in children more often the rash is the first sign of the disease.

Papules occur first but quickly become vesicular. Vesicles appear first in the mouth and throat and soon rupture, leaving ulcers which may cause a good deal of pain and difficulty in swallowing. The skin rash, unlike that of smallpox, is most profuse on the trunk and most sparse at the periphery of the limbs; and instead of all the lesions going through their various stages together, the spots appear in a succession of crops over several days, so that at any one time papules, vesicles, pustules and crusts can be seen together. The papules develop within a few hours into small round vesicles containing clear fluid set in the superficial layers of the skin. Within two or three days they become pustules and then dry up into crusts. The crusts fall off without scarring unless the lesions become secondarily infected.

Constitutional upset is usually slight, though the enanthem (mucosal lesions) may cause much discomfort and the exanthem (skin rash) much itching. The disease is more severe in adults, who may develop pneumonia and subsequently may be found to have scattered small calcified opacities on chest radiograph.

Complications

Complications are unusual. A haemorrhagic, vasculitic form is seen occasionally in adults. Secondary skin infection may lead to boils, impetigo, cellulitis or conjunctivitis. More serious are encephalitis, polyneuritis or transverse myelitis. Chickenpox and herpes zoster can be very serious infections in immunosuppressed patients because the disease can become generalized.

Diagnosis

The diagnosis is based on the clinical picture, and the virus can be isolated from the vesicular fluid. Smallpox is now eradicated so that the traditional comparisons have little relevance now.

Treatment

This is purely symptomatic. Irritation of the skin can be relieved by the application of calamine lotion containing 1–2% phenol, or by warm boracic baths, and antihistamine tablets may be helpful. Acyclovir is used for generalized disease and pneumonia or in herpes zoster when, started early, it speeds resolution.

Skin infections

Herpes simplex (see also page 221)

This is a DNA virus. Most infections are produced by the serotype HSV1, but genital herpes (see page 434) is more often caused by HSV2. The infection is characterized by periods of latency and recurrence of local lesions. Infection is by droplet spread or contact.

Clinical features

Herpetic stomatitis is usually the primary infection. It occurs most often in children with painful mouth ulcers, fever and local lymphadenopathy.

Cold sores are the subsequent recurrent form of herpes simplex. They occur on mucocutaneous junctions, usually around the mouth. Recurrence may be precipitated by trauma, ultraviolet light or infections, particularily pneumococcal pneumonia. Vesicles appear and heal with crusting in one or two weeks.

Corneal ulcers (dendritic ulcers) cause a painful red eye. The branching ulcer fluoresces yellow-green with fluorescein drops.

The cutaneous variety produces vesicular lesions most common on the face or finger pulp.

Diagnosis

This is usually obvious from the site and vesicular appearance. It can be confirmed by growing the virus in tissue culture.

Treatments are shown in Table 14.3.

Table 14.3 Treatment of herpes simplex infections

Stomatitis	5% acyclovir applied five times daily
'Cold sores'	Efficacy of antiviral agent unproved; other methods include 1% prednisolone ointment or ice cubes applied locally when symptoms develop
Corneal ulcers	3% acyclovir eye ointment five times daily or 0.5% idoxuridine eye ointment
Herpetic Whitlows	oral acyclovir 200 mg five times daily for five days
Genital herpes	oral acyclovir 200 mg five times daily
Herpes encephalitis	Intravenous acyclovir

Herpes zoster (shingles)

Shingles occurs when varicellar-zoster virus, latent in sensory ganglia, is reactivated. This reactivation may occur spontaneously or be associated with some underlying illness or immunosuppression.

Clinical features

Skin involvement occurs in a single dermatome unilaterally. The lesions go through the same stages as those in chickenpox, usually healing in one or two weeks. In immunosuppressed patients the rash may be more widespread or even generalized.

Complications are secondary infection and postherpetic neuralgia. In the latter condition pain persists for months or years after the vesicles heal and is often difficult to treat. Involvement of the ophthalmic division of the trigeminal nerve may cause iridocyclitis leading to formation of synechiae if the pupil is not dilated.

Treatment

Acyclovir is used in severe cases and is effective if introduced early enough. With ophthalmic involvement the pupil must be kept dilated. Acyclovir (800 mg five times daily) should be considered when:

1 the attack is widespread and particularly painful;
2 the face is involved;
3 treatment can be started within 48 hours of the onset of the rash.

Upper respiratory tract infections

Streptococcal sore throat, scarlet fever

This is caused by Lancefield group A streptococci, which are often found in asymptomatic subjects and spread by droplet infection.

Clinical features

After two or three days incubation, fever and sore throat develop. The tonsils are enlarged with yellow-white exudate, and local lymph nodes become enlarged and tender.

Complications

Scarlet fever may occur if the streptococcus produces a special erythrogenic toxin. In the first half of this century scarlet fever was a serious disease with a high mortality, but it is much less of a problem today. The tongue is initially covered in white 'fur' which peels off to leave a clean surface with enlarged red papillae – the 'strawberry' tongue. The rash (a punctate erythema) appears on the second day. The skin is bright red with minute darker red spots and enlarged palpable hair follicles. It is more marked in the flexures (Pastia's sign) and spares the perioral area. After about a week desquamation of the skin occurs.

Quinsy is a peritonsillar abscess caused by local spread of infection. Swelling involves the soft tissues around the affected tonsil and bilateral quinsies may cause respiratory obstruction. Similar local spread can cause retropharyngeal abscesses, sinusitis and cervical adenitis.

Rheumatic fever can occur 2–3 weeks after group A streptococcal tonsillitis, most commonly in chidlren between 5 and 14 years. Two-thirds of patients with rheumatic fever give a recent history of an upper respiratory tract infection, and in 20 per cent streptococcus still grows from throat culture at presentation. Clinical features of rheumatic fever are dealt with on page 39.

Acute glomerulonephritis is another late complication of streptococcal infections, but unlike rheumatic fever the initial infection may be of the skin as well as the pharynx.

Diagnosis

The beta-haemolytic streptococcus will grow from throat swabs, although this may be found in the absence of disease. When infection occurs the serum antistreptolysin-O titre (ASOT) rises, and a titre above 250 μ/ml signifies recent infection.

Treatment

Mild disease can be treated with oral penicillin (phenoxymethyl penicillin; 250 mg four times daily). More severe infections require intramuscular penicillin six-hourly for the first two days followed by oral penicillin. Treatment should continue for ten days to eradicate the streptococ-

cus and reduce the risk of glomerulonephritis and rheumatic fever. Alternative treatments are a single injection of benzathine penicillin or, in those allergic to penicillin, oral erythromycin (500 mg 6-hourly) for ten days.

Diphtheria

Diphtheria is an infection of the throat, nose or larynx (or occasionally the skin), and although the organism *Corynebacterium diphtheriae* (a Gram-positive rod) remains localized to this site, it produces a powerful exotoxin which becomes widely distributed and may cause serious or fatal effects on other parts of the body. The amount of exotoxin produced by different strains of the organism varies a good deal, and that is one reason why some patients are much more severely ill than others. Another reason for the variation in clinical severity is the state of the patient's immunity at the time of infection.

Immunity

Immunity to diphtheria may be acquired in three ways:

1 after recovery from an attack of the disease;
2 after repeated subclinical infection (that is, as a result of coming into contact from time to time with organisms in sufficient numbers or virulence to cause a full-scale attack of diphtheria);
3 as a result of childhood immunization which is safe and effective and largely responsible for the marked decline in the incidence of diphtheria.

The *Schick test* is used to detect whether an individual has immunity against diphtheria, but it is largely of historical and theoretical interest. Diphtheria toxin (0.2 ml) is injected into the skin of the left forearm and inactivated toxin (0.2 ml) into the right forearm. The result is read in five days.

Clinical features

Diphtheria is classified clinically according to the exact site of infection. The commonest variety is *faucial diphtheria*, in which the characteristic membrane of the disease forms in the throat. There is a short incubation period of only three or four days from exposure to infection. Points which help to distinguish diphtheria from streptococcal tonsillitis are:

1 The throat is not so sore and the temperature usually not so high, but the general exhaustion and toxaemia are much greater.

2 The lymph nodes in the neck are usually enlarged to a greater extent, in severe cases causing a collar of swelling sometimes referred to as the 'bull-neck'.

Complications

Myocarditis may occur during the second week but leaves no permanent damage. Demyelination can cause paralysis, most often of palate or extraocular muscles, rarely larynx, respiratory muscles or limbs.

Treatment

Upper airway obstruction is a potentially lethal hazard and emergency tracheotomy or tracheostomy may occasionally be necessary. Antitoxin is given to neutralize circulating toxin, together with benzylpenicillin or erythromycin. Carriers should be treated with oral erythromycin and eradication checked with nose and throat swabs.

Pertussis (whooping cough)

Whooping cough is an infection of the respiratory tract caused usually by *Bordetella pertussis* or, in a minority of cases, adenovirus, influenza virus or by respiratory syncitial virus. In this country at the present it is the most serious of the acute specific fevers of childhood, not only causing many deaths in young children, particularly under the age of 12 months, but occasionally leading to serious damage to the bronchi and lungs (see bronchiectasis, page 113). Infants receive no passive immunity from the mother and are therefore susceptible to the infection from birth.

Clinical features

After an incubation period of about 7–14 days the child develops what is thought at first to be an ordinary cold with a cough, but within a week of onset the paroxysms of coughing have usually become so severe and typical that the diagnosis is obvious. A characteristic paroxysm consists of a deep inspiration followed by a rapid series of explosive coughs during expiration. The tongue protrudes, the face and lips become cyanosed and the attack may end with the inspiration of air through a partially closed glottis, producing the classic whoop. Paroxysm may follow paroxysm until a little sticky mucus is expectorated or until the child vomits and sinks back exhausted. During the spasms of coughing the tongue may be abraded against the lower incisors, causing a traumatic ulcer on the fraenum; rectal prolapse, hernia and haemorrhage, particularly under the conjunctiva, may also be induced. The preliminary catarrhal stage is short in duration but highly infectious, the paroxysmal stage and whooping may continue for many weeks but the infectivity is now very slight. The weeks of coughing and poor feeding can lead to exhaustion of the parents as well as the child.

In young infants, however, cough is often not such a prominent symptom. Instead, procedures such as feeding or changing may induce cyanotic attacks, in which the child becomes flaccid, blue and alarmingly lifeless. There may also be frequent vomiting. Furthermore, immunized subjects may have a mild form of the disease without the typical paroxysmal cough or whoop. The diagnosis may remain very obscure until the appearance of a few feeble whoops at the end of attacks.

Diagnosis

The paroxysmal coughing with vomiting is virtually diagnostic, but bacteriological confirmation may be obtained by isolation of *B. pertussis* on 'cough plates' (a Petri dish held in front of the patient's mouth) or, better, by taking a post-nasal swab. *B. pertussis* does not grow readily, however, and special culture media are essential. Patients with negative cultures probably have a similar virus infection. The blood count shows a lymphocytosis, but young children have a high lymphocyte count in health so that no significance should be attached to a count of less than 70 per cent of 20 000.

Complications

Acute bronchitis and bronchopneumonia are the most serious complications and account for most of the deaths that occur in infancy and in old age. Collapse of bronchopulmonary segments, or less often of lobes of the lung, from plugging of bronchioles or bronchi by sticky mucus may lead to bronchiectasis if allowed to persist. A radiograph should be taken, therefore, and appropriate physiotherapy instituted if necessary. Otitis media is the other common infective complication. Convulsions occur more often in whooping cough than in any of the other specific fevers and anoxic cerebral damage can occur. Spontaneous pneumothorax is another complication.

Treatment

Antibiotics make no difference to established illness, but oral erythromycin (12.5 mg/kg four times daily) is usually given in the first week of infection in an attempt to attenuate the symptoms and should be given to infants under one year old. Feeding is often a problem; the diet is most likely to be retained if given after an episode of vomiting. Cyanotic attacks in infants should be treated by freeing the upper airway of mucus and re-establishing breathing by gentle pressure on the chest. It may also be advisable to nurse such a child in an oxygen tent. Nebulized salbutamol can help to reduce coughing. Opinions vary on the usefulness of giving erythromycin to contacts.

Prophylactic inoculation

Suspended whooping cough vaccine may be given subcutaneously or intramuscularly. It is given as a combined triple vaccine against diphtheria, whooping cough and tetanus (see page 414). Pertussis has become more common with the fall-off in immunization rates associated with worries about the vaccine. However, the morbidity and mortality of the disease are greater than any risks from the vaccine, although care is necessary in some circumstances (see page 414).

Influenza

There are three strains of the myxovirus producing influenza; A is more common than B, and C is rare. There is no correlation between the clinical severity of the illness and the strain of virus and no cross-immunity between the strains. Variation in the antigenic structure of the virus occurs from time to time, particularly in influenza A, and limits the effectiveness of vaccines. Epidemics of influenza A tend to occur every two or three years and influenza B every four or five years. The antigenic shift in influenza A produced occasional pandemics, as in 1918 and 1957 (the 'Asian flu'). Between epidemics the virus is probably kept going in a chain of sporadic infections in man; some of these may be subclinical. Transmission is by droplet infection.

Clinical features

The incubation period is 1–3 days. The severity of the illness varies from a mild upper respiratory tract infection to the sudden onset of fever, shivering, headache, profound malaise, and severe aching in the back and limbs. Cough, sneezing and upper respiratory catarrh are usually relatively slight. Remittent fever and general prostration continue for up to a week. Meningitis and encephalitis are rare complications. In some patients con-

valescence is very slow and post-influenzal debility and depression may persist for months. Primary influenzal pneumonia is a serious condition with a high mortality. Outbreaks of influenza may also be associated with secondary bacterial pneumonia, particularly staphylococcal.

Treatment

There is no specific treatment, although the appropriate chemotherapy should be given for any bacterial complication. Analgesics and antipyretics help to relieve symptoms during the febrile stage.

Prophylaxis

Vaccines containing inactivated strains of A and B virus give partial immunity and are worth administering to patients with chronic respiratory disease.

Infectious mononucleosis (glandular fever)

Infectious mononucleosis is caused by primary infection with the Epstein–Barr virus, a herpes virus. Reactivation of the virus is associated with Burkitt's lymphoma in Africa and nasopharyngeal carcinoma in the Far East.

It is a common disease, seen mainly in young adults. Its infectivity is low, although small outbreaks occur quite often in hostels and similar institutions. There is evidence that the virus is transmitted in saliva, either by kissing, or sharing of drinking vessels.

Clinical features

The main symptoms are fever, which is usually low and long-continued, lassitude, general malaise, and sometimes sore throat; but the severity and course of the disease are very variable. Some patients simply feel a little tired for a week or two, while others are gravely ill with high fever, headache and severe sore throat. Although this acute stage does not usually last for more than a week or so, general debility and depression may persist for months. The prognosis, however, is excellent. Examination usually reveals enlarged lymph nodes in the neck and elsewhere, and the spleen is palpable in around 50 per cent of patients. Vigorous attempts at palpation are to be avoided because of the possibility of rupture of the congested spleen. Many patients have a transient macular rash, and petechiae at the junction of hard and soft palates are common. A rash almost always occurs if ampicillin is given to treat the sore throat.

Subclinical hepatitis is very common, but actual jaundice infrequent. ECG evidence of myocarditis has been reported in 16 per cent of patients, but clinical evidence of myocarditis is rare. Acute abdominal pain simulating appendicitis, benign lymphocytic meningitis, mononeuritis, haemolytic anaemia, transient thrombocytopenic purpura and rupture of the spleen are rare manifestations.

Diagnosis

The white blood count, after an initial leucopenia, is usually raised with an excess of monocytes and T-lymphocytes, many of which are seen in the stained film to have a characteristic abnormal appearance ('glandular fever cell'). Abnormal cells take up to two months to disappear. Mild thrombocytopenia is common.

The Paul–Bunnell test is usually positive after the first week, but occasionally a positive response is delayed. It depends on the fact that in glandular fever the serum contains an antibody which agglutinates sheep's red cells. Occasional false-positive results occur, but a titre of 1:64 or higher, and particularly a rising titre during illness, is significant. If the Paul–Bunnell test is negative, the possibility of toxoplasmosis or cytomegalovirus infection should be considered. The test may remain positive for up to a year.

Antibodies against the EB virus found in the IgM fraction of the plasma proteins are evidence of recent infection by the virus and are found in a high proportion of cases.

Treatment

The duration of fever and debility may be reduced by a week's course of prednisolone, starting with 40 mg daily; but this should be reserved for severely ill patients and those with neurological complications. There is no specific treatment, and prolonged convalescence is often necessary.

Gastrointestinal infections

Enteric fever (typhoid and paratyphoid)

Enteric is the name applied to a group of diseases that consists of typhoid fever and paratyphoid A, B and C. They are due to closely related organisms – short, thick, motile Gram-negative bacilli that can be distinguished from most of the non-pathogenic organisms by their inability to ferment lactose. Typhoid and paratyphoid B occur all over the world, the latter being the most common of the enteric fevers in this country; paratyphoid A is found mainly in the East; paratyphoid C is rare.

Method of spread

Enteric fever is spread by contamination of food or water by excreta from carriers or from patients with the disease. It is, therefore, prevalent in countries whose standards of sanitation are low. The sharp reduction in the incidence of the disease in the UK at the end of the nineteenth century was due to the introduction of methods of sewage disposal which prevent access to the water supplies. In countries with good sanitation, outbreaks can usually be traced to unsuspecting carriers of the disease who are engaged in the handling of foodstuffs.

Clinical features

1 Typhoid

There may be an initial mild bout of diarrhoea followed by an incubation period of about a fortnight before the gradual onset of headache, aching in the limbs, tiredness, cough, constipation and fever, which typically rises in 'step-ladder' fashion by about half a degree Celsius daily to reach a height of perhaps 39–40 °C towards the end of the first week. For the next week, or sometimes much longer, the temperature continues at this high level, showing very little variation throughout the 24 hours. The pulse usually does not show the increase in rate that accompanies most febrile illnesses, a relative bradycardia of less than 100 per minute being frequently maintained through the whole course of the illness. Cough and signs of bronchitis or even bronchopneumonia are common in the first few days and may dominate the clinical picture at this stage.

In suspected cases watch must be kept about the end of the first week for the appearance of the characteristic rash. In typhoid this consists of a few 'rose-spots', which can easily be overlooked but which nevertheless are very typical of the disease. They occur particularly on the abdomen or chest and appear for a few days in a succession of crops of tiny pink spots, which blanch on pressure and are not more than 1–2 mm in diameter; each one lasts for only 24 hours or so. It is useful, therefore, to make a ring with a skin pencil around each spot so that the next day it is clear at a glance if any new ones have appeared. The spleen often becomes palpable at about the same time as the rash appears.

Most patients are constipated during the first few days, but towards the end of the second week the abdomen becomes distended and diarrhoea sets in. By this time, if the attack is a severe one, the patient is very gravely ill and may pass into the 'typhoid state', in which he remains throughout the 24 hours in what has been called a 'coma-vigil' – drowsy and confused but continually muttering to himself, plucking at the bedclothes, and groping for non-existent objects. The faeces are now fluid and greeny yellow in colour ('pea-soup stools') and up to twenty may be passed in 24 hours.

Gradual improvement usually occurs during the third and fourth weeks; the temperature settles by lysis, the diarrhoea stops, the mind becomes clearer and the other symptoms also slowly disappear. However, this is also the time that complications arise. Very occasionally relapse occurs in convalescence.

2 Paratyphoid

The incubation period is shorter and the disease milder and shorter than typhoid. Diarrhoea is often evident from the start. In paratyphoid B the rash is often more profuse and may coalesce to give an eruption similar to measles.

Complications

The two most serious complications of typhoid are liable to occur during the third week of illness, when sloughs separate from the Peyer's patches in the ileum leaving deep ulcers which may perforate or cause serious hae-morrhage. Such perforations are easily overlooked clinically. By the time they occur the patient is in such a weak state that very little peritoneal reaction takes place; the only clue may be a sudden worsening of the general clinical condition, with a fall in the temperature and a rise in the pulse and respiration rates and the appearance of minimal abdominal tenderness. Small perforations without generalized peritonitis can usually be treated conservatively. Haemorrhage is more common than per-foration; it is diagnosed by sudden faintness, pallor and sweating, and the appearance of bright-red blood in the next stool passed. Transfusion may be necessary. Bronchitis, pneumonia and venous thrombosis may occur.

Cholecystitis, with the subsequent formation of gallstones containing *Salmonella typhi*, and acute arthritis, are rare complications.

Typhoid abscesses in bone and periostitis causing the stiff and painful typhoid spine are very rare sequelae which may appear years after the original infection.

Diagnosis

Blood culture is the best way of establishing the diagnosis, and as the organisms circulate in the blood only during the first week it is extremely important that blood should be taken for culture as early as possible, preferably during the first three days.

The blood count typically shows a leucopenia, but this is not a constant finding, particularly in paratyphoid, and in the presence of bronchitis or other complications there may even be a slight leucocytosis.

As a rise in the agglutinating antibody titre during the illness is evidence of active infection, blood should be taken for this estimation at the same time as the initial blood culture during the first few days, and again during the second week (the *Widal test*). Quite high titres of 'H' (flagellar) agglutinin may be found in the blood of healthy people who have been inoculated with TAB, but a rising titre of 'O' (somatic) agglutinins is usually indicative of enteric infection. A high titre of 'Vi' (virulence) agglutinin is also usually significant.

Treatment

Patients with typhoid must of course be nursed with strict barrier precautions. The prognosis of typhoid has been greatly improved since the introduction of chloram-phenicol, which is usually very effective. A satisfactory scheme of dosage for an adult is 1.5 g twice daily for the first five days, then 0.75 g twice daily for a week, and finally 1 g daily for a few more days. Co-trimoxazole in high doses for two weeks is an alternative treatment. Excretion of the organism often continues after recovery, but if it continues for longer than a year this is regarded as a carrier state. Clearance of the stool and urine needs to be checked, particularly for those involved in preparing food. Subsequent development of the carrier state is no commoner in treated than in untreated patients, but chloramphenicol usually fails to eradicate the organisms from the carriers. High-dose ampicillin for four weeks may clear carriers but in the presence of gallstones cholecystectomy is usually necessary.

Prophylactic immunization against the enteric fevers is achieved using an inactivated vaccine. It should be given to those visiting endemic areas.

Salmonella enteritis

This organism is a common cause of 'food-poisoning' from contaminated meat or fish.

Clinical features

The incubation period is 12–24 hours. Symptoms are diarrhoea, usually with some vomiting and fever. These usually resolve in three or four days, but sufferers may continue to excrete the organism. Those who work in jobs where others are at risk from faecal–oral transmission should be shown to have three negative stools before returning to work.

Diagnosis and treatment

Stool culture may grow one of the many serotypes of *Salmonella enteritidis*. Treatment is based around careful maintenance of fluid balance.

Viral gastroenteritis

Various viruses can be responsible for outbreaks of gastroenteritis. These include rotaviruses, adenoviruses and astroviruses.

Clinical features

The incubation period is around 24 hours. Predominant features are diarrhoea and vomiting. *Epidemic vomiting* or *winter vomiting* occurs in small outbreaks often within a family. It lasts one or two days with little or any diarrhoea and is caused by a calcivirus.

Diagnosis and treatment

It is possible to isolate virus particles from the stool. Treatment is symptomatic, maintaining the fluid balance.

Escherichia coli gastroenteritis

Although *E. coli* is a part of the normal bowel flora, some serotypes produce an enterotoxin.

Clinical features

The incubation period is two days. Symptoms are vomiting, diarrhoea and fever of varying severity.

Diagnosis and treatment

E. coli can be isolated from stool cultures and distinguished from non-pathogenic serotypes. Treatment involves appropriate fluid replacement.

Shigella dysentery

Shigella flexneri and *Sh. dysenteriae* cause severe diarrhoea with fever, abdominal pain and bloody stools for weeks.

They are common in parts of Asia, Africa and South America. Treatment with trimethoprin or ampicillin is effective in most cases, with the addition of fluid replacement. Resistance occurs in some areas (see page 441).

Sh. sonnei and *Sh. boydii* occur world-wide and cause a milder illness lasting two or three days and not usually requiring antibiotic treatment.

Campylobacter enteritis

Now recognized as a common cause of diarrhoea, this Gram-negative microaeropholic bacteria usually comes from meat, pets or contaminated water.

Clinical features

The incubation period is up to one week. The symptoms are fever and malaise followed by diarrhoea with severe, cramp-like abdominal pain. Red blood cells and neutrophils may be prominent in the stools. The symptoms usually settle in 4–5 days, but on occasions it can be prolonged and will then respond to oral erythromycin.

Yersinia enteritis

Yersinia enterocolitica is a Gram-negative bacillus which can contaminate milk or water.

Clinical features

Symptoms are usually diarrhoea, fever and abdominal pain. The picture may mimic appendicitis and lead to appendicectomy.

Erythema nodosum occurs in around 20 per cent of patients, and arthritis, thyroiditis and Reiter's syndrome may also develop. Yersinia can be grown on stool culture.

Treatment

Antibiotics may help when the cause of an outbreak has been recognized. Most isolates are sensitive to tetracycline, co-trimoxazole, chloramphenicol and aminoglycosides.

Cholera

Cholera is associated with poor hygiene and contamination of water supplies. John Snow recognized the association in 1849 and reduced the incidence by removing the handle of the Broad Street water pump. Today cholera is mainly a disease of underdeveloped countries. *Vibrio cholerae* produces a toxin which acts on the bowel mucosa. Other strains, non-01 *V. cholerae* or atypical *V. cholerae* 01, may cause mild diarrhoea but not epidemics and are not notifiable.

Clinical features

The incubation period varies from a few hours to a few days before abdominal fullness and diarrhoea develop. Loss of fluid in the 'rice-water' stools may be very severe, leading to dehydration and death. The vital mainstay of management is careful adequate fluid replacement parenterally, although tetracycline may help to reduce the length of the illness.

Giardiasis

This is discussed on page 442.

Cryptosporidium

This is an organism of the toxoplasma group which produces occasional outbreaks of diarrhoea and gives particular problems in immunocompromised patients.

Amoebiasis

Amoebiasis is most frequent in the tropics. The protozoan *Entamoeba histolytica* is usually transmitted by contaminated water. For a further discussion, see page 442.

Clinical features

The initial illness consists of diarrhoea, occasionally with vomiting and fever and often with abdominal pain and urgency. Complications include the development of chronic diarrhoea, amoebic masses (amoebomas) in the colon, amoebic abscesses in the liver and occasionally, by direct extension, in the lung or pleura.

Diagnosis

This requires the examination of a fresh stool sample to look for amoebic cysts or trophozoites. These may also be found in the large bowel mucosa on biopsy. Serological diagnosis is also possible.

Treatment

Metronidazole is the mainstay of treatment, although large liver abscesses may require aspiration or surgical drainage.

Some subjects may pass amoebic cysts and be asymptomatic but a source of infection. They should be treated with metronidazole and diloxanide since metronidazole fails to clear the stool in 15 per cent of patients.

Clostridium difficile

The toxin produced by *Clostridium difficile* produces pseudomembranous colitis. This condition develops usually after antibiotic therapy. The symptoms are profuse diarrhoea together with abdominal pain, fever and leucocytosis. The diagnosis is made by finding the organism and its toxin in the stool and by identifying the typical yellow adherent pseudomembrane on sigmoidoscopy. Treatment is with oral vancomycin, tetracycline or metronidazole.

Viral hepatitis

This is discussed on page 177.

Respiratory disorders

The various causes of pneumonia are dealt with in Chapter 3.

Neurological infections

Meningitis (see also page 220)

Many organisms are capable of causing inflammation of the meninges. In some cases this is associated with inflammation of the brain substance: encephalitis. Viruses are the most common cause of meningitis, particularly coxsackie, mumps and ECHO viruses. Amongst the bacteria, *Haemophilus influenzae*, *Neisseria meningitidis* and *Streptococcus pneumoniae* are the three commonest pathogens. In neonates, Gram-negative organisms are another cause. Tuberculous meningitis should always be remembered, particularly as the diagnosis may be more difficult because of the slower, atypical presentation. Other unusual organisms occur, particularly in immunosuppressed patients.

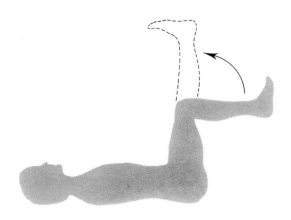

Figure 14.1 *Kernig's sign. The thigh is flexed to 90° from the abdomen; the knee cannot be extended passively owing to hamstring muscle spasm.*

Clinical features

In viral meningitis the other features of the viral infection may be present, often preceding the meningeal signs. The symptoms of meningitis are headache, photophobia, nausea and vomiting. Fever occurs and meningeal irritation is shown by neck stiffness or by *Kernig's sign* in children (Fig. 14.1).

If there is encephalitis then changes in conscious level and personality and focal neurological signs develop.

1 Neisseria meningitidis (meningococcus)

The condition occurs sporadically or in epidemic form. The incubation period is two or three days before fever, severe headache and signs of meningeal irritation develop. Convulsions are common in children. Most patients have a petechial rash sometimes preceded by a macular eruption. Occasionally a fulminating form of meningococcal meningitis develops, with acute meningitic signs and a profuse purpuric rash proceding to coma within a few hours and death in 24–48 hours. Other complications are endocarditis, septic arthritis and the *Waterhouse–Friderichsen* syndrome. The latter condition often involves bilateral adrenal haemorrhage, but the problems relate more to septic shock and only large doses of steroids rather than adrenal replacement doses are likely to be helpful.

Chronic meningococcal septicaemia occurs occasionally with bouts of low fever accompanied by headache, joint pains and a maculopapular rash on the trunk and limbs. The diagnosis is confirmed by finding the meningococcus on blood culture.

In meningococcal meningitis close contacts should also be treated with rifampicin (600 mg twice daily) for two days.

2 Streptococcus pneumoniae

Pneumococcal meningitis occurs mainly in adults. Predisposing causes are sinusitis, otitis media or any lesion disrupting meningeal continuity. Complications are more common with pneumococcal meningitis and include abscess formation and neurological defects such as cranial nerve palsies or intellectual impairment.

3 Haemophilus influenzae

This occurs mostly in children below three years of age. The onset is often slow.

Diagnosis

The white cell count usually shows a neutrophil leucocytosis in bacterial meningitis but not with a viral aetiology. Blood cultures are often positive in bacterial disease. Whenever meningitis is under consideration it is essential to perform a lumbar puncture and to examine the fluid for

Table 14.4 Typical cerebrospinal fluid findings in meningitis

Appearance	Normal	Viral	Bacterial
	Clear	Clear	May be opague or purulent
Protein (g/l)	0/1–0.4	0.5–0.9	> 0.9
Glucose (mmol/l)	1 mmol below blood level	Normal	low (> 1.5 mmol below blood level)
Cells (× 10⁶/l)	< 6 lymphocytes	20–100: usually lymphocytes but neutrophils early	Often > 400 neutrophils

protein, glucose (with simultaneous blood glucose), cells and organisms. The typical features in viral and bacterial meningitis are shown in Table 14.4.

Treatment

Analgesia and rest in a darkened room are the only treatments necessary for viral meningitis. In bacterial meningitis treatment should be started as soon as possible. Blind antibiotic therapy may well be necessary before a precise bacteriological diagnosis has been made. Suitable treatment regimens are shown in Table 14.5. In meningococcal meningitis carriers should be given rifampicin for two days after penicillin.

Poliomyelitis

This is discussed on page 221.

Post-infectious encephalitis and encephalomyelitis

This condition is a very rare sequel to acute specific fevers such as whooping cough, measles and mumps, and less often to others such as chickenpox, rubella, scarlet fever and infectious mononucleosis; it is no more common after severe than mild attacks.

It also sometimes follows vaccination and other immunizing procedures. It has been suggested that the underlying cause may be an antigen–antibody reaction, and sometimes improvement does seem to follow treatment with ACTH or cortisone.

Clinical features

Symptoms appear within a week or two of the onset of the original infection or vaccination. Headache, malaise,

Table 14.5 Treatment of bacterial meningitis

Meningococcal	IV benzylpenicillin, 1.2–2.4 g 4-hourly
Pneumococcal	IV benzylpenicillin, 1.2–2.4 g 2-hourly
Haemophilus influenzae	IV chloramphenicol, 500–1000 mg 6-hourly initially, then reduced
Organism unknown	Chloramphenicol + benzylpenicillin (chloramphenicol alone if penicillin-sensitive)
Tuberculosis	Triple or quadruple therapy including pyrazinamide

vomiting, irritability, drowsiness or coma are common; other patients present with fits or sudden paresis mimicking a cerebral vascular accident; while in others the clinical picture is dominated by signs of meningitis, cranial nerve palsies, and transient lower motor neurone weakness in the limbs. Mortality is around 10 per cent. Moreover, many of those who recover are left with a disability such as hemiplegia, cranial nerve palsies, mental defect, or a Parkinsonian syndrome.

General infections

Cytomegalovirus (CMV)

Maternal infection early in pregnancy leads to fetal infection and subsequent abnormalities. Later in pregnancy there may be no symptoms. Infection in childhood or adult life is common but usually remains subclinical. However, immunocompromised patients do have problems with CMV infection.

Clinical features

Congenital infection may produce severe generalized disease at birth or mental retardation, chorioretinitis and cardiac abnormalities.

Children and adults may develop a mild illness with fever and lymphocytosis, while immunosuppression can result in a severe CMV pneumonia with a high mortality.

Diagnosis

Antibody can be detected on serological testing, and the organism may be grown from sputum or urine. Characteristic intracellular inclusion bodies may be present on lung biopsy specimens.

Treatment

No reliable treatment is widely available, but the problems of CMV in acquired immunodeficiency syndrome are producing speedy improvements in diagnosis and treatment (e.g. Foscarnet).

Leptospirosis (Weil's disease)

The causal organism, *Leptospira icterohaemorrhagica*, is excreted in the urine of infected rats. Man acquires the infection either by ingesting food or drink contaminated by rat urine or by immersion in contaminated water, since the spirochaete is able to gain entry through the nasal mucosa or through minor skin abrasions. In this country leptospirosis is therefore mainly seen as an occupational disease of people working in damp, rat-infested places, notably sewer workers, miners, canal and dock workers, farm hands and fish cleaners. A milder disease (*canicola fever*) is produced by *L. canicola* from the urine of dogs.

Clinical features

After an incubation period of around two weeks there is a rapid onset of fever, headache, pains in the back and limbs. Injection of the conjunctivae is often a very striking feature. The name 'icterohaemorrhagiae' implies jaundice and purpura, but clinical jaundice is seen in only about 75 per cent of patients; it appears during the first week. Features which help in distinguishing the disease from infective hepatitis are the profound prostration, heavy albuminuria, purpuric rash, and sometimes haemoptysis, haematemesis, melaena, or bleeding from the gums. There is usually a leucocytosis. Some patients develop signs of meningeal irritation, and some proceed from oliguria to anuria and uraemia; the mortality rate is about 15 per cent.

Diagnosis

This is established by identifying the spirochaete by dark-ground illumination of specimens of blood taken during the first few days or urine during the third week. The organism can also be isolated by intraperitoneal inoculation of guinea-pigs with blood or urine. A rising titre of serum agglutinins also occurs but does not give diagnostic information until the clinical illness is more or less over.

Treatment

To be effective, benzylpenicillin must be given early in the illness, in large doses (e.g. 1.8 g 6-hourly). If there is no improvement after three days, or with penicillin sensitivity, oxytetracycline (1.5 g 6-hourly) should be used.

Brucellosis (undulant fever)

The causative organism is a Gram-negative coccobacillus which infects animals and is transmitted to man in infected milk. In this country the usual infecting organism is *Brucella abortus*, which is prevalent throughout the world and is transmitted in cow's milk. *Brucella melitensis* is transmitted in goat's milk and is found particularly in the Mediterranean area. *Brucella suis* infects pigs and is rarely transmitted to man.

The disease is an occupational hazard of farm workers and slaughter-men since infection can be aquired through skin and mucosae, but others may be infected by drinking unpasteurized milk. Cases in the UK have decreased markedly in relation to the reduction in infected animals.

Clinical features

Typical acute brucellosis has an incubation period of between one and three weeks, followed by headache, malaise, anorexia, constipation, and a bout of fever which usually settles by lysis after about ten days. Cough and profuse sweating are common and the spleen is usually palpable. After the temperature has been normal for a few days another bout of fever begins, and these febrile episodes may continue recurring at short intervals for some months. During the course of the illness arthritis is common. One joint is usually affected at a time, the pain and swelling subsiding after a few days and then appearing elsewhere. The joints most often affected are the hip, knee, shoulder, ankle and wrist, but occasionally the small joints of the fingers and toes or of the spine may be involved. Peripheral neuritis, orchitis and albuminuria are less common complications.

Chronic brucellosis may or may not be preceded by the acute disease. Recurrent bouts of drenching night sweats without serious general ill-health should always suggest this diagnosis. Fatigue, arthralgia, myalgia and depression are the commonest features.

Diagnosis

Blood culture is the most satisfactory way of establishing the diagnosis, but the organism is difficult to isolate (even under increased CO_2 tension) and slow to grow, so that sterile cultures do not rule out this disease. Urine culture is occasionally positive. A rising antibody titre during the illness is helpful; dilutions up to 1:5000 should be tested, since agglutination may be found in the higher dilutions but not in the lower ones. Serology may be only weakly positive or even negative in the chronic form. The blood count usually shows a leucopenia and perhaps mild anaemia.

Treatment

Tetracycline (0.75 g 6-hourly) with or without intramuscular streptomycin is the treatment of choice and should be given for four weeks. A second course of treatment is given after two weeks to prevent relapse. Chronic brucellosis will require more prolonged treatment.

Tetanus

Clostridium tetani is a normal inhabitant of the alimentary tract of horses and sheep, so that its spores are particularly prevalent on cultivated land; and as it is a strict anaerobe it thrives especially in deep penetrating wounds contaminated with soil or road dust. The wound, however, may be a trivial one which heals before the tetanic symptoms appear. These are due to a powerful exotoxin which is absorbed by muscle end-plates at the site of infection and travels along motor nerves to the central nervous system.

Clinical features

The incubation period is very variable and is important in prognosis. Tetanus appearing within a few days of a wound is usually fatal, while if symptoms are delayed for two or more weeks the disease is likely to be mild. Local muscular weakness near the site of infection, attributable to the action of the toxin on the motor end-plates, may precede the generalized spasms. These are usually heralded by trismus (hence the term lockjaw), which may be accompanied by spasm of the facial musculature causing the classical risus sardonicus. Tonic spasm spreads to the trunk, causing opisthotonus and board-like rigidity of the abdomen. Fever is commonly present.

The paroxysmal stage starts in severe cases within two days of the appearance of trismus; the longer it is delayed the better the prognosis. Paroxysms are precipitated by stimuli such as feeding and other nursing attentions, clinical examination or even simply external noises. The whole body is thrown into painful spasm, with arching of the back, extension of the limbs and clenching of the teeth, this may subside after a few seconds or persist for several minutes. In severe cases the paroxysms recur with increasing frequency and interfere with swallowing and respiration. Autonomic dysfunction produces instability of pulse rate and blood pressure.

The diagnosis is based on the clinical picture.

Treatment

Specially staffed and equipped tetanus units have been established in Britain, and in most cases the patient should be transferred without delay to the nearest of these. The patient should be nursed in a quiet room with shaded light.

1 Antitoxins

Human tetanus immunoglobulin is the antitoxin of choice since it avoids the serious allergic reactions that may follow horse serum antitoxin; the dose is 30–300 units/kg body weight given intramuscularly. Even though neurotoxin is fixed to the nervous tissue by the time clinical signs of tetanus appear, it is important to give antitoxin to deal with toxin still circulating in the blood or being produced at the wound site.

2 Wound toilet

An hour after the antitoxin has been given, surgical debridement of the wound should be carried out under light general anaesthesia.

3 Antibiotic therapy

Intravenous benzylpenicillin is given to eradicate the organism.

4 Control of muscular spasms

For successful management of severe cases, continuous skilled medical supervision for 24 hours is necessary. Diazepam may help in mild cases but, in severe cases, neuromuscular blockade and mechanical ventilation are necessary. Sedation and feeding will be necessary. Overall mortality is around 10 per cent. Beta blockade may help the cardiovascular instability.

Prophylaxis

Active immunization with tetanus toxoid should be given to all children in the combined triple vaccine with diphtheria and pertussis. Booster doses should be given every ten years, especially to those at greatest risk such as farmers. If an individual actively immunized in this way receives a wound he should be given a further dose of toxoid instead of anti-tetanic serum.

Non-immunized patients with tetanus-prone wounds should be given human tetanus immunoglobulin (250 i.u. IM). At the same time the first immunizing dose of absorbed toxoid should be given.

Cat-scratch fever

This disease is transmitted by the scratch of apparently healthy cats.

Clinical features

A few days after the scratch a small indolent ulcer or sore may appear at the site of inoculation and a week or two later the regional lymph nodes become very enlarged. There may be some fever at this stage but constitutional upset is slight. The affected lymph nodes sometimes suppurate, but recovery without serious complications or sequelae is the rule, though adenitis may persist for some months. The white blood count is normal and aspirated pus is sterile.

Treatment

A course of tetracycline (250 mg 6-hourly) for five days may prevent suppuration.

Actinomycosis

The organism *actinomyces bovis* occurs in pus as 'sulphur granules' of up to 1 mm in diameter and is anaerobic. The disease is much more common in men than in women.

Clinical features

1 Actinomycosis of the jaw
This is the most common clinical type. Infection through the mucous membrane of the gum leads gradually to woody induration of all the tissues of the jaw and overlying skin, through which multiple sinuses eventually discharge. There is little pain or constitutional upset and the regional lymph nodes are not usually involved.
2 Ileocaecal actinomycosis
This causes a hard, irregular mass in the right iliac fossa, and in time fixation to the overlying skin and sinus formation occurs. The disease may spread to the liver, spleen and other organs and is frequently fatal.
3 Actinomycosis of the lung
This is the least common type. Cough, dyspnoea, fever and pain in the chest occur. The radiograph may show periosteal duplication in the ribs. Later, induration and sinuses appear in the chest wall.

Diagnosis and treatment

This depends on identification of the 'sulphur granules' in the pus; these contain the Gram-positive branching organisms. The treatment is amoxycillin (1 g 8-hourly) for a prolonged period (e.g. three months).

Toxoplasmosis

Infection with the protozoon *Toxoplasma gondii* is common, but only rarely causes clinical disease. It is acquired by eating undercooked meat from infected animals or by contact with infected cats.

Clinical features

1 Congenital toxoplasmosis
This may lead to choroidoretinitis, or less often to lesions in the brain which may calcify and may cause hydrocephalus.
2 Aquired toxoplasmosis
There are few if any symptoms. It may produce lymphadenopathy, particularly cervical, malaise and occasionally uveitis. The diagnosis may be suspected from the histology of a node removed by biopsy.

Diagnosis

Antibody tests, particularly the dye test, confirm the diagnosis. Atypical mononuclear cells are seen in the blood.

Treatment

Spiramycin (50–70 mg/kg daily) may give good results in children with ocular infections, but has little effect on lymphadenopathic toxoplasmosis. No treatment is necessary for the malaise and lymphadenopathy which resolve spontaneously. When treatment is required high-dose co-trimoxazole is of benefit.

Infection in the immunocompromised host

Many factors may interfere with the normal defence functions of the body. For many years occasional toxic effects of drugs and rare hereditary diseases have resulted in suppression of the immune system allowing infection with unusual organisms. The emergence of drugs acting specifically on the immune system and diseases such as acquired immunodeficiency syndome (AIDS) has increased greatly the importance of such *'opportunist' infections*. Some of these organisms are not usually pathogenic and are capable of producing disease only when resistance is lowered. However, in the management of such patients it is important to remember that most of their infections are caused by common pathogens rather than the more obscure opportunist agents.

Septicaemias are common, arising from the urinary tract, the intestines or the skin. The likely organism will depend on the site of entry but is usually one of the common Gram-positive organisms, *E. coli* or pseudomonas.

Table 14.6 Immunosuppression and opportunist infections

Condition	'Opportunist' organisms
Splenectomy Agammaglobulinaemia Lymphoma, Lymphocytic leukaemia Treated leukaemias	Pneumococcal infections Bacterial infections Tuberculosis; herpes virus (zoster and simplex); cryptococcal meningitis Bacterial septicaemias; *Pneumocystis carinii;* Cytomegalovirus
Transplants Acquired immunodeficiency	Fungal infections; Cytomegalovirus *Pneumocystis carinii;* tuberculosis *Pneumocystis carinii;* Cytomegalovirus; *Mycobacterium avium – intracellulare*

The most frequent causes of immunosuppression and their associated opportunist infections are shown in Table 14.6.

Clinical features

A common site for such infections is the lung. Pulmonary shadowing in such cases is not always infective. For example, a patient with leukaemia may develop radiological pulmonary shadowing because of drug toxicity, intrapulmonary haemorrhage from thrombocytopenia, or leukaemic infiltration as well as pneumonia.

Infections such as fungal pneumonias, cytomegalovirus or the protozoal *Pneumocystis carinii* pneumonia usually require a procedure such as fibreoptic bronchoscopy and alveolar lavage or transbronchial lung biopsy to confirm the diagnosis. There may be more than one pathogen involved in the infection.

Treatment

The range of potential organisms is very wide and treatment is often guided by the clinical situation and local prevalences. Unless there is a specific indication it is usual to start with broad-spectrum combined antibiotic therapy while awaiting the results of bacteriological investigations.

Pneumocystis carinii pneumonia usually responds to treatment with high-dose co-trimoxazole (trimethoprim 20 mgkg per day). An alternative therapy is pentamidine isethionate. In some high-risk groups, particularly where pneumocystis has been a local problem, low-dose co-trimoxazole or nebulized pentamidine is used as prophylactic therapy.

Sexually transmitted diseases

Syphilis and gonorrhoea were originally the main target of venereal disease clinics. The renamed departments of genitourinary medicine (GUM) are still involved with these diseases but see more cases of viral, fungal and chlamydial infections. Genitourinary medicine clinics have usually a large number of homosexual males who are at risk of acquiring human immunodeficiency virus (HIV, HTLV III). A substantial number of these patients will develop the acquired immunodeficiency syndrome (AIDS) dealt with on page 395. An important part of the work of GUM clinics involves contact tracing, education and counselling, designed to control the spread of sexually transmitted diseases. This function has become particularly important with the advent of AIDS; an untreatable fatal disease where prevention is vital.

Gonorrhoea

Neisseria gonorrhoeae is a delicate organism which does not survive for long outside the body, and gonorrhoea is almost invariably acquired by coitus with an infected person. Recovery confers no immunity and it is therefore possible for the same individual to have repeated attacks of the disease.

The organism is identified in smears of purulent exudates as a Gram-negative kidney-shaped diplococcus which must be seen within the cytoplasm of polymorph leucocytes before the diagnosis can be made. It is rather difficult to grow in culture unless special media and increased carbon dioxide tension are employed.

Between the mid-1950s and mid-1970s numbers of cases increased steadily in the UK, with a reduction in the male to female ratio. Since the late 1970s the number of cases appears to be steady or decreasing.

Clinical features

1 In men

Within about 3–10 days of exposure to infection the first symptom is usually slight scalding on micturition, soon followed by a purulent urethral discharge; and there may be tender swollen lymph nodes in the groin. If treatment is not given the infection tends to spread to the posterior urethra, and may produce periurethral abscesses. Infection of the prostate may follow and may cause acute retention of urine, while involvement of the seminal vesicles causes severe local pain and fever.

Stricture in the posterior urethra is now a rare late complication. Acute epididymitis, indicated by severe pain, swelling and tenderness which often spread to involve the testicle on the same side, is a serious complication. With modern treatment spread beyond the anterior urethra is rare. A small minority of infected males are asymptomatic. Rectal and oropharyngeal disease occur in homosexual males.

2 In women
After a similar incubation period the disease may present with painful, frequent micturition, and vaginal discharge, although there may be no symptoms of the infection in around 50 per cent of women. Most women seek medical advice as contacts of symptomatic males. Involvement of Skene's or Bartholin's glands may lead to large, painful abscesses, although in fact Bartholin's abscess is much more often of streptococcal origin. If untreated the infection may spread to the uterus and Fallopian tubes, leading to the formation of a pyosalpinx. This presents with severe lower abdominal pain and fever and a tender adnexal mass can be felt on one or both sides on pelvic examination. It may be possible to demonstrate gonococci in cervical smears. Involvement of the tubes usually leads to permanent sterility.

Complications

Metastatic lesions due to transient bacteraemia are now very rare, but a purulent arthritis is occasionally seen. Gonorrhoeal rheumatism, however, is usually not due to bacteria *in situ* and may be in fact an associated Reiter's syndrome (see page 247). It may take the form of a flitting polyarthritis coming on a month or so after infection, or a single joint may be involved, particularly the knee, wrist or ankle. Associated tenosynovitis is common and iritis and skin rashes may occur.

Diagnosis

Gram stain and microscopy of a urethral smear is usually positive in men, but cervical smear and culture are often necessary in women.

Treatment

A single oral dose of 3 g ampicillin or a single injection of procaine penicillin of 2.4 million units combined with 1.0 g of probenecid is usually adequate treatment of uncomplicated gonorrhoea. There are now strains of gonococci relatively resistant to penicillin. In areas where these are frequent, treatment consists of a single injection of spectinomycin given intramuscularly or cefuroxime and probenicid. In penicillin-sensitive subjects suitable

treatment is co-trimoxazole 4 tablets twice daily for four days. This drug will not mask the appearance of syphylis. It is important to remember that the treatment of gonorrhoea with penicillin and some other antibiotics may suppress the appearance of a syphilitic lesion acquired at the same time, and serological tests for the latter disease must always be made three and six months after the gonorrhoea has been treated.

Syphilis

As a result of improved treatment and the consequent reduced infectivity of patients with the disease, syphilis is much less common. It remains very important, however, because of the serious lesions that may appear in almost any organ of the body many years after the primary infection.

The causative organism, *Treponema pallidum*, is a thin, actively motile spirochaete from 6 to 14 μm in length, which can be recognized by its characteristic movements in preparations of the serous discharge from the early infectious lesions examined by the microscopic technique known as dark-ground illumination (DGI). It cannot withstand drying and is transmitted only by direct contact.

Congenital syphilis is contracted by the fetus through the placenta in the later months of pregnancy; *acquired syphilis* is nearly always the result of sexual intercourse with an infected person, though occasionally extragenital infection may be acquired, for example, by doctors or nurses handling syphilitic lesions. Congenital syphilis is fortunately extremely rare nowadays. It is a preventable disease, since if a woman with syphilis is given adequate treatment before the fourth month of pregnancy the child is not affected. Routine serum tests are made on all women on their first attendance at antenatal clinics.

Clinical features

1 Congenital syphilis
This may cause intrauterine death and result in miscarriage or stillbirth; or the child may be born apparently healthy only to develop various stigmata of the disease during childhood. Early manifestations are failure to gain weight in the first month or two of life, and an infection in the nose (snuffles) which interferes with the development of the nasal bones and leads eventually to the depressed bridge of the nose which is one of the most characteristic signs of the disease. A scaly yellow or copper-coloured rash is also common. Among the many lesions which may appear later in childhood are notches

in the incisor teeth of the second dentition, which also tend to be widely spaced and to taper from the gum margin to the cutting edge (Hutchinson's teeth); scars known as rhagades radiating from the margins of the lips; and opacity of the cornea due to interstitial keratitis. Aortic lesions are very rare in congenital syphilis, but juvenile forms of tabes and general paresis are occasionally seen.

2 Acquired syphilis

This passes through three stages, primary, secondary and tertiary. The secondary stage occurs within a few months of primary infection, but many years may elapse before a tertiary lesion appears.

Primary syphilis is characterized by the appearance of a hard chancre about a month after exposure to infection. In men the chancre usually occurs on the penis or in the anal canal. In women it appears most often on the labia or cervix and in the latter situation readily escapes notice. More rarely the primary sore may be on the lip, tongue, tonsil or nipple. The chancre is a hard, painless ulcer about 1 cm in diameter, has a thin, serous discharge and is accompanied by painless enlargement of the regional lymph nodes. Diagnosis depends on identifying the *Treponema pallidum* in the exudate with the use of the dark-ground microscope.

Secondary syphilis may cause some constitutional disturbance with sore throat, low fever and generalized lymph node enlargement, but usually its manifestations are confined to the skin and the mucous membrane of the mouth. Various types of skin rash are seen, all having in common a symmetrical distribution including the palms and the soles, absence of irritation, and a colour usually likened to raw ham. In the mouth painless, slimy, greyish patches known as 'snail-track ulcers' are the typical lesions. Warty lesions known as condylomata may appear in the perianal and vulval regions. The cutaneous and mucosal lesions of the secondary stage are highly infective and the serum tests for antibody are invariably positive.

In the *tertiary stage*, a localized swelling known as a gumma may appear anywhere in the body many years after the primary infection; these lesions differ from those of primary and secondary syphilis in containing no spirochaetes and being therefore non-infective. In certain situations such as the liver, the lung or the stomach, a gumma may be mistaken for a carcinoma. The centre of a gumma often breaks down and leads to the formation of an ulcer with sharply punched out margins. This may cause perforation of the nasal septum or hard palate.

Syphilitic aortitis is discussed on pages 49, 73 and *neurosyphilis* on page 222.

Diagnosis

Tests for syphilis can be divided into those that test for reagin, a non-specific plasma protein fraction which is elevated in syphilis together with a number of other diseases, and other more specific tests for anti-treponemal autobodies. It is usual to perform one non-specific and one more specific test to confirm syphilis.

Non-specific tests

The VDRL (Venereal Disease Research Laboratory) test is a flocculation test for reagin, and it can be quantified. The RPR (rapid plasma reagin) test is similar.

These tests are sensitive, cheap and easy to perform and are very useful for screening large numbers of specimens. Their disadvantage is that false-positive reactions may be found in patients with immune disorders such as lupus erythematosus, in conditions in which there is increased destruction of cell nuclei and occasionally in healthy people.

2 Specific tests

It is usual to perform also one of the specific tests employing *T. pallidum* as the antigen.

The *fluorescent antibody (absorbed) test* is the first serological test to become positive in primary syphilis. It is expensive and tedious to perform and is not used for routine screening, but is very useful if dark-ground microscopy cannot be performed. False-positive reactions are rare.

The *Treponema pallidum haemagglutination assay* (TPHA) can be quantified, is highly specific and can be automated and used for large-scale screening.

The *Treponema pallidum immobilization test* (TPI) is specific but expensive and complex.

In most patients the reagin tests become negative one year after treatment for primary syphilis and two years after treatment for secondary syphilis, but the specific tests may remain positive for many years. The reagin tests are therefore more useful than the specific ones for evaluating the result of treatment.

In general the serological tests for syphilis are also positive in patients with other treponemal infections such as yaws. When such a patient develops syphilis a rise in the reagin titre may give a clue to the diagnosis.

Treatment

1 Early syphilis

Procaine penicillin injection BP (900 mg; 900 000 units) should be given daily for eight days. Alternatively itinerant or uncooperative patients may be given a single intramuscular injection of benzathine penicillin (2.4 g; 2.4

million units) as this will maintain the necessary blood level (at least 0.03 units per millilitre) for about two weeks. Patients who are sensitive to penicillin should be given tetracycline (500 mg 6-hourly) for 14 days with a repeat course after three months, or erythromycin (1 g twice daily) for two weeks. Those with early infectious syphilis should be kept under observation for two years, by which time serological tests should have returned to normal. Sexual intercourse should not be resumed until the course of treatment is finished and lesions have healed. Cure is achieved in 90 per cent of patients.

2 Late syphilis

Procaine penicillin (900 000 units daily) for 14 days is satisfactory treatment. Prednisolone (30 mg daily) should be given to cover the first few days of treatment to ameliorate a Herxheimer reaction (see below).

Complications

Acute symptoms consisting of fever, shivering, headache and malaise, and lasting for a few hours, may occur within a day or two of starting treatment. This is known as a *Herxheimer reaction* (or Jarish–Herxheimer) and is thought to be caused by release of endotoxin from killed spirochaetes. The Herxheimer reaction may have serious effects in patients with syphilitic neurosyphilis aortitis or gummata in special situations such as the larynx; penicillin therapy should be started under steroid cover in such patients.

Non-specific urethritis (NSU)

About 50 per cent of patients presenting with NSU (i.e. with bacteria in urethral pus) have urethritis due to *Chlamydia trachomatis*, which is now by far the most common sexually transmitted disease in the West. The D–K serotypes of *C. trachomatis* primarily infect the genital tract; the A, B, Ba and C serotypes cause trachoma in developing countries. There is a huge reservoir of D–K serotypes in the genital tract of both men and women.

Clinical features

Men complain of dysuria, urethral discharge and difficulty in micturition. Women often have few or no symptoms so that the infection may be discovered only when some complication appears or an infant develops ophthalmia neonatorum, which is now seven times more often due to chlamydial than to gonococcal infection. Similar urethritis may occur with myocoplasmal and trichomonal infections.

Complications

Chlamydial infection may be complicated by acute epididymitis and prostatitis in men; Bartholinitis, cervicitis and salpingitis in women; and in both sexes proctitis, conjunctivitis (due to contamination of the eye with genital secretion), perihepatitis and Reiter's syndrome (see page 247).

Treatment

Oral tetracycline or erythromycin (500 mg four times daily) for 14 days (21 days for complications) is effective. Tetracycline should be taken two hours after meals, which should not include milk or milk products.

Genital herpes

Genital herpes is due to infection with HSV2 or more rarely HSV1, aquired by sexual intercourse.

Clinical features

The incubation period is 2–4 days. Primary infection may be heralded by malaise, fever, headache and pain in the back and buttocks, but the main symptoms are usually in the glans penis and frenal area in men and in women severe dysuria and vaginal discharge. Proctitis may follow anal intercourse in either sex. Examination reveals groups of papules which become vesicular in a day or two and then rupture forming painful ulcers. Spread of infection from the posterior ganglia to the sacral nerve roots may cause transient impotence and impairment of micturition.

Recurrent infection occurs in about half the patients. The relapses, which are shorter and less severe than the first attack, may be precipitated by fever, exposure to UVL, trauma, menstruation or stress.

Treatment

Neonatal herpes occurs in 50 per cent of babies born to women with active genital herpes. Caesarean section should be considered to reduce this risk.

The antiviral drug acyclovir shortens individual attacks (see page 418) and prolonged treatment may reduce the frequency of recurrent attacks.

Molluscum contagiosum

Genital molluscum contagiosum has shown an increase in genitourinary medicine clinics over the last ten years. It is caused by a poxvirus. Small papular lesions occur and are self-limiting. However, it may act as a marker for other more serious sexually transmitted diseases.

Chancroid

Chancroid is very rare in Britain, though it is occasionally seen in seaports. The causative organism in *Haemophilus ducreyi* (Ducrey's bacillus), a Gram-negative bacillus about 1–2 μm in length. It is very common in Africa and South-East Asia.

Clinical features

After an incubation period of 2–14 days one or more small red papules appear on the genitalia or surrounding skin. Within a few days these develop into necrotic ulcers with undermined edges surrounded by an area of erythema and oedema. The inguinal lymph nodes enlarge and sometimes suppurate. The important distinction from syphilis is made by the shorter incubation period, the absence of induration in the lesions, the failure to demonstrate spirochaetes on dark-ground illumination, and identification of Ducrey's bacillus in stained smears and on culture.

Treatment

Tetracycline or sulphonamides are appropriate treatment.

Lymphogranuloma venereum

This is very rare in Britain and is caused by strains of *Chlamydia trachomatis*.

Clinical features

The incubation period is up to three weeks. The initial lesion may be a small vesicle or ulcer on the genitalia, but more often the first evidence of the disease is enlargement of the inguinal lymph nodes. The swelling may become quite massive and eventually suppuration may occur with the discharge of yellow pus through multiple sinuses in the skin. There is often severe constitutional reaction with high fever. In women proctitis and subsequent rectal stricture may occur; sequelae in men include scarring and elephantiasis of the genitalia.

Diagnosis

A positive intradermal Frei test indicates that the patient now has or has had the disease. The *Chlamydia* may be seen in infected tissue or grown on tissue culture and antibodies can be found in the serum.

Treatment

Some success may be achieved with either the sulphonamides or the tetracyclines, or the two drugs may be combined. Fluctuant buboes should be aspirated.

Granuloma inguinale

This is caused by *Calymatobacterium granulomatosis* which produces Donovan bodies in mononuclear cells in the genital lesions. It is endemic in areas of Southern India and the Caribbean. A papule on the penis or labia ulcerates. This ulcer gradually enlarges and local inguinal granulomas occur.

Diagnosis depends on finding Donovan bodies, and then *treatment* is tetracycline, streptomycin or co-trimoxazole.

Further reading

Bannister, B. (1983) *Infectious Diseases*. Baillière Tindall, London.
Christie, A.B. (1980) *Infectious Diseases: Epidemiology and Clinical Practice*, 3rd edn. Churchill Livingstone, Edinburgh.

15
Imported and Tropical Diseases

Over the past few years there has been an increase in the number of patients with imported diseases, and in particular malaria, in the United Kingdom. This increase is related to increasing numbers of people travelling to the tropics, people seeking the sun in winter, immigrants returning to their former homes for holidays, and business travellers. Many travellers to tropical Africa do not appreciate that there is as great a risk of contracting malaria for the unprotected traveller as in the days of David Livingstone and that poor hygienic conditions may expose them to a wide variety of infections. Exotic infections often give rise to symptoms that are indistinguishable from those of common conditions such as influenza. Only the doctor who asks 'Where have you been?' is likely to avoid the occasional disastrous misdiagnosis.

Information on the necessary immunizations and prophylaxis for different countries can be obtained from Tropical Diseases Centres. Some conditions common in the tropics are dealt with elsewhere in this book; for example, AIDS (page 395), tuberculosis (page 108), typhoid (page 422) and venereal diseases (page 431).

Protozoal diseases

Malaria

At present there are about two thousand patients with malaria diagnosed each year in England and Wales. Each year there are several deaths from *falciparum malaria* among non-immune travellers who have failed to come for treatment early enough or whose doctors have not recognized the infection.

Aetiology

Four varieties of malaria parasite infect humans (Table 15.1). The parasites (male and female gametocytes) are taken up in the blood meal when a female *Anopheles* mosquito bites an infected person. The parasites multiply in the mosquito and after eight or more days are transformed into sporozoites in the salivary glands of the mosquito and are capable of transmitting infection when the mosquito bites again. Sporozoites injected into a person pass into the blood stream and are rapidly removed by the liver. Within an hepatocyte the parasite multiplies again to form a shizont. When the shizont is mature it ruptures and releases large numbers of merozoites into the blood stream. Merozoites enter red cells where they grow and multiply to form shizonts which in turn rupture to release merozoites which infect more red cells. After a few days some of the intraerythrocytic parasites differentiate to form gametocytes capable of infecting a mosquito.

Vivax and *Ovale* parasites differ from the other varieties in that some of the sporozoites infecting liver cells may enter a dormant phase for some months (hypnozoites) before they multiply and infect red cells.

Symptoms of malaria only occur when there is a sufficiently heavy infection in red blood cells, this often takes about twelve days from the infected bite with falciparum malaria and rather longer for the other varieties. Because of dormant hypnozoites some strains of Vivax malaria or Ovale malaria produce symptoms eight or more months after infection.

The severity of falciparum malaria is related both to the parasites tendency to produce massive infections involving 20 per cent or more of the patients red cells and the site of shizogony in the small blood vessels of many organs including the brain resulting in anoxia and tissue damage.

Falciparum malaria

Patients with falciparum malaria present with fever and headache and occasionally with vomiting or diarrhoea.

Table 15.1 Malaria parasites

	Hypnozoites	Shizogony in deep tissues	Blood shizogony cycle and fever in late cases
Plasmodium falciparum (malignant tertian)	–	+	36–48 hours
P. vivax (benign tertian)	+	–	48 hours
P. ovale (ovale tertian)	+	–	48 hours
P. malariae (quartan)	–	–	72 hours

The fever is usually irregular and the symptoms are identical with those of influenza during the first few days. After a few days without treatment the patient may suddenly deteriorate with mental confusion progressing rapidly to coma, cough, diarrhoea, the development of slight jaundice and severe anaemia, oliguria or shock.

Whilst falciparum malaria is usually straightforward to treat if diagnosed sufficiently early, once the diagnosis in the non-immune patient has been delayed for a few days the patient may be very difficult to rescue.

On examination the patient is usually febrile or becomes so if the temperature is followed for a few hours. There may be anaemia or jaundice, signs of altered consciousness or an enlarged spleen or liver. In severely ill patients haemorrhages are sometimes found in the optic fundi. Hypoglycaemia is a frequent complication particularly in childhood and gram negative septicaemia occurs ocassionally.

Because of the non-specific nature of the symptoms of falciparum malaria it is essential to have blood films examined at once in any ill person who has been exposed to infection. Thick blood films have the advantage of concentrating parasites so that light infections are much easier to recognize but the most important point is for the examination to be undertaken by someone with experience in recognizing malaria parasites. Haemoglobin values may be low if the infection has been progressing for several days: white cell counts are usually normal but blood platelets may be much reduced.

People who have been heavily exposed to falciparum malaria over many years, usually in childhood, develop a partial *immunity* to the parasite. Thus many adult Africans have only a mild illness when they get falciparum malaria and are termed semi-immunes. Immunity is gradually lost during residence outside a malarious area for longer than a year or two and the person may then develop a sharp attack of malaria if he returns home.

Vivax and ovale malaria

These varieties of malaria are rarely lethal but they do make people feel extremely ill. After a few days of irregular fever the temperature may begin to show a regular pattern of peaks every 48 hours (tertian fever). The febrile periods being with intense feelings of coldness, soon accompanied by shaking chills which may last for several hours, and are followed by a feeling of heat with vasodilatation with which the fever falls accompanied by intense sweating. Between the febrile periods the patient may feel fairly well.

Examination of the patient may show some pallor or splenomegaly but diagnosis is dependant on examination of blood films. It is characteristic of these forms of malaria that they recur weeks or months later if the patient is treated only with a blood shizonticide drug such as chloroquine since these drugs do not deal with hypnozoites in the liver.

Malariae malaria

This is an uncommon imported infection but can persist at a very low level in the blood stream for 40 years. It may cause blood transfusion transmitted malaria long after infection.

Treatment of malaria

Unfortunately falciparum parasites readily develop resistance to antimalarial drugs. Resistance to chloroquine first recognized in South America and South-East Asia is now common in much of East and Central Africa and has been reported from West Africa also. Patients with falciparum malaria who are not immune should therefore be treated with quinine. Quinine may be given by mouth in a dose of 600 mg of salt every eight hours for five days and this is followed by a single dose of pyrimethamine (75 mg) with sulfadoxine (1.5 g; 3 tablets of Fansidar). Patients who are vomiting or show evidence of severe malaria should be given quinine (10 mg/kg) diluted in 250 ml of saline intravenously over about two hours every eight hours until they are well enough to continue treatment by mouth. Patients with highly resistant parasites from Thailand may require a loading dose of 20 mg/kg initially. Patients ill with falciparum malaria are best cared for in an intensive care unit where they can be monitored closely for anaemia, fluid and electrolyte balances, renal failure, hypoglycaemia, respiratory failure and state of consciousness.

Semi-immune patients from West Africa can still be safely treated with chloroquine by mouth; 600 mg chloroquine base is given initially followed by a further 300 mg after six hours and then 300 mg daily for three days.

Patients with vivax or ovale malaria are first treated with chloroquine in the same dose as above, this is sufficient to kill the blood stages of the parasite and hence cure the current symptoms. However the malaria may well relapse unless the patient is also given a course of primaquine. Before giving the primaquine the patient's blood should be tested for glucose-6-phosphate dehydrogenase deficiency (G6PD) since deficient patients may develop severe haemolysis with this drug. The usual adult dose of primaquine is 7.5 mg twice daily for 14 days by mouth. Patients infected in the Pacific islands or South-East Asia are given treatment for 21 days. Chloroquine alone is sufficient to treat patients with malariae malaria.

Malaria prophylaxis in travellers

People travelling to malarious areas must be protected against malaria. With increasing resistance of malaria parasites to drugs (Fig. 15.1) it is now much more difficult to ensure freedom from malaria, and travellers to such areas as East Africa or rural South East Asia must understand that no drug combination is now certain to protect them and they must therefore take simple precautions against mosquito bites and must report quickly for medical attention should they develop a fever. Precautions against mosquito bite include sleeping in a screened room or using a bed net, wearing trousers and long sleeves if out of doors after dusk, and using an insect repellant on any exposed skin.

In most malarious areas at present the best balance of safety and protection is given by taking both chloroquine and proguanil together. Chloroquine is given as 300 mg base once a week and proguanil as 200 mg daily after food. Chloroquine prophylaxis should be started at least a week before exposure and both drugs must be continued for at least four weeks after the last exposure. A new drug, mefloquine, may soon become available in the UK and shows promise of greater protection against falciparum malaria in areas resistant to other drugs.

Some of the other tropical infections which may cause fever are summarized in Table 15.2.

Trypanosomiasis

Trypanosomes are *flagellate* protozoa which produce two main types of disease, African trypanosomiasis (sleeping

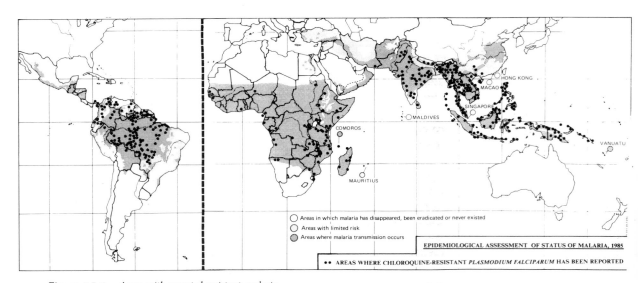

Figure 15.1   *Areas with reported resistant malaria.*
Based on: WHO, Vaccination Certificate Requirements and Health Advice for International Travel, 1987

Table 15.2 'Tropical' fevers in travellers

Disease	Epidemiology	Clinical features	Tests
Malaria	Tropics, bite of anopheline mosquito	Undifferentiated fever, later stupor, anaemia, shock (falciparum) regular rigors (vivax)	Blood films
Dengue viruses types 1–4	Tropics, bite of Aedes mosquito; sometimes epidemic; incubation period 5–6 days	Fever for about 5 days; severe headache; retro-orbital pain; lymphadenopathy; skin rash on third day; rarely haemorrhages and shock	Leucopenia Serology
Lassa fever virus	Rural West or Central Africa or hospital workers exposed to rodent urine or blood of patients; incubation period 6–21 days	Persistent fever with severe malaise; pharyngeal exudate; swollen face, stupor and hypotension. ISOLATION NEEDED	Leucopenia Virus isolation, or serology. DANGER
Tick typhus *Rickettsia conori*	Mediterranean, South and East Africa; bite of hard tick	Small black ulcer where tick bit; generalized maculopapular erythematous rash from fourth day	Serology
Typhoid fever	Worldwide	Headache; persistent fever; abdominal discomfort; splenomegaly; rose spots	Leucopenia Blood culture
Amoebic liver abscess	Worldwide but chiefly tropics	Persistent fever; right upper abdominal pain and tenderness signs at right lung base	Polymorph Leucocytosis Ultrasound of liver. Serology
African trypanosomiasis *Trypanosoma rhodesiense*	Vistors to African game parks; tsetse fly bite	Tachycardia, lymphadenopathy, splenomegaly, transient oedema and erythematous skin rashes anaemia, encephalopathy	Thick blood films Serology
Visceral leishmaniasis *Leishmania donovani*	Mediterranean Middle East, India, East Africa, and South America. Sand fly bite	Persistent fever and wasting in a relatively well person Progressive splenomegaly; Anaemia and lymphadenopathy; Infants affected in Mediterranean countries	Leucopenia Bone marrow Microscopy and culture serology
Acute schistosomiasis mansoni	Bathing in infected fresh water	Persistent fever; urticaria diarrhoea; liver and splenic enlargement; cough	Eosinophilia Ova in stool serology

sickness) and American trypanosomiasis (Chaga's disease).

African trypanosomiasis (sleeping sickness)

There are two clinical varieties of sleeping sickness caused by subspecies of *Trypanosoma brucei*. Gambian sleeping sickness caused by *T. brucei gambiense* is found in West and Central Africa from Sudan to Angola, it is a slowly developing illness. Rhodesian sleeping sickness due to *T. brucei rhodesiense* is usually an acute illness and occurs in East Africa from Ethiopia to Botswana. These trypa-

nosomes are transmitted from the bites of infected tsetse flies, with different species of fly involved with the two varieties.

Trypanosomes are injected into the skin where a boil-like chancre sometimes forms a few days after the bite. Trypanosomes quickly spread to the blood and reticulo-endothelial tissues. Recurrent fever, enlargement of lymph nodes especially those at the back of the neck, transient oedematous swellings and erythematous rashes are features of this stage of the disease. Invasion of the central nervous system may present years after the initial infection. At this stage complaints are of headache, depression, daytime sleepiness or intellectual deterioration. With rhodesiense infections the disease is acute with high fever, anaemia, hepato-splenomegaly and myocarditis and the rapid development of meningo-encephalitis.

The diagnosis is suggested by the patient having lived in or travelled to an endemic focus and by a positive fluorescent antibody or card agglutination test. Confirmation by finding trypanosomes in the blood, lymph node aspirate or cerebro-spinal fluid is necessary.

Pentamidine is an effective *treatment* for gambian disease and suramin for either variety provided invasion of the central nervous system has not taken place. Once there are signs of neurological disease, or a raised protein content, or cell count in the cerebro-spinal fluid, cure depends upon the use of the toxic arsenical preparation melarsoprol.

American trypanosomiasis (Chaga's disease)

Chaga's disease is widespread in South and Central America where in some foci it is the commonest cause of heart disease. *Trypanosoma cruzi* is transmitted to humans in the faeces of cone-nosed triatomid bugs which live in roofs and walls of houses. Infection enters via the conjunctiva or by scratching through the skin.

Most *T. cruzi* infections are asymptomatic but some, especially in children, cause an acute illness with a local swelling or periorbital oedema at the site of entry, lymphadenopathy, fever and in a minority of cases meningo-encephalitis. Trypanosomes are present in the blood at this stage.

Chronic Chaga's disease involves the myocardium producing ECG abnormalities, arrhythmias, heart failure, systemic emboli and sometimes sudden death. In other patients the myenteric plexus of the gut is involved and mega oesophagus or mega colon may ensue. Diagnosis in the chronic stage chiefly depends upon positive serological tests such as complement fixation or ELISA tests.

The *treatment* of Chaga's disease remains unsatisfactory. In the acute disease nifurtimox or benznidazole are useful but anti-parasitic treatment is ineffective in the chronic stage.

Leishmaniasis

Leishmaniae are protozoa which are spread by the bites of sandflies. The main forms are visceral leishmaniasis and cutaneous leishmaniasis which has several varieties.

Visceral leishmaniasis (kala-azar)

Visceral leishmaniasis is caused by *Leishmania donovani* and is found in parts of Asia including Bihar State, India, the Mediterranean coast, East and North Africa and parts of South America especially Brazil. Mediterranean visceral leishmaniasis is chiefly a disease of infants. Occasionally there is a small skin lesion at the site of the infected bite but more usually the first sign of disease is a continued fever which develops months or even years later. The parasites are taken up in the reticulo-endothelial system and progressive splenic enlargement is characteristic. The liver enlarges more slowly and sometimes lymph nodes are also involved. Anaemia, cough, diarrhoea and weight loss are frequently present. Sometimes after treatment skin lesions known as post kala azar dermal leishmaniasis appear.

There is usually a striking leucopenia and serological tests including indirect immunofluorescence or ELISA tests are very helpful. However a definite diagnosis depends upon finding the rounded amastigote form of the parasite within macrophages. Sometimes amastigotes can be found in buffy coat preparations of the blood but more often prolonged search of the bone marrow aspirate (80 per cent positive) or splenic aspirate (95 per cent positive) are necessary.

Treatment is with pentavalent antimony preparations such as sodium stibogluconate given intravenously.

Cutaneous leishmaniasis

In parts of the Middle East, Mediterranean countries and Central Asia *Leishmania major* causes a slowly growing papule which ulcerates and eventually heals spontaneously. Multiple lesions and local lymphadenopathy are common. *L. aethiopica* in North East Africa causes similar lesions or occasionally very chronic diffuse cutaneous lesions. When *treatment* is needed local excision or pentavalent antimony is used.

Cutaneous leishmaniasis in Central and South America is a complex of different infections but most are related to *L. mexicana* which causes ulcers like those of the Old World leishmanias except when it involves the cartilage of the ear when very chronic destructive lesions occur. *Leishmania braziliensis* parasites are also widespread and are noted for causing muco-cutaneous leishmaniasis or espundia with 'metastases' to the muco-cutaneous junctions of the nose and mouth sometimes many years after an apparently innocent self-healing leishmanial ulcer on a limb. This late involvement of the naso-pharynx causes slowly progressive tissue destruction which can be very mutilating and lead to death from aspiration

Table 15.3 Causes of diarrhoea in travellers

	Fever	Abdominal pain	Other features	Diagnostic tests
Simple diarrhoea				
Enteropathogenic E. coli	+/−	+/−	−	Stool culture
Giardiasis	−	−	Gaseous distension; frothy stool	Stool microscopy
Campylobacter	+/−	+	Sometimes blood in stool	Stool culture
Salmonella enteritis	+/−	+/−	'Food poisoning'; may be others affected	Stool culture
Falciparum malaria	++	+/−	−	Blood film
Viral infection (especially rotavirus)	+/−	+/−	Usually in young children	Stool electron microscopy or serology
Cholera	−	−	Rice water stools; muscle cramps; severe vomiting; shock	Stool culture
Dysentery				
Shigellosis	+	+	Rapid onset; frequent stools and tenesmus	Stool culture
Amoebic dysentery	−	+/−	Slow onset; often mild but recurrent	Stool microscopy of fresh, warm specimen
Schistosomiasis (mansoni or japonicum)	+/−	+	Only in heavily infected individuals	Stool microscopy or rectal snip
Trichuris infection	−	+/−	Rare; seen only in heavily infected children who are also anaemic	Stool microscopy

penumonia. At this stage amastigotes are usually impossible to find in the tissues but serological tests are positive.

Treatment of the American forms of cutaneous leishmaniasis is also with pentavalent antimony preparations.

Diarrhoeal diseases

Diarrhoea is an extremely common symptom among travellers returning from the tropics especially among those who have visited Asia. Some of the common causes are shown in Table 15.3.

Traveller's diarrhoea

Many travellers experience the sudden onset of diarrhoea with stomach cramps and often brief fever at the onset, together with nausea and/or vomiting. Colourful names such as Delhi belly or Montezuma's revenge attempt to disguise the misery these attacks cause.

A variety of organisms may cause attacks, including viruses such as rotavirus and food poisoning organisms such as Salmonellae; but most often they are due to enteropathogenic strains of *Escherischia coli*. The attacks are usually self-limiting and the only *treatment* needed is maintenance of hydration by drinking a glucose electrolyte solution with the use of an anti-diarrhoeal drug such as loperamide if needed for social convenience.

Culture of the stool will sometimes show other bacteria, such as a *Campylobacter* or *Shigella*, which may require specific treatment.

Prevention of traveller's diarrhoea depends upon careful avoidance of foods or fluids which are likely to be contaminated, including unboiled water, ice in drinks, salads, cold meats and shellfish; and sticking to bottled or boiled fluids and hot foods. Prophylactic antibiotics will often reduce the incidence of traveller's diarrhoea by about a third but they carry risks of the development of bacterial resistance and of toxicity. They are probably not advisable for the great majority of travellers.

Bacillary dysentery (shigellosis)

Infection with dysentery bacilli often leads to an acute febrile illness with severe abdominal colic, tenesmus and the passage of frequent stools which are watery at first but later contain fresh blood and mucus. The patient may be ill and toxic with a rapid pulse and signs of dehydration. Young children often suffer from convulsions. There are four groups of dysentery Shigellae: group A, *Shigella dysenteriae*, group B *S. flexneri*, group C *S. boydii* and group D *S. sonnei*. Severe attacks of dysentery are most often associated with organisms in the first three groups and in particular with *S. dysenteriae* type 1.

Sonnei dysentery is common among British children especially among pre-school and nursery classes. It usually gives rise to mild watery diarrhoea without blood in the stools.

The dysentery organisms are spread by the faeco-oral route and especially by unwashed hands, so they spread very readily in unhygienic conditions. Infection can be initiated by as few as 100 organisms. The incubation period is usually 1–3 days.

Antibiotic *treatment* is needed in severe infections and may help to render the patient non-infectious in milder cases also. Unfortunately Shigellae easily acquire resistance to many antibiotics and during the last decade there have been very severe epidemics of multiple antibiotic-resistant shigellosis in a number of developing countries with many deaths. Whilst some Shigellae remain sensitive to ampicillin or co-trimoxazole, others will only respond to treatment with nalidixic acid or ciprofloxacin. Rehydration by mouth is also needed.

Giardiasis

Giardia lamblia is a single-cell flagellate organism which lives in the human small intestine attached to the mucosa by a small sucking disc. It produces resistant cysts which are passed in the faeces and infect others through contaminated water or food. Giardia infection is sometimes found in people who have been infected in Britain but it is much commoner among travellers; Leningrad is a city where many travellers have been infected in recent years.

Many Giardia infections are asymptomatic, but people commonly develop diarrhoea a week or two after infection. There is often gaseous distension of the abdomen and the passage of stools which are frothy or sometimes fatty in consistency. Some patients may lose a considerable amount of weight, although most will recover spontaneously over a period of several weeks or months.

Diagnosis is by finding the cysts in fresh stool specimens but cysts are sometimes only passed intermittently and are not always present in the stools at the onset of symptoms. Duodenal intubation to find the active trophozoites, small bowel biopsy or serological tests are sometimes used.

Treatment with metronidazole at a dose of 2 g once daily for three days in an adult is usually successful. Remind anyone taking metronidazole to keep off alcohol as severe reactions like those experienced with antibuse are common.

Amoebiasis

The single-cell organism *Entamoeba histolytica* lives in the human large intestine where it is usually harmless. Certain strains of this organism, in association with colonic bacteria, can invade the wall of the gut causing submucosal necrosis and flask-shaped ulcers with amoebae in their walls. On occasion amoebae are carried in the portal vein to the liver where they may cause hepatic necrosis and a *liver abscess*. Infection is spread by the formation of cysts in the large gut; these cysts are quite resistant in the environment and if hygiene is poor they are able to infect food or water.

Amoebic dysentery

We do not understand why previously harmless amoebae decide to stop browsing on the surface of the gut and invade the mucosa. Invasion seems to be limited to certain types of parasite, as shown by biochemical tests; but it is sometimes induced by immunosuppressive drugs such as prednisone, and may occur in pregnant women or severely malnourished children.

The symptoms of amoebic dysentery usually consist of episodes of rather mild diarrhoea with blood and mucus in the stool, without fever, alternating with periods of constipation. Sometimes there is fulminating dysentery with fever and a very ill patient who may die from perforation of the large gut.

The condition must be differentiated from bacillary dysentery due to *Shigellae* which usually begins abruptly and causes severe abdominal pain with tenesmus (painful defaecation) and high fever. The other chief differential diagnosis is ulcerative colitis.

The diagnosis of amoebic dysentery depends upon examining very fresh warm specimens of faeces under the microscope. The presence of active amoebic trophozoites containing ingested red blood cells is diagnostic. The presence of cysts of *E. histolytica* in the stool is not sufficient evidence to diagnose invasive amoebiasis since they are present as commensals in so many patients.

Amoebic liver abscess

Patients with an amoebic liver abscess often give no history of dysentery, but rather present with fever and pain over the liver or referred to the shoulder tip because of diaphragmatic irritation. The chief physical sign is the presence of a point of tenderness over the liver either beneath the costal margin or intercostal. If no such tenderness can be elicited a slight jarring impact to the chest wall may induce pain. There is usually a polymorphonuclear leucocytosis, and if the abscess has been present for long the patient may be anaemic.

A chest X-ray will frequently show a raised right hemidiaphragm with an overlying area of pleural reaction, and an ultrasound examination of the liver will usually show an abscess cavity. The most useful specific test is a serological test for amoebic antibodies, such as an indirect immunofluorescence test which nearly always shows a high titre.

A neglected amoebic abscess can rupture into any contiguous structure. Rupture into the pericardium or peritoneum is often life threatening. Rupture through the diaphragm into the lung often results in the patient coughing out large quantities of amoebic 'pus'—pinkish brown necrotic liver tissue which is traditionally likened to anchovy sauce. Rupture outwards through the intercostal spaces looks at first like a large subcutaneous abscess, but should the amoebae invade the skin a foul spreading ulcer can result.

Treatment of amoebiasis

Amoebic dysentery responds to treatment with oral metronidazole (800 mg 8-hourly) for five days, but since metronidazole acts best against those amoebae which are invading the tissues and is less effective against amoebae free in the gut lumen, it is wise to follow this course with 5–10 days of diloxanide fuorate (500 mg 8-hourly) by mouth. In patients with severe dysentery a short course of oral tetracycline helps to produce rapid improvement. Patients without symptoms who wish to be cleared of infection may be given diloxanide alone.

Amoebic liver abscess also usually responds promptly to treatment with metronidazole. Occasional patients who do not respond fully to metronidazole will need the more toxic drug emetine hydrochloride by intramuscular injection. It is always wise to clear the gut of any possible amoebic infection as well, since rarely there are recurrences of amoebic abscesses. A 10-day course of diloxanide is usually given.

Table 15.3 (page 441) summarizes some of the important causes of diarrhoea and dysentery.

Chronic diarrhoea

Persistent diarrhoea in people returning from the tropics is often due to giardiasis or amoebic infection. Sometimes it results from lactose intolerance following an acute attack of enteritis, in which case the patient may notice that his diarrhoea worsens after drinking milk; the stools tested for reducing substances with Clinitest will give a positive result for lactose. Persistent dysentery is sometimes due to inflammatory bowel disease which has been unmasked by an acute infection; but this diagnosis must only be made after firmly excluding amoebiasis, since steroids may cause a severe exacerbation of amoebic infections. Tuberculous enteritis is a diagnosis to consider in an immigrant with persistent diarrhoea; there may be evidence of pulmonary or lymph node tuberculosis. A barium follow-through examination of the small gut will show the tuberculous involvement.

Steatorrhoea in people who have travelled in Asia or the West Indies is occasionally due to tropical sprue. This condition of uknown cause must only be diagnosed if there is definite evidence of malabsorption of at least two substances, such as fat, xylose or vitamin B_{12}, and if other causes of malabsorption, including gluten enteropathy, have been excluded.

Helminth infections

Schistosomiasis

Schistosomiasis or Bilharzia is an infection with a fluke which lives in the blood stream and produces eggs. Immunological reactions to the eggs and their products cause symptoms. There are three varieties of schistosomes: *Schistosoma haematobium*, which causes urinary schistosomiasis and lives in the vesical venous plexus; *S. mansoni*, the cause of intestinal schistosomiasis, which lives in the portal venous system; and *S. japonicum*, the cause of oriental schistosomiasis, the last is somewhat similar to mansoni infection, but is rarely imported into the UK and will not be considered further.

All varieties are acquired by bathing in fresh water, where the infective cercarial forms of the schistosomes are released by their snail intermediate hosts and swim to penetrate the skin. Both *S. haematobium* and *S. mansoni* infections are prevalent in tropical Africa and the Middle East, and the latter infection is also found in parts of South America.

Urinary schistosomiasis

This usually presents as haematuria. The patient complains of passing blood at the end of micturition and sometimes of some frequency and pain on passing water. Obstructive uropathy from granulomatous masses in the bladder can occur but is unusual in the lightly infected traveller. Diagnosis is by finding the terminal spined eggs in centrifuged urine. The urine is best collected around mid-day.

Intestinal schistosomiasis

This sometimes causes a febrile illness with vomiting, diarrhoea, enlargement of liver and spleen and marked eosinophilia in the recently infected expatriate. Many light infections are asymptomatic, but heavy infections may cause a chronic dysenteric illness with large gut polyps or portal fibrosis of the liver which presents very like cirrhosis with portal hypertension, bleeding oesophageal varices and ascites.

The diagnosis is made by finding eggs with a spine at the side in concentrated faecal specimens, or by taking a small specimen of rectal mucosa and pressing it between two microscope slides which will allow any eggs to be seen under the microscope. Immunological tests such as ELISA are often helpful.

Treatment of schistosomiasis is now straightforward since all varieties respond to the oral drug praziquantel.

Intestinal worms

Most worm infections are asymptomatic. They are only of much importance if many worms are present, and since travellers are usually only lightly infected their chief impact is psychological rather than medical. The chief exception to this statement is with *Strongyloides stercoralis* which can cause autoinfection of the host and is thus both capable of maintaining itself in people for at least 40 years, and is also able to kill immunosuppressed individuals by massive generalized infections and consequent gram negative septicaemia. Strongyloides infections are found throughout the tropics and are especially prevalent among former Far East prisoners of war of the Japanese who were infected whilst working on the notorious Siam–Burma railway during the Second World War. People who have lived in the tropics must be carefully screened before undertaking organ transplantations because of the immunosuppressant drugs used.

Strongyloides infections are often asymptomatic, but they can cause abdominal pain similar to that of a peptic ulcer, diarrhoea which is sometimes fatty, and most commonly in the former traveller a characteristic skin rash. This rash, which is due to migrating larvae, presents as an itchy erythematous or urticarial serpiginous moving track which elongates by about 1–2 cm per hour and lasts for a day or two only to recur weeks or months later.

Infections with strongyloides are diagnosed by finding active larvae in the stool on microscopy or simple culture or, since larvae are often only intermittently present, by serological tests for antibodies. Strongyloides infections are usually treated with thiabendazole by mouth.

Enterobius vermicularis, the common threadworm, is found in many British people who have never been abroad. The female adult worms lay eggs on the skin around the anus and these eggs easily contaminate dust or fingers and are then passed on to others by mouth or inhalation. Intense anal itching especially at night is the main symptom but sometimes parents see the threadlike females on their children's anal area. Diagnosis can be confirmed by applying sticky Scotch tape to the anal area and then examining the tape microscopically for the characteristic eggs. This infection is nearly always present in the entire family even though only one person has symptoms. The whole family needs treatment: a single dose of mebendazole (100 mg) by mouth is effective, but should be repeated after a fortnight. This drug may be embryotoxic, so it should not be given to pregnant women or children under three years of age.

In many areas of the world worms such as the roundworm *Ascaris lumbricoides*, the whipworm *Trichuris trichiuria* and hookworms *Necator americanus* and *Ancylostoma duodenale* are very common. Light infections such as those often picked up by visitors to the tropics very rarely cause any symptoms, though on rare occasions a roundworm may migrate into the biliary tree and cause biliary colic. Heavy infections with roundworms can cause intestinal obstruction in young children and heavy hookworm infections cause iron deficiency anaemia because the worms suck blood.

Some details of intestinal worm infections are given in Table 15.4.

Filariasis

There are several varieties of filariasis caused by different filarial roundworms. Biting insects are the vectors.

Lymphatic filariasis is caused by *Wucheraria bancrofti* or *Brugia malayi*. Attacks of fever with lymphangitis and painful lymphadenopathy develop after an incubation period of about a year. Chronic infections can cause fibrosis obstructing the lymphatics and result in

Table 15.4 Intestinal worms and clinical features

	Mode of infection	Position of worm	Clinical features	Diagnosis
Ascaris lumbricoides (large roundworm)	Faeco-oral	Small gut	Colic, biliary obstruction	Stool microscopy
Trichus trichuria (whipworm)	Faeco-oral	Large gut	Dysentery, anaemia	
Necator americanus (hookworm)	Larval skin penetration	Small gut	Anaemia	
Ancylostoma duodenale				
Strongyloides stercoralis				
Enterobius vermicularis (threadworm)	Faeco-oral	Rectum	Diarrhoea, rash Anal itching	Stool culture Scoth tape
Taenia saginata (beef tapeworm)	Eating undercooked beef	Small gut	Passage of segments per anum	Stool microscopy
Taenia solium (pork tapeworm)	Eating undercooked pork	Small gut	Passage of segments per anum; danger of self-infection and cerebral cysticercosis presenting with fits	Stool microscopy

hydrocoele or chronic lymphoedema and elephantiasis of the leg. Diagnosis depends upon finding a marked eosinophilia and the demonstration of microfilariae in blood specimens taken during the night when they are released into the bloodstream. Treatment is with diethylcarbamazine.

Tropical eosinophilia (see page 99) is also due to the lymphatic filariae and presents with bronchospasm and pulmonary infiltrates. There is a very high eosinophil count.

Loa loa infections occur only in West and Central Africa. The adult worms live in the subcutaneous tissues and can sometimes be seen crossing the conjuctiva of the eye. Microfilariae are seen in daytime blood specimens. Calabar swellings are warm irritating subcutaneous swellings often occurring on the limbs where adult worms are passing.

Onchocerciasis occurs in tropical Africa and in foci in Central and South America. Adult worms live in the subcutaneous tissues and sometimes cause painless subcutaneous nodules. Microfilariae occur in the skin and the eye. Severe skin itching which results in lichenification and skin atrophy is common but the importance of the infection is that it is a major cause of blindness.

Hydatid disease

Hydatid disease results from the development in man of the larval or intermediate form of the dog tapeworm, *Echinococcus granulosus*. It is found throughout the world, mostly in association with sheep or cattle farming (patients are sometimes infected in Wales). Adult worms live in the intestine of dogs. Eggs are passed out in dog faeces and ingested by sheep, cows or other animals. Cysts develop in the tissues of these animals and when they are eaten by dogs the cycle is complete.

People are infected by eating vegetables contaminated by dog faeces or from eggs adhering to the hands after stroking a dog. Eggs hatch in the intestine and larvae pass through the portal system to the liver. Most cysts develop in the liver but cysts may also grow in the lung, kidney, bone, brain or other organ. Cysts grow slowly and are often asymptomatic but may produce symptoms from local pressure. Rupture into the peritoneal or pleural cavity sometimes occurs.

A calcified round lesion in the liver or lung may be seen on routine radiological examination and may be diagnostic. Ultrasound examination of the liver is very helpful. There is sometimes an eosinophilia and serological tests including complement fixation and immunodiffusion tests are usually positive. Aspiration of cysts is dangerous because it may spread daughter cysts and because there is sometimes an anaphylactic reaction to release of cyst contents.

Drug *treatment* is still uncertain in its effects but prolonged courses of albendazole are promising and this drug is also used to cover surgical treatment. Operative treatment is warranted only in symptomatic disease of the liver or for lung involvement.

Table 15.5 Tropical skin rashes

	Geography	Mode of infection	Clinical features	Tests
Rashes with itching: Fungal infections	All	Contact	Plaque with raised margin	Skin scrape, microscopy and culture
Scabies (*Sarcoptes scabei*)	All	Contact	Burrows; papules of fingers; genitalia and buttocks	Needle burrow for mite, response to benzyl benzoate or malathion 0.5% solution
Larva migrans	All	Larval skin penetration	Slowly moving red track; usually on foot	Response to 10% thiabendazole cream
Strongyloides rash	All	Larval skin penetration	Rapidly moving red or urticarial track on trunk	Stool microscopy or culture serology
Onchocerciasis	Africa; C. and S. America	Bite of Simulium black fly	Subcutaneous nodules; skin atrophy; eye corneal opacities and microfilariae	Skin snips for microfilariae
Itching not prominant: Leprosy (*Mycobacterium leprae*)	All	Inhalation	Tuberculoid form: anaesthetic patches; enlarged nerves. Lepromatous form: thickened or nodular skin	Slit skin smears for bacilli, biopsy
Leishmaniasis	Middle-East; N. Africa; C. and S. America	Bite of sand fly	Single or multiple nodules which slowly ulcerate to give ulcer with raised edge	Smears from edge of ulcer for amastigotes

Leprosy

Leprosy is caused by the acid fast bacillus *Mycobacterium leprae* and is contracted by exposure to people with multibacillary disease probably by inhalation of material from nasal secretions. This bacillus can still not be cultured on artificial media. Leprosy is widespread in the tropics but fortunately it is not as infectious as many other diseases.

The incubation period varies from a few months to more than ten years. The response to leprosy infection depends greatly upon the persons cell-mediated immune defences; with excellent defences no recognizable disease results.

Tuberculoid leprosy

This occurs when there is a reasonable immune response and few leprosy bacilli survive. There are small numbers of well demarcated skin patches which appear reddish in light skinned people but pale in those with darker skins. These patches show reduced sweating and loss of temperature and pin prick sensation. Nerves near the skin patches or other superficial nerves are often enlarged.

Skin smears are usually negative for acid fast bacilli but skin biopsies show typical granulomatous changes.

Lepromatous leprosy

This occurs in people who are unable to mount an effective immune response, and vast numbers of leprosy bacilli can be found throughout the body. Diffuse symmetrical skin lesions occur; these may be poorly defined macules, diffuse infiltrates or nodules. The nodules are often best seen on the face or around the ear lobes. The nasal mucosa and the eyes are often involved. Nerves although infected with many bacteria do not show evidence of damage until late in the disease.

Borderline leprosy

This is intermediate between the other two forms and is the commonest variety of leprosy. There are moderate numbers of bacilli in the skin lesions and nerve involvement is often prominent.

Various forms of immunological reaction occur in leprosy and produce worsening of skin lesions and more importantly often rapidly progressive nerve damage. *Erythema nodosum leprosum* is a type-III immunological reaction which occurs in about 50 per cent of patients with lepromatous leprosy during treatment and causes fever, joint pains and painful red skin nodules.

Lepromatous leprosy is *treated* with a combination of rifampicin, dapsone and clofazamine for at least two years and preferably until all skin smears are repeatedly negative. *Tuberculoid leprosy* may be treated with dapsone (100 mg) daily and rifampicin (600 mg) once a month for six months. The early recognition of nerve lesions, giving steroid treatment for acute reactions and education of the patient to avoid damage to anaesthetic extremities is also extremely important.

Table 15.5 gives a summary of some of the commoner skin infections seen in travellers from the tropics.

Rabies (see also page 222)

Rabies is caused by a rhabdovirus which causes an encephalomyelitis which is nearly always fatal in humans. It is widespread throughout most of the world but in the United Kingdom only occasional imported cases occur. Transmission is through the bite of an infected animal, usually a dog, but in some areas wild animals such as foxes, skunks and bats.

The incubation period varies from a few weeks to several years and the initial symptoms include renewed discomfort at the site of the bite, fever, myalgia and headache. 'Furious rabies' is the commonest form with agitation and painful spasms of the pharynx and larynx on attempting to drink (hydrophobia). Hallucinations and confusion ensue and, on examination, there is spasticity and sympathetic overactivity. Death usually occurs in about two weeks from respiratory or cardiac arrest. Paralytic rabies presents a progressive ascending paralysis from the site of the bite. It is the usual form seen after the bite of an infected bat. Spread occurs to involve all voluntary muscles.

Diagnosis depends on the history of a bite and the clinical picture. Fluorescent antibodies can be used to demonstrate rabies antigen in tissues or secretions.

Prevention depends upon careful cleansing of any animal bite and the use of human diploid cell rabies vaccine for anyone who may have been exposed to the virus through a bite or saliva contaminating a skin defect. Any person who had such exposure to a known rabid animal or who has severe wounds or wounds involving the face or hand should also be given rabies immune globulin. A dog which has bitten a person should be kept under observation for at least ten days and not killed immediately. If the dog survives and remains well it is unlikely to have rabies and the immunization series can be stopped.

There is no satisfactory treatment for rabies. Sedation is needed and ventilatory support may keep the patient alive for a while but very rarely saves him.

Rickettsial infections

The small bacteria of the Rickettsia group are spread by ticks, lice and fleas. The most important condition is epidemic typhus. It is characterized by fever, headache, malaise. A macular rash develops and becomes purpuric. After 5 to 7 days central nervous system features develop with stupor and coma. Other organs such as the heart, lungs and kidneys may be involved.

Other rickettsial infections are Rocky Mountain spotted fever, scrub typhus and rickettsial pox. The related organism *Coxiella burnetti* produces Q fever in which the main features are fever, pneumonia and endocarditis. Spread between animals, i.e. by ticks but spread to man, i.e by aerosol or infected milk.

Diagnosis

This is made serologically (the Weil-Felix reaction for Rickettsia).

Treatment

Chloramphenicol is used for Rickettsial infection or tetracycline which is the first choice for Q fever.

Further reading

Manson-Bahr, P.E.C., Bell, D. *Manson's Tropical Diseases*, 19th edn. London: Baillière Tindall.

16
Psychiatric Disorders

Introduction

Psychiatry is concerned with difficult, distressing or eccentric behaviour viewed from a medical aspect. The term 'behaviour' is broad, including everything people do, think and say, and behaviour problems may arise in connection with any illness. There is no absolute division between those problems that count as 'psychiatric' and others dealt with within other branches of medicine; but psychiatrists tend to be asked to deal with the more spectacular or difficult behaviour problems. The separation of part of medicine with special interest in this field is an ancient practice that began when primitive medicine-men tried to explain odd or eccentric behaviour as punishment inflicted by the Gods for misdeeds. In ancient Greece and Rome 'madness' was regarded as illness; but this idea was lost in the Middle Ages when insanity was attributed to demonic possession. By the nineteenth century humane views had revived, and deluded and disturbed people were again seen as ill and in need of care.

During the past century knowledge of psychiatric disorder has increased enormously, being derived from several separate but complementary points of view. The description of clinical symptoms and signs, based on careful observation in the Hippocratic tradition, led to the identification of syndromes by Kraepelin, Bleuler and others which form the basis of current psychiatric classification. Psychological understanding was increased by the work of Freud, Jung and other psychoanalysts and latterly by contributions from social, behavioural and experimental psychologists. At the same time, developments in neurosciences have greatly increased knowledge of biological aspects of psychiatry and of drugs that may affect psychiatric illness. There has also been continuing interest in the ways in which a psychiatric patient may respond to his environment—for better or worse—both in hospital and in the community, where treatment efforts are increasingly directed.

Psychiatric assessment

General considerations

In psychiatry the task is to understand the patient and his problem, and to make sense of his behaviour. This is done by history taking and examination as elsewhere in medicine, except that in psychiatry, examination is principally by observation during clinical interviewing. Clinical interviewing skills are therefore especially important in psychiatry.

Psychiatric assessment, based on history taking and examination, has four parts which then together form the basis of management.

Description

This is a summary of the significant symptoms and signs (often called phenomena in psychiatry) noted on psychiatric examination. It comes first because description should precede explanation. It is not very sensible to try to explain something without clearly defining what it is that has to be explained. Thus a complaint of 'depression', for example, should not just be taken at its face value, but explored in detail. It might refer, among other things, to tearfulness, worrying thoughts, indecisiveness, constipation, disturbing memories, etc. To put it another way, what the problem behaviour *is* should be clearly identified before attempts are made to account for it. What the symptoms are and how they are elicited are discussed later.

Diagnosis

This comes next because diagnosis in psychiatry is based on the identification of syndromes according to agreed rules of thumb (set out in various official diagnostic manuals in general use). Syndromes are collections of phenomena, so that the psychiatric diagnosis represents a further summary of examination findings. Psychiatric diagnosis is important because it (a) is a communicable summary of examination findings, (b) can indicate important things that the patient does not have, and (c) can provide some (even though often limited) pointers towards treatment and prognosis. Diagnosis has sometimes been devalued in psychiatry by people who expect it to do what the problem formulation more appropriately does.

Problems

One purpose of the psychiatric interview is to arrive at statements of the patient's problems which are useful in that they suggest and inform action. A similar principle underpins the problem-oriented approach developed in internal medicine by L. Weed in the USA in the early 1970s. In psychiatry the idea is to find the form of words that makes most sense of present problems to both patient and interviewer. The psychiatric interviewer should be able flexibly to approach the patient's problems in psychological, biological or social terms as seems most appropriate, and to talk about problems in ordinary language intelligible to the patient. No single conceptual framework (brain chemistry, psychoanalysis, etc.) is appropriate in all psychiatric circumstances.

In a way, the problem formulation is like the descriptive one, in that each problem statement is a summary of observable 'things that happen'. 'Problems' are, however, broader than symptoms and signs, and although a descriptive diagnostic syndrome is sometimes also usefully called a problem (e.g. the problem of a depressive neurotic syndrome requiring treatment), many problems requiring clinical attention are not syndromes of illness. Thus a person with a depression problem may also have 'inadequate housing including poor washing facilities', 'the problem of coping with educationally backward child', and 'the problem of indecision about contraceptive preferences'.

Explanation

This is an attempt to account for the symptoms, signs and problems that have been identified, indicating how they have arisen and how they may be linked together. This account again often needs to include psychological, biological and social aspects. The explanatory account should make sense to the interviewer and to the patient, with whom it should often be shared. For instance, the 'explanation' in a patient with a 'depression problem' might note long-standing inferiority feelings derived from childhood experience, a genetic predisposition to depression evidenced by a history of depression in a parent and grandparent, and several stressful recent events implicating the idea of loss, such as the death of a pet dog, the departure of a grown-up child from home, and theft of the family car.

Management

The above four aspects of assessment together form a sound basis for a comprehensive plan of management. However, the preparation of a *comprehensive* management plan may take a considerable time, and require a range of investigations. But a key idea in the problem-oriented approach is that problem statements should be based on a specified database; if the database is incomplete then problems and action can usually only be specified generally and provisionally, with the first step of management being further investigation allowing more detailed action planning. When this has become possible, the database has become sufficient.

History taking

A psychiatric history is a careful account of the changes, problems and symptoms that the patient has experienced or encountered; it is as simple as that. Sometimes students feel that psychiatric symptoms are less well defined than physical complaints, so that psychiatric history taking must be correspondingly more difficult; but this feeling can be overcome by attending sufficiently to the details of the symptoms—what they are, when and where they occur, what the experience is like, and so on—to make them well defined. It is important to remember that sometimes patients (a) are unaware of problems altogether; (b) are unaware of the impact of their symptoms on others; (c) minimize or even conceal symptoms; and (d) have problems (impotence, for example) that are manifest within a relationship rather than 'possessed' by an individual. For all these reasons a psychiatric history based on self-report may need to be supplemented by an account from one or more other informants—a family member, spouse, friend, colleague, etc. Experience shows that it is unfortunately only too easy to fail to see an informant. Time and again a clinical mystery is resolved by a meeting with a previously unseen relative.

Psychiatric symptoms involve highly personal aspects of life and often touch on experiences associated with pain, embarrassment, shame and guilt. The interviewer needs a tactful, accepting and understanding approach which allows the patient to tell his story in his own way while preventing him from straying too much from the point, and avoiding putting words into his mouth. Time is therefore required. It is simply not possible to make a detailed psychiatric assessment in a few minutes.

The history should be *recorded* under headings in a formal way, but this does not mean that history taking should be a rigid procedure. It is usually best to allow the patient to talk as freely as possible at the start of the interview, leaving specific follow-up questions until later.

Reason for referral

Finding the reason for referral involves asking various questions:

What is the problem?
What are the symptoms that trouble the patient?
What led the patient to the doctor?

This should summarize both the presenting complaints and the means whereby the patient came to medical attention. For example, 'patient admitted to hospital after self-poisoning with aspirin, now complaining of persistent sadness, insomnia, and weight loss over three months'.

History of present problem

This account amplifies the presenting complaints. Special attention should be paid to details of the onset of symptoms as well as to their nature. The symptoms of psychiatric illness are often changes in degree from normal experience rather than qualitatively novel departures from it, and a degree of sadness, anxiety, etc. which may not appear excessive at interview may yet represent for the individual a change indicative of illness. Illnesses have onsets, and problems that do not have onsets (i.e. are more or less life-long) are usually best thought of as personality problems rather than as illnesses.

As well as enquiring about the onset, nature and development of symptoms, the interviewer should note their temporal relations to possible precipitants. This is important because many psychiatric problems occur at least in part in response to stressful life events. Social changes (for example, changes in interpersonal relationships and work efficiency) should also be asked for and recorded, for many psychiatric disorders lead to problems of social role performance. One helpful tactic is to ask the patient to describe in detail a typical day in his life.

Family and personal history

The disorder must be set in its personal and social context. This involves enquiring into family background and personal biography. This enquiry naturally cannot and actually need not be prolonged and exhaustive in every case—common-sense and the time available affect the extent to which particular items should be pursued. For instance, a much briefer history is obtained during a single outpatient consultation than following a full inpatient assessment; and details of early childhood experience are usually of less immediate relevance with elderly patients than in adolescents. Nevertheless, at least some mention should be made under each heading in the following lists:

Family
1 Parents: ages, state of health, occupations.
2 Siblings: ditto.
3 Family relationships: parental discord, divorce, separation, overall evaluation of home, present status of relationships.
4 Family health: psychiatric disorder in blood relatives.

Remember especially psychotic disorders; suicide; alcohol and drug abuse; deliquency, including domestic violence; epilepsy; and known inherited diseases.

Biography
1 Origins: where born and brought up, any known problems.
2 Education: age at which education stopped, academic and other attainments, general evaluation of schooldays, psychological/behavioural problems.
3 Occupation: work record since leaving school (number of jobs, length of and reasons for periods of employment, reasons for leaving), personal evaluation of career (satisfied, bored, ambitious, etc.). This is a most important section as much can be learned from performance in work-roles and situations, and time is invariably well spent on it.
4 Health: medical and psychiatric problems and treatment. For women, also menstrual and obstetric history.

5 Relationships: friendships, psychosexual history, marital history, present domestic arrangements and current pattern of relationships within family.

Personality

This term refers to 'the sort of person this is'. If the patient has experienced a novel set of symptoms amounting to an illness, then we are interested in what the person was like before the illness began; that is, in the premorbid personality. However, sometimes patients seek help for long-standing aspects of themselves, for personality attributes which seem unsatisfactory in one way or another.

The assessment of personality should cover habitual patterns of personal and social behaviour, including sociability, gregariousness and interests, and emotional responsiveness, stability, ability to cope with stressful events, general levels of drive and energy, ambitions and moral standards. A person's self-description is often complemented usefully by the descriptions of others who know him well.

Examination of mental state

The assessment of mental state is based on the patient's self-report and on the observations made by the interviewer of the patient's behaviour. It is set out here under five headings.

General behaviour

When this is extravagantly abnormal it is not hard to see that something is amiss! Often, however, behavioural changes are less obvious, or reported by relatives rather than by the patient personally.

The observer should attend to the patient's dress, gestures, facial expression, and level of general activity, which may be increased as in states of excitement or agitation, or diminished or slowed, as in severe depression. Also, much may be learned by noting the appropriateness of the patient's behaviour to the interview situation—a patient may be flippant, aloof and unconcerned, or suspicious and on his guard. The examiner should note any failure to develop a customary sense of contact with the patient. While by no means pathognomonic, this may arise from the lack of human relating capacity found in schizophrenia, and therefore point to the possibility of this diagnosis. Schizophrenic patients sometimes display odd mannerisms (habitual

expressive movements), grimace in unusual ways, or adopt odd postures.

Thought and talk

Notice how the patient talks, and his language. Is the talk fast or slow? Is the patient evasive or reluctant to talk? Is he circumstantial, does he drift off into irrelevancies or does he stick to the point? Is he over-talkative, or does his talk contain oddities such as puns or rhymes? Grossly abnormal speech amounting to incoherence is found in severe organic disorders and in severe schizophrenia, where talk is sometimes fragmentary and disconnected or contains words invented by the patient (neologisms).

Disorders of thought have four aspects.

1 Stream

The stream or flow of thought may be accelerated, as sometimes happens in states of agitation or anxiety; or slowed (e.g. in depression); or interrupted, as in schizophrenic thought blocking where a train of thought stops and after a gap is replaced by a new one on a different topic. (A superficially similar experience of thought stoppage occurs in normal people under stress—in oral examinations, for example—and in anxiety states.) The flow of thought is usually accelerated in agitated depression and slowed in retarded depression.

2 Possession of thought

Some patients have disturbances of the control (or possession) of thought. Normally people feel their thoughts are their own, and are controllable; but schizophrenic patients may feel that their thoughts are inserted into their minds from without, or removed from them, or that their thoughts are known to others, or being broadcast. (These symptoms of thought insertion, withdrawal and broadcasting indicate that the individual is not experiencing the self as distinct from the outside world, as people normally do; the 'ego boundary' is impaired.)

3 Form

The form or structure of thought may be distorted. This can occur, of course, as a consequence of organic brain disease; but among the 'functional' psychiatric disorders it is seen most characteristically in schizophrenia. A patient with this illness may lose the ability to use concepts clearly and consistently, particular difficulty occurring in the handling of abstract ideas. Trains of thought may merge imperceptibly into others, forming a sequence which leads nowhere. This is often accomplished using sentences of normal structure. A sequence of normally arranged words which convey little meaning and yet are delivered earnestly has a disconcerting effect on the listener.

4 Content

Things people think about a lot are called preoccupations. Sometimes people are preoccupied with something to an unusually intense extent, or with something which most people are unlikely to think much of; these are called overvalued ideas. They are not in themselves signs of mental illness, although psychiatric patients may have them. Overvalued ideas lack the qualities of delusions, although this is not always easily established. A delusion is a demonstrably false belief, held with absolute conviction, which is inappropriate to the person's socio-cultural background. Delusions are *primary* when they arise spontaneously and cannot be understood empathic-ally; primary delusions always suggest the diagnosis of schizophrenia, even though they may occur in some other illnesses. Sometimes delusions arise as a consequence of some other experience, most commonly a severe mood disturbance; these are *secondary* delusions. They can be understood empathically, given that the person has the prior emotional disorder. In severe depression the patient may have nihilistic delusions, believing he has no worth (worst person in the world, even) or no bowels (body being eaten away by maggots, perhaps). Persecutory and grandiose delusions of exalted status are referred to as paranoid. Paranoid delusions may occur in many illnesses, including organic disorders, affective illness and schizophrenia; 'delusion' (or even 'hallucination') should never be equated with 'schizophrenia'.

Emotion

Feelings are notoriously hard to describe; the range of words applicable to feeling is so great that it is rarely possible to sum up a patient's feelings in a single sentence. The most useful tactic is to gauge the prevailing emotional state of the patient. Many psychiatric syndromes are associated with extensive change of mood. Sadness, misery, dejection, pessimism and an overall feeling of unhappy wretchedness are common-place in psychiatric disorders, particularly depression; but they are also found in other syndromes (in organic mental states, for example).

It is important to assess whether the ·patient's emotional state is appropriate to the rest of his mental condition and whether it is constant or variable. Shallow emotional responses and lability of mood are other features to look out for—they can occur in organic mental states and in schizophrenia. Many patients are apathetic and say that they have lost all feeling. Others may be unnaturally elated, breezy or euphoric, whilst others may describe states of bliss or ecstasy. These latter exalted feelings are found in mania and in schizophrenia, whilst episodic ecstatic states must raise the suspicion of temporal-lobe epilepsy.

It is helpful to think of feelings as having three components. When they speak about feelings, people sometimes refer to *behaviour*, sometimes to *physiology*, and sometimes to *cognitive–subjective* aspects. They may also refer simultaneously to any two components, or to all three. Hence 'depression' may mean sadness and hope-lessness (subjective); immobility and gloomy expression (motor–behavioural); constipation, insomnia and suicidal thoughts (physiological and subjective). In assessing mood the examiner should note which components of emotion are involved, and how they contribute to the clinical picture.

Perception

The collection of sense data from all modalities is the basis of interaction with the environment. Perceptions may be heightened or dulled as in some toxic and delusional states, as under the influence of hallucinogenic drugs. Illusions are distortions of environmental stimuli that can occur in states of fatigue and drug intoxication as well as in organic mental states and in schizophrenia. *Hallucinations* are perceptions that occur in the absence of an outside stimulus. Hallucinations do not always signify mental illness—they can, for instance, occur after prolonged sensory deprivation and while going to sleep (hypnogogic) and waking up (hypnopompic).

Hallucinations may arise in any sense modality, but hallucinations of taste, smell and touch are much less common than auditory and visual ones. Visual hallucina-tions suggest an organic mental disorder, although they also occur in schizophrenia. Auditory hallucinations occur in many mental illnesses; but complex voices, including third-person conversations about the subject, or commen-taries on his actions, are uncommon except in schizoph-renia.

Cognitive functions

Cognition is the means by which information is stored and retrieved. To test it involves giving simple formal tests of memory, general information, concentration and orientation for time and place. Cognitive function is always impaired in organic mental states. If there is disorientation and loss of recent memory, then the patient has some cerebral malfunction.

1 Orientation

This includes orientation for time. for place and for person. Test it by asking the patient to give the day, date and time of day. Also make sure that he knows where he is. Remember that disorientation often fluctuates in organic states and may be marked at one assessment and absent a few hours later. Repeated observations are therefore very useful. In hospital cases, nurses' records are invaluable.

2 Memory

Give the patient a name and address. Ask him to repeat it and then ask him to reproduce it in five minutes. This is a simple and useful test of the ability to register, retain and reproduce recently learnt material. Ask about the activities of the day before.

3 Concentration

Ask the patient to subtract 7 from 100 and go on subtracting—again a simple but useful test.

4 General information

Usually this can be assessed in interview, but if there is any doubt a good simple test is to ask the patient to name the capitals of six countries, the names of six large cities, the names of prominent public figures, etc.

5 Intelligence

This can also usually be assessed in interview, and educational attainment is a pointer; or tests of intelligence may be informative.

6 Insight

Ask the patient if he feels that he is ill in any way. The object is to find out not only whether the patient is aware of his illness, but also to find out whether he has a reasonable idea of its extent and implications. The importance of this heading is to draw attention to the way the patient's view of the problem(s) resembles or differs from that of the examiner.

Comment. Not every patient needs full cognitive assessment, but it is essential when there is any suspicion of physical illness. So, of course, are physical examination and whatever medical investigations may be indicated by it.

Psychiatric investigations

Initial psychiatric history taking and examination may suggest the need for medical, psychological or social investigations in order to clarify the nature of the problem. Sometimes, the examiner thinks that an organic disorder is likely to be present but no localizing neuropsychiatric signs are evident; in such cases investigations appropriate to the circumstances—following, of course, a

Table 16.1 Psychiatric indications for medical tests

(a)	Disorientation ± loss of recent memory ± clouded consciousness
(b)	Lability of mood Fluctuating state generally Paranoid ideas without prehistory Variable delusions of any sort Visual hallucinations
(c)	Failure of depression to respond as hoped to physical treatment Hysteria or hypochondriasis arising over age 40 for first time

thorough physical examination—may be important. In other instances, localizing clues may be available (the patient is alcoholic, for instance, and has some symptoms suggesting liver disease), and the appropriate medical system tests are required. *Psychiatric* indications for medical investigation are shown in Table 16.1.

Psychological and social investigations are often invaluable. Standard tests are available to allow estimates of intelligence, including verbal, conceptual and performing abilities which together contribute to this complex notion. Intelligence levels are often presented in terms of the intelligence quotient (IQ), which is based on the subject's test performance in relation to population norms for the test. Results for adults are presented as 'IQ' even though this idea was originally based on work with groups of children which allowed the calculation of 'mental age' divided by the true age. IQ measures may be useful when a person seems not to be living up to their intellectual potential, or when performance has fallen off recently.

Depressed, anxious and other moods can be measured, often by interviewer-completed rating scales or from self-report questionnaires completed by the patient; these give numerical estimates of mood severity which can be repeated and are therefore useful guides to progress. Examples are Beck's Depression Inventory, a self-report instrument, and Hamilton's Rating Scale for Depression, based on a standard interview.

Personality and disability inventories are also available and may be very useful in aiding assessment. Careful assessments of behaviour excesses or deficits in chronic patients are particularly helpful in informing on their placement outside hospital; a standardized interview, with behaviour tasks scored on rating scales, is an excellent method.

Home visits, interviews with informants, and joint

Table 16.2 Possible classification principles

Symptoms
Syndromes
Disease entities:
   aetiology
   clinical features
   prognosis
Dimensions

meetings with family members, are all procedures whose importance *cannot be overestimated*. First-hand knowledge of the patients' living conditions and social relationships is invaluable.

Diagnosis: classes of disorder

In the past there has been considerable disagreement about psychiatric diagnosis and classification. However, the situation was improved by the publication of successive editions of the *International Classification of Diseases*, whose eighth and ninth editions are based on the principle that psychiatric disorders should be defined as syndromes (collections of clinical phenomena). Table 16.2 lists possible classificatory principles.

Syndromes are an advance on *symptoms* only, for classification in terms of the latter gives a myriad of 'conditions' without reference to any general principles which help order a vast mass of data. The systematic delineation of disease entities is not possible in the present state of knowledge, in psychiatry. In some instances, notably organic conditions such as alcoholic hallucinosis, we can add an aetiological statement to a phenomenological one; but outside the organic field we cannot. A modern American diagnostic system, the *Diagnostic and Statistical Manual* third and third revised versions, DSM III and DSM IIIR, attempts narrower definitions of syndromes than does the *ICD*, which is more popular in the UK.

For completeness, Table 16.3 lists dimensions as a possible classificatory principle. This means that people are classified in terms of their position on continuous variables—analogous to height, or weight, for instance

Table 16.3 Classes of disorder

Organic disorders
The schizophrenias
Affective disorders
Neuroses
Personality disorders
Behaviour disorders

—rather than into categories which imply qualitative differences (discontinuities) from normal. For instance, depressive illness may be like severe prolonged sadness, into normal grades of which it shades imperceptibly. For practical purposes, categories are easier to use provided one remembers that they may represent oversimplications of the problems.

Table 16.3 lists the broad classes of disorder which constitute the subject matter of Psychiatry dealt with in this chapter.

General issues in psychiatry

Psychiatry in the community and in medicine

Most psychiatric morbidity is to be found outside hospitals in 'primary care' settings—places where people *first* receive professional help for health problems. In Great Britain this usually means general practitioners' surgeries. Table 16.4 shows just how small is the number of hospital psychiatric patients as a percentage of all those who consult family doctors. Most of the more severe, rarer, disorders *are* referred to hospital specialists; by far the commonest disorder in general practice psychiatry is mixed anxiety and depression which is usually bound up with family or social problems, lasts weeks or months, and often responds to simple counselling and pleasant changes in life circumstances. These problems represent a great deal of misery, and so treating them quickly and effectively is one of the most important and potentially rewarding tasks for the modern general practitioner. Specialist psychiatrists often work directly with GPs in the management of these patients, and in improving referral procedures so as to make best use of the specialist

Table 16.4 Psychiatric disorder and referral

Level	Psychiatric morbidity (%)	Action determining movement to next level
Community	100	Personal appraisal
Primary care	92	GP detection
total morbidity		
detected	56	GP referral decision
Psychiatric clinics	7	Specialist decision
Psychiatric inpatient	2.5	

After Goldberg, D.P. and Huxley, P. (1980), *Mental Illness in the Community*. Tavistock, London.

service, which can only deal with a small proportion of all the psychiatrically ill.

Many patients with a psychiatric disorder are referred from general practice to non-psychiatrist specialists. This happens because somatic symptoms of anxiety and depression are extremely common presentations of these disorders to GPs, who may tend to refer to the specialist concerned with the part(s) affected by important symptoms, failing to notice the emotional origin of the problem. To learn to recognize somatic symptoms which issue from anxiety or depression associated with life problems, and to refer for medical investigation only those cases which truly warrant it, is to acquire a very important skill.

Of course, physical illness should be recognized and treated; but there are psychosocial aspects to all illness and people do not function as either 'bodies' or 'minds'. It is easy to forget that emotion colours all illness and that emotions affect all doctors when they try to help patients.

Some 'physical' illnesses seem to have particularly important psychological aspects and have been called 'psychosomatic'. Examples are rheumatoid arthritis, peptic ulcer, asthma, ulcerative colitis, and hypertension. Nowadays it is accepted that these and many other illnesses—myocardial infarction, for instance—may be precipitated by stressful life events (see later) or made worse by psychological stresses, and psychosomatic medicine emphasizes these kinds of relationships rather than the idea that these illnesses have primarily psychological causes, for which there is no strong evidence. Psychosomatic medicine also covers the effects on health of social disadvantages such as poverty, bad housing and poor education, and the damaging effects of smoking, eating or drinking alcohol to excess, and taking insufficient exercise.

Nowadays a sensible view of psychosomatic medicine includes:

(a) remembering to assess psychological and social factors in every clinical situation (for they may be relevant to any disease whatsoever);
(b) being able to examine a patient's mental state as necessary in any clinical setting; and
(c) seeing patient's relatives as often as is necessary.

In addition, the student should be aware that an important growing point is the application of psychological principles of behaviour analysis and modification beyond psychiatry elsewhere in medicine (for example, eating behaviour problems including obesity, the modification of headaches, insomnia, blood pressure).

Ideologies

The ways in which a doctor thinks about people as psychological, moral and spiritual as well as physical beings inevitably affects the way patients are dealt with. This happens throughout medicine but may be especially important in psychiatry when patients' behaviour may arouse emotional or moral responses which the doctor finds hard to cope with. So the doctor needs to be aware of his or her personal attitudes and how they may obtrude in dealings with patients.

The set of ideas, feelings and attitudes which a person has about a field of activity is called their *ideology*. Doctors of all kinds naturally have a substantial biological component to their ideology, thinking automatically of bodily origins, manifestations, and consequences of disease processes. Also, everyone uses psychological notions about people in ordinary life—for instance, explaining behaviour in terms of supposed personality characteristics like 'being reliable' or in terms of dispositions like 'willpower' or 'courage'. There are many more technical psychological theories that can inform a more professional understanding of people; psychoanalytic ideas are popular, but there are many others, including notions derived from learning theory and theories of cognitive (information processing) activity. Social theories emphasize environmental causes and cures. In medicine generally, and in psychiatry in particular, biological, psychological and social ideas are all relevant, and a mixed (or eclectic) ideology is recommended.

Aetiological principles

Some general aetiological principles apply to all psychiatric illnesses (Table 16.5). First, and most important, aetiology is multifactorial: *always* enquire about biological, psychological and social factors. Some factors are predisposing; that is, they make more likely the occurrence of disorder, given certain other factors required to precipitate or 'bring on' the illness.

Types of predisposing and precipitating factors are listed in Table 16.6. 'Epidemiological' factors are population and geographical or ecological influences, and include different frequences of particular illnesses in men rather than women, particular age groups or social classes, immigrant status, rural compared with urban settings, etc. These headings are discussed below in relation to different disorders.

The distinction in Table 16.5 between individual and systemic factors refers to the importance of family,

Table 16.5 Aetiological principles

1	Remember multifactorial in nature
2	Distinguish predisposing and precipitating factors
3	Identify individual and systemic factors
4	Life events are very often, *though not always*, important
5	Disorder always occurs at some life-cycle stage, which may be important

Table 16.6 Aetiology of psychiatric disorder

Predisposition (risk factors)
  'epidemiological' factors
  genetic constitution
  early childhood experience
  personality
  aspects of current psychosocial environment
  current biological status
Precipitation
  acute life events
  biological factors

marital and other social relationships as well as individual characteristics in causing ill-health. 'Systemic' means that families work as systems, a system being something which functions as more than the sum of its parts. For instance, in a marital 'system', husband and wife influence one another in sequence and there is no starting point, such as when an illness starts with the introduction of a germ which produces effects by what is called 'linear' causality. In family and marriage systems causality is 'circular'.

Principles 4 and 5 in Table 16.5 are easy to understand but readily forgotten. Principle 4 reminds the doctor not to jump to the conclusion that a life event has precipitated an illness, because there are *always* events in people's lives and the attribution of an illness to an event may not be correct. A largely endogenous illness (for example, a depression due to hypothyroidism) might appear to be due to what was actually a purely coincidental domestic stress. The importance of principle 5 is that the life-cycle stage a person is at often contributes to illness—particularly when at a *transition* between stages such as at late adolescence, at the birth of the first child, or when the last child leaves home.

Principles of treatment

(a) Psychological treatments

Psychological effects

Psychological influences are operative whenever patient and clinician meet. Hence doctors have psychological effects on patients in every clinical setting, as do nurses, social workers, psychologists and occupational therapists. These psychological influences accompany pharmacological, surgical, nursing and other medical procedures, and are neither negligible nor unimportant. They affect patients' compliance with technical procedures and physical treatments, and often affect responsiveness to physical treatment. For example, relieving preoperative anxiety tends to reduce postoperative pain intensity and analgesic intake, increase the benefit from postoperative physiotherapy, and reduce length of stay in hospital.

Treatments

A psychological treatment is a procedure whose aim is to achieve therapeutic goals by psychological means in prescribed treatment activities.

1 Types of treatment

One easy way of distinguishing different sorts of psychological treatment (synonym: 'psychotherapy') is in terms of the personnel involved. Thus we can speak of three main varieties of psychotherapy.

(a) *Individual.* The therapist treats one patient.
(b) *'Natural group' treatment.* This means treating the patient as part of some group of which he or she is a member in ordinary life. This includes marriage therapies where treatment is of marriage partners, and family therapy involving the whole domestic unit.
(c) *Group therapy.* Treatment involves a therapist (sometimes two therapists) and several patients. Small-group therapy includes 4–10 patients; large groups are less popular but can involve 30–50 patients or even more. Therapeutic groups can be usefully set up for outpatients, on wards for inpatients, or in day-hosptial settings.

2 Length of treatment

Psychological treatments may be brief or prolonged, and time-limited or indefinite. Individual segments of treatment ('sessions') may also vary in length, from a few minutes to $1-1\frac{1}{2}$ hours, with about 50 minutes being most popular for formal individual treatment sessions; groups usually last 60–90 minutes.

Brief procedures require up to 10–15 meetings. Time-limited treatments take about 3–6 months. Treatments requiring not more than ten sessions over three months are particularly important in busy health-service settings where time and therapist personnel are scarce resources.

Therapists

Doctors can readily gain psychological treatment skills. So can members of other health professions, and the doctor interested in psychotherapy learns to work in a multidisciplinary team of which the doctor may not always be the leader.

Aims and approaches

The goals of psychological treatment are relief and/or behavioural change.

1 Relief

The aim is the relief of unpleasant feelings, or the cessation of other disagreeable experiences—to make the patient 'feel better'. The general approach is to encourage the patient to talk about his problems and express distressing feelings, the therapist being attentive, accepting and ready to articulate his understanding of what the patient is communicating. That ventilation and communication bring relief is a cardinal principle of counselling both by professionals and by ordinary people seeking to aid their fellows in distress.

Naturally, such relief of distress occurs informally as 'psychological effects'. But treatment whose goal is relief is frequently indicated as a formal procedure, usually brief and time-limited.

2 Behavioural change

This heading includes three treatment categories of differing conceptual and procedural complexity. There is a general shared aim of facilitating the occurrence of new behaviour of some sort.

Simple measures are often derived from common-sense notions of what the patient should do, or represent professional opinion of effects of illness on personal life. Thus simple measures designed to evoke behavioural change include giving advice about the effects of illness or operation; providing health-related information on sexual matters or the dangers of cigarette smoking; and helping a patient to resolve indecision or conflict about marriage, abortion or child rearing.

More complex measures include formal psychological treatments. They are all derived with varying degrees of cogency from one or other of the available theories applicable to behaviour. At the present time most treatments are either *psychodynamic* (based on psychoanalytic theory or its derivatives) or *behavioural* (based on learning theories); although there is an increasing tendency for treatments to be derived from other psychological approaches—personal construct theory, Gestalt psychology, a range of cognitive theories, and client-centred approaches.

Personality change is sometimes the declared aim of intensive, indefinite treatments, especially psychoanalytic ones. These procedures are too costly of time and people, and their results too uncertain, to be of any great health-service relevance. However, 'personality change' means 'extensive behaviour changes which persist and affect the subject's view of self and others and the world'; in this sense measures aimed at 'more complex' behaviour changes sometimes produce personality change.

Indications and applications

In general the aim is to fit the treatment to the individual patient's needs, and not to think of particular treatment techniques for particular illnesses. It is, however, possible to suggest guidelines for aiding choice of psychological treatment.

A 'relief' procedure should be considered when (a) the distress is intense, or (b) feelings are unexpressed, or (c) the patient is unable to think coherently about specific life problems or, more specifically, (d) when the patient has not worked through bereavement or other personally significant loss. The loss of a job, limb or pet, for instance, may cause grief-like states in people particularly sensitive to loss.

Simple behaviour-change measures are always potentially relevant in medicine. Provision of information, advice and education should always be considered.

Behaviourally based treatment programmes should always be considered with phobias, obsessions and sexual dysfunctions. They are often useful for patients with other disorders, too, and the question the clinician has to ask himself is: 'What might a behavioural approach have to offer in this case?'

Treatment programmes for interpersonal relationship problems, and for conflicts indicating difficulty in becoming mature, usually require some psychodynamic basis. This applies whether the treatment is brief or more prolonged, and individual, or group.

Brief, time-limited, treatments focusing on specific goals are preferable whenever possible.

Family treatment not infrequently leads to improvement when more traditional treatments have failed. Family therapy should not, however, be considered only as a last resort; it should be considered as a possible initial treatment of choice when problems are closely involved with what is happening at home (for example, for many middle-aged women with depression, patients with anorexia nervosa, and adolescent patients with severe psychiatric or behavioural problems). A family meeting is often of great *diagnostic* help, too. While family therapy may be inappropriate, there are no contraindications to a diagnostic family meeting.

Couple treatment (included above under 'natural

groups') is the approach of choice for marital problems, including sexual problems in married people.

A group approach is often helpful for people with interpersonal difficulties, for whom a group may offer greater opportunities for interpersonal learning than an individual approach. Groups are also helpful for patients who intend to become overly dependent in one-to-one situations.

(b) Biological treatments

Psychopharmacology

This relatively new science is concerned with the structure and mode of action of drugs that alter the mental state. These drugs can be broadly classified as psychotropic drugs in that they alter feeling, behaviour and perception without any significant change in consciousness, unlike sedatives and hypnotics which produce an altered mental state by dulling consciousness.

Psychotropic drugs include three main groups, and lithium. A fifth category—psychedelic (hallucinogenic) drugs—is not of practical importance now but has stimulated research into the nature of the psychoses.

1 Neuroleptics

These are antipsychotic drugs. Interest dates from 1952 when the antipsychotic action of chlorpromazine was demonstrated. In general the neuroleptics slow psychomotor overactivity, damp down feeling and block hallucinosis. This is probably related to their ability to diminish CNS arousal via the reticular activating system. There is little or no alteration in consciousness, though there is some sedation; and for this reason the neuroleptics are most valuable antipsychotic drugs. Mention is made here of the two most important groups, the phenothiazines and the butyrophenones.

Of the *phenothiazines*, chlorpromazine (75–400 mg daily) is the most widely used. Thioridazine (30–600 mg daily) has some antidepressant effect, and trifluoperazine (3–40 mg daily) has some alerting effect. Fluphenazine is most frequently used as the decanoate ('Modecate') and is given as a long-acting intramuscular injection; it is very useful in the maintenance treatment of chronic schizophrenia.

All phenothiazines have the capacity to cause extrapyramidal side-effects, which range from acute Parkinsonian symptoms (treatment by anti-Parkinsonian drugs such as procyclidine) to chronic syndromes, of which tardive dyskinesia is disabling and difficult to treat. As its name suggests, tardive dyskinesia is slow to develop; it includes complex involuntary movements involving the face, tongue and/or limbs. Phenothiazines may cause other side-effects, such as hypotension, jaundice ('chlorpromazine jaundice'), rashes and blood dyscrasias.

Of the *butyrophenones*, haloperidol is the most widely used. It may effectively calm acute excitement in hypomania and schizophrenia in small doses of about 15 mg daily, but sometimes much larger doses may be effective. Extrapyramidal side-effects are, however, common.

2 Antidepressants

The availability of antidepressant drugs has greatly reduced the need for electroconvulsive therapy (ECT). These drugs are in two main groups, tricyclic antidepressants and MAOIs.

More than 30 *tricyclic antidepressants* (as well as other compounds in more or less closely related categories) are available for prescription. The student should be familiar with the two that are of most proven value—imipramine and amitriptyline. Both are given in a dose of up to 150–250 mg daily. Amitriptyline is more sedative and may be preferred in more agitated patients; most of the daily dose may be given at night and will then aid sleep. All tricyclics take up to three weeks to act, and a tricyclic should not be rated 'ineffective' until the patient has had it in reasonable dosage for a month.

With all tricyclics, atropine-like side-effects are common; they include dry mouth, constipation, delayed micturition and erectile difficulties. They should be used cautiously in the elderly and in patients with glaucoma or prostatism. They may affect cardiac function and are dangerous in overdose. One of the newer compounds such as mianserin is to be preferred in depressed patients with heart disease. Tricyclics should not ordinarily be combined with MAOIs (see below) and may interact adversely with some drugs that lower blood pressure.

Monoamine oxidase inhibitors (MAOIs) were the first antidepressants. There are several monoamine oxidases, and this fact contributes to the uncertainty of action of these drugs. MAOIs may be very useful in phobic anxiety and in depressive neurosis. However, the usual practice in treating these disorders is to begin with a tricyclic because patients on MAOIs must observe very strict dietary restrictions which many find tiresome. The problem is that, when monoamine oxidases are inhibited, serious hypertensive crises may arise if the patient eats tyramine-containing foods. Some foods that must be restricted are cheese, yeast and beef extracts, broad bean pods and some red wines. MAOIs also potentiate sedatives, alcohol, narcotics and anaesthetics.

Popular MAOIs include phenelzine (30–60 mg daily) and isocarboxazid (20–30 mg daily).

3 Lithium

This element has mood-stabilizing effects and is a most important part of the treatment of manic-depressive disorders. It is somewhat toxic, and therefore requires specialist supervision. Serial blood lithium measures are essential to monitor therapy. Hypothyroidism and renal damage may occur but the danger of these toxic effects is not dose-related.

4 Tranquillo-sedatives

These are the anxiolytic or minor tranquillizers. They are very widely prescribed—far too widely given, in fact, because they cause dependence and foster ideas in society that pills can relieve unhappiness and life stress.

Most popular in this group are the benzodiazepines, such as diazepam (daily dose 5–30 mg). They calm anxiety in the short term but should be used cautiously because of the risk of dependence—and because they may cause disinhibition and hence contribute to outbursts of aggressive behaviour. Anxiolytic drugs should only be given for short periods of acute anxiety, never for chronic problems on a long-term basis.

Benzodiazepines are believed to act on the limbic system. Excessive doses cause drowsiness, ataxia and dysarthria, and fits can occur in abrupt withdrawal. Intravenous diazepam is a treatment of choice in status epilepticus and in any state of wild, uncontrolled behaviour.

Beta-blocking drugs such as propranolol can control some of the somatic concomitants of anxiety.

Cautionary notes

1 All psychotropic drugs are powerful. Dosage levels should always be kept at the minimal effective dose.
2 Interaction with alcohol is common—patients should be warned of this.
3 A good rule is to use one drug at a time, rarely two, and never three.
4 Patients taking MAOIs should carry a card with the drug dose and a list of food and drugs to avoid.
5 Weight gain on tricyclics can be very heavy. This puts people off taking them.

Other treatments

Electroconvulsive treatment (ECT) consists of inducing a fit by passing a 100 V alternating current across the head. This is done while using thiopentone anaesthesia and muscle relaxants to avoid muscle or bone damage.

It is used in affective disorders, where it can be life-saving, and to a limited extent in schizophrenia.

Psychosurgery (for example, the severing of connections between the frontal lobes and the thalamus) is used occasionally in cases where patients are in states of chronic tension, either through chronic depression or obsessional disorders.

(c) Social and rehabilitation treatments

The relevance of social factors for illness is increasingly appreciated. Recognition of the harmful effects that may be brought about in susceptible patients by prolonged exposure to an unstimulating institutional environment has led to the current emphasis on community-based care for psychiatric patients. For patients with chronic illnesses, this becomes essentially a matter of teamwork. To manage a chronic schizophrenic patient at home, for instance, may require regular home visits from a community psychiatric nurse, regular meetings between a social worker and the patient's relatives, attempts to improve behavioural skills by a clinical psychologist, occupational retraining by rehabilitation therapists, and medical supervision of the whole package.

Rehabilitation means maximizing the patient's assets and minimizing the effects of disabilities on personal and social life. A rehabilitation programme requires proper assessment of these disabilities, which may be *primary* (directly due to the illness itself), or *secondary* (effects—social stigma, or family rejection, for instance—consequent upon having had the illness).

(d) Service organization

Nowadays a comprehensive psychiatric management plan must take account of the way services are organized in the locality. This varies considerably from place to place. Not only are different professionals often involved, but different employing authorities (social services, health authorities, for instance) may contribute varying amounts to the plan. Doctors sometimes find it tiresome to learn all this; but in practice it is essential, and it can be very rewarding to be able to link effectively and coordinate all the agencies that may contribute to a comprehensive treatment plan.

Affective disorders

These illnesses all have a primary disturbance of mood, with symptoms in the areas of cognition, behaviour and body functioning. The basic abnormal mood is elation in mania and depression in the other illnesses.

In *depression* a person becomes persistently sad and unhappy but the disturbance exceeds in intensity and duration the everyday shades of feeling and emotional response that colour human life. The abnormally depressed mood is disproportionate to any cause, real or fancied. The intensity or duration of the feeling may lead family and friends soon to recognize that something is wrong, perhaps before the patient does. Depression may come on suddenly or insidiously; and it may become chronic.

Depression occurs in three major kinds of illness: in *bipolar affective disorder*, in *unipolar affective disorder*, and as *depressive neurosis*. The diagnosis of bipolar illness cannot be made until and unless hypomanic and depressive episodes have both occurred. Patients with depression only may be classified as having either unipolar affective illness or depressive neurosis. These can be defined as distinct syndromes, but many patients are difficult to allocate to one or other category, and seem to have characteristics of both. (The student may encounter the terms 'endogenous depression' and 'psychotic depression' and should regard these as synonyms for 'unipolar affective disorder'.)

Although neurotic depressives are often extremely distressed, most severely depressed (and never manic) patients tend to be classed as having unipolar affective disorder, because the marked biological and cognitive phenomena often thought to be characteristic of 'endogenous' depression are actually largely a consequence of the severity of the mood disturbance. Some clinicians prefer a single diagnostic category, 'depressive illness'. However, the trouble with such a broadly defined class is that distinct depressive syndromes certainly occur. The writer's approach is to reserve 'unipolar' depression for patients in whom cognitive and biological features (see below) are marked, and to refer to other illnesses as neuroses, recognizing that distinct syndromes may be recognizable within this class (also see below). (It is important to remember that the term 'reactive', which often enters this discussion, applies equally to manic-depressive, unipolar and neurotic depressions, in the same sense that episodes of all of them may be precipitated by —'reactive' to—stressful life events.) Depressions that are *secondary* to stroke, Parkinsonism, cancer or other medical illness, or to schizophrenia, alcoholism, anorexia nervosa or other psychiatric illness, may be severe, painful to experience, and treatable.

Aetiology

Depressive illnesses are more common in women than in men, about 15 per cent of women having significant clinical depression (often unrecognized by doctors and untreated) in some community studies. These depressions are more common in working-class than middle-class women; and childbirth is often followed by some degree of depression, sometimes reaching an 'illness' level of intensity. Depression occurs throughout the life-cycle, and is more likely at life 'transitions' when these signify 'loss' of something or someone important; for example, retirement can mean loss of status and friends.

A genetic factor operates in unipolar and in bipolar (i.e. manic depressive psychoses) affective disorders. These psychoses breed true, show a definite family incidence and a high concordance rate in monozygotic twins. Certain races (the Irish and Jewish people, for example) are more prone to affective disorders than others.

As regards family and personality factors, it is known that the loss of a parent in early childhood increases the chances of depression much later. Probably this is because the child becomes sensitized to the effects of loss. A strict and repressive family climate can mould children into depression-prone adults whose aggressive feelings cannot be expressed but can only be turned inwards. This 'depressive' way of dealing with aggressive impulses is one kind of personality factor predisposing to depression. Another is low self-esteem which can arise from early experiences which convey a sense of failure and personal worthlessness to the individual.

Chronic relationship difficulties, especially marital stress and poor affectionate communication between partners, even without troubles such as violence, or alcohol, gambling or sexual excesses, greatly increase the chances of depression. Often an acutely stressful event, signifying loss to the individual, precipitates depression in a setting of chronic difficulties.

Physical 'events' can also precipitate depression in predisposed people. Examples are some illnesses such as jaundice and other virus infections, and some drugs, including methyldopa, phenobarbitone and reserpine (formerly often used as an anti-hypertensive).

Biological status has been of great recent interest in depression. Current theory stresses the importance of CNS transmitters—the catecholamines, dopamine and noradrenaline and the indoleamine, 5-hydroxytryptamine (5HT or serotonin)—as being involved in depression when their concentration in the hypothalamus and brainstem is decreased. Medication produces higher concentration and relief of depression, but the mechanism is not fully understood.

Clinical features of depression

1 Mood

Mood disturbance is usually prominent and may be described in terms of despair, pessimism, sadness, gloom, solemnity, apathy, hopeless self-scrutiny and tearfulness —a range of feeling that cannot easily be summarized. Mood change may be constant or may show diurnal variation, and the subject may have lost the responsiveness of normal moods to outside events.

2 Behaviour

This is often slow, faltering and weary. Psychomotor retardation refers to a slowing of movement (and thought processes) issuing from what amounts to inhibition of cerebral control processes. Retardation is shown by slowing of all movements and by delay in producing answers to all questions—the answers when they do come are to the point, if brief. Retardation is roughly opposite to agitation, wherein psychic and motor processes are accelerated, leading to restless pacing, continual wringing of hands, pressured distressed talk, and so on; psychomotor agitation amounts to half-organized, worried overactivity.

3 Thought process

This is slow in retardation, and accelerated in agitation. Slowness is usually associated with poverty of thought (i.e. thinking few thoughts). In depression, concentration is poor because the patient is preoccupied. The memory performance may be poor, either because the patient feels too wretched to pay attention to what is going on, or because memory function has actually been impaired. This is particularly likely in elderly depressives, who often give the impression of being demented.

4 Thought content

There is a cognitive triad in depression of helplessness, hopelessness and worthlessness, representing negative attitudes to one's capacity to act effectively on the environment, to the future and to self-evaluation. These negative attitudes should be sought whenever depression is in question, for they not only occur in response to disturbing life events, but also tend to prevent the person from helping himself. The thought content of the depressive should be thought of as a long list of negatives —no help, no worth, no hope, no good, no health, no future, no interest, no energy, no God, no bowels, no enjoyment. Severely depressed patients may develop delusions, which may be hypochondriacal (delusions concerned with health matters), nihilistic ('nothing' ideas, as above, taken to a delusional degree), of guilt, or (less commonly) paranoid. Happily, the severest depressions in which these delusions arise are not often seen nowadays. Querulous and hypochondrial behaviour in depression may obscure the real diagnosis. It is the sense of badness about the self, and perhaps about others and the world, which may lead to suicidal thoughts and intent in depression.

5 Perception

In depression a person sees the whole world in a dull light. In severe psychotic depression the patient can experience auditory hallucinations, usually voices that condemn him—the voice of the devil, etc. These symptoms are rare, since nowadays treatment starts early, but they occasionally occur in elderly people.

6 Insight

This is always impaired in depression. No depressed person is able to judge himself sensibly. He may appear to agree that he is ill, while knowing how bad it all is and that the doctor is wrong. This type of insightlessness can lead to suicide.

7 Other symptoms

Depression can affect any aspect of personal functioning. Hence a wide range of symptoms can arise. Remember to inquire about:

(a) sleep disturbances, particularly early waking and lying awake;
(b) loss of energy, interest, volition—apathy and inertia;
(c) loss of appetite;
(d) hypochondriacal bodily complaints, especially involving bowels, abdominal churning, pains and headache;
(e) sexual dysfunctions and loss of sexual interest;
(f) irritability, anxiety and tension;
(g) indecision and self-doubt;
(h) deteriorating personal relationships and work performance;
(i) general malaise;
(j) self-neglect;
(k) suicidal thought, talk and behaviour;
(l) recent abuse of alcohol or drugs.

These symptoms are easily overlooked. Many are non-specific in that they are found in physical illness, but when viewed as a whole they add up to the picture of depression. It is still the case that a patient can be extensively investigated while the diagnosis of depression is missed, because the one symptom is followed up and the patient is ignored.

Clinical features of mania and hypomania

1 Mania

This is a state of high elation and uncontrollable

Table 16.7 Clinical features of affective disorders

	Hypomania	Depression
Cognitive/experience		
Mood	Elevated	Lowered
Thinking		
speed	↑	↑ or ↓ *
amount	↑	↑ or ↓ *
form	Flight of ideas	Normal
content	Positive	Negative
Secondary delusions	Grandiose/paranoid	Nihilistic/hypochondriacal/paranoid
Suicidal ideas		Frequent
Behaviour		
Motor activity	↑	↑ or ↓ *
Social behaviour	Disinhibited	↓
Interaction	↑	↓
Expression	Happy-looking	Sad-looking
Suicidal acts		Frequent
Physiological		
Sleep:		
amount	↓	↓ or ↑
insomnia	Early or late	Early or late
waking	May be early	May be early
Diurnal mood variation	Absent	Present
Appetite/food intake	Often ↓	↓ or ↑
Sexual interest/activity	Often ↑, may be ↓	Often ↓, may be ↑
Autonomic arousal signs	↑	↑

*Increases in these variables occur in agitation, decreases in psychomotor retardation

excitement. The patient is noisy, bounds with energy and ebullient high spirits. Grandiose delusional ideas are common and the patient's clothing may be covered in fantastic decoration. Often there is a paranoid colouring and the breezy elation turns to rage. Talk is so fast and overloaded with content as to be disorganized, though connected by rhymes, puns and jokes. Nowadays, morbidly elevated mood rarely reaches the level of mania.

2 Hypomania

This is less severe than mania and more common. The onset may be sudden, or gradual and hard to date. The symptoms are sometimes an exaggeration of the patient's personality characteristics—he may always be more cheery and energetic than his fellows, gregarious, hard-working and the 'life and soul of the party'. In hypomania acceptable levels of energy, self-confidence, elation and wakefulness develop into restless overactivity. Patients may need to be protected from the socially damaging consequences of hypomanic disinhibition which can lead to financial, sexual or occupational indiscretions.

Clinical features of depression and mania are contrasted and summarized in Table 16.7.

Diagnosis

1 Depression

Apart from mood disturbance, the key symptoms to look for include general symptoms of lost function as outlined above. Depressive states are inevitably coloured by the individual's premorbid personality; the irritable person gets more irritable, the histrionic person becomes more demonstrative and unstable. The history should point out any precipitating events. Bereavement is a typical and important example. Normal mourning is a healthy reaction to loss but is generally self-limiting in that people come to accept loss and adjust to normal living. However, if mourning extends for more than six months it is more than likely to be abnormal and depression should be considered.

In chronic and painful physical illness, true depression is hard to diagnose, since anyone in pain feels unhappy and lacks zest—a state of unhappy malaise that is sometimes called dysphoria.

The first and most important step in diagnosing depression is to check on the history of an onset of changed personal functioning, for this indicates that an illness of some kind is present. This is usually clearer when onset is acute rather than insidious. Depressive symptoms, especially cognitive ones (pessimism, low self-esteem, for example), without an 'onset', often reflect personality traits rather than illness.

Next, the observer must decide if the state indicates an episode of normal sadness or one of clinical depression. This decision is based on the onset, the quality, intensity and duration, judged intuitively in relation to common-sense ideas of what a person should feel in the patient's circumstances, and 'environmental associations', meaning judging whether or not the 'state' has reasonable temporal relations with a triggering event (for example, sadness starting immediately rather than six months after bereavement).

After a depressive state has been identified, the next step is to decide which variety of depression is being dealt with. The important historical aspects here involve a history of mania, a positive family history and a past history of previous episodes, because these point to bipolar and unipolar depressions; the presence of relevant medical illness (stroke, hypothyroidism, etc.); and the presence of other psychiatric illness.

2 Hypomania

The differential diagnosis of mania includes any cause of excitement, including schizophrenia and organic states (including intoxications). In extreme excitement, peculiarly schizophrenic symptoms may be hard to elicit. In delirium, excitement is accompanied by clouding of consciousness; manic episodes may herald neuropsychiatric disorders such as general paresis or encephalitis. Intoxication with alcohol, barbiturate, hallucinogens (LSD) and amphetamine can cause states of excitement resembling hypomania.

It should also be noted that overactive excited states occur as stress reactions in some cultures in which vigorous physical activity is socially sanctioned. These acute disorders have been reported in some Asian cultures and in the West Indies, for instance, and immigrants in the UK sometimes present with acute, noisy, excited overactivity superficially resembling hypomania or schizophrenia when the diagnosis is really a culture-influenced stress reaction.

In cases of hypomania where elation is not obvious, a change in the person's energy output and activity level may give a clue. Social behaviours that are out of character for the individual, but not abnormal in themselves, are characteristic but may easily be missed, especially by those who have not previously known the person.

Treatment

1 Depression

Hospital treatment is most appropriate for suicidal, elderly and physically neglected patients. The most severely depressed patients require inpatient admission, but many severe depressives are better treated as day patients, so long as the domestic environment is supportive. Many depressives can be treated as outpatients or by general practitioners.

The basic physical treatments of depression used nowadays have been described in the foregoing.

Sympathetic supportive acceptance of the depressive's painful predicament is essential. While depressed, people are often intensely sensitive to the feelings and attitudes of others. Breezy admonitions to 'pull yourself together' are unhelpful and usually interpreted by the depressive as lack of understanding and real concern.

Apart from this general psychological approach, which is always important, specific psychological treatments are sometimes indicated. These are sometimes called 'cognitive therapies' because they focus on ways of altering the depressive's negative ideas and attitudes. Also, marital or family therapy may be indicated where depression is intimately related to domestic or relationship problems. At present, all these specific therapies are applied to cases referred to specialist centres rather than to those treated in general practice.

Social acitivity of any kind tends to help depressives. Encouraging subjects to take small steps themselves to help put right any environmental precipitant problem, as they begin to improve, is especially important as this helps to counter the sense of helplessness.

Naturally concurrent medical disease must, of course, be treated.

2 Mania

Manic patients need admission to hospital because of their wild, exhausted state. Compulsory admission may be needed under the Mental Health Act because manic and hypomanic patients are often unwilling to accept help.

Physical treatments are obligatory. For the acute attack, the neuroleptics are the first line of treatment—usually the phenothiazines and haloperidol. For prophylaxis, continuous lithium therapy is vital.

Prognosis

In general the prognosis for *episodes* of affective disorder is good. Regrettably, recurrence is frequent in bipolar and unipolar disorder, but lithium prophylaxis can alter this. The probability of recurrence or relapse in depressive neurosis increases with poor social support and unrewarding or absent close relationships; psychological and social treatment after drug reponse may reduce the likelihood of relapse.

Schizophrenia

'Schizophrenia' is a term referring to a group of illnesses in which occur, in clear consciousness, disturbances of thought, perception, mood, behaviour and personality, symptoms which may be associated with multiple severe disabilities and many deeply distressing experiences, indicating that these illnesses are some of the most serious scourges of mankind.

Aetiology

Schizophrenia is likely to be a heterogeneous class of illness with differing sets of causes, many of which are as yet poorly understood.

1 Epidemiology
The incidence in the general population is 0.85 per cent. This figure is pretty constant world-wide, although there is a slightly increased rate in some countries (e.g. Ireland); and allowance must be made for the tendency of schizophrenic people to migrate into cities from rural areas, so that the incidence is usually greater in urban than in rural areas. The migration basically issues from the 'role function' problems (i.e. in working, social relationships, domestic life) of chronic schizophrenic people.

Schizophrenia is equally common in males and females. Very many are unmarried; this often issues from a mixture of personality, role function, and sexual problems. There is a relationship with season of birth, schizophrenics including an excess of people born in the winter months. The reason for this is unknown.

Schizophrenia is predominantly a disease of the young, many cases beginning in late adolescence. Illnesses starting after age 35 (into the 60s and 70s sometimes) usually have predominantly paranoid symptoms.

2 Genetics
Genetic factors are undoubtedly important in schizophrenia. In twin studies the concordance rates for monozygous twins are around 50 per cent, pointing to *both* genetic and environmental factors. The incidence of schizophrenia in the relatives of patients with the disease is increased beyond the 1 per cent general population level to approximately 10 per cent in parents, children and siblings. However, there is no family history in about half the cases—in these it may be that perinatal influences, possibly mediated by brain injury, may be more important.

3 Psychodynamics
Eccentric parent–child communication in early life has been thought to be an important cause of schizophrenia; while parents and others often communicate oddly with people who already have schizophrenia, and although we know that constant emotion-laden criticism ('expressed emotion') from family members can precipitate relapse, there is no good evidence that so-called 'double-bind' communication causes the illness (as precipitant or in any other way) in the first place.

4 Consitution and personality
Many have commented on the asthenic body-build of schizophrenics, and have commented that premorbid 'schizoid' personality traits (aloofness, seclusiveness, shyness, emotional coolness, detachment, eccentricity) are commonly found. However, no anomalies of body-build or personality are to be found in approximately 50 per cent of cases. Other theories involve slow virus infection or abnormalities of autonomic control.

5 Biochemical and metabolic factors
Despite intensive searching for toxic, metabolic, serological and endocrine factors, there are really few hard data. Much contemporary research involves brain biochemistry. One hypothesis is that in schizophrenia the brain produces an abnormal central transmitter in response to stress stimuli and that the build-up of the substance causes the symptoms in the same way that hallucinogenic drugs and amphetamines trigger off 'model' psychoses. Temporal lobe epilepsy is frequently associated with schizophrenic psychoses. Disturbances of cerebral dopaminergic neurones definitely occur in schizophrenia, and some of the benefits of neuroleptic drugs such as chlorpromazine are due to drug effects on dopamine systems.

6 Psychological factors
In schizophrenia there is defective information processing, and some symptoms are perhaps a consequence of faulty filtering of peripheral sensory input at brainstem level, causing overload at higher centres. This might underpin perception problems which are common in schizophrenia. In the established illness, learning is impaired and patients take longer to learn new skills than they did premorbidly.

7 Threatening life events
Stressful life events occur with increased frequency in the year before schizophrenic relapse (contrasting with three months for depressive illness) and may act as precipitants. Their role in *initial* illness onset is less clear.

Clinical features

Schizophrenic symptoms can never be understood in the same empathic way as depressive symptoms and are never a logical reaction to a life experience—indeed, an impression that the patient's predicament cannot be understood can be a useful pointer to schizophrenia.

Schizophrenic patients have specific symptoms, and these phenomena are often accompanied by disabling changes in the way the person functions as a whole human being. The personality changes, giving the impression of fragmentation of mental faculties that, in health, functions as a unity. Drive and impetus may be lost, and the person fails to initiate or complete sequences of goal-directed behaviour, so that purposeless social drifting ensues.

1 Disturbances of thought

Formal thought disorder refers to a basic flaw in conceptual thought which impairs reasoning. There may be thought blocking, knight's-move thinking indicating abnormal connections between concepts, and the introduction of neologisms (new words invented by the patient). Thought disorder may be more evident in writing than in speech.

A *delusion* is a false belief out of keeping with the person's social situation. A primary delusion may arise out of the blue or be preceded by a premonitory feeling or unusual awareness of impending revelation or disaster. Once established, it is maintained with extraordinary conviction. Schizophrenic primary delusions may be grandiose, paranoid or hypochondriacal, and are sometimes bizarre. There may be a conviction of being singled out in a special way.

Problems with *possession* of thought (the subjective sense of thoughts being one's own) are characteristic of schizophrenia. The boundary between the self and outside world becomes blurred and as a result the patient may experience his thoughts shared, put into his mind, or taken away by others (thought broadcasting, insertion, withdrawal). The patient may also experience his bodily movements and willed acts as in the control of outside agencies or other people.

2 Perception

Perceptual disturbances occurring in schizophrenia include distortions and misinterpretations of sensory stimuli, and hallucinations. Auditory hallucinations are the most common (though schizophrenics may also have visual hallucinations, even though these should suggest the possibility of organic disorder). Auditory hallucinatory phenomena include whispers, whistles and murmurs, as well as the more familiar 'voices'. Voices may be instructive or abusive, but these are not specific and it is voiced thoughts (hearing one's own thoughts spoken aloud), voices commenting on one's actions, and voices referring to the self in the third person, which should particularly suggest schizophrenia.

3 Emotional disorders

Often in the early stages a patient feels unaccountably anxious and vaguely depressed. Others feel strangely blissful or ecstatic or feel that something is about to happen or be revealed. During the acute attack mood may be intensely anxious, depressed, ecstatic, or mixed and fluctuating wildly. In the chronic stage common problems are *incongruity* between feeling and experience and *blunting* of emotional responses, the intensity of feelings being less than premorbidly. The patient becomes detached, cool, aloof, uninvolved and totally absorbed in his inner life. This comes across as a lack of empathy—like a pane of glass between him and others.

4 Behaviour

Many patients develop stiff, awkward movements and strange, symbolic movements which they repeat (stereotyped movement). They may become mute and stuporose (this is rarer since physical treatment has been possible). Excitement and uncontrolled aggression can also occur (again, rarer nowadays). Rarely, too, a schizophrenic can get fixed in a weird posture with sluggish stiff limbs (waxy flexibility). Again, some schizophrenics may behave impulsively and act in an inexplicable way without warning.

5 Social 'symptoms'

Traditional descriptions of schizophrenia emphasized clinical mental state abnormalities found in hospital patients. More recently it has become clear that the 'clinical' state of the schizophrenic is in part a response to the social environment. Schizophrenics are prone to demoralization, social withdrawal and careless personal care as a response to a dehumanized environment, as can exist in a large institution such as a hospital or prison. Patients are also prone to acute symptomatic outbursts in response to socially over-stimulating situations, as can arise with relatives with whom they are in serious conflict. A demoralized institutionalized state can persist in schizophrenics who are not in any institution but at large in communities in which they find they cannot fit. Much of the continuing distress of schizophrenics and their relatives derives not from 'mad' experiences, but from social difficulties. Assessment of a schizophrenic must include evaluating functioning at work and at home, in relationships with family and friends, and in relation to accepted norms of good manners and self-care.

Occasionally, a psychiatric illness has many features of

both mania or depression and schizophrenia. In these cases a diagnosis of *schizoaffective disorder* may be made.

Clinical types

The contrast between the frenzied derangements of many acute schizophrenic illnesses and the burnt-out aimlessness of many chronic patients' lives is striking. *Positive* symptoms such as delusions and hallucinations tend to coexist, and so do negative ones, such as blunting and incongruity of affect and volitional failure. The distinction between positive and negative is useful because these groups of symptoms require different management emphasis.

Traditionally, four types are described: simple, hebephrenic, paranoid and catatonic. Patients may show features of different types at different phases of a continuing illness.

1 Simple schizophrenia

This type starts early and insidiously. Florid symptoms are few; the usual picture is of a fall-off in activity, thought and feeling. The patient is unaware of symptoms; it is the family who complain that he has slipped into inert self-neglect. Talk is sparse, answers are scanty or abrupt, and there is a general impression of poverty of thought and emotion. The patient may end up as a long-term patient, or at best a rather dull, empty person doing simple jobs under careful supervision.

2 Hebephrenia

Onset is usually insidious in late adolescence. The clinical picture is dominated by severe thought disorder, emotional incongruity and auditory hallucinations. Personality disintegration is extensive. A typical end-point is one where the patient is fatuous, euphoric, buffoonish and thought-disordered.

3 Paranoid schizophrenia

Onset is usually late (30–45) with paranoid delusions often very complicated (systematized) in the forefront. The delusions are often persecutory, though grandiose and exalted ideas are also common. The personality is well preserved, so the patient is better able to survive in the community. Drive and energy may be high and encourage the patient to act on his delusions in a forceful way. Thought disorder is hard to detect and paranoid schizophrenics are skilful in concealing paranoid content. Survival in the community is less easy if the delusions become too forcefully expressed, leading to acute crises caused by psychotic outbursts. The prognosis is generally better than in other schizophrenias since the personality is relatively well preserved. Emotionally the paranoid schizophrenic may be remote, even callous, and may become absorbed in his delusions to the exclusion of everyone and everything else.

4 Catatonia

This type is comparatively rare nowadays. Onset is usually acute with either excitement or a quickly developing state of stupor. Early symptoms include odd gestures, stiff movements and weird postures. Catatonic excitement is severe to the extent of disorganized restlessness which may be aggressive or self-destructive. Bizarre acts and postures, and also echo reactions (mechanical repetition of the words or actions of the examiner), can occur as well as fixed rigid postures leading to stupor. This state requires total nursing care (feeding, washing, etc.), although ECT and neuroleptic drugs have made stupor and violent excitement short-lived and rare events.

Diagnosis

The diagnosis of schizophrenia need not be difficult. The first step is to see if characteristically schizophrenic experiences have occurred. These 'first-rank' symptoms include ego-boundary disturbances (thought withdrawal, etc.); passivity experiences; ideas of influence; and certain kinds of auditory hallucinations, as already noted.

If first-rank symptoms are present, then the patient has probably either an organic schizophrenia-like psychosis, or schizophrenia. Many organic illnesses can occasionally cause a schizophrenia-like state, but amphetamine intoxication and temporal lobe epilepsy are especially important. These physical disorders are investigated in the usual way. Clouded consciousness is a very important sign of organic schizophrenias.

If first-rank symptoms are absent, then the patient may still have schizophrenia. First-rank symptoms are positive, active experiences. Many schizophrenics have positive symptoms only episodically or transiently, the chronic clinical picture being dominated by negative phenomena such as loss of emotional responsiveness, apathy and social withdrawal. When a patient has negative symptoms, consideration of the course of the illness as a whole may clearly indicate the diagnosis.

Differential diagnosis

Affective illnesses may resemble schizophrenic pictures, but are recognized by the primary mood disorder, and delusions can be understood as secondary to this; the form of thought is not disordered. Acute psychotic episodes in people with personality disorder and in people from different cultures may also resemble schizophrenia. Emphasis is again on the understandability of the relationship between moods and symptoms, and between symptoms and environmental difficulties (life events). In old age, paranoid symptoms are common and may be caused by organic illnesses or depression rather than by paranoid schizophrenia. This last illness is often very indolent and chronic in elderly people and is sometimes called late paraphrenia. At any age, the occurrence of paranoid symptoms as the main mental problem should first suggest an organic psychiatric state rather than a schizophrenic illness. Crises in adolescence, where normal preoccupations with issues concerning the transition from childhood to adult life may be blown up out of all proportion, may sometimes resemble schizophrenia. In severe neuroses, particularly obsessional disorders, obsessional explanations and thoughts may seem very odd and difficult to distinguish from delusions.

Management

The first step is to ensure that the patient can in fact be treated. Many schizophrenic patients readily accept treatment, but for a minority compulsory treatment may be necessary.

Physical methods of management consist mainly of the use of neuroleptic drugs which calm agitation, block hallucinosis and help the person to think more clearly and feel more at ease (see page 458). ECT is used mainly to shorten periods of excitement or if there is associated depression. For maintenance treatment, long-acting depot injections of phenothiazines (page 458) are of value but require careful supervision.

Straightforward counselling of both patient and family about the disease is obligatory. Also, patients may have particular symptoms amenable to psychological treatments; for example, hallucinatory voices that are made worse with anxiety may be aided by relaxation therapy to reduce anxiety. Family help with patterns of communications between patient and relatives may reduce negative emotional conversation and hence the chances of relapse.

Resettlement means rehousing and is important in the many cases where the patient has become unable to live with the family, is drifting rootless in the community, or has been in hospital for a long time.

Rehabilitation involves helping the patient to make best use of this residual capacities and assets. A rehabilitation programme should be based on an assessment of capacities and disabilities. Some patients, for instance, find post-illness slowness a major work disability; others are greatly disabled by unrealistic aspirations to achieve goals which are no longer open to them.

There is no doubt that an over-long stay in hospital can be harmful, encouraging institutionalism. Maintaining patients in the community requires energetic treatment with coordinated hospital and community-based services and a high level of multiprofessional teamwork, often involving social worker, occupational therapist, community psychiatric nurse, clinical psychologist and doctor.

Prognosis

Acute onset, or onset following a life-event precipitant, are good points. An insidious onset and the presence of a schizoid premorbid personality are bad prognostic points. Prognosis for the acute episode is better in cases with marked affective symptoms. Relapse is more likely in families with high levels of 'expressed (critical) emotion' and in patients who do not take their pills or keep up their maintenance injections. Approximately 50 per cent of patients have no relapse after their first episode; of the remainder, half do relatively well and the rest do badly. For reasons that are not understood, outcome of schizophrenic illness is better in Third World countries than in industrialized ones.

Paranoid illnesses

Illnesses in which paranoid symptoms may occur are:

> Paranoid schizophrenia
> Paraphrenia
> Paranoia
> Induced (shared) paranoid disorders
> Morbid jealousy
> Organic paranoid states
> Paranoid affective disorder

Paraphrenia is like paranoid schizophrenia (see above), and probably a form of it, with hallucinations and delusions but no formal thought disorder, occurring in older people. Paranoia is rare and consists of delusions only. Sometimes a paranoid person dominates another member of the household, who then develops the symptoms (*induced paranoid disorder*). In couples jealousy can be delusional, one (more often the man) being deluded about the infidelity of the other. Paranoid symptoms can also occur in organic reactions and in affective illness.

Table 16.8 Organic psychiatric disorders: classification

Acute organic reaction
  confusional state
  delirium

Chronic organic reactions
  dementia
  amnesic syndrome
  personality change
  other focal syndromes

Organic states

Clinical outline

Organic psychiatric states are caused by dysfunction at cellular level, whether resulting from ischaemia, toxins, inflammation, tumour, trauma or degenerative disease. The clinical manifestations are a composite of the effects of the location and extent of cerebral damage, the acuteness of the affliction, and its medical nature. Clinical classification begins by distinguishing acute and chronic states (Table 16.8).

In all organic states, cardinal symptoms involve impairments of orientation, memory, intellect and, indeed, all cognitive abilities; of consciousness; and personality change. In addition, focal signs and symptoms may be present and abnormalities of emotion, perception and thought content may occur. However, the basic rule is that if the patient is disorientated and has disturbance of short-term memory then, even without impairment of consciousness or other symptoms, cerebral dysfunction is present.

Since organic states are caused by the malfunction or destruction of brain cells, they may result from any process which can so affect the brain. So, for instance, the causes of dementia include the causes of progressive brain-cell death: degenerative disease, chronic inflammation, tumour, and untreated metabolic disorder such as hypothyroidism. At the same time a tumour or cerebral infarct may be surrounded by partially damaged, recoverable cells, so that acute or subacute delirium may overlay dementia.

Clinical features of acute organic states

In the most acute disorders, often called 'delirium', consciousness is badly clouded, concentration and attention are fleeting and narrow. The patient is disoriented and the environment appears strange and frightening. In a sleepy state the patient misinterprets what is going on and may develop fragmentary delusions. The emotional state is usually fearful. Hallucinations often occur as well as illusions (perceptual errors). This general state of frightened uncertainty leads to excited overactivity and attempts to leave the ward. Onset of delirium is usually acute and the clouding of consciousness is worst at night when visual cues are less clear. Quiet calm nurses and doctors will do much to allay the frightened, delirious patient.

If the problem is subacute, then consciousness may be clear. In subacute illnesses disorientation is present and there is often also perplexity and incoherence of thinking, feeling and activity. The onset may be slow and the course prolonged. Subacute delirium is common in medical and surgical wards, and may not be spotted for days or weeks until the patient slips into frank delirium. Often the patient seems to be 'difficult' and 'uncooperative', but when examined carefully he is muddled and vague or flat and querulous—all based on his perplexity.

Clinical features of chronic organic states

1 Dementia (see also page 195)
This is a clinical syndrome defined as an acquired global impairment of intellect, memory and personality, without impairment of consciousness. Symptoms are in three broad areas (Table 16.9).

Cognition. There is failure to retain and remember recently acquired information, though past information remains untouched until the disease is more advanced. At first the patient cannot remember to keep appointments, but can get by with a notebook. This state of affairs worsens to the point where he gets lost while out shopping, or is so forgetful that everyone but he is concerned about it. Concentration falls off and thought is slow and muddled. Talk becomes sparse and repetitive. It

Table 16.9 Clinical features of dementia

Cognition
  poor orientation
  recent and, increasingly, distant
    memory fail
  vague, repetitive talk

Emotion
  lability; shallowness; irritability
  uncontrolled outbursts
  depression

Personality
  loss of self-control and self-care
  goal-directed acts fail
  social failure

is hard to shift from one topic to another; answers become non-committal. Flexibility of thought goes. As the process goes on disorientation in time and space, and personal disorientation, become more pronounced.

Emotion. Affective symptoms may come on, especially when the patient is *aware* of failing mental powers. Usually, however, the emotional change is caused by lack of higher cerebral control. Mood change is labile—tears and laughter may come easily but have little depth; and while sad family events seem to have no impact, irritability, distress and rage are sparked off by trivia. Later, 'emotional incontinence' occurs; there is no control over feelings, which are displayed noisily and without substance.

Personality. Change in personality is probably related to frontal lobe damage. There is loss of control of behaviour, which at first seems merely exaggeration of the normal self but soon tends to coarsening of behaviour: tactlessness and rudeness go beyond eccentricity and lead to social disgrace (examples are sexual acts with children, and shop-lifting). The end-point is fragmentation of the personality and babbling shadowing incoherence. Relationships fail as the patient becomes unable to recognize or remember past experiences with others, and to conceptualize his or her self in relation to another person.

2 Amnesic syndrome

This is a focal chronic cerebral disorder arising from damage to the parts of the brain subserving memory (including the mamillary bodies). The aspects of dementia arising from generalized brain damage may be largely absent. Severe loss of memory for immediate past events is the main symptom. A total failure to retain and recall immediate impressions is associated with disorientation for time and place and, most striking of all, a tendency to invent answers to make up for the memory defect (*confabulation*). The emotional state is flat and mildly euphoric. The classic amnesic picture is Korsakov's syndrome, where the amnesic syndrome and peripheral neuropathy occur in chronic alcoholism with thiamine deficiency (see page 345). A Korsakov-like picture can be caused by injury, ischaemic disease and various toxins.

3 Personality change and other focal syndromes

Frontal lobe damage (for instance after head injury or subarachnoid haemorrhage) may lead to personality changes similar to those found in dementia but without signs of damage to other parts of the brain. Focal damage to occipital, parietal and temporal lobes usually produces predominantly neurological symptoms and so are not discussed here.

Note that some symptoms in organic states express

the acuteness of the cerebral malfunction, while others express the extent or site of it. Thus clouding of consciousness occurs in acute states, while loss of recent memory and disorientation express general cerebral disturbance, acute or chronic. Organic syndromes indicate that the brain is malfunctioning, but not why this is so.

Diagnosis

This has two steps: identification of the existence of an organic psychiatric state, and the investigation of its cause(s).

The detection of an organic syndrome should not usually be difficult, provided the examiner remembers to enquire about orientation and memory and assess the level of consciousness. Depression may resemble dementia, especially in old people where slowness, forgetfulness and apathy can look like dementia (pseudodementia). Since depression is treatable, a confident diagnosis of dementia should always have excluded depression. Schizophrenia, particularly late onset and paranoid states, may appear to be organic states, but apparent clouding in schizophrenia is fleeting and there are no memory or intellectual defects. Personality disorders also sometimes give rise to diagnostic difficulty.

Investigations

These should follow the careful assessment of mental state. A routine physical examination may reveal systemic causes; for example, congestive cardiac failure causing subacute delirium or chest infection. Blood and serological tests may indicate macrocytic anaemia, systemic lupus, lead poisoning or neurosyphilis. A urine analysis may implicate various drugs, or porphyria.

Psychological testing is invaluable in establishing the extent of impairment. A *baseline* is useful because later retesting can indicate the rate of cerebral deterioration.

Recent developments in brain scanning techniques have greatly reduced the need for *invasive* cerebral investigations, but electroencephalography and lumbar puncture remain useful, indicated on neurological rather than psychiatric grounds.

Particular organic syndromes

Drug-induced states

A wide range of drugs, but especially alcohol, barbiturates and steroids, may cause clouded states.

1 Alcohol

In heavy doses, causing chronic intoxication, this can

produce a severe withdrawal syndrome of *delirium tremens*—tremors, hallucinosis and delirium. Onset is usually acute. Treatment includes chlormethiazole as an anticonvulsant and sedative, plus vitamin saturation and treatment of any associated infection. Tranquillizers such as diazepam are useful. Food, adequate fluids and good nursing are mandatory.

2 Barbiturates

In doses over 900 mg in 24 hours, these cause chronic intoxication (dysarthria, nystagmus, ataxia) and withdrawal fits. Acute withdrawal causes fits and a delirium which may be indistinguishable from delirium tremens. Treatment involves stabilizing the patient on a barbiturate such as pentobarbitone and reducing the daily dose progressively.

3 Corticosteroids

These can cause a wide range of psychiatric disturbances, though clouded states, excitement and labile mood disorder are the most common.

Infections

Acute infections produce delirium in high fevers, but these disappear when the infection is controlled.

Chronic infections such as neurosyphilis may present with a clouded state; the classic picture of general paralysis of the insane (GPI) is a late development (see page 223). Neuropsychiatric problems may develop in acquired immune deficiency syndrome (AIDS).

Metabolic disorders

1 Renal failure

This causes subacute delirium and coma.

2 Hepatic failure

This causes subacute delirium and coma as part of the syndrome of portal systemic encephalopathy; 'flapping tremor' and incoordination are well-known signs. The subacute delirious state may mimic irritable depression. Parietal dysfunction is common and for this reason a progress chart should always include the patient's writing and simple drawings.

3 Endocrine disorders (see Chapter 8)

These are frequently associated with psychiatric symptoms. *Hypothyroidism* is often accompanied by depression, which may fail to respond to antidepressive treatment if the diagnosis is missed, and may also cause a paranoid psychosis (myxoedema madness). *Hyperthyroid* patients often have very high levels of anxiety; less often there is here, too, a paranoid state. In *Cushing's syndrome*, as with exogenously administered steroids,

affective syndromes (including anxiety, depression and elation), delirious states and paranoid psychotic illness may all occur. In *Addison's disease* a neurotic picture may delay diagnosis or there may be a subacute delirious state; the psychiatric symptoms respond to steroid replacement therapy.

4 Electrolyte disturbances

Clouded states are the usual result and are most commonly seen after gastrointestinal surgery. Fluid and electrolyte replacement always correct the disorder.

5 Acute intermittent porphyria (see page 340)

This is a rare inherited metabolic disorder. Symptoms include peripheral neuropathy and mental symptoms whose real significance is overlooked. Abdominal pain, skin changes and fits are common, but the psychiatric symptoms may mimic neurosis or depression, though clouded states are common. Attacks are set off by drugs such as the barbiturates, ergot, alcohol, sulphonamides and chloroquine. The finding of porphobilinogen in the urine clinches the diagnosis.

Deficiency diseases

1 Pellagra (see page 346)

This is rare in the UK but is occasionally seen in alcoholics. The triad of 'diarrhoea, dermatitis and dementia' is classical, but psychiatric symptoms can mask everything by presenting as neurosis, depression or 'personality disorder'. Untreated cases pass through clouded states to dementia, coma and death. Treatment consists of replacing the deficient substance, nicotinic acid.

2 Pernicious anaemia (see page 360)

Anaemia and neurological signs usually present first, but some patients develop an organic mental state with a normal peripheral blood picture.

3 Folate deficiency (see page 360)

This may lead to a wide range of psychiatric symptoms. It should always be remembered in patients on barbiturates or anticonvulsants.

Intoxications

These are rare but should not be forgotten. For example, lead causes encephalopathy and dementia; manganese causes extrapyramidal signs and dementia; mercury causes tremor and dementia; carbon monoxide causes extrapyramidal signs and dementia.

Tumour

There is no simple rule that, when applied to an organic cerebral syndrome, will identify it as being caused by cerebral tumour. If there are focal signs, or if there are signs of raised intracranial pressure such as fits, vertigo, headache, nausea and papilloedema, then the diagnosis will be simpler; but 30 per cent of brain tumours start in 'silent' areas and 60 per cent start with psychiatric symptoms. There is no special 'tumour' syndrome, a fact which has always to be considered when assessing any organic cerebral syndrome. Fits are usually early symptoms, and often the earliest sign is personality change and memory defect; later more clear-cut organic changes appear.

Trauma

After open or closed head injury the immediate sequel is often delirium, and depending on the extent of brain damage the outcome may be permanent organic impairment. Progressive encephalopathy is found in boxers who have had repeated knock-outs ('punch drunk'). Subdural haematoma should not be overlooked as a cause of dementia, especially in elderly patients, alcoholics and anyone with a history of repeated head injury.

Cerebrovascular and degenerative disorders

1 Subarachnoid haemorrhage
This may be followed by depression, intellectual impairment, or personality change, especially if the frontal lobes have been affected.

2 Cerebral infarction and haemorrhage (see page 228)
Some degree of emotional, intellectual and personality impairment is frequent following strokes, especially when a large part of the brain has been damaged. Cerebrovascular disease may cause profound dementia without initial focal neurological signs—hypertension may cause this, and be more severe in younger patients. Depression may follow stroke and be severe and also treatable.

3 Presenile dementia
As already noted, dementia is a syndrome. Dementias are classified in terms of the age at which they occur: presenile dementias occur before age 65, and dementias of late life occur after this.

Possible causes of presenile dementia are legion—all the kinds of illness already discussed in this section. In addition, there are some special presenile dementias, all rare. Pick's and Alzheimer's diseases are clinically similar, though their pathologies are different. In *Pick's disease* frontal lobe signs are predominant, and the illness is probably inherited. In *Alzheimer's disease* the process affects the whole brain and there is a higher incidence of

fits and extrapyramidal signs. *Huntington's chorea* is a rare hereditary dementia (dominant). The onset is usually in the 40s or 50s. Early symptoms include involuntary and choreiform movements. Neurotic or depressive symptoms are inevitably followed by dementia. Survival rarely exceeds 10–15 years after diagnosis and the end is total helplessness and global mental deterioration. *Jakob–Creuzfeldt* disease is rare but of interest because it was recently shown to be due to a slow virus. Dementia is associated with myoclonus, epilepsy, extrapyramidal signs and a rapid downhill course. *Normal pressure hydrocephalus* is another rare cause of presenile dementia, but important because potentially curable.

4 Dementing illness in old age
This is now one of the major, and increasing, public-health problems in all countries where increasing numbers of people are surviving into their 70s and beyond. There are two common forms of dementia in old age.

Multi-infarct dementia (formerly 'arteriosclerotic') tends to start in the 60s rather than 70s or 80s. The onset may be insidious, or marked by an apparently recovered focal 'stroke', or by a delirious state. The course is typically progressively downhill, though marked by episodic worsenings ('little strokes') with partial recovery. Mental symptoms may include marked anxiety, hypochondriacal complaints, and paranoid, querulous ideas, though all accompanied by the signs of organicity—recent memory failure, disorientation, etc. Survival with established multi-infarct dementia is rarely beyond two years.

Alzheimer's dementia (see page 195) was formerly known as senile dementia, but it is now realized that the pathology is that of the presenile 'Alzheimer's disease' (see above). This is increasingly common over age 75 —upwards of one-quarter of the over 85s may suffer from it. There are more women than men with the disease because women tend to live longer. The pathological process has some similarities with normal ageing. There is progressive reduction in numbers of cortical cells, and consequent cerebral atrophy, and neurofibrillary tangles of the twisted fibrils of the degenerated nerve cells. The enzymes choline acetyltransferase and acetylcholinesterase are reduced in wide areas of the brain in this disease.

Clinically, the onset is usually insidious and the course progressive. Downhill progress may be slow and survival may be for 3–5 years or even longer, usually depending on the level at which the patient's physical health is maintained. The care of demented people often makes enormous demands on carers, most of whom are relatives who may make major sacrifices to look after their relatives in their own homes for as long as possible. Continual questioning, unpredictable wandering, incontinence, and restlessness at night are some of the behaviours which relatives find particularly difficult to cope with.

Psychiatric aspects of epilepsy

Psychiatric problems are particularly associated with focal epilepsy of temporal lobe origin (see page 224). Temporal lobe fits often start in early life following birth injury and may adversely effect psychosocial development, leading to personality disorder. Episodic aggression, ecstasy or excitement may indicate temporal lobe epileptic activity and fugue states (wanderings, losses of memory) may follow temporal lobe fits. Finally, a psychosis closely resembling paranoid schizophrenia occurs in a proportion of chronic temporal lobe epileptics.

The neuroses

Neuroses are very common. In a practice with 2000 patients, a general practitioner can expect about 20 new cases of depression in a year, and will probably have about four schizophrenics in the practice population. But he can expect roughly 10–20 per cent of all his consultations to be about neurotic disorders. These are often accompanied by social and family problems.

Neuroses can be extremely unpleasant and severe neurotic illnesses are among the most disabling afflictions to which man is heir. However, most neuroses are mild. Neurotic symptoms are part of everyone's experience, and the phenomena of neurotic illnesses are not qualitatively abnormal. What is meant by neurotic illness is that unpleasant experiences are more intense or more long-lasting than they are ordinarily. So neurotic illness feelings differ from normal ones in intensity and/or duration. As previously noted, only 5 per cent of all patients with psychiatric illness seen in general practice become psychiatric inpatients. Most of the general practice patients have neurotic *symptoms* and most commonly manifestations of anxiety and depression; but these symptoms are not always intense or long-lasting enough to be *illnesses*. When patients have neurotic symptoms not amounting to illness, this usually means they are attending the doctor because they cannot (or feel they cannot) cope with the level of symptoms they have, or some other aspect of their lives. This in turn is often because patients lack the sort of family and neighbourhood network which sustains most people in times of stress. Sometimes their personality seems less than averagely resistant to adversity.

Some symptoms are common to all neuroses: anxiety especially, but also low energy, a feeling of malaise, worries about coping, insomnia, aches and pains, and concern about relationships with others. Anxiety is an unpleasant experience like fear or dread related to the possibility, but not the certainty, of something happening. The behavioural features of anxiety include motor changes varying from tremulous restlessness to 'fight or flight' or being 'paralysed with fear'. Physiological accompaniments issue from autonomic activity and accordingly may include dry mouth, nausea and vomiting, or diarrhoea; tremor, muscular tension, numbness, dizziness; tachycardia, palpitations and chest discomfort; sensations of a lump in the throat, or of butterflies in the stomach; and anorexia, insomnia, frequency of micturation, and erectile impotence.

Anxiety is in itself normal, serving to mobilize the person's resources in response to some threat. Morbid anxiety is abnormal:

1 when it is a disproportionately intense or prolonged response to stress;
2 when it has no discernible relationship to stressful stimuli;
3 when it occurs in response to something which is objectively not at all threatening or dangerous.

The first two are varieties of 'anxiety neurosis'; the third is 'phobic neurosis'. Anxiety not associated with an object is 'free floating' or 'non-situational'. A phobia is an irrational (i.e. unnecessary) fear.

Normal and abnormal anxiety can be linked together and in a curvilinear relationship with performance in the so-called Yerkes–Dodson law; performance suffers if anxiety is *either* too low *or* too high.

Each neurosis is a syndrome defined by the phenomena

Table 16.10 Clinical features of anxiety

Cognition–experience
  mood: scared
  thinking: speed increased
  disjointed train of thought
  uncertainty about future
  preoccupation with objects of fear

Behaviour
  worried expression
  motor activity increased
  interrupted goal-directed activity
  avoidance of objects of fear

Physiological
  interrupted, restless sleep
  autonomic arousal increased

which dominate the clinical picture. The most important syndromes are anxiety and phobic neuroses; depressive neurosis; obsessional neurosis; and hysteria. There are also hypchondriacal, depersonalization and neurasthenic neurotic syndromes, but these are less important and are not considered further here.

In anxiety and phobic neuroses, the predominant symptom is free-floating anxiety; panic attacks (unexpected non-situation-related peaks of anxiety); or phobic anxiety. Commonly, all three kinds of anxiety are present to some degree. Symptoms may be in cognitive, behavioural or physiological domains (Table 16.10).

Types of neurosis

Anxiety neurosis

Free-floating anxiety is dominant, may be acute, disproportionately intense or prolonged in response to a stress, or without apparent relationship to stress; or chronic, when the major manifestations are often in the physiological domain.

Anxiolytic drugs play a part in the treatment of acute anxiety, but should be avoided in chronic cases, in which psychological treatments, especially behavioural psychotherapies, are extremely valuable. Supportive and intensive psychodynamic psychotherapy may also be useful.

Phobias

Mild phobias are very common, and normal, especially in children and in females. When severe they can be extremely disabling. They occur in three clinical groups: specific phobias, social phobias and agoraphobia. Specific phobias often date from early childhood and include fears of spiders, cats, mice, birds, snakes and dogs; specific phobias occur usually in women with no other significant psychological problems. They respond well to behavioural psychotherapy. Social phobias include fear of vomiting, speaking, eating, being seen, urinating, or drinking in public. Severe 'stage fright' is a social phobia. Social phobias are as common in men as women and are often closely linked with personality difficulties. Various psychological treatments may help.

Agoraphobia is the commonest severe phobic disorder. It occurs most often in young women aged 18–35. Its core symptoms are of anxiety in, and consequent avoidance of, situations which mean being away from home and safety. The typical agoraphobic is anxious about travelling by car, bus or train, or even on foot; about shopping or being in crowds; and perhaps about being trapped in enclosed places as well as exposed in open ones. Anxiety is usually reduced when the patient is accompanied by a trusted relative, friend or even by a pet or talisman. In addition to phobic anxiety, agoraphobics often also suffer 'free-floating anxiety', depression and panic attacks.

Treatment of agoraphobia includes drugs. Tricyclic or MAOI antidepressants may be helpful, and anxiolytics may aid behavioural progress, although they should not otherwise be given regularly (lest they lead to dependence). Psychological treatment is essential—behavioural, supportive and family treatments may all play their part. Day hospital attendance can be helpful. Agoraphobics often respond well to an enthusiastic 'total push' regime, and complete recovery is possible, even after years of disability.

Depressive neuroses

These are depressive illnesses which do not have a past history of hypomanic episodes or a family history of severe depressive episodes.

Within 'depressive neurosis', several sub-syndromes can be distinguished. Important ones are (a) anxious depression, (b) hostile depression, and (c) depression with personality disorder. Anxious depression seems related to agoraphobia, except that phobic foci are less evident; MAOIs may be helpful. Hostile and personality-disorder-related depressions are often more difficult to manage than other depressions because the hostility and personality characteristics are difficult for staff to cope with. Often, these depressions are viewed as responses to social difficulties requiring social remedies, marital or family therapy, rather than medical treatment.

Obsessional neuroses

Obsessions include words, ideas, phrases and actions which a person feels compelled to repeat against a feeling of inner resistance. Obsessions are always unpleasant for the sufferer and may cause anxiety and severe depression. Obsessions have a quality that is very like the common childhood experience of 'having to' avoid cracks between paving stones or like some everyday superstitions that people observe in an embarrassed way. Obsessional neurosis starts early in life and persists with remission well into middle and later years. Recent studies suggest that long-term prognosis is not as bad as had been suspected. Long periods of relative remission do occur and the end-point is likely to be a compromise with symptoms. Depression is a common complication as is a relentless state of shame and tension perpetuated by the obsessions and rituals.

Obsessions are regularly helped by treatment of any concurrent depression, and by admission to hospital (the obsessional benefits because hospital routine organizes his time for him, reducing his freedom to behave obsessionally). Behavioural psychotherapy often helps, at least in less severe cases, intensive psychotherapy aimed at analysing the symbolism of obsessions is of little value. Support is, however, invaluable. In severe, intractable cases, especially those in whom tension is considerable, psychosurgical intervention may be helpful.

Hysteria

Hysterial neuroses involve loss of function of some bodily part without structural damage to account for it. These states of 'conversion hysteria' can be thought of as caused by a dissociation of consciousness—a splitting off from consciousness of a function ordinarily under conscious awareness. Thus hysterical disorders include sensory and motor dysfunction as well as amnesia, trance-like states and fugues. Bizarre mental states that mimic psychosis can be hysteria, and usually occur in highly stressed situations. The same is true of amnesia and fugues. Paresis is much harder to evaluate, particularly when it is chronic. The diagnosis should not be made because no physical signs can be found. There should be some definite conflict situation which can be shown to present the patient with a gainful solution of an impossible problem.

The general theory is that states of conversion hysteria are the result of unacceptable conflict which causes intolerable stress which can only be dealt with by unconsciously simulating illness. The most extreme examples of this follow severe ordeals, as in wartime and disaster, but the theory hardly accounts for long-term follow-up of people diagnosed as suffering from 'hysteria', many of whom show a disturbingly high incidence of unrecognized organic disease, suicide and mental illness. Hysterical disorders are rarer than they used to be; this is possibly because a patient no longer has to complain of physical symptoms in order to receive help. On the other hand many physically ill people develop hysterical exaggeration of symptoms, and also organic brain disease can trigger off a hysterical reaction when higher control is impaired.

While 'conversion hysteria' is the most important professional use of the term 'hysteria', the word is a difficult one because it is used inconsistently in several ways and can therefore mislead. The term *'Briquet's syndrome'* has been used to describe a group of patients with multiple physical symptoms who attend many hospitals and doctors and, while not having paralyses or other clearly defined conversion symptoms, do have many bodily complaints. Sometimes these patients are described, vaguely, as hysterical. Hysterical personality is mentioned later. 'Anxiety hysteria' is a term coined by Freud to refer to patients with neurotic symptoms generally who would now be diagnosed as a more specific neurotic syndrome. 'Mass hysteria' occurs when a crowd or population seem to share the same distressing beliefs and begin to behave in unusual ways, including screaming, fainting, or behaving as if paralysed or otherwise incapable. These states often subside when the individuals disperse. Finally there are vague lay uses of the word 'hysteria'.

The acute hysterical reaction can usually be treated by heavy sedation followed by powerful suggestion and reassurance. Chronic hysteria tends to be propagated by diagnostic uncertainty. In general, vigorous and positive support and rehabilitation with the careful use of medication are the mainstays of treatment. The chronic hysteric will need careful and skilled psychotherapy to deal with conflict and encourage the return of lost function.

Syndromes related to neuroses

Sometimes people receive psychiatric help when distress is more intense than they can cope with and takes forms other than those described here; presentations of distress do not form convenient, neat, categories. Common are various combinations of somatic complaint with some components of arousal, often without the cognitive aspects of anxiety or other *emotional* state. Indeed the emotional nature of the problem is often vigorously denied by the sufferer who concentrates on physical causes. Every medical specialty has its syndrome of this kind—'spastic colon' in gastroenterology; 'hyperventilation' in thoracic medicine; chest pain with normal coronary arteries, and 'effort syndrome', in cardiology.

Sometimes syndromes of bodily ill-health are of more clearly psychiatric origin and their manifestations are better defined. Examples are anorexia nervosa and sexual dysfunctions, which are therefore discussed here.

Anorexia nervosa

This was first described by Sir William Gull in the late nineteenth century. It is a syndrome characterized by food refusal, weight loss and amenorrhoea. Most patients are girls, only about 10 per cent being males. It is important to stress the term 'food refusal' because usually the anorexic patient has a normal appetite; the problem is that he or she refuses to eat and adopts numerous devices to avoid it. These range from the obvious such as hiding food or throwing it away, to the less obvious such as self-induced vomiting and the use of excessive purgation. Self-induced vomiting can coexist with episodic bingeing, and eating behaviour is chaotic even though weight is maintained broadly within normal limits; this syndrome, called *bulimia nervosa*, is really rather separate from anorexia nervosa.

In anorexia nervosa, weight loss can be severe and extremely rapid leading in extreme cases to severe electrolyte depletion with dehydration and dangerously low potassium levels. Amenorrhoea is often simply a consequence of starvation but is an early symptom in a proportion of cases and may precede significant weight loss. Anorexic patients may show significant depression of mood and also be much distressed by obsessional symptoms.

Aetiology. Food refusal is often based on a fear of being fat. The anorexic sees herself (her 'self-image') as being fatter than she really is. The fear is partly determined by social pressures, including advertising which exhorts the virtues of slimness—social factors probably account for the recent increased incidence of anorexia nervosa. In a vulnerable individual conventional slimming gets out of control and becomes clinical anorexia nervosa. This vulnerability often includes maturational problems (changing from a child to an adult who is independent of parents, sexually mature, and socially competent). In a high percentage of cases disturbed family relations complicate the problem. By the time the patient is in hospital the whole topic of the patient's food refusal has become a matter of anxiety and concern within the family so that the parents will have overacted to an admittedly dangerous situation. Sir William Gull's original advice that the patient should be separated from the parents during treatment remains sound.

Management. Severe anorexia nervosa requires treatment in hospital, even though the patient may need much staff time and discussion before agreeing to it. The main object is to overcome the patient's food refusal and get her back to a reasonable weight which she can tolerate. In severe cases the patient may require enteral feeding or intravenous fluid and electrolyte replacement, particularly when potassium levels are low.

Drugs are of minor importance in this illness. The mainstay of treatment is supervised feeding with good support and encouragement from nursing staff. The patient learns to eat in order to achieve specific rewards or goals agreed beforehand in discussion with staff (e.g. being allowed out of bed, having visits from friends, etc.). It is usually necessary to involve the family in treatment at some stage.

Prognosis. Anorexia nervosa has a mortality of about 4 per cent and many patients require frequent readmission after speedy relapses. Some patients maintain a chronic anorexic state for years. Others recover to normal weight and mature both biologically and psychologically (periods return, sexual activity occurs, and so on).

Sexual dysfunctions

These are problems which make sexual intercourse difficult or impossible. In the male they include: erectile impotence (failure to achieve or sustain an erection sufficient for coitus); premature ejaculation (ejaculatory control being impaired so that ejaculation occurs before it is desired); and retarded ejaculation (ejaculation simply fails to occur—this is a rare dysfunction).

Female dysfunctions include: failure to respond early in the sexual arousal cycle, leading to dryness, pain (if coitus is attempted), and difficulty in going on to orgasm; anorgasmia, when arousal begins but does not lead on to orgasm; and vaginismus.

Many established dysfunctions become accompanied by loss of sexual interest and inclination as the sexual difficulty leads to accumulated argument, anxiety, guilt and failure.

Sexual dysfunctions can be caused by structural or functional interference with local nervous or vascular pathways. Possible causes here are legion—diabetic autonomic neuropathy, antihypertensive and antidepressant drugs, and spinal-cord tumour are but three examples. Hypogonadism is a rare hormonal cause. In about 80 per cent of cases of sexual dysfunction no significant organic factor is present, even though they should be sought in all instances. The most important factors are usually anxiety, especially fear of sexual failure and anxiety about sexual performance; and marital disharmony—few couples continue active sexual lives when their general relationship is bad. Of course, general and sexual aspects of the relationship tend to feed each other, both for better and for worse.

Treatment of marital sexual problems is best based on the methods which evolved from the pioneering work of Masters and Johnson. The key features of this approach are:

1 Both partners are involved.

2 It is time-limited.

3 'Homework' exercises for the couple to do at home are designed to achieve specified treatment goals.
4 The results are assessed at the end of treatment.

Results are often very good, provided both partners are involved and genuinely seek progress.

Sexual dysfunctions have obvious links with many branches of medicine, and many disciplines can contribute to sexual dysfunction treatment. The person treating sexual disorders may need access to physician, urologist, gynaecologist, family-planning expert, venereologist, clergyman, social worker, psychologist, marriage guidance counsellor, or psychiatrist. Provided such links are readily available, the ability to treat the majority of sexual dysfunctions is readily gained by students or general practitioners as well as by members of all these disciplines.

Personality disorders

As already noted, personality characteristics are relatively longlasting and unchanging, and are what people mean when they say 'what sort of a person is this?' It is helpful to think of personality as a coin with two sides—one is the individual's view of himself, the other is other people's view of him. The concept of abnormal personality is important in psychiatry, since it provides a way of explaining and understanding persistent modes of behaviour and emotional experience that puzzle society and distress the patient and his family. Some people behave in an odd way from childhood, and their oddities may cause problems, either for themselves by causing conflict and distress, or for others or society at large, especially if they offend moral codes or break the law in a relentless way that is unaffected by punishment or 'treatment'. Indeed, a popular definition of the term 'psychopath' is Schneider's . . . 'a psychopathic personality causes suffering to the person, to society, or both'. However, in Britain, 'psychopath' sometimes refers to people who show persistently antisocial conduct; but the original use of the term related it more widely to personality disorder.

The important point for the clinician is that personality abnormalities start early and persist. It is useful to identify syndromes of personality disorder, which when present in marked degree, represent extremes of variation from normal. People with severe personality disorders are unusual and often very eccentric and therefore often find it difficult to fit into society.

Schizoid personality

The schizoid personality has been likened to an abortive form of schizophrenia; this is offset by the fact that only 50 per cent of schizophrenics have a premorbid personality that could be fairly described as schizoid. Schizoid people are inward-looking and tend to be shy, quiet, self-absorbed and withdrawn. They usually have been 'model' children, being quiet, obedient and bookish. They cannot relate easily with others, tending to be seclusive and aloof. On the other hand their dreamy detached intellectualism may be advantageous and many go through life unscathed. If schizoid traits are marked with fanatical zeal, the patient may get into difficulty if he neglects himself or adopts a crankish diet or takes hallucinogenic drugs in a search for cosmic revelation. If he becomes depressed, the schizoid person may have atypical symptoms.

Obsessional personality

Obsessional people are excessively perfectionistic and over-conscientious. Obviously to be conscientious is a valuable social trait, but the obsessional personality tends to possess these traits to a degree that imposes handicap, since his exalted standards of perfection can never be attained. A moderate degree of obsessionality is useful in any professional or skilled person, but when excessive it becomes a hindrance. Obsessionals make good subordinates but bad leaders. They tend to be indecisive and glum and over-concerned by bureaucratic trivia. Conscientiousness may be carried to absurd lengths; everything is listed and checked in a stultifying way. They suffer from guilt and self-doubt and are prone to depression and hypochondriasis. They are easily upset by changes in routine and are usually loyal, diligent but rather dreary people whose talk is larded with qualifying phrases and apology. Often one parent has shown similar traits, providing a strict upbringing with undue emphasis on self-control and keeping feelings out of sight.

Paranoid personality

The paranoid personality is unrealistic often to the extent of being near deluded. He is suspicious, touchy and over-sensitive, and over-reacts to criticism, real or fancied. This makes it hard for him to settle in a job or relate with other people. Paranoid personalities often channel their basic sense of injustice into the support of a 'cause' but can prove to be an embarrassment to their associates by becoming fanatical. The paranoid tendency to overvalue ideas and resent criticism can build up into bitter, even violent feeling. In their most extreme forms certain paranoid personalities have influenced world history in a disastrous way.

Hysterical personality

The criteria of maturity include stability, the ability to adjust to change and the ability to handle relationships in a sensible, undemanding way without having to manipulate others to meet some patholgical need. Mature people can accept success, failure, frustration and disappointment with relative equanimity. Immaturity is a state of emotional childishness. Children react stormily to frustration and the failure to achieve gratification of immediate needs. Growing up and maturation modify this response and encourage a state of independent self-reliance. Some never grow out of this infantile response pattern and become egocentric, immature adults. Applied to personality, the term 'hysterical' means 'histrionic' rather than 'excessively prone to conversion hysteria', which it is not. Histrionic people are usually emotionally labile—sudden bouts of desperate gloom pass quickly and are replaced by some capricious infatuation or enthusiasm which is dropped as quickly as it is taken up. Behaviour tends to be dramatic and the person is importunate and cannot tolerate frustration. The emotions are shallow—effuse demonstrations of feeling mean nothing and relationships with others are never stable. Sexual behaviour is often flirtatious, with a facade of empty, provocative eroticism.

Antisocial (psychopathic) personality

The antisocial personality presents society with many problems, mainly because of repeatedly antisocial behaviour. The psychopath seems unable to control his impulses, learn from mistakes or show any foresight about the consequences of his actions. The impulsiveness of the psychopath is like that of a child who flies into a rage when an immediate wish is not granted. The failure to learn from experience suggests arrested emotional development—a failure in social learning. Many have commented on the youthful appearance of certain psychopaths and on the presence of immature patterns in the EEG. This does not apply to all psychopaths, but suggests that at least some of them are people who have a constitutional abnormality. Some psychopaths have emotional shallowness which can extend to callous brutality.

In general the antisocial psychopath is unreliable and untruthful, with little regard for laws and moral codes and a nonchalance that society may find inexplicable.

Treatment as if his personality were an illness is a mistake which can seriously damage further the psychopath's precarious sense of responsibility for his acts.

Antisocial psychopaths are sometimes called sociopaths in the USA. Family studies of these individuals suggest an interplay of genetic and environmental factors. There is an increased incidence of parental alcoholism, psychosis, criminality and neglect in such families. Truancy, early institutionalization and early delinquent behaviour all add up to a background that breeds psychopathy.

Inadequate personality

This applies to people who cannot cope with life at any level. They are usually passive and submissive with a history of repeated failure at school, in work and in relationships. They drift from one job to another, are easily led and deceived. Often they are vaguely but persistently hypochondriacal and attend their doctor very frequently. They are usually feckless and may drift into minor criminality or the abuse of alcohol or drugs. Their lives are a catalogue of repeated mistakes and well-intentioned failure. They fill the ranks of recidivist offenders and often find a haven in institutional life, be it hospital or prison. Mood disturbance is labile.

Conclusions

The antisocial psychopath presents the biggest problem because of his effect on society. There is good evidence to suggest that even severe psychopathic offenders improve as they grow older. Group therapy in prison or in hospital may help the patient to some awareness of the impact of his acts on others. Also, regular supervision by probation officers can provide a stabilizing influence. Other personality disorders can be helped by simple psychotherapy and guidance through periods of crisis.

Personality and its disorders are of considerable clinical importance for the following reasons:

1 Personality disorders cause much personal, family and social suffering.
2 They tend to make psychiatric diagnosis more difficult.
3 A person's personality characteristics affect the content of any psychiatric illness he may have, and how well he copes with the illness and complies with treatment.
4 Psychiatric illness may occur in response to (i.e. be precipitated by) personality problems.

5 Personality disorders predispose (i.e. increase the likelihood of) psychiatric illness and behaviour difficulties.

Personality problems predispose to two kinds of behaviour difficulty of especial medical and public concern—alcohol and drug abuse, and sexual deviations. These are therefore discussed next.

Alcohol and drug dependence

Human beings have an enormous capacity for damaging themselves in the pursuit of pleasure, whether through taking alcohol or drugs, riding fast motor-cycles or smoking heavily. In the case of alcohol and drug abuse and dependence, the doctor is presented with a condoned toxin (alcohol) and a proscribed or restricted group of toxins, namely 'drugs'. Drug misuse does not necessarily offend society, and much of it is at least partly caused by medical prescribing habits (e.g. iatrogenic analgesic or hypnotic dependence).

Alcohol abuse

Alcohol is condoned by society and is potentially very dangerous, but at the same time provides revenue as well as profit. Chronic alcoholism is a state in which a person is unable to control the amount he drinks and so develops physical, psychiatric and social handicap in consequence. It is vital to obtain a full psychiatric, family and social history in anyone suffering from an alcohol-related illness.

The harmful effects of chronic alcohol abuse are listed in Table 16.11. Many general medical admissions are associated with alcohol-related problems. Withdrawal symptoms occur when alcohol intake ceases in someone who is physically dependent. Of course social, psychiatric and physical problems are closely linked and often coexist.

Severe alcoholism is not really hard to diagnose; but doctors still sometimes have a blind-spot for someone whose drinking is getting out of control, especially someone reasonably high in the social scale, such as another doctor. The signs of developing alcohol dependence include telling lies about alcohol intake that is steadily creeping up, avoiding the topic of drink, becoming preoccupied with having enough drink readily available at home or elsewhere. The drinker who is losing control starts drinking earlier in the day and always has an excuse for a drink. Binges leading to total drunkenness *may* be frequent, although many alcoholics space their

Table 16.11 Harmful effects of chronic abuse of alcohol

Medical
Increased mortality from increased incidence of many diseases
Cardiac: heart muscle disease
Gastrointestinal: pancreatitis, peptic ulcer, cirrhosis
Neurological: peripheral neuropathy, cerebellar failure, amnesic syndrome, dementia, subdural haemorrhage, Wernicke's encephalopathy
Thoracic: liability to tuberculosis
Withdrawal phenomena: tremor, memory lapses, delirium tremens, epileptic fits, auditory hallucinations
Alcohol-induced hypoglycaemia

Psychiatric
Depressive illness
Suicide
Morbid jealousy
Sexual dysfunction

Social
Road accidents
Marital distress, violence, breakdown
Child violence
Absenteeism, loss of job
Financial difficulty
Criminal offences: acquisitive, traffic, violence

drinking throughout the day and never get insensibly drunk. Physical dependence is indicated by the development of withdrawl symptoms (see above) of which morning shakes usually develop first. These are temporarily relieved by alcohol, so the history is of 'liveners' to get going in the morning. Tolerance for alcohol varies, so there are individual differences in dose resistance, although anyone will become dependent if he takes enough for long enough. Some alcoholics find they can tolerate less alcohol once they become dependent on it.

Drug abuse

'Non-medical use' is a term which distinguishes casual drug abuse and dependence from therapeutic drug abuse and dependence. The former is related to the use of drugs for pleasure or to relieve distress, while the latter is related to the 'accidental' discovery by a patient that a drug makes him 'high'. Drug abuse means taking a drug in a way that exceeds its proper medical use. Dependence means the development of a state in which a person has to go on taking a drug (or alcohol, itself a drug) because he needs to get high on it or because he becomes sick if he stops.

There is no need to distinguish too carefully between physical and psychological dependence, except in two

Table 16.12 Classification of drug dependence

	Physical dependence	Psychological dependence
Central stimulant dependence	Nil	Severe
Opiate dependence	Severe	Severe
Alcohol/barbiturate dependence	Dose-related Severe	Usually severe
Hallucinogenic	Nil	May be severe

instances that are clinically important. The first is in the case of opiate drugs, where physical dependence usually is severe, though it presents no hazard to life. The second is in the case of alcohol/barbiturate dependence, where chronic dependence produces a state of intoxication in which acute withdrawal can cause fits which can be fatal (if vomit is inhaled, for example).

There are fashions in drug dependence depending on their availability and on media and other social influences. In the 1980s barbiturates became less common and cocaine more so.

Types of drug dependence

These are often classified according to the type of drug involved. This is currently unhelpful, since the last ten years have shown that multiple-drug use is likely to be the rule. A simple way of classifying the problem is as shown in Table 16.12.

Assessment

As noted, the assessment of individuals with alcohol and drug-related problems requires adequate physical, psychiatric and social evaluation. Often, this is particularly difficult because the person is secretive, not easily trusting of others, defensive, and at best ambivalent about giving up his habit. It is best to be cautious about accepting too readily what the patient says about his alcohol (or drug) consumption. It is very important, though often difficult, to see the patient's close relatives, both to obtain further information and to enlist cooperation and perhaps participation in treatment plans.

Personality is particularly important in the case of alcoholism and drug dependence. These habits often develop as attempts to cope with life problems or stressful environmental events. If the personality has few weaknesses or vulnerabilities, then it will take more external pressure (plus social opportunity) to push the person into alcoholism or drug dependence. People with personality disorders are more vulnerable. The stronger the personality, and the greater the environmental contribution to the alcohol or drug dependence, the better the prognosis.

Treatment

In both cases the objectives are the same, namely abstinence and normal social functioning. In alcoholism, withdrawal is relatively easy and abstention is encouraged by social pressures and by the use of drugs such as disulfiram which cause severe symptoms if alcohol is taken. Patients should be encouraged to join AA (Alcoholics Anonymous), which promotes abstinence through self-help and the recognition that alcohol has defeated the individual.

In the case of drugs the principles are the same, except that in the case of opiate dependence maintenance prescription of an opiate drug has been used as a medical–social measure aimed at limiting illicit drug traffic. In the UK methadone is used, given in special drug-dependency clinics. However, this practice may not always be best, and total withdrawal, covering 'withdrawal symptoms' with clonidine, may be better.

Withdrawal from drugs may require admission to hospital, though the patient's motivation is the key to success and people can be encouraged to stop drugs as part of an outpatient treatment programme. Continuing abstention can be encouraged by involvement in educational and readjustment groups, often run by former drug-users and including a residential component. Some of these programmes are hospital-based, while others have little to do with medical treatment. The aim is to help adjustment to a more realistic life-style, and to the acceptance that a useful and satisfactory life can be lived without resorting to mind-altering drugs as a barrier between oneself and reality.

Sexual deviations

'Sexual deviation' is a statistical term. That is, sexual deviations represent erotic preferences differing from those of the majority who prefer sexual activity with adults of the opposite sex. In this sense only can homosexuality be regarded as a deviation. Recent estimates suggest that in current Western societies perhaps 10 per cent of males have almost exclusively homosexual erotic preferences, while a much larger number (maybe 50–70 per cent) are capable of homosexual and heterosexual responses, while usually preferring the latter.

Other variants from the majority pattern include

paedophilia (sexual interest in children), and bestiality (interest in animals). These are naturally not socially acceptable forms of sexual expression.

Some sexual deviations are like part of the normal love-making process taken out of context and made ends in themselves. Dominating or submitting to a sexual partner become sadism or masochism when inflicting or enduring pain or cruelty become the means of attaining sexual gratification. Interest in possessions or representations of a loved one becomes fetishism when the boots, handkerchief or whatever become the vehicles for orgasm independently of the person. Transvestism implies wearing clothing of members of the opposite sex, again as a means to sexual gratification.

Sometimes transvestism is fetishistic (the clothing represents a preferred sexual partner in some way). It is not usually associated with any doubt in the mind of the transvestite that he (most transvestites are male) is male. Therein transvestism differs from transsexualism in which condition there is a clear conviction of being psychologically of the gender opposite to one's external genital sex. Transsexuals usually request, often with great earnestness, surgical treatment to make the body more appropriate to someone of the experienced gender. Operations such as penectomy and vaginoplasty may play a helpful part in the complex treatment programme required for someone seeking gender reassignment.

Serious sexual deviations often require specialist advice or treatment. However, it may not be easy to decide whether or not any treatment is needed. A useful criterion for determining this is if the person is complaining about it or if the person's sexual partner finds it intolerable. Sometimes agents of society (courts, etc.) complain about behaviour which the individual has no wish to change; in such instances the chances of behavioural change are remote.

Doctors may be called upon to advise people suffering uncertainty, anxiety or distress about their sexual orientation or about relations between sexual and other characteristics of the personality (for example, inferiority feelings and low self-esteem associated with sexual failure and sexual guilt). General counselling principles apply.

Psychiatric emergencies

1 Acute excitement

This means excessive motor activity, often largely purposeless, and excessive noise, associated with much anxiety in subject and observers. It is a clinical situation which may occur in home or hospital. The main causes are:

Organic brain syndromes
Schizophrenia
Mania
Disturbed behaviour of a psychopath usually intoxicated with alcohol or drugs.

Usually time does not permit detailed mental state examination, but it is important to try to find out whether consciousness is clouded or not, for this would suggest an organic state. Treatment of the basic illness follows calming of the acute excited state. The patient should be approached in a calm and quiet manner and medication used effectively. The best medications to use are the neuroleptics such as chlorpromazine and thioridazine given by mouth or by injection. These are effective in all excited states. It is also possible to start with a tranquillizer such as diazepam by injection; this calms the patient and the neuroleptics can be given thereafter. In cases of delirium, chlormethiazole is especially valuable and is the treatment of choice in alcoholic or barbiturate delirium. It should be used with care, however, as it causes respiratory depression when given intravenously and long-term use leads to dependence.

Feeding and adequate fluids, plus good nursing, complete the management.

2 Suicide and attempted suicide

The correlates of completed ('successful') suicide include being male; aged over 50; social isolation (living alone, being widowed, divorced or separated); recent loss of personal significance (bereavement, retirement); presence of serious (especially painful) physical illness; history of depressive illness and perhaps also recent treatment for depression; and presence of alcoholism (and less commonly schizophrenia or Huntington's chorea).

There is partial overlap between the 'suicide' and 'attempted suicide' populations, for many patients who complete suicide have a history of unsuccessful attempts, and some attempters will later complete suicide. Nevertheless, the statistical associations of attempted suicide (which in the majority of instances means self-poisoning) differ from those of suicide. Suicide attempts correlate with being female; aged under 30; current interpersonal difficulties (e.g. arguments with parents or boyfriend, or unwanted pregnancy), and social unsettlement (no steady job or stable living arrangements); and personality disorder rather than psychiatric illness. Only a minority of attempted suicides have depressive illness, alcoholism or schizophrenia. Most attempted suicides are best understood as maladaptive responses to stressful life events.

Admission after self-poisoning is the commonest medical emergency under age 30. Each patient requires psychiatric assessment, which should be a collaborative affair between medical and psychiatric teams. Intensive treatment is likely to be needed for patients who, after self-poisoning, articulate suicidal intentions; are found to be alcoholic, significantly depressed, or possibly psychotic; are judged to have significant problems of social adjustment (unsatisfactory home circumstances and work situation, and inadequate or absent network of supportive personal relationships); and disclose serious unresolved life crises (unwanted pregnancy, impending court appearance). The last two categories are highly correlated with personality difficulty and with the tendency to repeat self-poisoning. The social assessment is more important than the clinical one in many of these patients.

Some self-poisoning patients need only sensible counselling and advice, but admission and proper assessment are appropriate in all cases.

Pregnancy and the puerperium

Rarely (approximately after 1 in 500 births) a psychotic illness occurs. These so-called 'puerperal psychoses' are often episodes of affective illness or schizophrenia starting after, and probably precipitated by, some aspect of childbirth. They usually respond well to physical treatments.

Depressive neuroses are rather more common and occur in about 15 per cent of women during pregnancy or in the early postnatal months. Often they are precipitated by marital problems in depression-prone people.

Marital problems

Medical practice reaches beyond the diagnosis and recognition of various obviously physical or psychological disorders. Increasingly doctors are expected, and rightly, to be able to offer advice, comfort and counselling to people whose lives have become troubled and unhappy through disharmony in their relationships within the family. Relationship problems contribute not only to psychiatric illness but also to many other kinds of health problem, which are more prevalent in tense, stressed households than in calm, peaceful ones. Doctors should be aware of the common problems in marriage that may affect physical and psychological health.

Marital breakdown in the UK is on the increase, as it is elsewhere in the West. Divorce rates are, of course, partly an expression of the rigour or otherwise of divorce laws; but divorce is but a sign that marital breakdown has already occurred, and, where divorce is difficult to obtain, many broken marriages remain marriages only in name.

Factors contributing to marital disharmony and difficulty are many. Early age at marriage (age under 20) is highly correlated with divorce; often the partners in early marriage go on maturing from adolescence to adulthood after they are married and this leads them to grow apart.

Many marriages finally crumble after many years, in middle life. Sometimes this is associated for the husband with an excessive preoccupation and involvement with his work, leading him to neglect wife and family or even use his work as a way of avoiding a wife for whom he has grown to have little regard. On the other hand, a wife may have perhaps over-identified with the rearing of children and diverted less time and affection to her husband, or she may just find raising a family and looking after a house too stressful. A possible decline in sexual life, perhaps developing from sexual problems that have existed previously, adds to the factors potentially contributing to marital breakdown in the middle years. Alcohol problems, too, are frequent at this time of life.

A doctor consulted about marital disharmony needs to have a full and frank discussion with both partners if possible to find out exactly what is going on. Unhappily, however, one partner may be unwilling to participate in such a discussion. Sometimes it may be difficult to realize that a marital problem is present, for patients often present somatic complaints such as headaches, pains or tiredness instead of relationship difficulties about which they feel embarrassed or ashamed.

Once a marriage problem has been identified, and the willingness of both partners to be involved has been assessed, the doctor will need to decide whether he needs to refer for specialist guidance beyond his own counselling skills. Marriage guidance is available in some general practices and psychiatric departments, or from the various marriage guidance councils.

Psychiatric disorders in old age

People do not usually look forward to old age. The physical aspects—loss of elasticity, muscular weakness and stiffening joints—are hard enough to bear. The increased risk of poor health or serious illness is another burden of old age, and in addition there are psychological changes in old age which do not make for a happy life. As people grow older they tend to become more rigid in outlook, tend to lose the range of emotions and drives that formerly had kept them going, and this tends to produce an impatient and intolerant reaction amongst younger people so that it is easy for the elderly person to feel progressively more lonely and rejected. Important clinical points to remember include the following.

Organic cerebral syndromes in the elderly, whether caused by arteriosclerosis or senile dementia, may present as a subacute delirious state.

Affective disorder is common and may be misdiagnosed as dementia, especially where the picture is one of apathy and slowness. Elderly depressives respond very well to antidepressant treatment, either ECT or drugs.

Paranoid states are fairly common. These may be due to late-onset schizophrenia (paraphrenia), affective disorders with paranoid colouring, or they may be paranoid reactions in a life-long eccentric. The response to phenothiazines and antidepressants is very good.

Neuroses in the elderly are often overlooked. This

Table 16.13 The Mental Health Act 1983

Section	Purpose	Application made by	Medical recommendation	Comment
2	Admit for assessment	Nearest relative, or approved social worker	Two doctors, one recognized as having special experience under S.12 of Act	Lasts for 28 days
3	Admit for treatment	As above	As above	Duration 6 months, renewable 6 months and then yearly; patient and family may appeal to Review Tribunal
4	Emergency admission	As above	Any doctor	Lasts for 72 hours
5(2)	To detain a patient in any hospital for observation	Hospital doctor (consultant)	Lasts for up to 72 hours	
37	Provide compulsory treatment or guardianship for offenders	Two doctors: usually prison MO, hospital consultant	Order is made by Crown Court judge or magistrate; hospital doctor has right to discharge; duration after S.3; judge may recommend restriction of discharge under S.41	
136	To provide facility for examination of persons 'deemed' of unsound mind in public by police officer	Police may take such a person to a 'place of safety' to be examined by approved social worker and doctor; terminates at time of assessment, when options are release, informal admission, or admission under S.2 or S.4 as appropriate		

group of patients too easily misses out on sympathy and understanding, let alone psychiatric treatment.

Forensic aspects of psychiatry

Law and psychiatry interrelate in many ways. Laws are made to regulate society, to control criminality and to guarantee equity and justice for all citizens. Psychiatric aspects of the law that students should know about include civil and criminal responsibility, the Mental Health Act (England and Wales), and testamentary capacity.

Responsibility

In law it is assumed that a man is sane and responsible for his actions—he intends their result and must bear responsibility for their consequences. This is true for both criminal and civil matters. In criminal acts the law bases responsibility on actus reus (the guilty act) and mens rea (the guilty mind). Responsibility implies liability to punishment. The prosecutor has to prove the guilty act and the defence has to prove that there is no intent (no mens rea). Age is important: a person may be too young to form intent. Or intent may be said to be absent by reason of mental disorder. This used to be governed by the M'Naghten rules. M'Naghten was a schizophrenic who killed Sir Robert Peel's secretary, thinking he was Sir Robert, whom he believed was persecuting him. The rules said insanity was a defence if the accused was 'labouring under such a defect of reason from disease of the mind as not to know the nature and quality of the act; or if he did know it, that he did not know that what he was doing was wrong'. The rules were hard to apply and led to the legal concept of Diminished Responsibility for Homicide stated in the Homicide Act 1957, whereby a person is not convicted of murder if he 'was suffering from such abnormality of mind...as substantially to impair his mental responsibility'. Such a plea, if accepted, reduces the charge to manslaughter.

1   Civil responsibility
Sanity and responsibility are assumed. An anomaly here is that a drunk man can make a valid will, sign a valid contract or get married as long as he is not so drunk that he does not know what he is doing.

2 Absolute liability
For some offences liability is determined by scientific tests. For example, a blood alcohol level over a certain threshold means unfitness to drive and loss of licence.

Mental health legislation

The Mental Health Act of 1959 was replaced by that of 1983. The aim is to provide safeguards for the mentally ill against illegal detention; and to allow compulsory treatment in a fair and human way. The Act has various sections as summarized here in Table 16.13.

Testamentary capacity

Anyone can make a valid will as long as he is of 'sound disposing mind'. Incapacity may be in question in cases of mental illness, especially organic states. The criteria for capacity are that the person should know the implications of the act of making a will, and know the extent of the estate and the likely beneficiaries. His judgement should not be impaired. Severe mental illness such as schizophrenia or dementia does not automatically make someone incapable, since there are often large islands of lucidity. Doctors should never witness a will made by a patient, over and above the obvious bar to witnessing a will of which the doctor is a beneficiary.

Further reading

Bloch, S. (ed.) (1985) *An Introduction to the Psychotherapies*, 2nd edn. Blackwell, Oxford.
Granville-Grossman, K. (ed.) (1979, 1982 and 1985) *Recent Advances in Clinical Psychiatry*, vols. 3, 4 and 5. Churchill Livingstone, Edinburgh.
Gelder, M.G., Mayou, R. and Gath, D.H. (1983) *Oxford Textbook of Psychiatry*. Blackwell, Oxford.
Lishman, W.A. (1987) *Organic Psychiatry*. 2nd Edition Blackwell, Oxford.

17
Medical Genetics

There are some people whose failing health in early life is determined at conception. All the intrauterine influences, the dietary, infectious and toxic factors that contribute to the child's environment after birth, including at present the efforts of his doctors, do little to alter the course of *Duchenne muscular dystrophy*. At his conception his single X chromosome is carrying the Duchenne muscular dystrophy mutation, either inherited from his mother or arriving as a new mutation in the ovum before fertilization; and this alone is sufficient to cause him to be chairbound by the end of his first decade and dead by the end of his second. The tragedy for the family is compounded by the fear that subsequent boys will also be affected. The actual risk of this may be very high or low depending on the relative probability of either his mother being a carrier or his disease being the result of a new mutation. As with other genetic disorders clinical geneticists are likely to become involved in estimating this risk of recurrence, and then discussing this risk and the various options available to the couple involved. Certain principles of human genetics assist the doctor in this task. This chapter recalls some of these principles and describes their application in clinical medicine.

Genetic variation

In a sense genetically determined diseases like Duchenne muscular dystrophy are just part of the spectrum of genetic variation in human populations. With the exception of identical (monozygotic) twins, we all differ genetically, and these differences account not only for much of the variation in physical attributes like height, but also for some of the differences in the susceptibility to disease. Most common diseases are the result of a complex interaction between environmental and genetic influences, the latter being the result of many genes each having a small effect. Most of these genes cannot be regarded as abnormal in the sense that the gene for blood group O is no more abnormal than for blood group A. Here we are dealing with specific alternative genes which in most circumstances provide for adequate health. The variation is due in part to natural selection on our ancestors who faced environmental pressures different from today. By contrast, much of what follows in this chapter concerns changes in genes that are harmful, mutations that completely disrupt the normal functioning of the gene so that their effect generally overrides all other genetic and environmental influences.

Now that so much is known about the actual structure of genes and how they are encoded in the chromosomal DNA (deoxyribonucleic acid), it is helpful to explain some of the classic genetic concepts (derived from the study of the pattern of inheritance of characters) in simple structural terms. In females the 46 chromosomes are present in homologous pairs, and thus there are two copies of every gene, one maternal and the other paternal in origin. It is the same in males except for the difference in the sex chromosome pair X and Y.

A structural gene is made up of the DNA nucleotide sequences that code for a single polypeptide chain synthesized at the ribosomes in the cell cytoplasm. The polypeptide chain may subsequently be modified, or more than one type of polypeptide chain may associate to make a macromolecule; α globin and β globin chains go to make up adult haemoglobin, HbA. Each structural gene has a specific site on the DNA of a particular chromosome; there is one β globin gene on each of the pair of chromosomes 11. The two β globin genes together constitute the β globin gene *locus*. Alternative genes at a single locus are called *alleles*. One of the nucleotides in one of the two β globin genes is altered in people with the sickle-cell trait, and therefore the sickle,

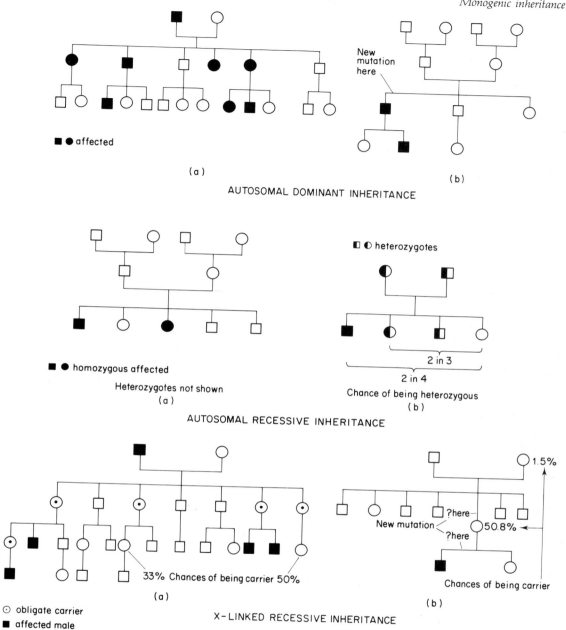

Figure 17.1 *Pedigrees illustrating Mendelian inheritance. Autosomal dominant (a) On average 50 per cent of the offspring of an affected individual are affected; there is male to male transmission. (b) In severe disorders new mutations will be frequently encountered. Autosomal recessive (a) Affected individuals usually confined to one sibship, with a 1 in 4 recurrence risk if both parents healthy. (b) The healthy sibs of an affected individual have a 2 in 3 chance of being a carrier X-linked recessive (a) No male to male transmission; daughters of an affected male and females in the direct line between two affected males are obligate carriers. For other females the chance of being a carrier is influenced by the number of normal sons. (b) In X-linked lethal disorders one-third of affected males and half of carrier females represent new mutations. The probability of this being the case is influenced by the number of normal males in the pedigree.*

or β^s, gene and the normal β gene are alleles. Obviously with only two DNA sites any one individual can only have two alleles at any one locus. However, in the population there may be numerous alleles, and indeed over 100 β globin chain variants have been described.

An individual with two different alleles at a particular locus is *heterozygous* for that locus. Where both alleles are the usual ones, we refer to *normal homozygous*, and where both are the same harmful alleles, the term *abnormal homozygous* can be used. Genes on the X chromosome are not one of a pair in males, and when such a gene is abnormal in a male the term *hemizygous* is sometimes used.

Monogenic inheritance

See Fig. 17.1.

Autosomal dominant disorders

In medical genetics the term autosomal dominant refers to the situation where a monogenic disorder is manifest clinically in the heterozygous state. In Britain the overall incidence of autosomal dominant disorders is about 7 per 1000 live births; some of the more common conditions being *polycystic kidney disease* (mutation on chromosome 16), *monogenic hypercholesterolaemia* (chromosome 19), *neurofibromatosis* (chromosome 17), and *Huntington's chorea* (chromosome 4). Appreciating that each parent passes on only one chromosome of each pair to the child, it can be simply deduced that any child of a person with an autosomal dominant disorder has a 1 in 2 chance of being affected. On average half will inherit the chromosome carrying the abnormal gene, and half the chromosome carrying the normal gene. Thus given enough offspring the condition can manifest in each generation and in both sexes, with only affected individuals able to pass it on.

Unfortunately in clinical practice the matter is complicated by two things, variation in the expression of the gene and new mutation. Both points are illustrated by neurofibromatosis, which has an incidence of about 1 in 3000. The manifestations in someone carrying the gene vary from just a few characteristic pigmented patches on the skin, so-called 'café au lait' spots, to gross disfigurement with a mass of cutaneous and subcutaneous tumours, and mental handicap. In neurofibromatosis as in many autosomal dominant disorders, a mildly affected person has to be warned that any child inheriting the gene may not be so lucky as they have been. It can also be seen that a person with minimal manifestations may be

regarded as normal, and give rise to the view that the condition has 'skipped a generation'. Taking variation in the expression of the gene one stage further, one can argue that in some situations there will be no manifestation of the gene carried by some family members; that is, the gene has less than 100 per cent penetrance. Reduced penetrance as a concept distinct from variable gene expression is not very helpful in practice. The important message is that you cannot advise someone until you have performed a careful physical examination, a general rule in clinical medicine. If they are clear one may be reassuring about risks to their children, but you can never give an absolute guarantee.

It is important, of course, to know the usual age of onset of the disease because quite a proportion of autosomal dominant disorders only manifest later in life, often after the carrier of the gene has completed his family. Huntington's chorea is a degenerative disorder of the brain, particularly of the basal ganglia, with an average age of onset of about 42 years. The close linkage of this mutation to a chromosome 4 DNA marker has opened up the possibility, in some families, of presymptomatic detection of those carrying the mutation with all its attendant psychological and management problems.

All dominant disorders have to start at some time as new mutations in the ovum or sperm, and obviously the more severe the type of disease, the less likely the patient is to reproduce, and the greater proportion of affected individuals will be the result of a new mutation. In the mild dominant disorders, or those of late onset, the vast majority of patients have inherited it from an affected parent. New mutations and the variable gene expression can combine to create difficult clinical decisions. If a single child in the family has overt neurofibromatosis, the apparently healthy parents will want to know the risk to further children. If it is decided the child is the result of a new mutation, then the risk of recurrence is very low. However, if an examination reveals convincing minimal signs of neurofibromatosis in one parent, then the couple face a 1 in 2 risk with each pregnancy. This demonstrates the importance of knowing what are the minimal signs of the disorder, and the difficulties that could arise in doubtful cases.

It is estimated that about half the cases of neurofibromatosis are due to new mutations, and this represents an estimated mutation rate of about 10^{-4}; that is, 1 in 10 000 germ cells mutate per generation, or 1 in 5000 babies have neurofibromatosis as a result of a new mutation. This is one of the highest mutation rates in man, and estimated mutation rates for dominant (and X-linked conditions) usually lie between 10^{-5} and 10^{-6}.

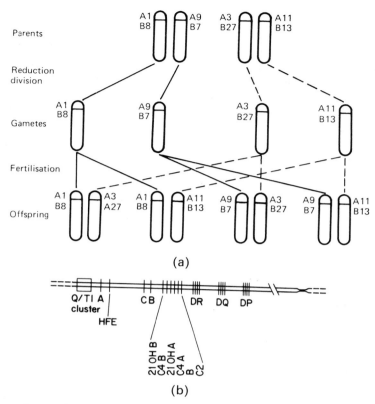

Figure 17.2   *(a) Chromosome diagram showing the usual segregation of HLA haplotypes with no crossover between loci A and B. (b) Genetic map of the major histocompatibility complex. Each vertical line represents a gene locus for a different HLA chain or some other protein as indicated. HFE, haemochromatosis; 21OH A, 21-hydroxylase (inactive gene); 21OH B, 21-hydroxylase; C4 A, C4 B, B, C2, complement components.*

Autosomal recessive disorders

In autosomal recessive inheritance the disorder is only manifest clinically when the patient has a double dose of the abnormal gene (i.e. in the homozygous state). The patient has no normal allele at the particular locus involved, having inherited one abnormal gene from each parent. Usually both parents are heterozygous for the gene in question, and are clinically normal, the action of their normal allele at the locus being sufficient to compensate. Rarely one or even both parents are themselves affected homozygotes. In the usual situation, where both parents are heterozygous, a child has a 1 in 4 chance of being an affected homozygote, there is a 2 in 4 chance of being a heterozygote like the parents, and a 1 in 4 chance of being normal.

In Britain the overall incidence of autosomal recessive disorders is about 2.5 per 1000 live births, and the commonest is *cystic fibrosis* (mutation on chromosome 7). About 1 in 2000 are affected and about 1 in 22 people are heterozygotes, or carriers of the gene. The exact bio-

chemical defect in cystic fibrosis is unknown, but there is a generalized alteration in mucus, with blocked pancreatic ducts leading to digestive problems, and blockage in the bronchial tree causing recurrent chest infections. A great number of autosomal recessive disorders are caused by an absent or inactive enzyme, preventing a step in a critical metabolic pathway—the so-called 'inborn error of metabolism' first elucidated by Garrod in the early years of this century. One fairly common example is a form of *adrenal hyperplasia (adrenogenital syndrome)*. The deficient enzyme is 21 hydroxylase, the gene for which happens to be situated on chromosome 6 (Fig. 17.2). The resultant metabolic block causes increased activity in an alternative pathway leading to the excess production of androgens. These result in 'virilization' of the female fetus with enlargement of the clitoris. More importantly the 21 hydroxylase deficiency interferes with the production of important cortical steroids. The clinical features of many inborn errors of metabolism are the result both of the accumulation of substances before, and a deficiency of substances beyond, the enzyme block.

The heterozygous state can be detected by biochemical tests in many autosomal recessive disorders and this can play an important part in genetic counselling. This fact also raises the question of whether a condition is truly recessive, if the gene produces a detectable effect in the heterozygous state. In practice the heterozygote is generally healthy, and there is such a vast difference between the clinical manifestation in the heterozygous and the abnormal homozygous state that the use of additional categories such as intermediate or codominant disorders is unhelpful. *Sickle-cell anaemia* and *β-thalassaemia major (Cooley's anaemia)* can be regarded as autosomal recessive disorders even though the heterozygote or sickle-cell trait may have some *in vivo* sickling of the red cells with extreme anoxia, and people with *β*-thalassaemia trait may be slightly anaemic.

The incidence at birth of a recessive disorder in a population depends primarily on the incidence of the heterozygous state. Obviously early death will modify the frequency with which it is encountered in an older population, and a changing rate of cousin marriage can also have an effect. The extent to which new mutations maintain the frequency of heterozygotes for different recessive disorders is difficult to estimate, but natural selection has played the predominant role in sickle-cell disease and the thalassaemias. The sickle-cell trait affords some protection against malaria, and analysis of DNA around the sickle-gene locus indicates that about 80 per cent of West Africans with the sickle-cell trait inherited the gene from a common ancestor.

First cousins share one-eighth of their genes in common and therefore they have a slightly increased chance of having children with recessive disorders compared with unrelated parents in the same population. Direct comparison between populations is not valid because a high cousin marriage rate over many generations tends to reduce the frequency of harmful recessive genes by natural selection.

X-linked recessive disorders

X-linked recessive inheritance produces a characteristic family pedigree, where males are affected and the gene is passed on by unaffected females. Using simple diagrams of the X and Y chromosome it is easy to satisfy oneself that an abnormal gene carried on one of the X chromosomes in a female will be passed on to half her daughters, who would be heterozygous like herself, and to half her sons who would manifest the disease because they have no compensating X. An affected male would produce only heterozygous daughters, but cannot pass the gene on to his sons, who only receive his Y chromosome. In a population where the X-linked red-cell enzyme defect *glucose-6-phosphate dehydrogenase* (G6PD) *deficiency* is common, an affected man may have an affected son, but only because his wife is also a heterozygote. Such a mating results in half the girls being affected homozygotes.

In some X-linked disorders a proportion of female heterozygotes are mildly affected, and this is the case with G6PD deficiency. Cytochemical staining of the red cells shows that about half are G6PD-deficient and half are normal. The explanation (the Lyon hypothesis) lies in the fact that only one of the X chromosome pair is active in any one cell. The random inactivation of one or other X chromosome occurs in each cell early in embryonic development, and thereafter the descendants of a particular cell have the same inactive X. By chance some women heterozygous for G6PD deficiency have the normal X chromosome inactivated in 80–90 per cent of their cells, and can therefore develop haemolysis, like the affected hemizygous males, when exposed to certain drugs such as sulphonamides and anti-malarials.

In Britain the incidence of X-linked disorders is about 0.9 per 1000 total male live births, excluding *fragile X mental retardation* considered later, which has an incidence of about 1 in 1500 males. *Duchenne muscular dystrophy* has a birth incidence of about 1 in 4000 males. As we saw earlier, when there is an isolated affected male in the family, one of the clinical problems is to establish the probability of his disease being due to a new mutation. One can take the number of healthy males on the mother's side of the family into account, as well as the mother's plasma creatine kinase level. The enzyme leaks out of dystrophic muscle fibres and very high levels are found in the plasma of affected boys. The creatine kinase level tends to be increased in women heterozygous for the muscular dystrophy gene, but the distribution of values overlaps with the distribution of values from normal women, so that whilst a very high level confirms the carrier state, a low level cannot completely exclude it. Similar problems arise when counselling families with *haemophilia* (two distinct genes: one causing factor VIII, the other factor IX deficiency). This general problem with biochemical carrier tests in X-linked recessive disorders is a reflection of random X-inactivation. Fortunately gene tracking within the family using gene-specific or linked DNA probes has proven particularly valuable in carrier exclusion, releasing such women from the fear of affected boys.

The term *X-linked dominant* has been used for the very

few rare conditions where the heterozygous female is regularly affected. However, the hemizygous male is always more severely affected, and in some instances, such as *incontinentia pigmenti* or the X-linked form of *oral–facial–digital syndrome*, affected males rarely survive gestation to be born, so only female patients are encountered in clinical practice.

Reference is made to the X-linked form of the oral–facial–digital syndrome, because an almost identical syndrome can be caused by an autosomal recessive gene. There are quite a number of disorders that are virtually indistinguishable on ordinary clinical examination, but are caused by different genes, often with different patterns of inheritance.

Genetic linkage and disease associations

At meiosis homologous chromosomes pair up, and there is often exchange of a length of chromosome between the pair: so-called crossing-over. Thus the single set of chromosomes that ends up in an ovum or sperm carries an assortment of the genes from both sets of chromosomes in the parent. If crossing-over did not occur, all the genes on a particular chromosome would always be inherited *en bloc*, the characteristics they determine being coinherited together generation after generation in the family. Crossing-over results in some genes that are carried on the same chromosome assorting independently, but obviously the closer two genes are situated on a chromosome, the less likely they are to be separated by crossing over and the more likely they are to be inherited together. Two such genes loci are said to be linked, and the genetic linkage could be demonstrated in a family, if it happens that different alleles are present at each of the two loci. In other words, one needs a tag on the four bits of chromosome one is interested in, to know what is going on. Detectable chromosome-site specific variations in DNA sequences are now the most abundant type of genetic marker, and are discussed later.

The genes involved in the HLA system of tissue types also illustrate some of these points. There is a large number of different histocompatibility antigens, which amongst other things are involved in rejection of foreign-tissue grafts. Although there are many genes loci involved, as shown in the gene map in Fig. 17.2, discussion will be confined to the four different HLA loci named HLA A, B, C and DR. There are about 10 alleles at locus A, 26 for B, 8 for C and 10 for locus DR. It will be recalled, however, that an individual can only have 2

alleles at each locus, as illustrated in Fig. 17.2, which for simplicity just gives the HLA A and B specificities.

The particular combination of alleles (and the specific antigens they determine) on a single chromosome is called a haplotype, and because the HLA A and B loci are closely linked, the parental haplotypes are generally passed on unchanged. However, during meiosis about one time in a hundred a cross-over between the two number 6 chromosomes occurs at a site between loci A and B, and the ovum or sperm will then carry a recombinant haplotype. A particular haplotype is not 'fixed' for ever, even if it is transmitted unchanged for many generations. Given enough time and random mating, every combination of alleles at loci A and B should arise; and in theory the frequency of the combinations, or haplotypes, should be a reflection (actually the product) of the frequencies of the individual alleles. Where this is the case the alleles are said to be in linkage equilibrium.

When two alleles occur together more frequently, or less frequently than expected from the individual frequencies, they are said to be in linkage disequilibrium. Linkage disequilibrium can arise in a variety of ways. One allele may have arisen by mutation relatively recently (on the evolutionary time scale) and not yet achieved equilibrium, still reflecting the original combination. A particular combination may have a selective advantage or disadvantage and achieve disequilibrium by natural selection. The same principles of equilibrium and disequilibrium can apply to alleles of any two linked gene loci. The haplotype A1B8 occurs more frequently than the individual frequencies would predict, and therefore these two alleles show linkage disequilibrium.

A mild dominant disorder, the *nail patella syndrome*, shows genetic linkage with the blood group ABO locus, both the ABO and the disease gene locus being situated on chromosome 9. If the nail patella syndrome gene happens to be on a chromosome 9 that carries the allele for group A, then the disease and the blood group A will tend to be inherited together. However, because of eventual crossing-over, or independent mutations leading to different affected families, the nail patella syndrome may be linked with blood group O in another family or group B in a third family. Thus there is genetic linkage, but no association with a particular blood group. Genetic linkage is a phenomenon demonstrable within families. By contrast, association is a phenomenon demonstrated by comparing a population of affected individuals with a control population. People with blood group A are more likely to get cancer of the stomach than people of blood group O. This is an association between the group A allele and the cancer, but this does not necessarily mean that a cancer susceptibility gene is situated on chromosome 9 close to the ABO gene locus.

Confusion between genetic linkage and the disease associations arises because, in cases of an association between a particular HLA antigen and a disease, one of the explanations for the association is genetic linkage between the HLA loci and a disease susceptibility gene *plus* linkage disequilibrium involving the particular allele at an HLA locus. Linkage disequilibrium is an essential part of this explanation, for as we have already seen with the nail patella syndrome and the ABO blood groups, genetic linkage alone does not result in a general association.

It should be realized that transplantation is not the only reason for the clinical importance of the HLA genes. These and other genes in the histocompatibility region (MHC) are concerned with the immune response. It is reasonable to guess that some common chronic diseases may be due, at least in part, to an abnormal immune response to certain infectious agents. It is these ideas that have given added significance to the associations that have been observed between certain HLA specificities and some diseases. By far the best example, and one of the strongest association, is between *idiopathic ankylosing spondylitis* and *HLA B 27*. Over 90 per cent of Europeans with ankylosing spondylitis have HLA B 27, compared with only about 9 per cent of the general population. HLA B 27 alone is not sufficient to cause the disease; for if it were, the disease would show an autosomal dominant pattern of inheritance, which it does not. Environmental factors are obviously also important.

Multifactorial inheritance

The correlation between the height of parents and their children's eventual height is clear for all to see. The inheritance of quantitative characters, like height, has been the subject of careful study for over a century, and it can be shown that the correlation between various relatives can be explained on the basis of many genes each of small effect segregating in a normal Mendelian fashion (i.e. obeying the same rules described so far in this chapter).

There is a significant genetic contribution to the cause of some common congenital malformations like *spina bifida*, *cleft lip ± palate*, or *congenital heart disease*, and it appears that this is mainly on the basis of many genes each having a small positive or negative effect on the susceptibility of the fetus to the malformation. First-degree relatives (brothers and sisters or children) of an affected person have a considerable risk of being affected, but this increased risk diminishes rapidly when one moves to second-degree relatives (nephews, nieces and grandchildren) and is almost back to the general-population incidence for third-degree relatives (cousins). This general point about multifactorial inheritance is illustrated by cleft lip ± palate which has incidence of about 1 per 1000 live births in Britain. In first-degree relatives of an affected case the incidence is about 40 per 1000, but falls to 7 per 1000 for second-degree relatives and 2–3 per 1000 for third-degree relatives. When a couple has had two affected children, the risk to a further child is higher, about 14 per cent. In reality, of course, the risk has been the same for each pregnancy; what has increased is our information about how susceptible the children of this couple are to the malformation. It must be emphasized that largely unknown environmental factors also play an important part in the cause of these common malformations, and 'preventative measures' around the time of conception and in early pregnancy might be possible in the future. There is increasing evidence that maternal multivitamin and folic acid supplementation is associated with a reduction in the recurrence risk for spina bifida and anencephaly.

Many common disorders of adult life, such as *diabetes mellitus, arterial hypertension, epilepsy* or *schizophrenia*, have a significant genetic component with close relatives having an increased risk of developing the disease. However, it is becoming clear that there are probably several causes of these conditions, some largely environmental, some genetic, whilst others are multifactorial, involving both the action of several genes and environmental factors.

Type I or insulin-dependent diabetes mellitus appears to be usually the result of virus-triggered autoimmune destruction of the β-islet cells in genetically susceptible individuals. The main susceptibility gene(s) are located on chromosome 6 within or close to the HLA gene complex. Much of the genetic susceptibility is dependent on the absence of aspartic acid at residue 57 of the DQβ chain. Overall a sibling of an index case has a risk of about 5–6 per cent of developing diabetes mellitus by the age of 16 years. However if the sibling has inherited the same two number 6 chromosomes as the index case (that is, they are HLA identical), the risk is much higher, perhaps 30 per cent by the age of 30; and it is correspondingly very low if the sibling has no chromosome 6 in common with the index case.

Type II or maturity-onset diabetes shows close to 100 per cent concordance in monozygotic twins (compared with just under 60 per cent concordance in monozygotic twins where one has type I diabetes), indicating almost complete genetic determination. Obesity clearly contributes in some way; and if the index case with type II diabetes mellitus is obese, the risk to a non-obese sibling is about 5 per cent whilst with a non-obese index case the risk to an obese sibling is about 25 per cent. This brief account is obviously an oversimplification, for there is almost certainly further heterogeneity within the general description diabetes mellitus.

Chromosome abnormalities

Chromosome abnormalities fall into two broad categories: disorders of chromosome number, and rearrangements or changes in chromosome structure. The overall incidence in live births is about 5–6 per 1000, and it is estimated that about 50 per cent of early spontaneous abortions are chromosomally abnormal, and of 1000 recognized pregnancies there are about 75 fetal or neonatal deaths due to chromosome abnormalities, the great majority arising as new mutations in the ovum, sperm or early zygote.

Fragile X syndrome

Simple monogenic disorders are not usually associated with any chromosomal change using routine karyotype analysis. However, an X-linked form of mental handicap affecting 1 in 1500 boys, the Martin Bell or fragile X syndrome, features an unstainable gap or 'fragile site' at the end of the long arm of the X, in 5–50 per cent of cells, when lymphocytes are cultured in folic-acid-deficient or other special medium (Fig. 17.3).

This represents the commonest cause of mental retardation in males after Down's syndrome, and about one-third of the female carriers are also clinically affected, although on average the intellectual deficit is less than in males. Whilst the clinically affected carriers show fragile sites, only about half the unaffected carriers are detectable cytogenetically, which creates difficulties in genetic counselling. Further difficulties are caused by the fact that quite often it is found that affected cousins have inherited the condition from the maternal grandfather who is fragile-site-negative and clinically normal. This irregular X-linked inheritance is best explained by a stepwise progression of the mutation over three generations. Affected males have large rather than small heads, and large testes after puberty. Behaviour problems are common in childhood and some 20 per cent have grand mal seizures.

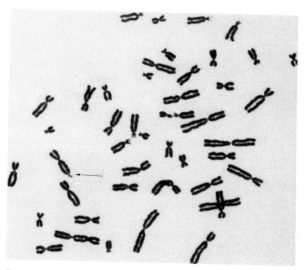

Figure 17.3 *A chromosome metaphase spread (simple unbanded stain) showing the appearance of the fragile site (arrowed) of Xq27.3 associated with the fragile X mental retardation syndrome.*

Disorders of chromosome number

During meiosis, the reduction division that leads to the ovum and sperm having a single, haploid, set of chromosomes, homologous chromosomes pair up before moving apart to the opposite poles of the dividing cell. Failure of the pair to associate in the first place, or failure to dissociate, can lead to an ovum or sperm with an extra chromosome, or one missing. The term non-disjunction, which assumes the latter mechanism, is often used for this error of chromosome segregation. The causes of non-disjunction are largely unknown, but the chance of it having occurred in the ovum increases with age. The resulting fetus will either have three copies of a particular chromosome (*trisomy*) or only one (*monosomy*). In practice the trisomies are the most important, monosomies in general being non-viable.

In some individuals the non-disjunction occurs after zygote formation, and in this case there are two cell lines each with a different chromosome complement. Such cases, which when they do occur often involve the sex chromosomes, are called *mosaics*. Overall, mosaics tend to manifest fewer abnormalities of development than the full trisomy, although this is not necessarily so and prediction of the clinical outcome when mosaicism is found on a prenatal test is not possible.

Anomalies of sex chromosome number

Trisomies involving the X or Y chromosome are

relatively common and lead to surprisingly minor physical abnormalities considering the size of the X chromosome and the many genes it carries. The explanation resides in the phenomenon of X chromosome inactivation described earlier. Only one X chromosome remains active in any one cell beyond an early stage of development, and the inactive X chromosome becomes the X chromatin body (formerly known as the Barr body) which is visible close to the nuclear membrane in a proportion of cell nuclei in females. XXX females have two X-chromatin bodies in their cell nuclei, and the much rarer XXXX females have three X-chromatin bodies.

About 1 in 700 newborn males has the chromosome complement 47XXY, is X-chromatin positive, and has the clinical picture of *Klinefelter's syndrome*. Twenty per cent of Klinefelters are mosaics (e.g. 47XXY/46XY, etc.). Those affected are outwardly nearly normal males, but the testes are always small after puberty with complete, or almost complete, azoospermia. In 30 per cent there is enlargement of the breasts, termed gynaecomastia, and concern about this, or infertility, are common ways for these patients to present. About 50 per cent have delayed language development, and although the IQ is below 90 in 30 per cent, only a few have an IQ below 80.

About 1 in 1000 newborn females has the chromosome complement 47XXX. Although disturbances of menstruation and fertility are common, many are essentially normal, fertile females. About 50 per cent have delayed language development and the IQ is below 70 in 15 per cent. Theoretically a proportion of their ova would carry two X chromosomes, leading to XXX or XXY offspring. This event has been observed, but there is probably selection against the abnormal ova.

With the relatively high incidence of 47XXY and 47XXX newborns, one would expect the complementary product of the non-disjunction, the 45X individual, to be common. It probably is at the time of conception, but about 98 per cent are lost as early abortions and only about 1 in 10 000 female births has the 45X chromosome complement with the associated clinical picture of *Turner's syndrome*. Affected females are short and fail to menstruate, their ovaries being replaced by streaks of connective tissue. There are often associated physical abnormalities, such as neck webbing, renal malformations, deafness and coarctation of the aorta, but intelligence is usually normal. Twenty per cent with Turner's syndrome have an isochromosome X, where a maldivision of the centromere has led to two long arms and no short arm.

The XYY complement is found in about 1 in 700 newborn males. Usually tall (at least 180 cm) and fertile, the great majority remain undiagnosed leading normal lives. There is language development delay in 30 per cent and the IQ is below 90 in 30 per cent with few below IQ 80. Some with mental retardation have antisocial behaviour leading to an over-representation in institutions for dangerous mentally ill subjects.

Down's syndrome due to primary trisomy 21

Down's syndrome (mongolism), always due to an extra chromosome 21, is the commonest viable autosomal trisomy, presumably because of the small size of the chromosome involved. Overall about 96 per cent are due to a primary non-disjunction, and about 80 per cent involve errors in the formation of the ovum rather than the sperm. In the other 4 per cent the extra chromosome 21 is attached to another chromosome and will be discussed in the next section. The incidence of Down's syndrome increases from about 1 in 1200 in mothers under 30 years to about 1 in 100 at the age of 40 years, and at present accounts for about a third of all cases of severe mental handicap at school age.

Chromosomal translocations and other structural abnormalities

With the change from simple staining (Fig. 17.3) to banding of chromosomes (Fig. 17.4) it became possible to identify individual chromosomes and parts of chromosomes, and to describe regions and bands (Fig. 17.5).

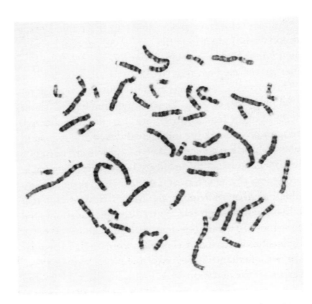

Figure 17.4 *A chromosome metaphase spread of a normal female stained with one of the Giemsa banding techniques.*

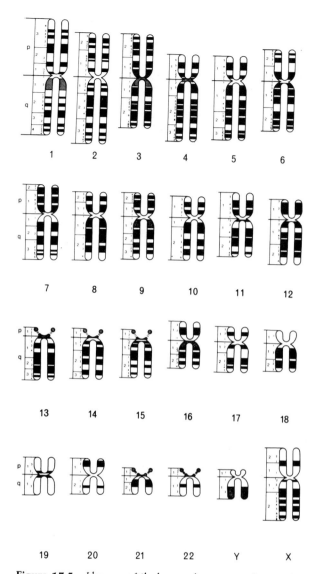

Figure 17.5   *Ideogram of the human chromosomes showing the banding pattern that allows each one to be identified. Chromosomes are analysed during division and each chromosome is shown divided into two daughter chromatids but attached at the centrometer. Chromosomes 13, 14, 15, 21 and 22 are termed acrocentric, with only ribosomal genes encoded on the short arms.*

This has allowed the accurate description of translocations and structural changes like small deletions. The condensed chromosomes in Fig. 17.3 show the two chromatids and centromeres where they are joined. These are less obvious in the longer chromosomes analysed earlier in cell division (Fig. 17.4).

An internationally agreed shorthand for describing a karyotype is as follows: 'p' indicates the short arm, 'q' the long arm, and 't' a translocation. The total chromosome count is written first followed by the sex chromosome complement. A gain or loss of a whole chromosome is indicated by '+' or '−' before the number of the chromosome involved; for example, 47XX + 21 = female Downs. A balanced reciprocal translocation between 1 and 3 would be written 46XXt(1; 3)(q32; q25), the position of the break points being described by arm, region and band for 1 and 3 respectively.

A *reciprocal translocation* occurs when two different chromosomes break simultaneously and a portion of one joins up with a portion of the other, and vice versa. Such a person has 46 chromosomes but part of two chromosomes, say a number 1 and a number 3, have been rearranged. There is no loss of genetic material and the carrier of this balanced reciprocal translocation is healthy. However, trouble can occur at meiosis, for normally just one of each homologous pair is passed on by the ovum or sperm. If the normal chromosome 1 and the normal chromosome 3 are passed on, a child with a normal chromosome complement will result. If the chromosome 1 carrying a bit of 3 and the chromosome 3 carrying a bit of 1 are passed on, a healthy child with a balanced translocation, like the parent, will result. However, if either of the other two combinations are passed on the child will have an unbalanced translocation and development can be severely disturbed. Risks vary with the particular translocation involved. A male or female carrier of a balanced reciprocal translocation ascertained because of an abnormal child has about a 20 per cent chance of a subsequent child having an unbalanced translocation. The risk is about 5 per cent if the carrier was picked up in some other way.

The effect of certain small constitutional deletions within a chromosome are now being delineated. Deletion of the band 11p 13 is associated with *aniridia* and *Wilms' tumour*; 13q 14 with retinoblastoma; and 15q 12 with the *Prader–Willi* syndrome.

Translocation Down's syndrome

We have seen that primary non-disjunction is the main cause of Down's syndrome and increases with maternal age. However, in about 8–10 per cent of the subjects with Down's syndrome born to mothers under 30 years, the extra 21 chromosome is attached by its short arm to the short arm of another acrocentric chromosome (13–15 or 21–22), usually chromosome 14. This type of fusion of two acrocentric chromosomes is termed a *Robertsonian translocation*. Thus the Down's syndrome child has 46 chromosomes, but one in fact is a composite chromosome 14^{21}.

In about a third of cases one or other parent carries the 14^{12} Robertsonian translocation. However, they have only 45 chromosomes, including a normal 14, a normal 21 and the composite 14^{21}; and since they have the right amount of chromosome material they are healthy. The short arm material can be lost without ill effect. Again the problems arise at meiosis, when the 14, the 21 and the 14^{21} chromosomes have to associate together and then segregate. Normal ova or sperm can be formed leading to normal offspring. The ova or sperm may carry the composite 14^{21} without the other 21 or 14, and produce healthy offspring carrying the translocation. Finally, both the composite 14^{21} and the other 21 may pass into the ovum or sperm and a child with Down's syndrome will result. There is selection against the unbalanced gametes and a woman carrying a 14^{21} translocation has a risk of about 1 in 8 of producing a child with Down's syndrome, whilst for a man the risk is about 1 in 50.

Direct analysis of DNA

Until recently the letters DNA in a patient's notes meant 'Did not attend'; increasingly it will indicate a test involving direct analysis of some of the patient's genes! The impact of the so-called 'new genetics' on clinical medicine stems from three main components: (a) the ability to isolate or construct specific sequences of DNA and clone these by exploiting the rapid replication of bacteria; (b) the fundamental discoveries concerning the organization of human chromosomal DNA, or genome, made possible by (a); and (c) the ability to analyse certain specific genes in any individual using DNA from any tissue.

The 46 chromosomes represent a 6 000 000 000 long string of the nucleotide bases guanine, cytosine, adenine and thymine; but probably only a mere 3 per cent or so represent coding sequences for the body proteins. A coding sequence is 'read' in base triplets, or codons. Codons exist for the 20 amino acids and also for initiation and termination of translation. Each coding sequence for a polypeptide chain is interrupted by non-coding regions (*introns* or *intervening sequences*) which range in number from 2 in many genes to about 50 in one of the collagen genes. The blocks of coding sequence are called *exons*. The exons and introns plus short sequences at either end of the gene are all transcribed into a single stranded nuclear RNA (ribonucleic acid) molecule. Next the introns have to be carefully spliced out before the definitive messenger RNA, now with a continuous coding sequence, can move into the cytoplasm (Fig. 17.6). The

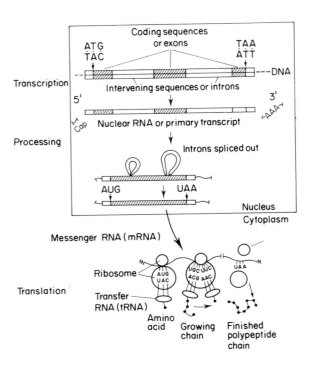

Figure 17.6 *Diagram illustrating the main features of transcription of a gene into a nuclear RNA molecule, the addition of a cap and a poly-A tail, the splicing out of the introns to produce the definitive messenger RNA molecule, and the translation of the mRNA into a polypeptide chain. The position of the translation initiation codon (AUG) and the termination codon (UAA) is indicated on both the DNA and RNA level.*

term 'gene' is usefully applied to the whole transcription unit (plus sequences necessary for the initiation of transcription) for mutations anywhere in this DNA can cause a deficiency or abnormality of the gene product. In sickle-cell anaemia there is a point mutation (single base change) in the β-globin gene with the codon corresponding to the sixth amino acid GAG (glutamic acid) changed to GTG (valine). β^0-thalassaemia (complete absence of β-globin) can be due to point mutations that result in premature termination of translation; point mutations that prevent splicing out an intron; or a base deletion leading to a disasterous shift in the reading frame during translation, to name just some of the causes. β^+-thalassaemia, producing just a few normal β chains, can be due to a point mutation in the middle of the first intron that results in ambiguous splicing with some mRNA molecules correctly assembled but with the majority incorrectly spliced.

The discovery of this heterogeneity at the DNA level, which is likely to be just as marked in most autosomal-dominant and X-linked disorders, poses some problems for identification of genetic defects by direct analysis of the DNA using a DNA probe. In this context, a DNA probe is a single stranded length of DNA labelled with ^{32}P that will hybridize with a unique complementary sequence from the human genome. The fragment with which it has hybridized can be revealed by autoradiography. A DNA probe can be either gene-specific (often derived originally from mRNA for the gene product in question), or chromosome-region specific. Elucidation of the exact point mutation or deletion in one family may tell one very little about the exact DNA defect in another family with the same clinical condition. A large deletion of all or part of the gene, such as often occurs in alpha-thalassaemia, can be simply detected by restriction fragment analysis and a gene-specific DNA probe (Fig. 17.7). If the exact point mutation is known as in sickle cell anaemia then tailor-made probes of 19 nucleotides in length can detect a single base mismatch.

Gene tracking

Fortunately for the families with inherited disorders where the gene involved or exact mutation is unknown, there is an alternative approach called gene tracking. Rather than define the DNA defect within the gene, one tracks the inheritance of the particular region of chromosomal DNA that includes the gene locus. Beta-thalassaemia always involves the β-globin gene locus, which is situated on the short arm of chromosome 11. A homozygous affected child has inherited two number 11 chromosomes from his parents (each carrying some form of beta-thalassaemia mutation); so if these two chromosomes can be distinguished from the parents' other two number 11 chromosomes, then transmission of the beta-thalassaemia genes can be predicted in a future fetus. What are required are common genetic markers closely linked to the disease gene locus; in the same way that different HLA alleles can act as markers of that part of chromosome 6 that carries the 21-hydroxylase gene locus (Fig. 17.2). Naturally occurring variations in DNA sequence are exploited as DNA markers for chromosomal bands or specific gene loci.

Restriction fragment length polymorphism (RFLP)

It will be recalled that only a very small percentage of total genomic DNA is actually coding sequence for proteins. The non-coding regions that flank genes, the intergenic DNA and to some extent the intervening sequences, are less conserved during evolution and point

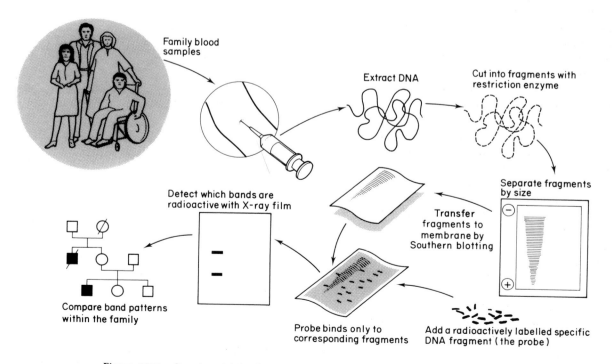

Figure 17.7   *Steps in restriction fragment analysis by Southern blotting for gene tracking.*

mutations are tolerated and become established in populations. The experience so far suggests that on average 1 in 100 to 200 nucleotide bases differ between the chromosome pair. A number of these DNA sequence polymorphisms involve the recognition sequence of 4 or 6 bases of a particular restriction enzyme, and this results, on digestion, in different size restriction fragments from each of the homologous chromosome pairs. Restriction enzymes are naturally occurring enzymes from bacteria that cut DNA at only very specific sites. Thus an RFLP is a relatively common change in DNA sequence that either destroys or creates a restriction enzyme recognition site, or alters the distance between two sites. In anyone who is heterozygous for an RFLP one restriction band pattern corresponds to one chromosome and the other band pattern to the other chromosome of the pair. This allows one to track the transmission of a single chromosome region through a family, and to see if a particular monogenic disease co-inherits with the polymorphic site; in other words, perform classical linkage studies. Once linkage is proven or if a gene-specific probe is used, genetic prediction (prenatal diagnosis or carrier detection) becomes possible in many families (Fig. 17.8).

Genetic prediction

Gene tracking within families is now becoming an established clinical service. Table 17.1 lists those common disorders that at the time of writing make up most of the clinical demand for DNA analysis.

Molecular genetics in non-Mendelian diseases

Although the 'new genetics' is having an immediate impact as expected on the investigation of monogenic

Table 17.1 The most common diseases for which prenatal diagnosis or exclusion is possible in selected families using DNA analysis

Huntington's disease
Myotonic dystrophy
Adult polycystic kidney disease

Beta-thalassaemia
Alpha-thalassaemia
Sickle cell anaemia
Cystic fibrosis
Alpha-1-antitrypsin deficiency
Phenylketonuria
Congenital adrenal hyperplasia
    (21-hydroxylase deficiency)

Duchenne muscular dystrophy
Haemophilia A
Haemophilia B

disorders, it would be wrong to imagine that its influence is limited to this group of disorders. There will be opportunities to define the main susceptibility genes in common multifactorial disease like *atherosclerosis* or *schizophrenia*, principally by asking the question: 'Which bit of DNA is common to affected sibling pairs but not inherited by the unaffected siblings?'

Another area where molecular genetics is making a dramatic contribution is in the field of cell division and proliferation, which has implications for cancer. The life-cycle of RNA viruses includes a phase of integration into the DNA of the infected cell and it appears that, whilst roaming around the collective mammalian genome, certain viruses have picked up some cellular genes, that after various modifications, bestow the virus with tumorigenic properties. The viral DNA sequences necessary for transforming cells into a neoplastic state are called *oncogenes*. Thus with most oncogenes there are corresponding but somewhat different genes in the human genome performing their regular function, presumably

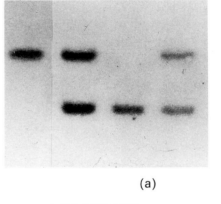

(a)

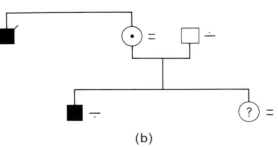

(b)

Figure 17.8 *Autoradiograph of DNA tracks from four family members digested with restriction enzyme Bgl II, and hybridized with probe DX13 that is closely linked to haemophilia A. The RFLP (see text) is represented by the polymorphic bands 5.8 kb and 2.8 kb. It will be seen that the 5.8 kb appears to be co-inheriting with the haemophilia mutation and the sister has inherited this band from her mother and the 2.8 kb band from her father. Barring an error due to recombination, she is therefore a carrier.*

related to cell division. They have been termed proto-oncogenes or cellular oncogenes (with the abbreviation of the viral oncogene often being preceded with a 'c', e.g. *c-abl*). Some 30 or more cellular oncogenes have been identified, but mutations in them have so far been implicated in very few human cancers. Mutant *H-ras* and *K-ras* cellular oncogenes from human tumours will transform the unusual cell line NIH3T3, indicating that certain mutations in these genes represent one step in the multi-step path to neoplasia. The structure or activity of cellular oncogenes could be altered by chromosomal translocations, and in this respect the association of a malignancy with a specific translocation is interesting. For example, patients with chronic myeloid leukaemia have a specific chromosome abnormality called the Philadelphia (Ph¹) chromosome, which usually results from a translocation between chromosomes 9 and 22 with breakpoints at 9q 34 and 22q 11. This translocation involves the movement of an oncogene, *c-abl*, which is normally situated on chromosome 9. The breakpoint of this deletion has been analysed in detail. It turns out that it involves the juxtaposition of a region of chromosome 22 to sequences near the 5' end of *c-abl*. The region on chromosome 22 has been called *bcr* (breakpoint–cluster region). The translocation creates a fused *bcr–abl* gene which, after some different splicing of the RNA, generates a novel protein with transforming activity. In *Burkitt's lymphoma* the cancer cells have specific chromosome changes; 90 per cent of patients have an 8/14 translocation, while others have 8/2 or 8/22 translocations. Chromosomes 14, 2 and 22 carry the genes encoding the immunoglobulin heavy chain, and κ and λ light chains respectively. The cellular oncogene *c-myc* is located on chromosome 8. It turns out that the breakpoint of all three translocations is at the site of the *c-myc* gene. Thus the important regulatory gene is transposed directly into regions of the genome which are undergoing major rearrangements during B-cell maturation.

It is important to emphasize that viral infections *per se* have only been implicated in Burkitt's lymphoma and a rare T-cell lymphoma. Viruses led to the discovery of cellular oncogenes, and the study of these will be important for our understanding of the regulation of cell growth and proliferation in general, not just malignant change.

Genetic counselling and prenatal diagnosis

The great majority of people seeking genetic counselling are couples who have had one child with an abnormality and want to know the risk to further children, and perhaps the risk to their affected child's offspring. Sometimes it is another relative, whose probability of being at risk has to be assessed from a combination of pedigree data and test results (often a complex calculation). The first responsibility is to give them as reliable an estimate of the risk as possible, and put it into perspective. In any random pregnancy the risk of any serious error of development is about 1 in 40 and this is a useful yardstick for the couple in assessing the degree of risk. Whether or not to go ahead with planning further children is clearly, in the end, the couple's own decision. The clinical geneticist should discuss the various options available, including prenatal diagnosis followed by selective abortion of an affected fetus. There are some couples who will not entertain an abortion on any grounds, but there are many who see this as a way of having a healthy family. Most prenatal tests are specific, and for this reason it must be clear for what particular abnormality the fetus is at risk. In metabolic genetic disorders a precise biochemical diagnosis on the affected relative is essential before embarking on prenatal diagnosis.

Amniocentesis is done at about 16 weeks gestation, and ultrasound examination is an integral part of the process and is increasingly used to detect anatomical defects. Amniotic fluid contains cells of fetal origin and these can be cultured for chromosome, biochemical or DNA analysis. Sometimes the amniotic fluid can be used directly, for example, when measuring the α-fetoprotein level for the detection of open spina bifida. *Chorionic villus sampling* is rapidly replacing amniocentesis, especially in high-risk situations. It can be offered from 9 weeks of pregnancy and usually yields 10–20 mg of cellular material that can be used for chromosome or DNA analysis or metabolic studies. The transcervical approach is limited for safety reasons to about 9–11 weeks gestation, but the transabdominal approach does not appear to have such limitations.

Fetoscopy plays a role in prenatal diagnosis in the mid-trimester of pregnancy. Carried out at a few specialized centres, it allows direct vision of the fetus, and facilitates sampling of fetal blood from the umbilical cord. The latter is now possible under ultrasound guidance only. In common with all medical practice, the risk of the investigative procedure has to be taken into account and discussed fully with the patient.

In addition to prenatal diagnosis in specific families at risk, there are now two prenatal screening procedures that are available in many centres to women who wish to have them. Pregnant women of 38 years or over can be offered mid-trimester amniocentesis for chromosomal prenatal diagnosis, particularly for the exclusion of Down's syndrome. Spina bifida and anencephaly are relatively common congenital malformations in Britain, and a woman carrying an affected fetus tends to have a higher than normal serum α-fetoprotein level. Taken at 16–17 weeks gestation, the maternal serum α-fetoprotein level can be used to define an 'at risk' group, who can then be offered the definite prenatal diagnostic tests, measurement of amniotic α-fetoprotein, detection of a specific neural cholinesterase in amniotic fluid and careful ultrasound examination.

18
Adverse Reactions to Drugs

Introduction

Drug reactions are becoming increasingly important as the range of substances used for diagnostic and therapeutic purposes multiplies. Probably about 10 per cent of hospital inpatients suffer some sort of adverse drug reaction. Drug-induced disease is usually short-lived, about 80 per cent lasting less than a week, and over 80 per cent of patients recover without sequelae. The classification of these reactions is difficult, for their underlying mechanism is often not fully understood.

A useful classification originally proposed by Rawlins and Thompson is:

1 *type A reactions* which can be predicted from the known pharmacological action of the drug.
2 *type B reactions* which are unpredictable and include allergies, idiosyncratic reactions and those due to some genetically determined abnormal response to the drug.

Type A reactions

In this type of reaction the pharmacological effects of the drug are excessive. This can be due to *overdose* or to *undue sensitivity* of the patient to the drug's action—an example being the undue respiratory depression produced by morphine in a patient with long-standing respiratory disease. Pharmacokinetic factors may be important, usually because the patient is unable to eliminate the drug as a result of disease. A good example is the patient with renal failure who fails to excrete digoxin with subsequent toxicity.

Sometimes adverse effects are inherent in the action of the drug even when given in normal doses and without undue sensitivity on the part of the patient. Most people taking tricyclic antidepressants will complain of dry mouth and other anticholinergic effects, and about half the patients taking the vasodilator nifedipine will develop some ankle swelling. Generally this type of side-effect can be predicted and often avoided if the possibility is considered before prescribing.

Type B reactions

This is a more heterogenous group where the reaction is unrelated to the drug's pharmacological action and is usually unpredictable. They can be divided into drug allergies, idiosyncratic reactions and genetically determined reactions.

Drug allergies

Some reactions to drugs are known to be mediated by immune mechanisms. This means that the patient has been previously exposed to the drug or to some closely related substance. Most drugs are of a low molecular weight and are therefore not antigenic. They can, however, combine covalently with a large molecular substance, usually a protein, and the combination which is known as a *hapten* acts as an antigen.

Four types of allergic reaction are now recognized and it is possible for a single drug to cause more than one type of allergy.

Type I (immediate anaphylactic) reactions

This is due to the antigen/antibody reaction occurring on the surface of the mast cells and releasing pharmacologically active substances including histamine, bradykinin and 5-hydroxytryptamine. The antibody belongs to the IgE fraction of the immunoglobulins. This type of reaction is seen typically with penicillin, streptomycin and some other drugs, and antiserum raised in animals. It is not a problem with immunoglobins from human sources which are now widely used.

Clinical features

The reaction occurs within a few minutes of administration of the drug. The main features are chest pain, dyspnoea, cyanosis and a rapid fall in blood pressure with collapse. The attack may be fatal.

Treatment

1 Prophylaxis
It is important to ask the patient whether he is sensitive to the drug about to be given. It is also useful to know whether he suffers from hay fever, asthma, infantile eczema or urticaria as this type of reaction is more frequent in atopic subjects.

When serum obtained from animals is being given the following rules should be observed.

1 The patient should be asked whether he has had serum before or whether he suffers from allergic diseases such as asthma, hay fever, eczema or urticaria.
2 If the answer to these questions is negative, 0.1 ml of serum is injected subcutaneously. If there is no local or general reaction within half an hour, the full dose of serum is given intramuscularly.
3 If the patient has a history of allergic disease or has had serum before, 0.1 ml of serum diluted 1:10 is given subcutaneously; if there is no reaction within half an hour, 0.1 ml of serum is given subcutaneously; if after a further half an hour there is still no reaction, the full dose of serum is given intramuscularly.
4 Whenever serum is given it is essential that a syringe of fresh 1:1000 adrenaline solution be at hand and also an antihistamine suitable for intravenous injection (chlorpheniramine maleate 10 mg). Whenever patients are given serum they must be observed for half an hour after the injection and must be warned of the possibility of a delayed serum reaction.
5 Intravenous injections of serum should be avoided if possible. Where they are necessary, the same precautions should be adopted. Intravenous serum should not be given to those who have previously had serum or who have allergic disorders, and in addition a test dose of 0.1 ml of serum should also be given intramuscularly. As a general rule intravenous serum should be given only to patients in hospital.
6 Following the administration of serum the patient should be actively immunized against the appropriate

diseases. This should be delayed until at least one month after he has received the serum, as the circulating antibody from the serum may prevent the antigen from provoking active immunity.

2 Management of reaction
Adrenaline (0.5 ml of a 1:1000 solution) should be given intramuscularly together with an antihistamine (chlorpheniramine maleate 10 mg IV). Often hydrocortisone hemisuccinate (100 mg IV) is required.

Type II reactions

These are due to antibodies of class IgG and IgM combining with antigens on the surface of cells and fixing complement. Drug-induced haemolytic anaemia and transfusion reactions are of this type.

Type III reactions

These are responsible for several clinical syndromes which are believed to be due to circulating immune complexes consisting of antigen/antibody/complement.

Serum sickness is due to a circulating antigen/antibody/complement complex which causes transient damage to certain tissues. About a week to ten days after the patient has received serum he develops a rash, usually urticarial, pain and stiffness with some swelling in the joints, and usually a fever. Sometimes there is enlargement of the lymph nodes and a transient albuminuria. Rarely, a shock-like state develops with low blood pressure. This condition usually clears up in a few days. Local application of calamine lotion helps to relieve the itching. An antihistamine such as chlorpheniramine maleate (4 mg t.d.s.) shortens the duration of the illness. In severe or resistant cases, prednisolone (30 mg) for a day or two and then tailed off will usually relieve the symptoms.

A syndrome resembling *systemic lupus erythematosus* is caused by several drugs, including procainamide, hydralazine, anticonvulsants and isoniazid. It recovers on stopping the drug.

Type IV (delayed hypersensitivity) reactions

The typical example of this type of reaction is a contact dermatitis. When the drug is applied to the skin it forms an antigenic conjugate with the dermal proteins which stimulates the formation of sensitized T-lymphocytes. If the drug is applied again a rash develops.

Idiosyncratic reactions

Although it has been possible to demonstrate an allergic basis for a number of drug reactions, in many cases there is no evidence suggesting allergy and other mechanisms may be involved. It is therefore better to consider these reactions on a system basis. The drug reaction may not be due to the drug itself but to a metabolite or even to a non-drug component in its formulation.

Drug-induced liver damage is discussed in Chapter 4.

Blood dyscrasias (see also chapter 11)

Blood dyscrasias are among the most important drug reactions. It would seem that many of them are hypersensitivity reactions and are due to a combination of antigen, antibody and complement on the cell. Others are due to a direct effect on the blood cells or their precursors.

Agranulocytosis

This may occur with a number of drugs, including amidopyrine, the sulphonamides, thiouracil, carbimazole, tridione, isoniazid, phenylbutazone, chloramphenicol, gold, and arsenic. In addition large doses of most cytotoxic drugs will produce agranulocytosis as part of their pharmacological action. With most drugs the agranulocytosis is reversible, provided the drug is not continued for too long, but with chloramphenicol recovery may not occur.

There may be no symptoms and the depression in the granulocytes may be found by a routine blood count. Such patients are susceptible to infection and may present with general malaise, fever, and some infective process, usually a severe throat infection.

The patient should always be asked if he is susceptible to the drug before it is given. Certain drugs such as amidopyrine and chloramphenicol should be avoided if possible. It is doubtful if routine blood counts on patients taking drugs which may cause agranulocytosis are much help as the fall in granulocytes may be sudden. The patient must, however, be told to report to the doctor if he becomes ill, and in particular if he develops a sore throat; a blood count must then be performed.

When there is a reaction the drug must be stopped immediately. If the white count does not improve within a few days, prednisolone (30 mg daily) should be given. Infections should be treated as they arise with the appropriate antibiotic. The majority of patients will recover on this treatment. When granulocytopenia is due to heavy metals it should be treated with dimercaprol (see page 509).

Thrombocytopenia

This may occur as a result of drug administration. It has been described with sedormid, tridione, chloramphenicol, thiazide, gold, sulphonamides and quinine. It may occur with excessive dosage of cytoxic drugs. Clinical features include purpura and bleeding from various sites.

The drug should be stopped immediately. Prednisolone (30 mg daily) sometimes helps. Platelet transfusions will raise the plasma platelet count for a few days.

Aplastic anaemia

This is not common following the taking of drugs. It may occur with benzol and its derivatives, with chloramphenicol, and with a number of other drugs including gold and the sulphonamides. It may be associated with depression of other elements of the blood.

The drug should be stopped. Repeated transfusion may be required. Prednisolone is not usually very helpful, but it is worth a trial in patients who are not recovering. If poisoning is due to heavy metals, dimercaprol should be used. Provided the drug is stopped quickly, recovery usually occurs. The exception is chloramphenicol, which rarely causes bone-marrow dyscrasias and usually only after repeated courses; if they occur, however, they are usually irreversible and ultimately prove fatal.

Haemolytic anaemia

Drugs can occasionally cause haemolysis. It seems that a number of mechanisms may be responsible. Quinine has long been known to precipitate the acute haemolysis occurring in association with malaria and called *blackwater fever*.

Potassium chlorate in large doses will produce haemolysis by a direct action on the cell; occasionally this occurs with quite a small dose of the drug and it can then be classed as an example of intolerance.

In about 10 per cent of American negroes, a high proportion of Africans and some races in the Mediterranean littoral there is a *deficiency in glucose-6-phosphate dehydrogenase* which is normally responsible for the integrity of the red cells. This results in acute haemolysis when such subjects take primaquine, sulphonamides, nitrofurantoins and other drugs and is an example of a genetically determined reaction to a drug.

Methaemoglobinaemia and sulphaemoglobinaemia

These changes in the haemoglobin may occur with certain drugs, including phenacetin, potassium chlorate, and the sulphonamides. The patient appears cyanosed, but is not distressed or dyspnoeic. The diagnosis is confirmed by finding the absorption spectra of methaemoglobin or sulphaemoglobin in the blood. The only treatment usually required is to stop the offending drug. Methaemoglobinaemia can be temporarily reversed by giving methylene blue as a 1% solution intravenously, the dose for an adult being 5 ml.

Megaloblastic anaemia

Certain drugs including pyrimethamine and the anticonvulsants primidone and phenytoin may produce a megaloblastic anaemia which can be reversed by folic acid 10 mg daily.

Drug reactions and connective tissue disorders

Although some authors include a wide variety of syndromes under the term collagen diseases, this term should be confined to inflammatory disorders of connective tissues such as rheumatic fever, rheumatoid arthritis, systemic lupus erythematosus (SLE), polyarteritis nodosa, dermatomyositis, and giant-cell arteritis. There has been considerable discussion whether drug reactions can cause these conditions. There is no doubt that a clinical picture similar to that of SLE can be produced by hydralazine and by procainamide, but it differs from the true disease in that recovery occurs when the drug is stopped. It is of interest that the development of drug-induced SLE is also related to the sex of the subject, his/her acetylation status and tissue type. In addition, transient arteritis can occur in association with hypersensitivity reaction to a number of drugs, including penicillin and the sulphonamides. Whether such reactions play any part in the pathogenesis of true *polyarteritis nodosa* is more doubtful, and it is unlikely that drug reactions are causal to any of the other collagen diseases.

Other types of connective tissue disease can be drug-induced. *Methysergide* causes a retroperitoneal fibrosis which may affect the mediastinum. It is a rare cause of ureteric obstruction.

Other drug reactions

Fever is quite common and should always be remembered in patients with PUO.

Lymphadenopathy can be caused by drugs, particularly phenytoin, and the histological picture resembles a lymphoma.

Rashes are often caused by drugs and are considered on page 406.

Genetically determined drug reactions

Hereditary differences in response to drugs may be due to *polygenic influences*, when there is a continuous variation, as in the elimination of many drugs including aspirin and warfarin; or to *polymorphism*.

Genetic polymorphism can produce two distinct types of adverse effect. First, a specific deficiency of an enzyme concerned with drug metabolism results in a group of subjects in whom *elimination* of certain drugs is prolonged. The following are examples:

1 About 60 per cent of caucasian Britons are relatively deficient in the enzyme N-acetyltransferase and are therefore *slow acetylators*. They are more likely to develop peripheral neuritis when taking isoniazid, and an SLE-like syndrome from isoniazid, procainamide or hydralazine.
2 The muscle relaxant suxamethonium is inactivated by *cholinesterases*. In a small group of people with an inherited deficiency the paralysing effect of suxamethonium is greatly prolonged.
3 About 10 per cent of the population of the UK are deficient in *hydroxylating enzymes*. This was originally noted with the hypotensive drug debrisoquine, but it also applies to several others including metoprolol, propranolol, phenformin and nortriptyline.

Second, an enzyme deficiency can *alter the response to a drug*. Examples are:

1 *Glucose-6-phosphate dehydrogenase deficiency* leads to haemolysis with certain drugs (see page 368).
2 A wide range of drugs, including hypnotic anticonvulsants and oral hypoglycaemic agents, can precipitate *acute porphyria* in sensitive individuals (see page 340).

Drug interactions

The increasing use of drugs, particularly the prescribing of more than one drug at a time, has made interactions an important problem. For example, there is about a 20 per cent chance of an interaction if five drugs are prescribed together. However, many interactions are of little clinical importance, either because the variations in drug handling or action are small or because the concentration of the drug is not critical. The difficulty is to know which interactions are potentially dangerous in a particular patient. In general, serious adverse effects are more liable to occur if the therapeutic ratio of the drug is small.

Interactions may happen at several stages during the drugs' passage through the body.

1 The gastrointestinal tract

Drugs may combine or their physical state may be altered so that absorption is modified. For example, iron combines with tetracycline, decreasing its absorption and leading to lower blood levels of the antibiotic.

2 Competition for transport sites on the plasma proteins

Many drugs are transported to their sites of action partially or almost totally bound to plasma proteins. When bound in this way they cannot produce their pharmacological effects and are not available to be metabolized or excreted. The activity of the drug depends on the unbound fraction.

When two drugs compete for a limited number of protein-binding sites, there is a decrease in the bound fraction of each and an increase in the amount of free drug, with a corresponding enhancement of the pharmacological effect. Examples of this type of interaction are the displacement of bilirubin by sulphonamides in the newborn causing kernicterus, the displacement of tolbutamide by salicylates leading to hypoglycaemia, and the displacement of warfarin by salicylates causing haemorrhage.

3 Modification at sites of action

The pharmacological action of a drug can be modified in several ways by the concurrent administration of another drug. For example:

(a) Hypokalaemia produced by diuretics enhances the toxic effects of digitalis on the heart.
(b) Tricyclic antidepressants reverse the effect of adrenergic blocking hypotensive agents, possibly by increasing the amount of noradrenaline at the adrenergic nerve endings. They also enhance the effect of sympathomimetic amines which, for example, may be added to a local anaesthetic.
(c) The action of central nervous depressants such as barbiturates and alcohol is additive.
(d) Monoamine oxidase inhibitors interact in two ways. First, certain drugs, particularly sympathomimetic drugs such as phenylpropanolamine or tyramine, release the excess noradrenaline which accumulates in nerve endings of the subject taking MAO inhibitors, resulting in a hypertensive crisis. Tyramine is found in certain foods. Second, the effect of some central depressants, particularly pethidine, is enhanced.

4 Enzyme induction

Many drugs are metabolized by enzymes, usually in the liver. Certain drugs increase the activity of these enzymes so that drug breakdown is enhanced. For example, if a patient on an oral anticoagulant is given phenobarbitone the barbiturate increases the enzyme activity and the anticoagulant is metabolized more rapidly. An increased dose is therefore necessary to produce a satisfactory anticoagulant effect. Conversely, if the phenobarbitone is stopped enzyme activity decreases and signs of anticoagulant overdosage may appear.

5 Enzyme inhibition

Sulphonamides decrease the rate of breakdown of tolbutamide. Allopurinol decreases the rate of breakdown of 6-mercaptopurine.

6 Renal excretion

Competition for pathways in the kidney by two drugs given together may reduce the rate of excretion of both. Use is made of this phenomenon when probenecid is given with penicillin to reduce its excretion and so achieve a higher level of penicillin in the blood.

Further reading

Folb, P.I. (1984) *Drug Safety in Clinical Practice.* Springer-Verlag, Berlin.

Davies, D.M. (ed.) (1981) *Textbook of Adverse Drug Reactions*, 2nd edn. Oxford University Press, Oxford.

Stockley, I.H. (1981) *Drug Interactions.* Blackwell Scientific Publications, Oxford.

19
Poisoning

Introduction

Poisoning is responsible for about 10 per cent of all acute admissions to hospital in the UK. It may be due to self-poisoning, which may be a serious suicide attempt, or more often an attempt to draw attention of relatives, friends or doctors to some intolerable situation in the patient's life. It may alternatively be accidental, and rarely homicidal.

About 80 per cent of patients admitted to hospital with poisoning are not seriously ill and merely require observation until the poison has been eliminated, and any psychiatric problems have been investigated.

Preliminary assessment

When a diagnosis is made it is important to determine the following:

1 The nature of the poison or poisons; more than one poison has often been taken.
2 Any other complicating factors such as injuries, etc.
3 The severity of the poisoning.

The assessment of the severity of the poisoning will be based on three criteria.

Level of consciousness

This is usually divided into:
Grade I: drowsy but responds to mild stimulation
Grade II: unconscious but responds to mild stimulation
Grade III: unconscious but responds to severe stimulation
Grade IV: unconscious and unresponsive.

Circulation

Many drugs cause acute circulatory failure by depression of myocardial function and/or vasodilation. This can be assessed by the blood pressure and by the peripheral blood flow (the temperature of the extremities and urinary output). A normal blood pressure, however, may be associated with inadequate peripheral perfusion.

Cardiac arrhythmias are common in poisoning, as a result either of the action of the drug itself (e.g. tricyclic antidepressants) or to the associated hypoxia.

Respiration

Central depression of respiration is caused by many drugs. A crude assessment may be obtained from the respiration rate and the presence or absence of cyanosis. If there is any doubt, arterial blood gases should be measured.

Not only may respiration be suppressed; in the unconscious patient airway obstruction caused by the tongue blocking the pharynx and inhalation of vomit is a danger.

Treatments

In a few patients cardiac or respiratory arrest requires immediate resuscitation along the usual lines.

Certain non-specific measures are common to the management of most types of poisoning.

Ventilation

Maintenance of adequate ventilation includes keeping a clear airway in unconscious patients whose protective reflexes are absent, and preventing the inhalation of vomit by nursing in the semi-prone position until a cuffed endotracheal tube has been inserted. In severe respiratory depression the use of a ventilator is needed.

Fluids and electrolytes

Maintenance of correct fluid and electrolyte balances and nutrition is essential.

Support of the circulation

Hypovolaemia is treated by infusion of plasma or saline. This requires care as it is easy to overload the circulation, particularly if the cardiac function is compromised by poison, heart disease or old age. A central venous line is often desirable.

If cardiac function is depressed, dopamine and/or dobutamine may be helpful. Cardiac arrhythmias are treated in the usual way (see page 55).

Infections

These are common in severe poisoning (particularly pneumonia) and require prompt treatment with antibiotics.

Prevention of absorption

1 Emptying the stomach
In all patients who are conscious, except those who have taken corrosive poisons, emesis should be provoked by giving ipecacuanha paediatric emetic mixture (30 ml/adult, 10–15 ml/child). This will usually cause vomiting within half an hour. Whether this reduces drug absorption is uncertain.

In the unconscious patient gastric lavage should be used provided that:

(a) the poison has been taken within the previous four hours, exceptions being:
salicylates (up to 24 h)
tricyclic antidepressants (8 h)
methanol (8 h)
phenobarbitone (8 h)
dextropropoxyphene (8 h)
slow-release methylxanthines (8 h);
(b) a cuffed endotracheal tube has been inserted to prevent inhalation;
(c) a corrosive poison is not involved.

A 30 English gauge Jaques tube is passed and 300 ml of warm water is run into the stomach and siphoned out.

This is repeated at least three times. If the nature of the poison is known a suitable antidote can be left in the stomach. Finally, all vomit and the first return from the gastric lavage should be kept for further analysis.

2 Adsorbents
Activated charcoal given within an hour of taking the poison reduces the absorption of a number of drugs. Its use is under investigation at present.

Promoting elimination of poisons

Renal excretion of certain drugs is influenced by the pH of the urine. Elimination of weak acids (e.g. salicylates) is maximal if the urine pH is about 7.5; conversely, weak bases are better excreted in an acid urine. The use of forced diuresis is largely confined to serious overdose with salicylates.

To produce an *alkaline* diuresis, in the first hour infuse 1000 ml of 5% dextrose and 500 ml of 1.26% sodium bicarbonate. At the end of the hour a decision has to be made. If the urine flow is *below* 3 ml/minute, give frusemide (40 mg IV), but abandon diuresis if it fails to produce an adequate urinary output. If the urine flow is *above* 3 ml/minute, continue to maintain the urine flow and the urine pH at 7.5–8.5. Add 10 mmol of potassium to each 500 ml of infusion. This method requires careful monitoring to be effective and to prevent fluid overload and hypokalaemia.

Haemoperfusion, in which the patient's blood is passed over an adsorbent, and haemodialysis are used in some types of serious poisoning.

Centrally acting drugs

Sedatives and hypnotics are very commonly used in acute overdose. Previously barbiturates were most usually employed but they have been replaced by benzodiazepines, probably reflecting a change in prescribing habits.

Acute barbiturate poisoning

Barbiturates are usually taken in a deliberate suicide attempt; occasionally by accident. Barbiturate and alcohol poisoning may be combined; these two drugs certainly have an additive effect, and it is believed by some that their actions are synergistic.

The speed of action and duration of effect depend on the type of barbiturate used.

The symptoms of mild barbiturate overdosage are mental confusion with slurred speech, nystagmus and unsteady gait. These are followed by deep sleep from which the patient can be roused though perhaps with difficulty. The corneal and pharyngeal reflexes remain and respiration is not markedly depressed. A bullous rash occurs in about 10 per cent of patients with barbiturate overdosage.

In severe barbiturate overdosage there is deep coma, the patient cannot be roused and the reflexes have disappeared. Finally death occurs from respiratory depression complicated by circulatory failure. The diagnosis can be confirmed by finding the drug in the urine, blood or gastric contents.

The blood level of barbiturate is a poor guide as to prognosis as patients vary in their sensitivity to the drug and in the rate of its elimination.

If the patient is conscious, no treatment will usually be required unless a large dose has just been taken, when it should be removed by gastric lavage. In the unconscious patient management is:

1 Ensure a clear airway; if the cough reflex is absent an endotracheal tube should be introduced.
2 Ensure adequate ventilation; in a cyanosed patient with respiratory depression some form of mechanical ventilation will be required.
3 Gastric contents should be aspirated and the stomach washed out only if the drug has been taken within the previous four hours.
4 Maintain hydration by giving 2.0 litres of intravenous fluid in 24 hours (0.18% dextrose saline).
5 Treat intercurrent chest infections as they arise.

In severe intoxication, however (absent reflexes, depressed respiration), an attempt should be made to increase the rate of barbiturate elimination. Renal excretion of phenobarbitone can be increased by producing a high flow rate of alkaline urine. This is not, however, effective with the short-acting barbiturates which are largely broken down in the liver.

The death rate from hospital admission with barbiturate poisoning is about 2–5 per cent.

The benzodiazepines

This group of drugs, now widely used as anxiolytic agents and hypnotics, produces in overdosage a picture of general CNS depression, very similar to that caused by barbiturates. However, respiratory depression and circulatory failure are much less pronounced and the benzodiazepines are considerably 'safer' in overdose provided they have not been combined with other centrally acting drugs.

The duration of unconsciousness is approximately related to the half-life of the drug, and this varies considerably. The benzodiazepines are inactivated by biotransformation but some of them have active metabolites which prolong the duration of their action. The half-lives of some commonly used benzodiazepines are:

Temazepam: 5–20 hours
Nitrazepam: 15–24 hours
Lorazepam: 10–20 hours
Clonazepam: 30 hours
Diazepam: 20–50 hours

Desmethyldiazepam (active metabolite): 36–200 hours. Treatment is symptomatic and active intervention to support ventilation or circulation is rarely required. There is as yet no way to speed elimination.

Phenothiazines

The dose response curve of the phenothiazines is fairly flat so there is a wide safety margin. Overdosage produces unconsciousness associated with extrapyramidal signs and with torticollis. Cardiac arrhythmias, hypotension and hypothermia occur.

If the extrapyramidal signs are severe they respond to benztropine (2.0 mg IV), otherwise treatment is supportive.

Ethyl alcohol

Most subjects with acute alcoholic intoxication will sleep it off. Hypoglycaemia can be a complication, particularly in fasting patients or children. Lactic acidosis rarely develops in patients with liver disease or on biguanides (see page 318).

In severe cases the stomach should be washed out if the alcohol has been taken recently, and treatment continued as in barbiturate poisoning. Forced alkaline diuresis is not used. Various substances, including vitamins B and C and fructose, have been claimed to sober up a patient, but there is little evidence that they are of practical use in the treatment of acute alcoholic poisoning.

The combination of alcohol and other centrally acting drugs is additive and can be very dangerous.

Methanol

Methanol poisoning is serious with an overall mortality of 20 per cent. The lowest fatal dose is about 25 ml. It is metabolized to the toxic metabolites formaldehyde and formate and is thus associated with a metabolic acidosis.

The patient is confused, with abdominal pain and vomiting. Visual disturbances are common and examination of the retina may show pallor and oedema of the discs.

Treatment of acidosis, if severe, is with infusion of bicarbonate. Removal of methanol and metabolites and correction of acidosis is by haemodialysis; this will be required if there are visual symptoms or signs, severe acidosis or a blood methanol level above 0.5 g/litre.

It is common practice to give ethanol to reduce methanol metabolism. 50 g of absolute alcohol is suitably diluted and given orally or intravenously, and then the blood alcohol level is maintained at 1–2 g/litre by the infusion of 10–12 g/hour. Whether this is effective is not established.

Analgesics

Opioids

This term covers all drugs with opiate-like actions. Although morphine and diamorphine are classically used in overdose, several other powerful members of this group (e.g. pethidine, methadone, dipipanone, etc.) and even the weaker opioids (codeine, dextrapropoxyphene, diphenoxylate, etc.) are dangerous if the dose is sufficiently large.

The features of opioid overdosage are coma, very slow respiration and pin-point pupils. In addition the skin is cyanosed, cold and clammy. The blood pressure is low in severe poisoning. Fits or acute pulmonary oedema may be a serious complication. Death usually results from respiratory depression.

If respiratory or cardiac arrest has occurred this takes priority and should be treated in the usual way.

Naloxone competes for opioid receptors in the nervous system and is the specific antidote. The adult dose is 0.8–1.2 mg given intravenously. If this does not improve the patient's condition (respiration, level of consciousness or pupil size) in three minutes it should be repeated. Failure to respond suggests reconsideration of the diagnosis. The benefits from naloxone may only last for 10–15 minutes as it has a short half-life (about 30 minutes), so with long-acting opioids repeated doses may be required or an infusion of up to 5 mg/hour may become necessary. A number of patients suffering from opioid overdose are narcotic addicts, and then naloxone will not only reverse the effects of overdosage but will precipitate acute withdrawal symptoms. Partial agonist opioids may be partially resistant to the effects of naloxone.

Supportive measures such as oxygen, maintenance of the airways and, possibly, circulatory stimulants may be required.

Salicylates

Poisoning by salicylates (usually aspirin) is still common but its incidence is falling. It may be suicidal, or in children it may be accidental. The fatal dose in adults is in the region of 25 g. Doses of 2–4 g have proved lethal in children.

In mild cases the main symptoms are nausea, vomiting, tinnitus and increased respirations. After larger doses there is mental confusion, the patient is flushed and sweating with a full pulse and overbreathing is very striking. In the early stages hyperventilation lowers the PCO_2 of the plasma and leads to a respiratory alkalosis; with increasing absorption of salicylate there is a metabolic acidosis with a fall in plasma bicarbonate. In children acidosis is common, whereas in adults a raised blood pH is more usual. In addition vomiting and sweating lead to dehydration and oliguria.

In salicylate poisoning it is worth while washing out the stomach up to 24 hours after ingestion of the drug. It the patient is in coma a cuffed endotracheal tube should be passed beforehand to avoid possible aspiration of vomited material into the lungs.

In *mild* cases 5% sodium bicarbonate solution should be given orally in doses of 2 g four-hourly for 24 hours. Sodium bicarbonate, by making the urine alkaline, increases the rate of excretion of salicylate by the kidneys.

In *severe* cases (plasma salicylate level of more than 300 mg/litre in children and 500 mg/litre in adults) treatment is aimed at correcting dehydration and producing a diuresis of alkaline urine and thus rapidly clearing salicylate from the body. Owing to the complex acid/base disorder which occurs in salicylate poisoning, it is important to estimate plasma pH, bicarbonate and PCO_2. For the method of forced diuresis see page 505.

Phytomenadione (25 mg) should be injected intravenously to prevent bleeding. Monitor for hypoglycaemia and treat as necessary.

By this method a majority of adult patients with salicylate poisoning can be resuscitated. In a few patients with high plasma salicylate levels (over 1 g/l) and with renal or cirulatory failure, haemodialysis will be required. Children are more sensitive to the toxic effects of salicylate.

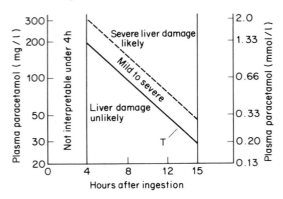

Figure 19.1 *Relationship between plasma concentrations, time after ingestion and liver damage after paracetamol overdosage. T, treatment line. Reproduced with permission of Dr J.A. Henry and the British Medical Journal.*

Paracetamol

Overdosage by paracetamol is dangerous and a single dose of over 15 g can produce serious liver damage and 25 g is usually fatal. With the normal therapeutic dose of paracetamol a toxic metabolite is produced which, however, is mopped up by glutathione in the liver. With overdose the glutathione mechanism is saturated and the metabolite combines with the liver cell macromolecules causing cell death. Liver damage is probable if the blood level of paracetamol exceeds 200 mg/ml at 4 hours or 50 mg/ml at 12 hours after ingestion (Fig. 19.1).

After ingestion of the drug there are few symptoms except for perhaps nausea and vomiting and some abdominal discomfort. In severe overdosage, signs of liver involvement start with pain over the liver after 24–36 hours followed by jaundice after 36–48 hours. Rarely, renal failure develops at this time. If death ensues it is usually within a week.

The stomach should be washed out up to six hours after ingestion of the drug.

The specific remedies are methionine or acetylcysteine. These substances increase the intracellular glutathione which inactivates the toxic metabolites of paracetamol. One or other should be given immediately to all patients suspected of having taken an overdose of paracetamol in the previous 12 hours. Methionine is given orally and is easier to use, but acetylcysteine may be needed if vomiting is a problem.

A blood sample is taken at this time and if blood levels are below the safety level no further treatment need be given.

Analgesic mixtures

Combinations of mild opioids with either paracetamol or aspirin are popular. In overdose they may show the toxicity of both drugs and thus produce a mixed clinical picture.

Coproxamol (Distalgesic: paracetamol + dextropropoxyphene) has achieved a reputation of being particularly dangerous in overdose. Within an hour or two of ingestion it may cause circulatory collapse, respiratory depression and occasionally pulmonary oedema, particularly if combined with alcohol. This is due to the dextropropoxyphene content of the mixture and will respond to naloxone. Evidence of paracetamol overdose may develop later.

Antidepressants

Tricyclic antidepressants

This group includes imipramine, nortriptyline and amitriptyline. These drugs have become common agents in attempted suicide. The clinical picture is the result of cholinergic blockade, increased adrenergic activity and direct cardiac and CNS depression. It is essentially one of excitement followed by coma.

In *moderate* poisoning the patient is flushed with hot, dry skin, tachycardia and dilated pupils. With more *severe* poisoning there is confusion leading to fits and coma. Reflexes are brisk and the plantar response may be extensor. Cardiac arrhythmias are common and the ECG shows prolongation of the QRS interval. Cardiac arrest may occur several days after severe poisoning. These drugs may be taken with other centrally acting substances such as ethanol or the benzodiazepines, and this produces a mixed clinical picture.

There is no specific antidote and symptoms must be treated as they arise. Gastric washout is useful up to eight hours after ingestion as emptying may be slow. This should be followed by oral activated charcoal which helps to reduce absorption.

Electrolytes should be corrected as necessary (particularly acidosis). Ventilation should be maintained, mechanically if necessary.

Arrhythmias are treated in the usual way, practolol being particularly useful. Hypotension is difficult to treat, and plasma expanders such as dextran can be combined with dopamine/dobutamine to raise cardiac output. Fits can be controlled by diazepam.

Physostigmine has been used to reverse the anticholinergic actions of tricyclics but it is of doubtful value. Forced diuresis and dialysis are not effective.

Monoamine oxidase inhibitors

Overdose with these drugs does not usually cause the hypertensive crisis which occurs when they are combined with certain amines in the diet.

The onset of symptoms is delayed about 12 hours, when tachycardia, sweating and muscle spasms develop. Hyperthermia may be dangerous. Agitation may be followed by fits.

Sympathetic blockade with labetalol may control symptoms, but *severe* poisoning requires muscle relaxants with ventilation to prevent hyperpyrexia due to excessive muscle contractions.

Other drugs

Beta-blocker poisoning

Bradycardia and a low cardiac output are the important signs. Bradycardia can be reversed by atropine (2.0 mg IV) or, if this fails, by a pacemaker.

In an attempt to raise the blood pressure, hydrocortisone (500 mg) is given intravenously, and various positive ionotropic agents can be used (i.e. isoprenaline or dopamine). If bronchospasm is a problem salbutamol should be given by nebulizer in high doses.

Arsenic poisoning

Inorganic arsenic, usually in the form of the oxide, acquired notoriety as a homicidal poison and is still sometimes taken with suicidal intent. Poisoning may also occur as a result of exposure to arsenical dusts which are produced in various industrial processes. It produces its toxic action by inhibiting the intracellular sulphydryl enzymes which are essential to metabolism.

The main symptoms of *acute* poisoning by arsenic are burning on the throat, vomiting, abdominal pain, and diarrhoea. In severe cases circulatory collapse and death may follow.

The stomach should be emptied and then washed out with freshly prepared ferric hydroxide, which is made by adding 45 g of ferric chloride to 15 g of sodium carbonate (washing soda) in half a tumbler of water.

Dimercaprol (BAL; 300 mg) in oily solution is given six-hourly intramuscularly for two days and then decreased over the next few days. The action of dimercaprol is to offer SH groups with which the arsenic combines; it is thus unable to combine with the SH groups in intracellular enzymes.

Ferrous compounds

This form of poisoning has become common; it is usually due to children eating sugar-coated ferrous sulphate tablets in mistake for sweets.

Initially there is vomiting and diarrhoea often associated with haematemesis and melaena. After a few hours the patient becomes confused, and this may be followed by coma, convulsion and shock. Acute liver necrosis can occur.

As the first line of treatment vomiting should be induced. The stomach should then be washed out with a solution containing 2.0 g of desferrioxamine per litre and 5.0 g in 50 ml should be left in the stomach in adults. Desferrioxamine is an iron chelating agent.

2.0 g of desferrioxamine are given intramuscularly twice daily. In severe cases desferrioxamine can be given intravenously in 5% glucose solution at a rate of 5 mg/kg/hour to a maximum of 80 mg/kg/24 hours.

The patient must be kept in bed and under observation for at least 48 hours after apparent recovery.

Anticholinesterases

A number of these substances are used in medicine and as insecticides. They also have a potential use in war, and are known as 'nerve gases'. They inhibit the enzyme cholinesterase either temporarily or for long periods, so that there is widespread overactivity of the parasympathetic nervous system and neuromuscular block in voluntary muscle. Symptoms may include colicky abdominal pain, excess salivation, respiratory paralysis and the pupils are constricted.

Atropine should be given in doses of 2.0 mg (IV or IM) and repeated as required. This will not, however, relieve neuromuscular block. Cholinesterase can be reactivated by pralidoxime (1.0 g in 5 ml of water IV or IM) and repeated at four-hourly intervals as required. In *severe* cases some form of assisted ventilation may be necessary.

Paraquat

Paraquat is normally used as a weed killer and is very toxic. More than 30 ml of the concentrated drug is dangerous. With *massive* overdosage, death may occur from acute renal failure; with *smaller* doses it is usually due to lung damage and may be delayed for one to two weeks. There is no known antidote.

Carbon monoxide

Carbon monoxide can be a cause of both accidental and

suicide deaths, although the increasing use of North Sea gas has made the latter less common than in previous times. Poisoning may result from the escape of carbon monoxide from gas lights or gas fires, from car exhausts, from combustion stoves in a poorly ventilated room or from coal-mine explosions.

Carbon monoxide is odourless and lighter than air. It has a far greater affinity for haemoglobin than oxygen and forms a compound, carboxyhaemoglobin, which is bright-red in colour. It cannot carry oxygen and tissue anoxia results.

Symptoms are minimal if less than 30 per cent of haemoglobin is combined with carbon monoxide, and consist of nausea, lassitude and headache. With higher concentrations the onset of symptoms is rapid. There is a transient increase in pulse rate and respiration followed by weakness, dimness of vision and finally coma, respiratory depression and death.

The patient with carbon monoxide poisoning is often pale and cyanosed. The typical cherry red colour due to carboxyhaemoglobin is usually only seen at post-mortem. The presence of this compound in the blood may be confirmed by its characteristic absorption spectrum.

The patient must be removed from the poisoned atmosphere. Artificial respiration should be started immediately. If possible, pure oxygen should be given by the best available method. Cerebral oedema may develop in severe cases. The diagnosis is suggested by papilloedema and it should be treated by 50 ml of 20% mannitol by infusion. Several days in bed are required after apparent recovery. Occasionally patients show evidence of permanent brain or cardiac damage after recovery.

Cyanide

Hydrocyanic acid and potassium or sodium cyanide are very powerful poisons. They act by inhibiting a number of enzymes, the most important of which is cytochrome oxidase. They are used as pesticides and in metallurgy.

The inhalation of hydrocyanic acid (which is a gas) results in death within a few minutes. After ingestion of cyanide salts, death may occur in anything from a few minutes up to several hours, depending on the dose. Generally speaking the absorption of about 1 mg of cyanide is fatal.

The aim of treatment in cyanide poisoning is to give substances which will combine with cyanide and prevent interference with enzyme systems. The following steps should be taken as rapidly as possible:

1 Crush ampoules of amyl nitrite and allow the patient to inhale the vapour; this will form some methaemoglobin which combines with cyanide. This should be followed by sodium nitrite (0.3 g in 10 ml of water) given intravenously over three minutes, to form more methaemoglobin.

2 Sodium thiosulphate (25 ml of 50% solution) should be given intravenously over 10 minutes; this also combines with cyanide.

3 The stomach should be washed out with 5% sodium thiosulphate.

4 Oxygen and artificial respiration may be required.

If available, 20 ml of a 1.5% solution of cobalt edetate given intravenously over one minute is a specific remedy. It can be repeated if the response is adequate. It should not be used unless the diagnosis is established, as side-effects can be unpleasant.

Bee and wasp stings

Bee and wasp stings contain a number of pharmacologically active substances. Some of these only produce local reactions with pain and swelling, but there are also allergens which can cause serious reactions with urticaria, bronchospasm, hypotension, visual disturbances, diarrhoea, vomiting and collapse. Most subjects only develop local swelling and pain, but sometimes repeated stings cause increasingly severe reactions until a severe generalized response occurs which may be fatal.

Bee stings can be removed and local swelling and pain can be treated with aspirin and local antihistamines.

If anaphylaxis develops, adrenaline (0.5 ml of 1:1000 solution) should be given intramuscularly together with chlorpheniramine (10 mg) intravenously. Subjects who have *severe* reactions should be given immunotherapy, which consists of increasing doses of venom given at intervals.

Adder bites

The adder is the only poisonous snake found in the UK, and its venom contains substances with anticoagulant and cardiotoxic properties.

Local signs are swelling and oedema with bruising. General symptoms include diarrhoea and vomiting and sometimes urticaria. In severe cases there may be collapse with low blood pressure and loss of consciousness. Death is very rare.

The immediate treatment consists of splinting the affected limb, analgesia for the pain and antihistamines if urticaria develops. Many patients are frightened and need reassurance. Most patients only require observation in hospital and symptomatic treatment for 48 hours.

Anti-venom is available, and the Zagreb anti-venom is less likely to produce anaphylactic reaction than previous preparations. Indications for giving anti-venom are:

(a) hypotension and/or coma;
(b) systemic bleeding;
(c) leucocytosis above $20\,000 \times 10^9$ per litre;
(d) acidosis;
(e) markedly raised CPK.

Great care should be taken with atopic patients as reactions are common.

A further possible reason for giving anti-venom is to reduce the local reaction which can be severe and persistent.

10.8 ml of anti-venom is diluted in 100 ml of saline and infused intravenously over one hour.

Lead poisoning

Lead poisoning may occur in a number of industries including lead smelting and lead burning, the manufacture of white and red lead and the making of accumulators. Children may also develop lead poisoning from sucking lead-containing paint. Poisoning is infinitely more probable when lead is absorbed through the lungs as dust or fumes rather than when taken by mouth. If lead is absorbed slowly it is stored in the bones. The development of the symptoms of lead poisoning depends not so much on the total amount of lead in the body, but on its rate of absorption or mobilization from the bones.

Generally speaking, a blood level of 100 μg of lead per 100 ml of blood (5 μmol/litre) or 200 μg of lead per litre of urine are associated with symptoms of lead poisoning. Levels above 60 μg/100 ml (3.0 μmol/litre) in lead workers necessitates withdrawal from exposure.

Acute lead poisoning

Lead salts are irritant and produce vomiting, diarrhoea and collapse. Organic lead compounds produce an acute confusional state with delusions and fits.

Chronic lead poisoning

1 Lead colic

Intestinal colic and constipation are the most common symptoms of lead poisoning. The pain is usually periumbilical and there are no abnormal signs in the abdomen.

2 Lead neuropathy

In lead poisoning, weakness develops in certain groups of muscles, usually the extensor muscles of the wrist and rarely of the foot. Sensory changes do not occur. The site of the lesion in lead neuropathy is not certain, but is probably in the muscles.

3 Lead encephalopathy

This manifestation of lead poisoning is rare and is usually seen in children. The patient complains of severe headaches, vomiting, restlessness, irritability and fits.

4 Anaemia

A normocytic hypochromic anaemia occurs in lead poisoning, usually with punctate basophilia. This is due to the inhibition of enzymes concerned with the synthesis of haem, and it is possible to measure haem precursors as an index of lead poisoning.

5 Gums

Patients with lead poisoning may show a bluish stippled line on the gum margin. It is only found in association with gingivitis and is due to the deposition of lead sulphide in the gums. The lead line may be found in patients without other manifestations of lead poisoning.

6 Renal involvement

This can cause tubular defects or an interstitial nephropathy.

7 Other symptoms

consist of weakness, loss of weight, joint pains, and a metallic taste in the mouth.

Treatment

Lead colic can be relieved by intravenous injections of 10 ml of a 10% solution of calcium gluconate. Lead can be cleared from the body by using a chelating agent. Certain of these substances form compounds with lead which are soluble and which are excreted by the kidneys. The agent of choice is sodium calcium edetate. The lead in the body displaces the calcium from this chelating agent and the resulting compound is excreted. The adult dose is 1 g twice daily, given by slow intravenous infusion in saline at intervals of 12 hours. Such treatment may be carried out for five days and then repeated if necessary. A high calcium diet should be given after treatment. *Prophylactic measures* include:

(a) avoidance of exposure to lead dust or fumes by ventilation, hygiene, and by wearing masks;
(b) avoidance of absorption from the intestine by personal cleanliness, including washing of the hands, etc., before meals;
(c) regular medical examination of those exposed to lead;
(d) a high calcium diet.

Food poisoning

Food poisoning may be due to bacteria or viruses (or their

products) in the food, to poisonous substances or to allergy to something ingested.

Bacterial food poisoning

Staphylococcal

Some strains of staphylococci produce an enterotoxin which is fairly stable to heat and will resist boiling. The chief symptoms, which start abruptly in from one to six hours, are nausea, vomiting, intestinal colic and diarrhoea. The attack is short-lived and is all over within a few hours. It is not usually serious, but rarely there may be collapse with dehydration and deaths have occurred, particularly in young children and the aged.

In most cases rest in bed with frequent sips of fluid and mist. kaolin and morphine (BPC) (15 ml 4-hourly) will control the symptoms. Rarely if there is collapse with severe dehydration and sodium chloride deficiency, intravenous fluids will be required.

Salmonella (see page 423)

Certain of the salmonella group of organisms produce specific diseases such as typhoid and paratyphoid fevers. Others of the group, particularly *S. typhimurium*, *S. newport*, *S. St. Paul*, *S. thompson*, and *S. dublin*, produce an acute gastroenteritis which presents as a food poisoning.

The onset is usually within 48 hours of eating infected food. The main symptoms are general malaise, headache and fever, combined with vomiting, intestinal colic and diarrhoea. Occasionally there may be high fever with rigors, suggesting a septicaemia, and the spleen may be palpable. The disease usually lasts several days.

The diagnosis is confirmed by culture of the pathogenic organism from the stools. This is important in indicating the most appropriate treatment and in helping to trace the source of infection.

General measures include rest in bed and sips of fluid by mouth. If the diarrhoea has been severe, the oral fluids should consist of 0.3% saline flavoured with fruit juice and added glucose. Occasionally when vomiting is severe and prolonged, fluids and electrolytes must be given intravenously, and this requires a daily estimation of the blood electrolytes and a full record of fluid balance. The diarrhoea and colic can be controlled by mist. kaolin and morphine (15 ml 4-hourly).

There is little evidence that antibiotic treatment modifies the course of salmonella gastroenteritis.

Campylobacter infections (see page 424)

This group of organisms usually causes an enteritis. *Campylobacter jejuni* and *C. coli* are associated with an illness characterized by diarrhoea, abdominal pain and sometimes fever. Rarely septicaemia can occur and the infection may involve other organs. It is commonest in the young child but may be seen at any age. In mild cases no treatment is required but more severe intestinal infection responds to oral erythromycin and the rare systemic infections to gentamicin.

Pseudomembranous enterocolitis

Diarrhoea is common after a number of antibiotics but is not usually severe. However, occasionally a much more serious clinical picture emerges and is particularly associated with clindamycin and lincomycin. It is believed to be due to superinfection with *Clostridium difficile*. The diarrhoea is profuse and may be associated with toxaemia and shock. Sigmoidoscopy shows whitish membrane adhering to the bowel wall.

Treatment consists of rehydration and combating infection with metronidazole (400 mg three times daily) or oral vancomycin (500 mg four times daily). Alternatively cholestyramine can be given which binds the toxin produced by the organism.

Viruses (see page 424)

There is no doubt that certain outbreaks of gastroenteritis are due to a virus. They are usually mild and respond to symptomatic treatment.

Mushroom poisoning

Mushroom poisoning is usually due to *Aminita phalloides*. This mushroom has a yellow or olive cap with white gills and there is a volva (cup) at the base of the stem.

There is often a delay of several hours before the onset of symptoms. This is followed by severe abdominal colic with bloody diarrhoea and vomiting. Death may occur from shock or collapse. If the patient survives this stage, acute liver necrosis may develop and prove fatal.

The stomach should be washed out. Atropine (1 mg) should be given intravenously and repeated as required. Fluid and electrolyte replacement will be necessary and this will have to be given intravenously. Anti-phallinic serum should be given if available. It has been suggested that mashed rabbit stomach and brain should be given as these animals are resistant to mushroom poisoning. Otherwise, treatment is symptomatic.

Adverse reactions to food

Some patients are hypersensitive to certain articles of food and may suffer from urticarial rashes, diarrhoea, and even attacks of asthma. Adverse reactions are not necessarily allergic. They may be related to enzyme deficiencies or direct toxic reactions. It is best to avoid foods that cause problems provided these have been convincingly identified and the diet is not left too limited.

An attack due to allergy to food is treated as a sensitization reaction (see page 500). If diarrhoea is a prominent symptom it can be relieved by a mixture containing morphine, such as mist. kaolin and morphine (NF) (15 ml 4-hourly).

Further reading

Henry, J. and Volans, G. (1984) *ABC of Poisoning. Part I: Drugs.* British Medical Association, London.

Vale, J.A. and Meredith, T.J. (1981) *Poisoning Diagnosis and Treatment.* Update Books.

20
Diseases Due to Physical Agents

Decompression sickness

Decompression sickness occurs when people who have been working at a high atmospheric pressure, such as workers in a caisson or diving bell, are suddenly decompressed. It may also occur in a subject who rises quickly to a height above 7500 m (25 000 ft). In both circumstances, nitrogen rapidly comes out of solution both in the blood and in the tissues and forms bubbles. Oxygen and carbon dioxide also come out of solution, but rapidly diffuse away. These bubbles occur particularly in the nervous system and in adipose tissue, as nitrogen is soluble in fat.

Within a few hours of decompression the patient complains of severe pain in the muscles and joints. This may be followed by evidence of involvement of the central nervous system, including vertigo, weakness of the limbs, and sphincter disturbances. Various skin rashes may develop.

Where possible workers should not be exposed to pressures greater than 124 kPa (18 lb/in^2), for below this pressure sickness does not occur. If they work under higher pressures they should be slowly decompressed. If decompression sickness develops the subject should be recompressed again and then very slowly decompressed.

Motion sickness

Motion sickness may occur as a result of sea, land or air travel. Although the exact mechanism is not known it would seem that repetitive stimulation of the vestibular apparatus plays a large part; it is not possible to produce sickness in animals who have had their vestibular apparatus removed, nor are deaf mutes seasick. Susceptibility to motion sickness varies, but is particularly common in migrainous subjects.

The victim of motion sickness complains of feeling unwell with nausea, headache, and sometimes faintness. Finally symptoms are such as to require a rapid withdrawal from company and terminate in severe vomiting. The duration of the attack is variable and may last only a few hours, although susceptible subjects may be prostrate for several days.

People susceptible to motion sickness should avoid undue movement. When at sea they should remain near the centre of the ship and if possible lie down with the eyes closed. In an aeroplane the head should be rested back on the head rest. Some food should be taken, and if this is not possible, barley sugar should be sucked.

Certain drugs diminish the liability to sea-sickness. They are the hyoscine group and the antihistamines. The most satisfactory drug is not decided, but there is a little evidence that hyoscine is better for short journeys and the antihistamines for longer ones. The doses are:

(a) Hyoscine (0.3–0.6 mg according to weight) taken 20 minutes before starting is suitable for journeys lasting up to four hours. Side-effects include dry mouth and paralysis of accommodation.
(b) Cyclizine (50 mg three times daily) or meclozine (50 mg daily) are suitable for longer journeys.
(c) Cinnarizine (30 mg) two hours before travelling (and then 15 mg 8-hourly) is also suitable but can cause drowsiness.

These drugs can be used for children in reduced dosage.

Anxiety even before the journey begins may upset some people and diazepam (2–5 mg) taken before setting out is sometimes helpful.

Disorders due to heat

A number of syndromes may appear in those exposed to

heat. They are more liable to occur in subjects who have had no opportunity to become acclimatized, in the very young, the elderly and in association with heavy exertion.

Heat stroke (heat hyperpyrexia)

Heat stroke signifies a raised body temperature because heat production exceeds heat loss. It occurs when:

(a) there is excessive heat production due to heavy exertion (marathon or 'fun' running), or to a feverish illness such as malaria;

(b) there is failure of heat loss, normally by evaporation of sweat combined with convection and radiation, resulting from a high ambient temperature and humidity.

Diversion of blood from the skin and muscles may also be a factor during severe exertion.

There is hyperpyrexia, often greater than 41°C, combined with headache, confusion, coma and fits. Initially there is a high cardiac output with full pulse but, terminally, output falls. Purpuric haemorrhage is common, probably owing to a failure to produce coagulation factors or, sometimes, to disseminated intravascular coagulation. The skin is hot and dry, the sweating mechanism having failed.

Heat stroke is a medical emergency. The body must be cooled as rapidly as possible until the rectal temperature is 39°C. This is best achieved by removing clothing and cooling in an ice bath. Alternately, the body surface should be kept moist by sprays of water and evaporation encouraged by means of fans.

The possibility of some precipitating infection must be remembered and the appropriate treatment given.

Various figures have been given for mortality, but it is probably about 25 per cent.

The condition can be prevented by avoiding dehydration, ensuring an adequate salt intake, and encouraging heat loss from the skin by suitable clothing, fans, etc.

Heat exhaustion

Heat exhaustion may occur for a number of reasons and has to be subdivided on this basis.

Salt-deficiency heat exhaustion

This is due to salt loss with inadequate replacement. The symptoms are those of salt deficiency (i.e. weakness, cramps, vomiting, and collapse with a low blood pressure). The plasma sodium and chloride levels are reduced and the urine may be low in chlorides.

Treatment is aimed at replacing the salt loss and this may be done by mouth, or by intravenous infusion if vomiting is troublesome.

Anhidrotic heat exhaustion

This form of heat exhaustion is usually associated with prickly heat. The symptoms are weakness and irritability and if exertion is attempted the patient may collapse. Examination shows that sweating is confined to localized areas, usually the face and axillae and sometimes the hands and feet. The condition may proceed to heat stroke.

In addition, heat exhaustion on effort may occur without clear evidence of either salt deficiency or anhidrosis.

The treatment is to remove the subject to a cooler environment.

Prickly heat

Prickly heat is due to excessive sweating. It is a fine papular rash which sometimes becomes vesicular and usually gives a sensation of prickling (thus the name). It may become infected.

The treatment is removal to a cooler and less humid atmosphere.

Sunburn

Sunburn is due to the ultraviolet fraction of sunlight. It may be merely an erythema, but if severe the erythema will be accompanied by some local oedema and sometimes headache and pyrexia.

Sunburn may be prevented by graduated exposure to direct sunlight and by applying creams containing aminobenzoic acid, which exclude part of the ultraviolet end of the spectrum. If sunburn has occurred further exposure to sunlight should be avoided and some soothing lotion such as oily calamine applied.

Disorders due to cold

They may be either local or general. Local effects in temperate climates are commonly chilblains or Raynaud's phenomenon (see page 77). If cold is extreme, then the tissues of the extremities may freeze, and frostbite results.

General effects result from the progressive cooling of the whole body, the syndrome of hypothermia.

Hypothermia

Hypothermia is defined as a deep temperature (usually measured rectally) of less than 35°C. It may occur under several circumstances.

In the UK it is most often found in the elderly and poorly nourished who may have insufficient means for adequate domestic heating. The crisis may be precipitated by an injury such as a fractured hip, a stroke or perhaps excessive alcohol or drug consumption. It may also complicate myxoedema.

Hypothermia can also occur in the young and active. It may succeed prolonged immersion in water, and every winter a few adventurous people die as a result of hypothermia, having been overtaken by a blizzard while walking or climbing. In this context it is important to remember that alcohol is dangerous when combined with exposure for it inhibits gluconeogenesis (causing hypoglycaemia), and by interfering with vasoconstriction increases heat loss.

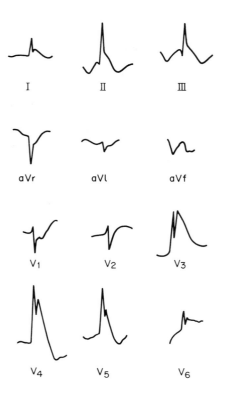

Figure 20.1 *Typical ECG of hypothermia. Showing J waves at end of QRS complex.*

Clinical features

As the body temperature falls below 35°C the patient becomes confused and sluggish and ultimately unconscious. The heart rate slows and the cardiac output and blood pressure fall. Various cardiac arrhythmias may develop. These include atrial fibrillation, ventricular ectopics or tachycardia leading eventually to cardiac arrest or, rarely, ventricular fibrillation. A typical ECG of hypothermia is shown in Fig. 20.1.

A diuresis occurs with decreasing temperature owing to depression of tubular reabsorption in the kidney. This is important as fluid replacement may be required during treatment.

Respiration is depressed but oxygen needs are reduced. There is excessive lactic acid production leading to acidosis.

Investigations and treatment

An initial blood count, urea and electrolytes, blood glucose and amylase, blood gases and thyroid function tests are required. The rectal temperature should be measured half-hourly.

1 Rewarming
There is some controversy about the speed of rewarming. Covering with a space blanket and allowing the patient to warm up at room temperature (about 1°C every two hours) is usually adequate. If intensive care facilities are available active rewarming may be used (i.e. 1.5°C/hour), but careful monitoring is required.

In the younger subjects suffering from hypothermia as a result of exposure rewarming can be more rapid. Immersion in a bath at 45°C followed by warm blankets is appropriate.

2 Fluids and circulation
In hypothermia a low cardiac output develops combined with hypovolaemia, and leads to hypotension. If the patient is hypotensive a CVP line should be inserted and plasma carefully infused. It is important not to overload the patient with fluid with resultant pulmonary oedema, as the heart's ability to respond to an increased load will be temporarily reduced.

Acidosis may require treatment with appropriate infusion.

Cardiac arrhythmias are common. Cardiac arrest or ventricular fibrillation are treated in the usual way (see page 63). Occasionally ventilation is required if respiration is suppressed.

Some authorities give hydrocortisone (100 mg 4-hourly), although the evidence that this is helpful, except in adrenal deficiency, is scanty. Finally, myxoedema may present as hypothermia and requires the usual treatment (see page 295).

Complications

Pneumonia develops frequently and should be treated with antibiotics (see page 103). Pancreatitis is a rare but well recognized complication.

The prognosis depends on the severity of the hypothermia, on how old or frail the patient is and on coincident disease, the overall mortality being about 30 per cent.

Altitude sickness

This is due to hypoxia as a result of the decrease in the partial pressure of oxygen in the atmosphere that occurs at high altitudes. It may arise from flying or mountain climbing, the latter becoming more frequent with the ever-increasing number of people climbing or trekking. Up to 2400 metres (8000 ft) no symptoms occur; over 3000 metres (10 000 ft) they begin to appear.

The incidence of symptoms depends on the altitude, the rate of climb, and the susceptibility of the individual. The young and healthy suffer less often than the elderly or those with cardiac or respiratory disease. It occurs in about 50 per cent of those climbing to 4000 metres.

Benign mountain sickness

This is probably due to salt and water retention. Symptoms include headache, nausea, vomiting and insomnia. The subject should rest and the symptoms usually disappear in about 48 hours.

Malignant mountain sickness

There may be acute pulmonary oedema with cough, frothy sputum and dyspnoea. There may also be acute cerebral oedema with disorientation, hallucinations and coma.

These very serious developments often ensue because the symptoms of benign mountain sickness were disregarded. The patient should be rapidly removed to a lower altitude. Oxygen (if available) helps, and frusemide should be given in doses large enough to produce a diuresis.

Prevention

Climb slowly: above 3000 metres, one day and two nights should be spent at each 300 metre increase in altitude. If benign mountain sickness occurs, the subject should rest until fully recovered. Acetazolamide (250 mg thrice daily) helps acclimatization.

Further reading

Editorial (1978) Treating accidental hypothermia, *Br. Med. J.*, **2**: 1383.

McLean, D. and Emslie-Smith, D. (1977) *Accidental Hypothermia*. Blackwell, Oxford.

Clowes, G. and O'Donnell, T. (1974) Heat stroke, *New Engl. J. Med.*, **291**: 564.

Milledge, J. (Ed.) (1983) Mountain sickness, *Thorax*, **38**: 641.

Wolfe, S. and Behrman (1981) Heat stroke and community runs, *Br. Med. J.*, **282**: 2060.

21
Medicine in Old Age

The elderly make up an increasing proportion of the population in Western society and their needs require particular attention. Many of the conditions from which they suffer are the same as those in younger patients, but there are particular illnesses limited to the old and the processes of ageing change the body's responses. The changes produce a reduction in the efficiency of many organs and result in altered responses to drugs as well as to disease and to the environment itself. Thermoregulation is often impaired, putting the elderly patient at risk from conditions of excessive heat or cold (see Chapter 20).

The specialty of geriatrics has developed to deal with many of these problems. However, a large part of the work of most general physicians and family doctors involves the care of patients over the age of 65 years and will continue to do so. An important part of this care is the development of a team approach, coordinating all the services both in the hospital and in the community which help in the care of the elderly. In the assessment of elderly patients failing memory and hearing mean that more time and consideration are often necessary to obtain a clear clinical history. It is usually advisable to supplement this with information from relatives. The home environment and potential support are important factors which need to be considered.

Much of what appears in the other chapters of this book is relevant to older people, and particular relevant points are mentioned under the body systems. This chapter will deal with some general features important in the management of disease in old age.

Mental disturbance and dementia

Confusion

Many aspects of dementia and of acute mental disturbance in relation to illness are dealt with in Chapters 5 and 16. Acute illnesses commonly precipitate confusion in the elderly, and this is likely to be exacerbated by changes in the environment such as admission to the strange surroundings of a hospital. One-third of patients admitted directly to geriatric beds are confused on admission.

Clinical features

The conditions that commonly precipitate confusion are those illnesses which are particularly frequent in old people; for example, cerebrovascular ischaemia, cerebrovascular accidents, infections, diabetes, drugs such as hypnotics, antiparkinsonian drugs and vasodilators. An especial look out should be kept for subdural haematoma. Old people tend to fall and bleed rather easily from their intracranial vessels. Subdural haematomas are rare, but since the confusion is reversible a high level of suspicion should be kept for this condition readily diagnosed by CT scan.

A careful history should be taken in the case of a confused old person. It will be particularly important to obtain information from relatives and others usually involved in caring for the patient. The rate of onset of the confusion should be ascertained and its relation to any drug therapy documented. Physical examination should include a careful neurological examination.

Treatment

The treatment of elderly confused patients presents great difficulties. It may sometimes be necessary to sedate the patient for their own safety; but in general sedation is likely to lead to an increase in the level of confusion or produce a very drowsy patient at risk of new problems such as venous thrombosis, falls and dehydration. The first part of the management is to look for an underlying cause and treat this if possible. It is best to carry out treatment in surroundings and with people familiar to the patient as far as possible.

Confusion is likely to be worst at night and the greatest trial to relatives at this time. Some form of hypnotic may help to provide a night's rest. Temazepam, chlormethiazole and thioridazine are sometimes helpful. They should be tested and the response carefully monitored since it is easy to exacerbate the confusion or to produce oversedation.

It is important to be aware of the possibility of depression in withdrawn old people since this may respond well to appropriate therapy.

Dementia

This is a frequent problem in the elderly. Over the age of 80 years around 20 per cent of patients have dementia. The causes, investigation and management of dementia are dealt with in Chapter 5. The management is difficult and often unrewarding; it involves practical problems of deciding where the patient is to be managed, working with other support services and even dealing with legal aspects such as the ability of the patient to cope with their financial affairs. These problems emphasize the importance of diagnosing and treating reversible causes such as hypothyroidism or vitamin B_{12} deficiency in the rare cases when these are present.

Drug treatments

There is a decline in renal function and in metabolic function of the liver with age so that old people handle drugs differently from the young. Renal function declines because of reduced glomerular filtration and reduced tubular reabsorption, and the half-life of renally excreted drugs lengthens. There are often changes in receptors on cell membranes and changes in body mass. Lean body mass declines and there is a relative or real increase in fat, leading to changes in distribution of drugs according to their fat solubility. Drug absorption is not changed significantly.

At all ages compliance with drug therapy is a factor which is often ignored. In older age groups compliance tends to decline, particularly if complicated regimens involving many drugs are prescribed. The situation is complicated by problems old people may have in reading the small print on instruction labels and in opening childproof containers. When drug therapy in the elderly fails to produce the expected response, compliance

should be checked rather than increasing the dose of the drug. Drug therapy in the elderly should be regularly reviewed. Continuation of drugs which could be stopped leads to the development of complicated multiple drug regimens. The elderly often suffer from a number of conditions, and care must be taken to avoid drug interactions related to several different prescribers and self-medication particularly with analgesics and laxatives.

Specific drugs

Digoxin is excreted mainly by the kidneys and requires a reduced dose in the elderly. It is usually only necessary as maintenance therapy in the presence of atrial fibrillation. Even then the ventricular response in the elderly is often reduced so that the rate is controlled even in the absence of digoxin therapy. The maintenance dose in the elderly is likely to be between 62.5 and 125 μg daily.

Diuretics are often used to control heart failure or hypertension. They are not usually advisable in the management of simple peripheral oedema. They may lead to potassium depletion, postural hypotension, magnesium depletion, exacerbation of diabetes or gout.

Beta-blockers and *vasodilators* are particularly likely to produce symptomatic postural hypotension in the elderly where responses of the sympathetic nervous system to postural changes may be impaired. Hepatic metabolism of drugs such as propranolol is reduced and treatment should start at a lower dose. A careful assessment needs to be made of treatment of hypertension in the elderly to ensure that the effects of the treatment are not more troublesome than the risks of the underlying disease. Falls in old people are generally the result of a combination of factors, and drug treatment may be the additional element which precipitates the problems.

Non-steroidal anti-inflammatory drugs are often prescribed for pain and arthritis. They can produce problems with indigestion, gastrointestinal blood loss and fluid retention.

Investigations

Laboratory investigations in the elderly need to be interpreted with care. The normal ranges of a number of tests are dependent upon age and in some cases the ranges in older subjects are poorly documented.

Biochemistry

In most cases normal values for routine biochemical tests do not vary with age. However, *blood urea* and *creatinine* do increase with age, and upper limits for the over-65 age group are around 10 mmol/l and 150 μmol/l respectively. *Glomerular filtration rate* declines by about 1 per cent annually after the age of 40. *Uric acid* also rises with age, particularly in association with diuretic treatment. Treatment for hyperuricaemia is not usually indicated without the combination of raised uric acid and clinical gout. Serum *cholesterol* rises with age, but its estimation is rarely indicated since treatment at this age is not likely to incur any benefit. Tests such as *alkaline phosphatase* and *calcium* may be raised because of Paget's disease or mild hyperparathyroidism. Minor elevations would not usually require further elaborate investigation.

Haematology

The *haemoglobin* level and red cell indices do not change significantly with age. However, the *white cell count* tends to be a little lower, so that the lower limit of normal can be taken as 3×10^9 per litre. The platelet count is unchanged. Normal ranges of *folate* and *vitamin B$_{12}$* are not changed by age, but the *erythrocyte sedimentation rate* (ESR) shows a distinct relationship to age. Estimations of normal values have varied mainly because of the problems of being sure that the subjects are free of any condition which might lead to a raised ESR. One attempt at establishing a normal range takes values up to half the age in men and up to half of the sum of the age plus 10 in women. Serum iron falls slightly with age.

Other tests

Tests such as *respiratory function tests* are sometimes difficult for elderly people to perform with full effort. The normal ranges are wide and it is therefore difficult to be sure of abnormalities. They are more useful in monitoring changes in the same patient over time to assess the progress of a disease or response to treatment.

Calcification in the costal cartilages is common and of no significance on *chest radiographs*. Calcification may also occur in the tracheal cartilages. It can often be seen outlining large vessels, particularly the aorta. Degenerative changes in vertebral bodies and intervertebral joints are common with age and bear little relationship to clinical symptoms, unless they are severe. Symptoms may occur without significant radiological change, limiting the usefulness of investigations such as cervical spine and lumbar spine radiographs, except in special circumstances.

Resting heart rate and maximal heart rate on exercise decrease slightly with age. The *electrocardiogram* shows no significant changes with age and can be interpreted in the usual way.

Rehabilitation

Bed is a dangerous place for the elderly patient, leading to a distancing from normal, active, ambulant life and increasing the risk of infections and thromboses. Rehabilitation aimed at returning the older patient to as independent a life as is safe and possible is a vital part of geriatrics. Much of this is a question of attitudes to what can be achieved, attitudes in the nursing and medical staff and in the patients themselves. Rehabilitation is most likely to be successful when there is a team approach of occupational therapists, speech therapists, physiotherapists, doctors and nurses trying to achieve this goal and when the ward environment allows the development of rehabilitation towards independence.

For common conditions in old age, such as cerebrovascular accidents, expert help is needed to cope with impaired balance and walking. Where disabilities are not reversible a good knowledge of available aids and appliances is necessary. This will need to extend into the patient's home, making suitable alterations to cope with new limitations.

In addition to dealing with adaptations at home and improving mobility, it is important not to lose sight of the patient's psychological needs. The motivation of the patient is of crucial importance in successful rehabilitation and the programme is not likely to be successful if this element is ignored.

All of medicine is concerned with the treatment of the whole person rather than a particular disease. Perhaps this is nowhere so important as in geriatric medicine where decisions on appropriate investigation and treatment and the wishes and dignity of the patient are paramount.

Further reading

Andrews, K. (1988) *Rehabilitation of the Older Adult*. Edward Arnold, London.

British Medical Journal (1985) *Medicine in Old Age*. British Medical Association, London.

Brocklehurst, J.C. (Ed.) (1985) *Textbook of Geriatric Medicine and Gerontology*. Churchill Livingstone, Edinburgh.

Brocklehurst, J.C. (1987) *Geriatric Medicine for Students*. Churchill Livingstone, Edinburgh.

Appendix
Normal Values

This section gives the results of tests in relatively common use. The values given can generally only be taken as the approximate normal range. There will be differences between techniques and machines used in the analysis. In many cases laboratories will build up their own range of normal values which should be used in preference to those given here.

Haematology

Total blood volume	65–85 ml/kg (male)
	60–80 ml/kg (female)

Red cells

Red cell mass	25–35 ml/kg (male)
	20–30 ml/kg (female)
Haemoglobin	13.0–18.0 g/dl (male)
	11.5–16.5 g/dl (female)
Red cell count	4.5–6.5×10^9/l (male)
	3.9–5.8×10^9/l (female)
Mean corpuscular haemoglobin (MCH)	27–22 pg
Mean corpuscular haemoglobin concentration (MCHC)	32–35 g/dl
Mean corpuscular volume	80–96 fl
Packed cell volume	0.40–0.54 l/l (male)
	0.37–0.47 l/l (female)
Reticulocyte count	0.2–2.5% of red cells

White cells

Total white cell count	4.0–11.0×10^9/l
Neutrophils	2.5–7.5×10^9/l
Lymphocytes	1.5–3.5×10^9/l
Monocytes	0.2–0.8×10^9/l
Eosinophils	0.04–0.44×10^9/l
Basophils	0–0.10×10^9/l

Coagulation

Prothrombin time	10–14 s
Partial thromboplastin time	30–40 s
Bleeding time (Ivy)	3–8 minutes

Other haematological values

Platelet count	$150–400 \times 10^9/l$
Serum folate	5–63 nmol/l
Red cell folate	> 160 μg/l
Serum B_{12}	150–675 pmol/l
Fibrinogen	2–4 g/l

Biochemistry

Acid phosphatase	1–5 U/l
Alanine aminotransferase	5–35 U/l
Albumin	30–46 g/l
Alkaline phosphatase	80–300 U/l
Alpha-fetoprotein	< 10 kU/l
Ammonium	37–84 μmol/l
Amylase	0–180 U/l
Aspartate aminotransferase	5–35 U/l
Bicarbonate	22–30 mmol/l
Bilirubin (total)	3–17 μmol/l
Bilirubin (direct)	0–3 μmol/l
Calcium (Calcium should be corrected for abnormal levels of albumin)	2.1–2.6 mmol/l
Carcinoembryonic antigen (CEA)	< 10 μg/l
Chloride	98–108 mmol/l
Cholesterol	3.4–6.5 nmol/l
Cortisol (09.00 h)	280–700 nmol/l
Cortisol (24.00 h and asleep)	140–280 nmol/l
Creatinine	50–130 μmol/l
Creatinine clearance	105–132 ml/minute per 1.73 m^2 surface area
Creatine phosphokinase (CPK)	24–195 U/l
Gamma glutamyl transpeptidase	10–40 iu/l
Globulin	25–35 g/l
Glucose (fasting)	4.0–5.8 mmol/l
Glycosylated haemoglobin (HbA1c)	3.8–6.4%
Hydroxybutyric dehydrogenase (HbD)	40–125 U/l
Iron	12–30 μmol/l
Iron binding capacity	42–80 μmol/l
Lactate	0.3–0.8 mmol/l
Lactic dehydrogenase (LDH)	240–525 U/l
Magnesium	0.7–1.1 mmol/l
Osmolality	280–296 mOsm/kg
Phosphate	0.8–1.5 mmol/l
Potassium	3.4–5.0 mmol/l
Protein (total)	60–82 g/l
Sodium	134–148 mmol/l
Thyroid function	
Thyroxine (T_4)	60–160 nmol/l
Triiodothyronine (T_3)	1.2–3.1 nmol/l
Free thyroxine (free T_4)	9–23 pmol/l
Free triiodothyronine (free T_3)	3–9 pmol/l

Thyroid stimulating hormone (TSH)	0.3–3.0 mU/l
Triglycerides	0.4–2.2 mmol/l
Urate	0.2–0.42 mmol/l
Urea	2.5–7.5 mmol/l

Urine

Values per 24 hours

Volume	600–2500 ml
Protein	< 150 mg
Potassium	80–160 mmol
Sodium	10–200 mmol
Calcium	2.5–7.5 mmol
Phosphate	16–48 mmol
Creatinine	9–17 mmol

Arterial blood gases

PCO_2	4.8–6.1 kPa (36–46 mmHg)
PO_2	10–13.3 kPa (75–100 mmHg)
pH	7.35–7.45
$[H^+]$	35–45 nmol/l

Cerebrospinal fluid

Pressure	70–160 mm of csf
Lymphocytes	0–5 mm^3
Polymorphs	0
Red cells	0
Protein	20–45 g/l
IgG	< 15% total protein
Glucose	> 50% blood glucose
Chloride	122–128 mmol/l

INDEX